INTERNATIONAL TRENDS IN GENERAL THORACIC SURGERY

INTERNATIONAL TRENDS IN GENERAL THORACIC SURGERY

INTERNATIONAL TRENDS IN GENERAL THORACIC SURGERY

VOLUME 3

BENIGN ESOPHAGEAL DISEASE

Edited by

TOM R. DeMEESTER, M.D.

Professor and Chairman, Department of Surgery,
Creighton University School of Medicine; Chief of Surgery,
Saint Joseph Hospital, Omaha, Nebraska

HUGOE R. MATTHEWS, F.R.C.S.

Senior Clinical Lecturer in Surgery,
Department of Surgery, University of Birmingham;
Consultant Thoracic Surgeon, Regional Department of Thoracic Surgery,
East Birmingham Hospital, Birmingham, England

with 190 illustrations, including 16 color plates

The C. V. Mosby Company

ST. LOUIS • WASHINGTON, D.C. • TORONTO   1987

A TRADITION OF PUBLISHING EXCELLENCE

Editor: Thomas A. Manning
Developmental editor: Elaine Steinborn
Assistant editor: Laurel Fuller
Project manager: Mark Spann
Manuscript editor: Stephen C. Hetager
Production: Radhika Rao Gupta, Donna L. Walls
Design: Gail Morey Hudson

VOLUME 3

Printed in the United States of America

The C.V. Mosby Company
11830 Westline Industrial Drive, St. Louis, Missouri 63146

Library of Congress Cataloging-in-Publication Data

Benign esophageal disease.

   (International trends in general thoracic
surgery; v. 3)
   Includes bibliographies and index.
   1. Esophagus—Surgery. 2. Esophagus—Diseases.
I. DeMeester, Tom R., 1938-   . II. Matthews,
Hugoe R. III. Series. [DNLM: 1. Esophageal Diseases.
W1 IN914 v.3 / WI 250 B467]
RD539.5.B46 1987   617'.548   87-20427
ISBN 0-8016-2471-1

T/MV/MV 9 8 7 6 5 4 3 2 1   01/C/011

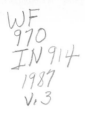
Contributors

IAN P. ADAMS, B.Sc.

Medical Physiologist, The Oesophageal Laboratory, Regional Department of Thoracic Surgery, East Birmingham Hospital, Birmingham, England

The laboratory in the diagnosis of esophageal disease

RAYMOND A. AMOURY, M.D.

Katharine Berry Richardson Professor of Pediatric Surgery, University of Missouri–Kansas City School of Medicine; Surgeon-in-Chief, Department of Surgery, The Children's Mercy Hospital, Kansas City, Missouri

Discussion: Children and reflux

JEAN PIERRE ANGELCHIK, M.D., F.A.C.S., F.A.C.G.

Department of Surgery, Phoenix Baptist Hospital, Phoenix, Arizona

Use of a prosthetic device to control gastroesophageal reflux

PAUL DAVID ANGELCHIK, M.D.

Surgical Resident, Department of Surgery, University of Wisconsin Hospital and Clinics, Madison, Wisconsin

Use of a prosthetic device to control gastroesophageal reflux

MICHAEL ATKINSON, M.D., F.R.C.P.

Special Professor of Gastroenterology, Department of Surgery, University of Nottingham; Honorary Consultant Physician, University Hospital, Queens Medical Centre, Nottingham, England

Discussion: Drug-induced esophageal injuries

FERNANDO AZPIROZ, M.D.

Chief, Section of Gastrointestinal Research, Department of Gastroenterology, Vall D'Hebron Hospital, Barcelona, Spain

Gastroesophageal reflux: the role of delayed gastric emptying and duodenogastric reflux

JOHN BANCEWICZ, Ch.M., F.R.C.S.(Glasg.)

Senior Lecturer in Surgery, University of Manchester, Manchester, England; Consultant Surgeon, Hope Hospital, Salford, England

Discussion: Principles of surgical treatment of gastroesophageal reflux

GILLES BEAUCHAMP, M.D., F.R.C.S.

Associate Professor of Surgery, Department of Surgery, University of Montreal, Maisonneuve-Rosemont Hospital, Montreal, Quebec, Canada

Discussion: Esophageal scintigraphy and tests of duodenogastric function

PAOLO BECHI, M.D.

Associate Professor of Surgery, Department of Surgery, Patologia Chirurgica I, Florence, Italy

Discussion: Gastroesophageal reflux: the role of delayed gastric emptying and duodenogastric reflux

RONALD H. BELSEY, M.S.

Visiting Professor of Surgery, Department of Surgery, University of Chicago, Chicago, Illinois

Personal reflections on standard antireflux procedures

ADOLFO BENAGES, M.D.

Professor of Medicine and Director, Department of Internal Medicine, University of Murcia; Head, Service of Internal Medicine, Department of Internal Medicine, Hospital V. Arrixaca, Murcia, Spain

Discussion: Pharyngeal dysphagia

BRUNO BERTHET, M.D.

Interne des Hôpitaux, Départment de Chururgie Thoracique, Hôpital Salvator, Marseille, France

Surgical management of caustic injuries to the upper gastrointestinal tract

J. BOIX-OCHOA, M.D.

Professor of Pediatric Surgery, Department of Pediatrics, Autonomous University; Chief, Department of Pediatric Surgery, Children's Hospital Vall d'Hebron, Barcelona, Spain

Children and reflux

ELFRIEDE BOLLSCHWEILER, M.D., Dipl. Math.

Department of Surgery, Technical University of Munich and Klinikum rechts der Isar, Munich, Federal Republic of Germany

Update on esophageal pH monitoring

CEDRIC G. BREMNER, M.B., Ch.B., Ch.M., F.R.C.S.

Professor and Chief Surgeon, The University of the Witwatersrand; Chief Surgeon, Department of Surgery, Hillbrow and the Johannesburg Hospital, Johannesburg, South Africa

Barrett's esophagus

DONALD O. CASTELL, M.D.

Professor of Medicine and Chief of Gastroenterology, Bowman Gray School of Medicine; Chief of Gastroenterology, Department of Medicine, North Carolina Baptist Hospital, Winston-Salem, North Carolina

Function of the normal human esophagus

ROBERT E. CONDON, M.D., M.S., F.A.C.S.

Ausman Foundation Professor and Chairman, Department of Surgery, Medical College of Wisconsin; Chief of Surgery, Department of Surgery, Froedtert Memorial Lutheran Hospital and Milwaukee County Medical Complex, Milwaukee, Wisconsin

Discussion: Management of failed Heller's operation

TOM R. DeMEESTER, M.D.

Professor and Chairman, Department of Surgery, Creighton University School of Medicine; Chief of Surgery, Saint Joseph Hospital, Omaha, Nebraska

Discussion: Update on esophageal pH monitoring
Definition, detection, and pathophysiology of gastroesophageal reflux disease

JACQUES Di COSTANZO, M.D.

Réanination Digestive, Clinique La Résidence du Parc, Marseille, France

Surgical management of caustic injuries to the upper gastrointestinal tract

R. DOM, M.D.

Professor, Department of Neuropathology, Catholic University of Leuven; Director, Laboratory of Neuropathology, Department of Neuropathology, University Hospital Gasthuisberg, Leuven, Belgium

Cricopharyngeal myotomy for pharyngoesophageal diverticula

ANDRÉ DURANCEAU, M.D.

Professor, Department of Surgery, University of Montreal; Head, Division of Thoracic Surgery, Department of Surgery, Hôtel-Dieu de Montréal, Montreal, Quebec, Canada

Recent advances in esophageal manometry
Discussion: Cricopharyngeal myotomy for pharyngoesophageal diverticula

J. E. DUSSEK, M.B.B.S., F.R.C.S.

Consultant Thoracic Surgeon, The Cardiothoracic Unit, Guys Hospital, London England

Discussion: Recent advances in esophageal manometry

F. HENRY ELLIS, Jr., M.D., Ph.D.

Clinical Professor of Surgery, Department of Surgery, Harvard Medical School, Boston, Massachusetts; Chief, Department of Surgery, Division of Thoracic and Cardiovascular Surgery, New England Deaconess Hospital and Lahey Clinic Medical Center, Boston, Massachusetts, and Burlington, Massachusetts

Discussion: Personal reflections on standard antireflux procedures
Diffuse esophageal spasm and related disorders

D. F. EVANS, Ph.D.

Lecturer in Surgery, Department of Surgery, The University of Nottingham, Nottingham, England

Discussion: Definition, detection, and pathophysiology of gastroesophageal reflux disease

FRANCOIS FEKETE, M.D.

Professor and Chairman,, Department of Surgery, University of Paris VII, Paris, France; Chief, Department of Digestive Surgery, Hôpital Beaujon, Clichy, France

Management of failed Heller's operation

MARK K. FERGUSON, M.D.

Assistant Professor, Department of Surgery, University of Chicago Pritzker School of Medicine; Attending Physician, Department of Surgery, University of Chicago Medical Center, Chicago, Illinois

Esophageal scintigraphy and tests of duodenogastric function
Principles of surgical treatment of gastroesophageal reflux

JACQUES FIGARELLA, M.D.

Professor of Surgery, Faculté de Médecine, University of Marseille; Head, Department of General Surgery, Assistance Publique, Marseille, France

Surgical management of caustic injuries to the upper gastrointestinal tract

ANDRÉ GAUTHIER, M.D.

Professor of Surgery, Faculté de Médecine, University of Marseille; Hépato-gastro-enterologie, Hôpital de la Conception, Marseille, France

Surgical management of caustic injuries to the upper gastrointestinal tract

HEIN G. GOOSZEN, M.D., Ph.D.

Department of Surgery, University Hospital Leiden, Leiden, The Netherlands

Discussion: Management of failed antireflux procedures

GEOFFREY M. GRAEBER, M.D.

Associate Professor, Department of Surgery, Uniformed Services University of the Health Sciences, Bethesda, Maryland; Director, Division of Surgery, Walter Reed Army Institute of Research; Staff Thoracic Surgeon, Walter Reed Army Medical Center, Washington, D.C.

Reflux control in operations for achalasia

JACQUES A. GRUWEZ, M.D., Hon.F.R.C.S.

Professor of Surgery, Clinical and Experimental Surgical Pathology; Head, Department of General Surgery, University Hospitals, Catholic University of Leuven, Leuven, Belgium

Cricopharyngeal myotomy for pharyngoesophageal diverticula

PAUL J. GUELINCKX, M.D.

Clinical and Experimental Surgery, Department of Developmental Biology and Surgical Pathology; Plastic and Reconstructive Surgery—Microsurgery, Department of General Surgery, U.Z. St. Pieter, Catholic University of Leuven, Leuven, Belgium

Cricopharyngeal myotomy for pharyngoesophageal diverticula

ROBERT D. HENDERSON, M.B., F.R.C.S.(C.), F.A.C.S.

Professor of Surgery, University of Toronto; Surgeon-in-Chief, Department of Surgery, Women's College Hospital, Toronto, Ontario, Canada

Extended esophageal myotomy in the management of diffuse esophageal spasm

LUCIUS D. HILL, M.D.

Clinical Professor of Surgery, Department of Surgery, University of Washington; Attending Staff and Teaching Staff, Department of Surgery, Swedish Medical Center and Virginia Mason Medical Center, Seattle, Washington

Discussion: Management of failed antireflux procedures
Discussion: Management of reflux strictures

Ö. P. HORVÁTH, M.D.

Department of Surgery, Medical University of Szeged, Szeged, Hungary

Discussion: Surgical management of caustic injuries to the upper gastrointestinal tract

GLYN G. JAMIESON, M.S., F.R.A.C.S., F.A.C.S.

Dorothy Mortlock Professor of Surgery, Department of Surgery, University of Adelaide; Professor of Surgery, Department of Surgery, Royal Adelaide Hospital, Adelaide, Australia

Recent advances in esophageal manometry
Discussion: Cricopharyngeal myotomy for pharyngoesophageal diverticula

LAWRENCE F. JOHNSON, M.D., F.A.C.P.

Professor of Medicine and Director, Digestive Disease Division, Uniformed Services University of the Health Sciences and F. Edward Hebert School of Medicine, Bethesda, Maryland; Attending Gastroenterologist, Department of Medicine, Walter Reed Army Medical Center, Washington, D.C.

Discussion: The laboratory in the diagnosis of esophageal disease

JACQUELINE JOUGLARD, M.D.

Centre Anti-Poison, Hôpital Salvator, Marseille, France

Surgical management of caustic injuries to the upper gastrointestinal tract

PHILIP O. KATZ, M.D., F.A.C.P.

Assistant Professor of Medicine, Department of Medicine/Digestive Disease, Johns Hopkins University; Division of Digestive Diseases, Francis Scott Key Medical Center, Baltimore, Maryland

Function of the normal human esophagus

EDWIN LAFONTAINE, M.D.

Assistant Professor of Surgery, Department of Surgery, University of Montreal; Attending Surgeon, Department of Surgery, Hôpital Hôtel-Dieu, Montreal, Quebec, Canada

Pharyngeal dysphagia

RÜDIGER LANGE, M.D.

Department of Surgery, Technical University of Munich and Klinikum rechts der Isar, Munich, Federal Republic of Germany

Update on esophageal pH monitoring

GERALD M. LARSON, M.D.

Associate Professor of Surgery, Department of Surgery, University of Louisville; Associate Professor of Surgery, Department of Surgery, Humana Hospital University, Louisville, Kentucky

Discussion: Reflux associated with other disorders or lesions

R. E. LEA, M.B., Ch.B., F.R.C.S.

Consultant Thoracic Surgeon, Wessex Regional Cardio-Thoracic Unit, Southampton General Hospital, Southampton, England

Discussion: Reflux control in operations for achalasia

GUIDO LEMAN, M.D.

Consultant Surgeon, Department of Surgery, Catholic University of Leuven and University Hospitals, Leuven, Belgium

Cricopharyngeal myotomy for pharyngoesophageal diverticula

TONI LERUT, M.D., F.A.C.S., F.A.C.C.P.

Associate Professor in Surgery, Department of Surgery, Catholic University of Leuven; Joint Clinical Head, Department of Surgery, U.Z. St. Rafael–St. Pieter, Leuven, Belgium

Discussion: Diffuse esophageal spasm and related disorders
Cricopharyngeal myotomy for pharyngoesophageal diverticula

ALEX G. LITTLE, M.D.

Associate Professor, Department of Surgery, University of Chicago Pritzker School of Medicine; Chief, Section of Thoracic Surgery, Department of Surgery, University of Chicago Medical Center, Chicago, Illinois

Proximal esophageal strictures

HUGOE R. MATTHEWS, F.R.C.S.

Senior Clinical Lecturer in Surgery, Department of Surgery, University of Birmingham; Consultant Thoracic Surgeon, Regional Department of Thoracic Surgery, East Birmingham Hospital, Birmingham, England

The laboratory in the diagnosis of esophageal disease

K. MOGHISSI, M.D., F.R.C.S.(Eng.), F.R.C.S.(Ed.)

Consultant Cardiothoracic Surgeon, Humberside Cardiothoracic Surgical Centre, Hull, England

Discussion: Proximal esophageal strictures

PHILIPPE MONNIER, M.D.

Associate, Department of Otolaryngology–Head and Neck Surgery, University of Lausanne School of Medicine; Chief Resident, Ear, Nose and Throat Clinic, University Canton Hospital (CHUV), Lausanne, Switzerland

New endoscopic techniques

F. MORA, M.D.

Assistant Professor, Department of Internal Medicine, Facultad de Medicina, University of Valencia; Medical Assistant, Digestive Motility Unit, Department of Digestive Service, University Hospital, Valencia, Spain

Discussion: Pharyngeal dysphagia

KEITH S. NAUNHEIM, M.D.

Assistant Professor, Department of Surgery, St. Louis University Medical Center, St. Louis, Missouri

Proximal esophageal strictures

MICHEL JEAN NOIRCLERC, M.D.

Professor of Surgery, Department of Thoracic Surgery, School of Medicine, University of Marseille; Chief Surgeon, Hôpital Salvator, Marseille, France

Surgical management of caustic injuries to the upper gastrointestinal tract

DAVID D. OAKES, M.D.

Associate Professor of Surgery, Stanford University School of Medicine, Stanford, California; Chief, Division of General and Thoracic Surgery, Santa Clara Valley Medical Center, San Jose, California

Drug-induced esophageal injuries

MARK B. ORRINGER, M.D.

Professor and Head, Section of Thoracic Surgery, University of Michigan Medical Center, Ann Arbor, Michigan

Management of failed antireflux procedures

PETER C. PAIROLERO, M.D.

Professor of Surgery, Department of Surgery, Mayo Medical School and Mayo Clinic, Rochester, Minnesota

Gastric secretion suppression and duodenal diversion: the Roux-en-Y principle in the management of complex reflux problems

F. PARÍS, M.D.

Titular Professor of Surgery, University of Valencia; Head of Thoracic Surgery Service, Department of Surgery, Hospital General "La Fe," Valencia, Spain

Discussion: Extended esophageal myotomy in the management of diffuse esophageal spasm

W. SPENCER PAYNE, M.D.

James C. Masson Professor of Surgery, Department of Surgery, Mayo Medical School; Consultant, Section of Thoracic and Cardiovascular Surgery, Mayo Clinic and Mayo Foundation, Rochester Methodist Hospital and Saint Mary's Hospital, Rochester, Minnesota

Gastric secretion suppression and duodenal diversion: the Roux-en-Y principle in the management of complex reflux problems

F. GRIFFITH PEARSON, M.D., F.R.C.S.(C.), F.A.C.S.

Professor of Surgery, Department of Surgery, University of Toronto; Surgeon-in-Chief, Department of Surgery, Toronto General Hospital, Toronto, Ontario, Canada

Discussion: Barrett's esophagus

JEFFREY M. PIEHLER, M.D.

Associate Professor of Surgery, Mayo Medical School; Consultant, Section of Thoracic and Cardiovascular Surgery, Mayo Clinic and Mayo Foundation, Rochester, Minnesota

Gastric secretion suppression and duodenal diversion: the Roux-en-Y principle in the management of complex reflux problems

HIRAM C. POLK, Jr., M.D.

Professor and Chairman, Department of Surgery, University of Louisville, Louisville, Kentucky

Discussion: Reflux associated with other disorders or lesions

JAMES W. RYAN, M.D.

Associate Professor, Department of Radiology; Associate Director, Section of Nuclear Medicine, Department of Radiology, University of Chicago, Chicago, Illinois

Esophageal scintigraphy and tests of duodenogastric function

BERNARD SASTRE, M.D.

Professor of Surgery, Faculté de Médecine, University of Marseille; Service de Chirurgie Générale et Digestive, Hôpital Sainte-Marguerite, Marseille, France

Surgical management of caustic injuries to the upper gastrointestinal tract

MARCEL SAVARY, M.D.

Professor and Chairman, Department of Otolaryngology–Head and Neck Surgery, University of Lausanne School of Medicine, Lausanne, Switzerland

New endoscopic techniques

JOHN P. SHERCK, M.D.

Clinical Associate Professor of Surgery, Department of Surgery, Stanford University Medical School, Stanford, California; Department of Surgery, Santa Clara Valley Medical Center, San Jose, California

Drug-induced esophageal injuries

J. RÜDIGER SIEWERT, M.D., F.A.C.S.

Professor of Surgery, Department of Surgery, Technical University of Munich, Munich, Federal Republic of Germany

Update on esophageal pH monitoring

DAVID B. SKINNER, M.D.

Dallas B. Phemister Professor of Surgery, Department of Surgery, University of Chicago Pritzker School of Medicine; Chairman, Department of Surgery, University of Chicago Hospitals and Clinics, Chicago, Illinois

Principles of surgical treatment of gastroesophageal reflux

ROBIN BARKER SMITH, M.D., Ch.M., F.R.C.S.

Consultant Surgeon, General Surgery, Royal United Hospital, Bath, England

Reflux associated with other disorders or lesions

JOHN SPENCER, M.S., F.R.C.S.(Eng.)

Reader, Department of Surgery, Royal Postgraduate Medical School; Consultant Surgeon, Hammersmith Hospital, London, England

Discussion: Gastric secretion suppression and duodenal diversion: the Roux-en-Y principle in the management of complex reflux problems

RAYMOND TAILLEFER, M.D., F.R.C.P.(C.)

Assistant Professor of Nuclear Medicine, Department of Radiology, University of Montreal; Specialist in Nuclear Medicine, Department of Radiology, Hôpital Hôtel-Dieu de Montréal, Montreal, Quebec, Canada

Discussion: Esophageal scintigraphy and tests of duodenogastric function

JOHN G. TEMPLE, M.B., Ch.M., F.R.C.S.(Ed.), F.R.C.S.(Eng.)

Senior Clinical Lecturer, Department of Surgery, University of Birmingham; Department of Surgery, Queen Elizabeth Hospital, Birmingham, England

Discussion: Use of a prosthetic device to control gastroesophageal reflux

J. L. TERPSTRA, M.D., Ph.D.

Surgical Department, University Hospital, Leiden, The Netherlands

Discussion: Management of failed antireflux procedures

GEOFFREY B. THOMPSON, M.D.

Fellow, Department of Surgery, Mayo Graduate School of Medicine; Senior Resident, Department of General Surgery, Mayo Clinic, Rochester, Minnesota

Gastric secretion suppression and duodenal diversion: the Roux-en-Y principle in the management of complex reflux problems

M. TOMAS-RIDOCCI, M.D.

Assistant Professor, Department of Internal Medicine, School of Medicine, University of Valencia; Head of Digestive Motility Unit, Department of Gastrointestinal Service, University Hospital, Valencia, Spain

Discussion: Extended esophageal myotomy in the management of diffuse esophageal spasm

VICTOR F. TRASTEK, M.D.

Assistant Professor of Surgery, Department of Surgery, Mayo Medical School; Consultant, Section of Thoracic and Cardiovascular Surgery, Mayo Clinic and Mayo Foundation, Rochester Methodist Hospital and St. Mary's Hospital, Rochester, Minnesota

Gastric secretion suppression and duodenal diversion: the Roux-en-Y principle in the management of complex reflux problems

J. VANDEKERKHOF, M.D.

Department of Surgery, Catholic University of Leuven and University Hospitals, Leuven, Belgium

Cricopharyngeal myotomy for pharyngoesophageal diverticula

G. VANTRAPPEN, M.D., Ph.D.

Professor of Medicine, Department of Medicine, University of Leuven; Head, Department of Medicine and Division of Gastroenterology, University Hospital Gasthuisberg, Leuven, Belgium

Discussion: Function of the normal human esophagus

ANTHONY WATSON, M.B., Ch.B., M.D., F.R.C.S.

Consultant Surgeon, Department of Surgery, Royal Lancaster Infirmary, Lancaster, England; Associate Professor of Surgery, Department of Surgery, Creighton University School of Medicine, Omaha, Nebraska

Management of reflux strictures

HANS-FRED WEISER, M.D.

Department of Surgery, Technical University of Munich and Klinikum rechts der Isar, Munich, Federal Republic of Germany

Update on esophageal pH monitoring

ROY K. H. WONG, M.D., F.A.C.P.

Assistant Professor, Department of Medicine, Uniformed Services University of the Health Sciences, Bethesda, Maryland; Director of Clinical Services, Department of Gastroenterology, Walter Reed Army Medical Center, Washington, D.C.

Reflux control in operations for achalasia

Foreword

General thoracic surgery already has a glorious past. It has given birth to the modern discipline of cardiovascular surgery and has seen the prodigious growth of that discipline. It has developed the fundamental techniques of intrathoracic operations. The time has come to recognize the specialty of general thoracic surgery as a full-fledged discipline that is in the process of becoming progressively more distinct and unique. In many teaching centers it is already separated from both general surgical service and cardiovascular disciplines. The separate status presently held honors the surgical pioneers who made this recognition inevitable. However, continuing advances will require effective exchange of new ideas and steady reinforcement of the sense of identity that must remain the cornerstone of the edifice that has earned these past accolades. By stimulating the dialogue necessary for these goals to be attained, the current series of books is designed to help in generating an equally bright future.

Although an enormous volume of information is available in textbooks, monographs, and journals concerning matters the practicing general thoracic surgeon may find of great interest, retrieval of information is not always simple. Textbooks may not contain the most up-to-date information because of their extended publication schedules. Relevant articles may be in journals that do not primarily relate to the individual specialty and therefore are overlooked. In addition, the language problem militates significantly against the ready transfer of information from one country to another. It was in an attempt to bridge these sorts of gaps that *International Trends in General Thoracic Surgery* was designed. We believe this forum will most effectively convey new information in relation to the practical aspects of actual patient care as well as emphasize the clinical application of the material.

This series of books was developed to deliberately foster international interplay on relevant topics as expeditiously as possible. Initially, biennial publication was planned, but the enthusiastic reception given the proposal led to an expansion of the horizons and an annual publica-

tion schedule. As the concept was refined, it was agreed that, as a general principle, an attempt should be made to cover major subjects in single-topic issues and provide a forum for discussion of other topics and diseases in multitopic volumes released in an alternating sequence. Editorial boards were chosen to ensure that attention would be drawn to new and important contributions from all geographic areas, thereby providing the broadest possible audience at the earliest possible moment. The contributors were asked to stress their personal concepts and proposals in order to engender a worthwhile exchange of opinions that would ultimately prove informative and stimulating for an international readership.

Coverage will be restricted to general thoracic surgical problems (including esophageal diseases), and no attempt will be made to include cardiovascular topics. Although emphasis will be placed on the practical aspects of patient care, an attempt will be made to review the relevant historical background whenever necessary for better understanding of complex issues. The application of new basic and clinical investigative studies will be discussed in their clinical contexts in order to maintain the emphasis on practical clinical issues.

We believe that by following the plan just outlined, this series of books will pay particular attention to the needs of the specific target groups for whom the books are intended: practicing general thoracic surgeons, general thoracic surgical trainees, referring physicians (including respirologists and gastroenterologists), and of course the reference resources housed in university, hospital, and inservice libraries. In most instances, the information presented will also be of particular interest to many other allied disciplines, notably oncologists, radiotherapists, otolaryngologists, emergency care physicians, and general internists.

North American and European editorial boards have been created to meet annually to select topics for consideration and choose knowledgeable authors who are best able to present the requested information from a broad base of clinical experience. An international advisory board has also been constituted to ensure an effective international approach to the process of topic selection and author choice. The editors-in-chief wish to ackowledge their indebtedness to the many members of these various boards, who have accepted their responsibilities conscientiously and effectively.

Undoubtedly, as time passes, the manner in which editorial policy is pursued in attempting to achieve these objectives may well change as part of a natural evolutionary process. Nonetheless, if the fundamental aim continues to represent the basis for future decisions, we feel that the developing series will provide a useful purpose—provided the books satisfy the requirements of the target audiences. The editorial boards are determined to make every effort to merit a continuing favorable reception, since it is clearly recognized that readership acceptance must be the final arbiter of the books' value.

The editors-in-chief would be remiss indeed were they not to express—on behalf of all the board members—their warm appreciation of the efforts made by the guest editors and those who have contributed in such willing fashion to ensure that the goals established for this ongoing series are met. Its eventual success will, assuredly, depend entirely on the dedicated fashion in which they have accepted their responsibilities.

The appearance of thoracic surgical units in teaching hospitals ensures the availability of consultative services that will provide knowledgeable advice regarding the indications for surgical investigation and treatment as well as experienced management of serious postoperative problems. It is to be hoped that the books in this series will support and strengthen the role of these units in clarifying those situations in which complex issues and unusual pathologic conditions require highly sophisticated—rather than routine or traditional—therapeutic approaches.

The W.B. Saunders Company published the first two volumes *(Lung Cancer* and *Major Challenges)*. With the release of volume 3, The C.V. Mosby Company takes on the responsibility for publication. The editors-in-chief join with the guest editors and their authors in expressing sincere appreciation to Thomas Manning and Elaine Steinborn for their enthusiastic support and knowledgeable guidance in the production of the current volume and for their sensible advice in the planning of future issues.

NORMAN C. DELARUE
HENRY ESCHAPASSE

Preface

Progress in surgery depends upon experience in the care of patients with diseases amenable to surgical therapy, accurate record keeping of the experience, reflection on the experience, structuring of subsequent clinical experience or laboratory models to answer questions raised by the reflection, and communication of the results of these inquiries to others in a convincing, rational manner.

Those experienced in this art realize that after all the effort, it takes years before their concepts are accepted, if ever, by their peers. We all are biased in favor of our own analytical abilities and become skillful in defending them, as well as in modifying the concepts of others in an effort to support our own thoughts. The process is called discussion, and is enjoyed by the spectator or reader as much as any sport. It is fueled by ego, jealousy, popularity, economics, altruism, and the love for travel. Hopefully what emerges is truth, and surprisingly it often is—if the point of view is pertinent, if there are no ongoing economic pressures to suppress it, and if those who have defended most eloquently their concepts, though erroneous, have reached ages at which they no longer have the energy or the desire to rise again.

What follows in this book reflects this process. The subject is benign esophageal disease, and the essayists and discussants come from around the world. As a consequence, the reader is exposed to various views, some conflicting, and to the current thinking regarding esophageal physiology, diagnosis of esophageal disease, gastroesophageal reflux disease, esophageal strictures, and motility disorders. The authors are well known, have first-hand experience with the issues they address or discuss, and are skilled in communication. The reader will be entertained while being instructed.

TOM R. DeMEESTER
HUGOE R. MATTHEWS

Acknowledgement

Chapter 5 of this text contains 34 four-color endoscopic photographs. The inclusion of these color illustrations was made possible by a generous grant from Storz Instrument Company. We appreciate its support for our educational endeavor.

Contents

PART III
REFLUX PROBLEMS

PART VI
THE UPPER ESOPHAGUS

PART I PHYSIOLOGY

1 Function of the normal human esophagus

Philip O. Katz and Donald O. Castell

The esophagus is a hollow, muscular tube, approximately 23 cm in length, extending from the level of the fifth cervical vertebra to the tenth thoracic vertebra, bordered at its upper end by a sphincter composed of striated muscle and at the lower end by a sphincter composed of smooth muscle. It lies in the middle of the chest until the carina (approximately T5), where it passes to the right of the midline. It passes posteriorly to the left atrium, turns left and posteriorly to pass beneath the left ventricle, and enters the abdomen at the diaphragm in a leftward and anterior direction, entering the stomach at the angle of His. The esophageal wall is composed of longitudinal and circular muscle; the upper third is primarily striated muscle and the lower two thirds smooth muscle. The esophagus is the only organ in the gastrointestinal tract that does not have a serosa, with its external support being provided by a layer of fibrous connective tissue. The epithelial lining of the mucosa is stratified squamous until its transition at the gastroesophageal junction.

In this chapter, we will discuss the available information on the normal function of the two esophageal sphincters and the esophageal body, and review the events occurring during a normal swallow.

UPPER ESOPHAGEAL SPHINCTER

The upper esophageal sphincter (UES) is a high-pressure zone, consisting of striated muscle, ranging from 2.5 to 5 cm in length, located between the fifth and seventh cervical vertebrae. It remains closed at rest, with a constant discharge of motor action potentials maintaining a state of contraction. Action potentials are inhibited when a swallow occurs, causing the UES to relax. The UES also opens during vomiting, belching, and gagging. The innervation of the UES is somewhat controversial. Animal studies suggest that the sphincter is innervated in part by motor fibers of the ninth, tenth, and eleventh cranial nerves, with the major supply being through a pharyngeal plexus having principal contribution from the pharyngeal branch of the vagus nerve.[1] Some of the nervous supply appears to be from both the superior laryngeal and recurrent laryngeal nerves as well.[1]

UES pressures are best measured by means of an oval catheter with recording orifices radially oriented at 90-degree angles. Posterior pressures are higher than anterior pressures, and both are higher than lateral pressures within the sphincter (see Table 1-1). This is referred to as radial asymmetry. Peak pressures do not occur at the same level in the sphincter. Peak anterior pressure occurs approximately 0.5 cm proximal to peak posterior pressures, so the sphincter exhibits axial asymmetry as well. Pressures can be measured with a pull-through technique or a continuous-recording sleeve device.

The normal high resting UES pressure serves to protect the esophagus from filling with air during inspiration. When a swallow occurs, the sphincter relaxes, allowing pharyngeal contractions to propel the bolus from the pharynx into the esophagus. Respiration is inhibited during this event, which is under central control of the swallowing center in the medulla.

Acid infusion into the upper esophagus, just below the UES, has a stimulatory effect on the UES, causing a rise in pressure.[2] This occurs

TABLE 1-1. Resting upper esophageal sphincter pressure (mm Hg)*

Orientation	Mean	Range
Posterior	101	(60-142)
Anterior	84	(55-123)
Lateral	48	(30-65)

*Data from 20 normal subjects.

with saline as well, but to a lesser degree. In addition, the closer the fluid is infused to the UES, the greater the pressure response.[2] This suggests that the UES acts as a barrier to the reflux of esophageal contents and helps prevent aspiration and regurgitation. This mechanism appears to be deficient in some patients with gastroesophageal reflux disease, who have UES hypotension and spontaneous regurgitation of fluid or food into the pharynx.[3] These patients have also been shown to have a decreased response to acid infusion, suggesting a link between UES malfunction and regurgitation.

UES relaxation is produced by inhibition of the tonic contraction of the cricopharyngeus and inferior and pharyngeal constrictor muscles. Some role may also be played by forward displacement of the larynx by the geniohyoid muscle. The UES will relax prior to the arrival of a pharyngeal peristaltic contraction. Resting UES pressure drops within 0.2 to 0.3 seconds of a swallow, and remains relaxed for 1.2 to 1.7 seconds.[4] UES relaxation occurs approximately 0.7 seconds prior to the onset of a pharyngeal contraction. The nadir of relaxation occurs just prior to the peak of the pharyngeal contraction. The sphincter remains relaxed for the entire pharyngeal contraction, with pressure returning to the baseline after termination of the contraction[4] (see Fig. 1-1). Relaxation appears to be mediated by a cholinergic nicotine-mediated mechanism, but little information is available to substantiate this.

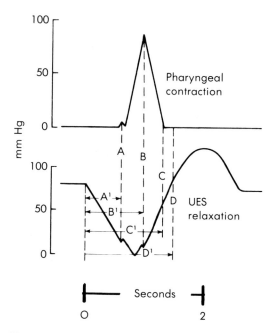

Fig. 1-1. Illustration of time intervals for upper esophageal sphincter relaxation in relationship to pharyngeal contraction in normal people. A^1, Time from onset of UES relaxation to onset of pharyngeal contraction; B^1, time from onset of UES relaxation to peak pharyngeal contraction; C^1, time from onset of UES relaxation to end of pharyngeal contraction; D^1, duration of UES relaxation.

LOWER ESOPHAGEAL SPHINCTER

Though an anatomically distinct lower esophageal sphincter (LES) has been difficult to identify in humans, there is little doubt that a physiologic sphincter exists. Manometric studies characterize the LES as a high-pressure zone, approximately 2 to 4 cm in length, located in the area of the diaphragmatic hiatus. It relaxes during esophageal peristalsis, vagal stimulation, and esophageal distention. It can be demonstrated radiographically by a muscular ring at its proximal end (A ring), an ampulla or vestibule in the middle, and a mucosal ring at the squamocolumnar junction at its distal end (B ring). It is innervated by efferent fibers from the autonomic nervous system, with parasympathetic and sympathetic input being provided by the vagus and thoracic greater splanchnic nerves, respectively. The resultant neurogenic control probably rests with a fine network of nerve plexuses in the muscle itself

(enteric nervous system). The LES has unique responses to drugs, hormones (peptides), and stretching that allow it to be distinguished from adjacent smooth muscle. Its major functions are to prevent reflux of gastric contents into the lower esophagus and to relax in response to a swallow. Failure of the former function results in gastroesophageal reflux disease, and ineffective relaxation results in dysphagia.

Although the LES was first identified manometrically by Fyke et al. in 1956,[5] accurate measurement of LES pressure was not possible until the development of perfused catheters in the 1960s.[6] Using radially oriented constantly perfused catheters, investigators have found radial asymmetry of the LES, with pressures on the left and posterior pressures being higher than those from other orientations in the sphincter. Published normal pressure values vary considerably from laboratory to laboratory. In our studies with 95 normal subjects ranging in age from 22 to 75 years, the LES pressure range was from 10 to 45 mm Hg, with a mean value of 26 mm Hg (Table 1-2). Pressure can be measured by a pull-through

TABLE 1-2. Comparison of lower esophageal sphincter pressure by two techniques ($\bar{x} \pm 1$ SD)*

Rapid pull-through	29.0 ± 12.1 mm Hg	p < .005
Station pull-through	24.4 ± 10.8 mm Hg	

*Data from 95 normal subjects.

technique—either a rapid method[7] or a station technique[8]—or with a stationary sleeve device. Pressure measurements are somewhat higher when the rapid pull-through method is used (mean = 28 mm Hg) and vary considerably in normal individuals, making an isolated sphincter pressure measurement difficult to interpret in the clinical situation.

The LES has been shown to contract in response to maneuvers that increase intraabdominal pressure, such as abdominal compression and the Valsalva maneuver. Isolated low LES pressures are often seen in patients with gastroesophageal reflux disease, particularly those with strictures, scleroderma, or Barrett's esophagus.[9] Studies in the mid-1970s by Johnson and DeMeester,[10] using 24-hour pH monitoring, suggest that normal people regularly reflux, although they do so infrequently. Recent studies by Dodds et al.,[11] using a sleeve device that allows continuous active recording of LES pressure, have given new insights into the role of the lower sphincter in gastroesophageal reflux. In these studies, done over 12-hour continuous recording periods, they found that both normals and patients with esophagitis developed transient complete LES relaxation in association with reflux episodes. Most of these relaxations occurred without any associated motor event in the stomach or esophagus, a so-called inappropriate LES relaxation. More than 60% of all reflux episodes in esophagitis patients were associated with these transient relaxations. More than 90% of reflux episodes in normals, those with "physiologic reflux," occurred during these periods of transient complete sphincter relaxation.

Three factors appear to be important in the control of LES pressure: nerves, muscle, and hormones. Neural control of the sphincter appears to be mediated by both excitatory and inhibitory nerves. Cholinergic stimulation with bethanechol has been shown to increase LES pressure, while atropine and other anticholinergic drugs decrease sphincter pressure.[12] LES pressure is decreased in response to beta-adrenergic agonists (e.g.,

isoproterenol)[13] and alpha-adrenergic blockers such as phentolamine. Dopamine has been shown to cause a decrease in sphincter pressure, while the dopamine antagonist metoclopramide will increase LES pressure.[13] The nerve poison tetrodotoxin does not appear to lower resting LES pressure in the opossum, suggesting that neural control is not important in maintaining resting LES pressure in this animal.[14] Agents that have been shown to experimentally change LES pressure are listed in the boxes on pp. 6 and 7.

LES relaxation appears to be controlled by nerve fibers carried in the vagus nerve and appears, from studies in the opossum, to be controlled by a nonadrenergic, noncholinergic mediator. If the vagus is cut in the neck of the opossum and the distal end electrically stimulated, LES pressure will decrease; that is, relaxation occurs. Neither cholinergic (atropine) nor adrenergic blockade inhibits this relaxation, but it can be abolished by tetrodotoxin.[14] Although the specific nonadrenergic, noncholinergic neurotransmitter is not known, current evidence suggests that the hormone vasoactive intestinal peptide (VIP) is the leading candidate.

The smooth muscle tone of the LES appears to be dependent on available calcium. In vitro studies in the opossum have shown that muscle strips from the region of the LES will demonstrate decreased peak force of contraction and velocity of shortening if the calcium concentration in the perfusing medium is decreased.[15] Other in vitro studies in the opossum have shown decreased tone and diminished "off" contractions in muscle strips exposed to a calcium-free solution.[16] Pharmacologic studies with verapamil and diltiazem—calcium channel blocking agents—in the baboon and the opossum have shown a decrease in LES pressure in response to intravenous infusion of both drugs.[17,18] Significant decreases in LES pressure have been found in normal subjects exposed to oral doses of nifedipine, another calcium channel blocking agent.[19] These studies support a role for calcium ions in maintaining basal sphincter pressure.

The effects of many gastrointestinal peptides (hormones) on LES pressure have been extensively studied. Gastrin has a stimulatory effect on the lower esophageal sphincter. Higgs et al. found increases in LES pressure following alkalinization of gastric contents in human volunteers, though they did not actually measure endogenous gastrin levels.[20] Another study, by Castell and Harris, did show an increase in LES pressure following injection of exogenous pentagastrin in normal subjects.[21] The release of endogenous gastrin from the antrum after the eating of meat

---

AGENTS THAT INCREASE LES PRESSURE

Hormones

Gastrin
Motilin
Substance P
Bombesin
Vasopressin
Angiotensin

Neurotransmitters

Alpha-adrenergic agonists (norepinephrine, phenylephrine)
Beta-adrenergic antagonists
Cholinergic drugs (bethanechol)
Anticholinesterase (edrophonium)

Other agents

Histamine
Antacids (gastric alkalinization)
Metoclopramide
Domperidone
Protein meals
Prostaglandin F
Indomethacin

---

extract causes LES pressure to rise. Also, the increase in sphincter response to a protein meal and gastric alkalinization is inhibited by somatostatin, suggesting that there is a definite hormone effect.[22]

The effect of gastrin on LES pressure has been shown to be inhibited by secretin, but physiologic doses of secretin do not lower LES pressure. LES pressures are lowered after a fatty meal, suggesting that cholecystokinin (CCK) may play a role in mediating LES pressure.[23] All members of the secretin family, including glucagon, gastric inhibitory peptide, and vasoactive intestinal peptide, have been shown to lower LES pressure in both humans and animals. VIP has been given the most attention, particularly as a possible chemical mediator for LES relaxation. Animal studies in awake baboons compared secretin, VIP, and glucagon and their effects on LES pressures, and found that VIP produced the greatest drop in basal LES pressure and was able to prevent the LES pressure rise with pentagastrin stimulation.[24] LES relaxation can be partially inhibited by intravenous infusion of antibodies to VIP.

Clinically, the most important hormonal action on the lower sphincter is probably that of progesterone. LES pressures are lowered during preg-

nancy and in women taking birth control pills containing progesterone.[25,26] Heartburn is seen to increase frequently during pregnancy and may be related to decreased LES pressure. Decreased sphincter pressures are not seen, however, during the normal menstrual cycle,[27] which casts some doubt on the ability of progesterone alone to decrease LES pressure. Other hormones or peptides that have been experimentally shown to change lower sphincter pressure are listed in the boxes above. The clinical importance of these findings is currently unknown.

MECHANISM OF A SWALLOW

A swallow has traditionally been divided into three phases. The first, or oral, phase is under voluntary control and involves the passage of food from the mouth to the pharynx. After food is moved voluntarily to the back of the mouth, the tongue forces food into the pharynx by pushing up and back against the palate. The tongue is then pushed posteriorly to the pharyngeal wall by the hyoglossus and styloglossus muscles. The nasopharynx is closed when the veli palatini muscles elevate the soft palate. The pharyngeal constriction raises the hypopharynx when the

AGENTS THAT DECREASE LES PRESSURE

Hormones

Secretin
Cholecystokinin
Glucagon
Gastric inhibitory polypeptide (GIP)
Vasoactive intestinal polypeptide (VIP)
Neurotensin
Progesterone

Neurotransmitters

Beta-adrenergic agonists (isoproterenol)
Dopamine
Anticholinergics (atropine)

Foods

Fat
Chocolate
Ethanol
Peppermint
Caffeine

Other agents

Theophylline
Gastric acidification
Smoking
Diazepam
Meperidine/morphine
Prostaglandins E, E_2, A_2, I_2
Nitrates
Calcium-blocking agents
Lidocaine

epiglottis closes over the larynx, preventing aspiration. It is at this point that voluntary control of swallowing ceases and reflex mechanisms take over. During the second, or pharyngeal, phase, food is transferred from the pharynx into the esophagus. The bolus in the pharynx stimulates afferent receptors around the opening of the pharynx to send impulses to the swallowing center in the brainstem. This area, located in the medulla and pons, controls the involuntary sequence of swallowing and simultaneously stops respiration by inhibiting the respiratory center in the medulla. The central nervous system areas initiate a series of involuntary responses. The soft palate extends upward, closing the posterior nares, and preventing expulsion of food through the nose. The palatopharyngeal folds are pulled medially, limiting the opening through the pharynx and preventing the passage of large boluses. The vocal cords are closed, and the epiglottis swings backward and downward to close the larynx. The larynx is pulled upward and forward by muscles attached to the hyoid bone, stretching the opening of the esophagus. At this point the upper esophageal sphincter relaxes and contraction of the superior constrictor muscle initiates a peristaltic wave, sending food into the esophagus. The third, or esophageal, phase is characterized by transport of the food bolus down the length of the esophagus by a progressive peristaltic wave, a process that normally takes 7 to 10 seconds.

A normal contraction wave, initiated by a swallow, is designated as primary peristalsis (see Fig. 1-2). A secondary peristaltic wave, caused by esophageal distention, may be initiated by an intraesophageal bolus or gastroesophageal reflux. Experimentally, secondary peristalsis may be induced by balloon distention. A tertiary contraction is a simultaneous wave that may occur spontaneously or after a swallow. The three parts of the peristaltic wave are seen on a motility tracing. The first phase occurs almost simultaneously with a swallow and is recorded as a 5- to

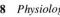

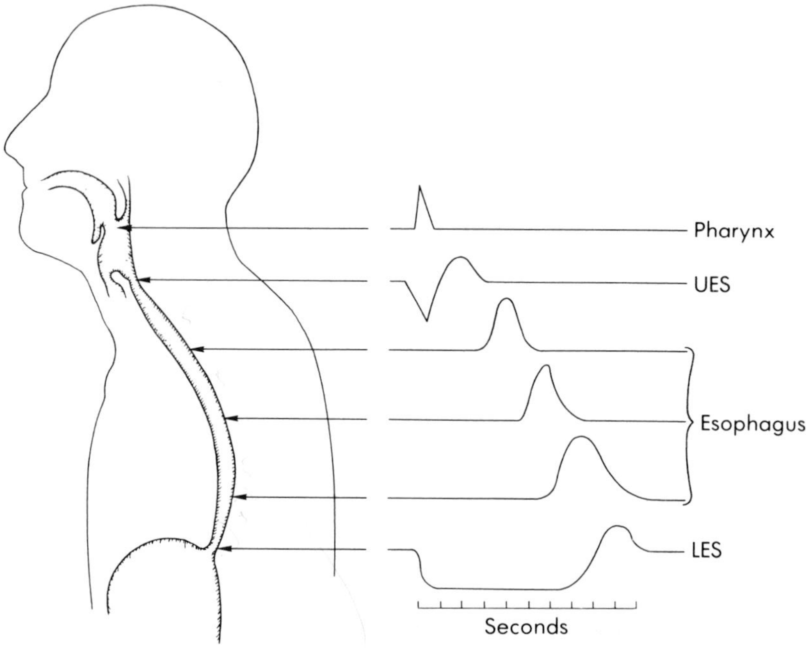

Fig. 1-2. Timing of pharyngeal contraction, UES and LES relaxation, and progressive peristalsis in the esophageal body in response to a single swallow.

10-mm Hg negative pressure. The second phase is a pressure rise to 5 to 10 mm Hg and occurs simultaneously throughout the esophagus. The third phase is the high-amplitude pressure wave seen to peak in sequence as the wave moves from the proximal to distal recording sites. (See Fig. 1-3.)

ESOPHAGEAL BODY

Despite the extensive use of esophageal manometry in evaluations of swallowing disorders, few data are available defining the normal ranges of contraction amplitude, duration, and velocity of a swallowed bolus. In our laboratory, we have studied 95 healthy volunteers during wet and dry swallows. Several important observations have been made. Amplitude is significantly greater when subjects are given wet swallows as compared to dry, while duration is unaffected. Contraction amplitude increases as the bolus proceeds from the proximal esophagus to the distal esophagus. There is a zone of low peristaltic pressure, 4 to 6 cm below the UES and about 2 to 3 cm in length, at the junction of striated and smooth muscle. Pressures in this area may be as low as 20 mm Hg. After wet swallows, mean distal esophageal amplitude and duration (measured at

3 and 8 cm above the LES) increased with age and peaked in the fifties. Normal subjects had average distal amplitudes ranging from 20 to 180 mm Hg and durations ranging from 2 to 6 seconds. Normal velocity with wet swallows averaged 3 to 3.5 cm/sec; velocity was slower with wet swallows than with dry. The velocity appeared to slow as the wave approached the distal esophagus, particularly the last 2 to 3 cm. Normal subjects may have double-peaked contractions and spontaneous activity during periods without swallows. Triple-peaked contractions and simultaneous contractions were extremely rare with wet swallows, but simultaneous contractions were seen in 12% of normals if dry swallows were used. Dry swallows underestimated amplitude and were associated with frequent abnormal contractions and, therefore, should not be used in assessing esophageal motility.

Bolus size, if greater than 2 ml, appears to have little effect on esophageal contractions.[28] Temperature, however, does affect response to swallows. Cold water (30° C)[29] or ice cream (−5° C)[30] decreases peristaltic frequency and contraction amplitude, prolongs duration, and slows the peristaltic velocity in the distal esophagus. Cold barium may result in aperistalsis and esophageal dilatation.[31] Warm water (58 to 61° C) appears to do the opposite.[29]

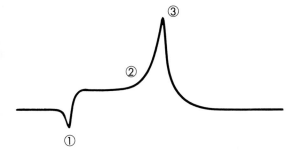

Fig. 1-3. Representation of pressure events during recording of normal esophageal peristalsis by intraesophageal catheters: **1,** onset of swallow, reflecting negative intrathoracic pressure; **2,** plateau response, approximately 10 to 15 mm Hg, that occurs simultaneously throughout the esophagus prior to phase 3; **3,** the progressive peristaltic wave seen in the esophageal body.

CONTROL OF ESOPHAGEAL PERISTALSIS

Although it is apparent that swallowing causes an esophageal contraction wave that starts proximally and proceeds distally down the esophagus in an orderly, peristaltic fashion, the mechanism of control of esophageal peristalsis is not completely known. Neural control of the esophageal body appears to be via both cholinergic and nonadrenergic, noncholinergic pathways. The cholinergic effects are the most clearly defined. The cholinomimetic agents edrophonium and bethanechol[32] increase peristaltic amplitude and duration in the distal esophagus, and peristaltic pressures are lower after administration of atropine.[33] The adrenergic nervous system appears to have little role in control of esophageal function. The information available suggests that alpha receptors are excitatory and beta receptors are inhibitory in the esophageal body.

Most of what is known about esophageal peristalsis has been derived from animal studies, particularly in the opossum. In 1969, Christensen and Lund[34] described three responses of the smooth muscle of the opossum esophagus to electrical stimulation in vitro. Two responses were seen in circular muscle: the "on-response," a contraction produced when the stimulus was applied to the muscle, and the "off-response," occurring after the stimulus was discontinued. A "duration response," occurring only in longitudinal muscle, was also described. In this original work, the on-response occurred immediately upon stimulation of the muscle, while there was considerable variation in the timing of the off-response following termination of the stimulus. This so-called "latency gradient" was shown to be directly proportional to the distance down the esophagus from which the muscle strip was taken —that is, longer latency in more distal esophageal muscle. In these experiments, the off-response but not the on-response was abolished by the nerve poison tetrodotoxin, suggesting neural control for the former but not for the latter. The off-response was not affected by phenoxybenzamine, tolazoline, hexamethonium, or methysergide, suggesting that this was a noncholinergic, nonadrenergic nervous pathway.

Recent data by Crist et al.[35] are in some conflict with those of Christensen and Lund. Using high-frequency electric field stimulation, this group demonstrated that there is a latency gradient for the on-contraction as well. This latency period increases in duration as one moves distally toward the LES. In contrast, the latency period for off-contraction did not change as the stimulus moved aborally down the esophagus. In these experiments, tetrodotoxin, at a concentration 1×10^{-7} M, abolished both the on- and off-contractions, suggesting that these are under neural control. Atropine antagonized the on- but not the off-contraction, raising speculation that both contractions are under neural control, and that the on-contraction is mediated by a cholinergic pathway.

The above studies have led to a conclusion that esophageal smooth muscle contracts in response to electrical stimulation, both during (on-response) and after (off-response) a period of stimulation. The off-response appears to be of greater amplitude and frequency and probably greater physiologic importance than the on-response. The off-response appears to be under neurogenic control through a noncholinergic pathway.

The duration response occurs in longitudinal muscle only. It occurs throughout an applied stimulus and is manifested by shortening of the esophagus. In the work of Christensen and Lund, the duration response was blocked by both atropine and tetrodotoxin, suggesting a cholinergic excitatory pathway mediating longitudinal muscle contraction. In a recent study by Sugarbaker et al.,[36] also in the opossum, the contraction pattern of longitudinal muscle was investigated. Vagal stimulation of the muscle produced a simultaneous contraction throughout the esophagus, with a short, constant latency period, while a stimulated swallow resulted in a sequential contraction with a variable latency period that increased aborally down the esophagus. The longitudinal muscle contracted before the circular muscle and had a greater velocity with contraction. It appears from these studies that the longitudinal muscle contraction is controlled by activation of vagally mediated neurons in the central nervous system.

Conflicting data make it difficult to develop a unified hypothesis as to the mechanism of control of esophageal peristalsis. It appears that both longitudinal and circular muscle play some role. Perhaps the longitudinal muscle provides form and rigidity to the esophagus during intraluminal bolus propulsion and helps to slide the esophagus over the bolus as it moves down toward the sphincter. The circular muscle appears to be under neural control by both cholinergic and noncholinergic, nonadrenergic mechanisms. Increased amplitude and predominance in number of off-contractions suggest that the predominant control of peristalsis is of an inhibitory nature.

REFERENCES

1. Ingelfinger, F.J.: Esophageal motility, Physiol. Rev. **38**:533-584, 1958.
2. Gerhardt, D.C., Shuck, T.J., Bordeaux, R.A., and Winship, D.H.: Human upper esophageal sphincter: response to volume, osmotic and acid stimuli, Gastroenterology **75**:268-274, 1978.
3. Gerhardt, D.C., Castell, D.O., Winship, D.H., and Shuck, T.J.: Esophageal dysfunction in esophagopharyngeal regurgitation, Gastroenterology **78**:893-897, 1980.
4. Knuff, T.E., Benjamin, S.B., and Castell, D.O.: Pharyngoesophageal (Zenker's) diverticulum: a reappraisal, Gastroenterology **82**:734-736, 1982.
5. Fyke, F.E., Jr., Code, C.F., and Schlegel, J.F.: The gastroesophageal sphincter in healthy human beings, Gastroenterology (Basel) **86**:135-150, 1956.
6. Dodds, W.J., Hogan, W.J., Stet, J.J., Miller, W.N., Lydon, S.B., and Arndorfer, R.C.: Rapid pull through technique for measuring lower esophageal sphincter pressure, Gastroenterology **68**:437-443, 1975.
7. Welch, R.W., and Drake, S.T.: Normal lower esophageal sphincter pressure: a comparison of rapid vs. slow pull-through techniques, Gastroenterology **78**:1446-1451, 1980.
8. Dent, J., and Chir, B.: A new technique for continuous sphincter pressure measurement, Gastroenterology **71**:263-267, 1976.
9. Knuff, T.E., Benjamin, S.B., Worsham, G.F., Hancock, J.E., and Castell, D.O.: Histologic evaluation of chronic gastroesophageal reflux, Dig. Dis. Sci. **29**:194-201, 1984.
10. Johnson, L.F., and DeMeester, T.R.: Twenty-four pH monitoring of the distal esophagus: a quantitative measure of gastroesophageal reflux, Am. J. Gastroenterol **62**:325-332, 1974.
11. Dodds, W.J., Dent, J., Hogan, W.J., et al.: Mechanism of gastroesophageal reflux in patients with reflux esophagitis, N. Engl. J. Med. **307**:1547-1552, 1982.
12. Lind, J.F., Crispin, J.S., and McIver, D.K.: The effect of atropine on the gastroesophageal sphincter, Can. J. Physiol. Pharmacol. **46**:223-238, 1968.
13. Dimarino, A.J., and Cohen, S.: Effect of an oral beta$_2$-adrenergic agonist on lower esophageal sphincter pressure in normals and in patients with achalasia, Dig. Dis. Sci. **27**:1063-1066, 1982.
14. Goyal, R.K., and Rattan, S.: Genesis of basal sphincter pressure: effect of tetrodotoxin on the lower esophageal sphincter in opposum in vivo, Gastroenterology **71**:62-67, 1976.
15. Cohen, S., and Green, F.: The mechanics of esophageal muscle contraction: evidence of an inotropic effect of gastrin, J. Clin. Invest. **52**:2029-2040, 1973.
16. deCarle, D.J., Christensen, J., Szabo, A.C., Templeman, D.C., and McKinley, D.R.: Calcium dependence of neuromuscular events in esophageal smooth muscle of the opossum, Am. J. Physiol. **232**:E549-E552, 1977.
17. Richter, J.E., Sinar, D.R., Cordova, C.M., and Castell, D.O.: Verapamil: a potent inhibitor of esophageal contractions in the baboon, Gastroenterology **82**:882-886, 1982.
18. Goyal, R.K., and Rattan, S.: Effects of sodium nitroprusside and verapamil on lower esophageal sphincter, Am. J. Physiol. **238**:40-44, 1980.
19. Blackwell, J.N., Holt, S., and Heading, R.C.: Effect of nifedipine on esophageal motility and gastric emptying, Digestion **21**:50-56, 1981.
20. Higgs, R.H., Smyth, R.D., and Castell, D.O.: Gastric alkalinization effect on lower esophageal sphincter pressure and serum gastrin, N. Engl. J. Med. **291**:486-490, 1974.
21. Castell, D.O., and Harris, L.D.: Hormonal control of gastroesophageal sphincter strength, N. Engl. J. Med. **282**:886-892, 1970.
22. Bybee, D.E., Brown, F.C., Georges, L.P., Castell, D.O., and McGuigan, J.E.: Somatostatin effects on lower esophageal sphincter function, Am. J. Physiol. **237**:E77-E81, 1979.
23. Snape, W.J., Jr., and Cohen, S.: Hormonal control of esophageal function, Arch. Intern. Med. **136**:538-542, 1976.
24. Siegel, S.R., Brown, F.C., Castell, D.O., Johnson, L.F., and Said, S.I.: Effects of vasoactive intestinal peptide (VIP) on lower esophageal sphincter in awake baboons, Dig. Dis. Sci. **24**:345-349, 1979.
25. Dodds, W.J., Dent, J., and Hogan, W.J.: Pregnancy and the lower esophageal sphincter, Gastroenterology **74**:1334-1335, 1978.
26. Van Thiel, D.H., Gavaler, J.S., and Stremple, J.: Lower esophageal sphincter pressure in women using sequential oral contraceptives, Gastroenterology **71**:232-234, 1976.
27. Nelson, J.L., Richter, J.E., Johns, D.N., and Castell, D.O.: Esophageal contraction pressures are not affected by the normal menstrual cycle, Gastroenterology **87**:867-871, 1984.

28. Hollis, J.B., and Castell, D.O.: Effect of dry swallows and wet swallows of different volumes on esophageal peristalsis, J. Appl. Physiol. **38**:1161-1164, 1975.

29. Winship, D.H., Viegas de Andrade, S.R., and Zboralske, F.F.: Influence of bolus temperature on human esophagus motor function, J. Clin. Invest. **49**:243-250, 1970.

30. Meyer, G.W., and Castell, D.O.: Human esophageal response during chest pain induced by swallowing cold liquids, JAMA **246**:2057-2059, 1981.

31. Respess, J.C., Ingelfinger, F.J., Kramer, P., and Hendrix, T.R.: Effect of cold on esophageal motor function, Am. J. Med. **29**:955, 1956.

32. Hollis, J.B., and Castell, D.O.: Effects of cholinergic stimulation on human esophageal peristalsis, J. Appl. Physiol. **40**:40-43, 1976.

33. Kantrowitz, P.A., Siegel, C.I., and Hendrix, T.R.: Differences in motility of the upper and lower esophagus in man and its alterations by atropine, Bull. Johns Hopkins Hosp. **118**:479-491, 1966.

34. Christensen, J., and Lund, G.F.: Esophageal responses to distention and electrical stimulation, J. Clin. Invest. **48**:408-419, 1969.

35. Crist, J., Gidda, J.S., and Goyal, R.K.: Characteristics of "on" and "off" contractions in esophageal circular muscle in vivo, Am. J. Physiol. **246**:6137-6144, 1984.

36. Sugarbaker, D.J., Rattan, S., and Goyal, R.K.: Swallowing induces sequential activation of esophageal longitudinal smooth muscle, Am. J. Physiol. **247**:G515-G519, 1984.

Function of the normal human esophagus

DISCUSSION

G. Vantrappen

Active transport of a bolus from the pharynx into the stomach requires the coordinated action of pharynx, upper esophageal sphincter, esophagus, and lower esophageal sphincter. Relaxation of the normally tightly closed upper and lower esophageal sphincters must precede the arrival of the bolus. The sphincters stay open until they contract in sequence with the pharyngeal and the esophageal peristaltic contraction waves.

Another important function of the esophagus and its sphincters is prevention of reflux from below. Gastroesophageal reflux is prevented mainly by a closed lower esophageal sphincter, which adapts its strength of closure to increases in intraabdominal pressure and other forces that tend to favor this reflux. Active closure of the upper esophageal sphincter prevents both esophagopharyngeal reflux and aspiration of air into the gullet. Since prolonged contact of acid gastric or alkaline duodenal contents with the esophageal mucosa may be harmful, the normal esophagus tries to keep the esophageal lumen empty. This esophageal clearing is brought about primarily by swallow-induced "primary peristaltic contractions" but may also result from "secondary peristaltic contractions," induced by esophageal distention.

The neuromuscular substrate and the physiologic mechanisms that enable the esophagus to perform these various functions are nicely described by Katz and Castell. They have succeeded in synthesizing a vast amount of experimental data into a simple, neat description of how the normal esophagus fulfills its rather complex mechanical functions. I agree with most of the views and interpretations of the authors. Therefore, in this discussion I will focus on some topics that, because of space limitations, could not be included in their chapter.

SENSORY INNERVATION OF THE ESOPHAGUS

The sensory innervation has attracted relatively little attention in the literature, despite the fact that afferent information has been shown to modulate the strength, the progression velocity, and other parameters of the deglutitive response and thus may be important in the pathogenesis of esophageal pain and esophageal motor disorders.[1] Recent studies show that both mechanoreceptor and thermoreceptor mechanisms can be identified in the esophagus in several animal species.[2] Vagal mechanoreceptors are concentrated at both ends of the esophagus. They are located not only in the muscular wall and mucosa, but in the serosa as well. The sympathetic mechanoreceptors are found mainly among the muscles, while some lie in the serosa. The anatomic substrate of the mechanoreceptors of the striated muscle layer is probably the richly innervated muscle spindles described in the canine esophagus. The mechanoreceptors in smooth esophageal muscles have not yet been clearly identified, but the intraganglionic laminar nerve endings (IGLEs) of Rodrigo[3] are the most suitable candidates. Being located within the intramural ganglia, these structures have been shown to be terminals of nerves arising from cell bodies in the nodose ganglion, the main sensory ganglion of the esophagus. Little is known about the mucosal and serosal mechanoreceptors.

Three types of vagal thermoreceptors have been described.[4] Warm receptors respond to temperatures between 39° and 50° C and cold receptors to temperatures between 10° and 35°C. Mixed receptors discharge at temperatures in both ranges. It was found that stimulation of warm receptors depresses and stimulation of cold receptors enhances proximal esophageal contractions. It is possible that the intraepithelial nerve endings that extend from the subepithelial plexus and terminate at various levels between the epithelial cells constitute these thermoreceptors.

Rodrigo et al. described yet another type of receptor-like structure.[5] In the submucosa of the midesophagus of cats and monkeys, nonvaricose nerve fibers formed a series of laminar structures on the surface of blood vessels. The function of these putative arterial receptors is unknown.

NEW METHODS OF STUDYING ESOPHAGEAL MOTILITY IN HUMANS

Radiology and conventional manometry, using a capillary-perfused catheter system, are established methods of studying esophageal transit and esophageal motor activity in humans. New techniques have been developed recently and are becoming available.

Radionuclide scintigraphy

Radionuclide scintigraphy not only allows the determination of total esophageal emptying time, but also the assessment of the dynamics of bolus passage through the esophagus. When the radioactivity in a liquid bolus is plotted against time for each of the three areas of interest (proximal, middle, and lower thirds of the esophagus), the resulting graphs describe bolus transit through each area. The normal radionuclide transit pattern consists of three distinct sequential peaks of activity. This pattern is markedly abnormal in patients with esophageal motility disorders, such as achalasia, diffuse esophageal spasm, and systemic sclerosis. However, the technique does not always allow identification of the various disease entities.

Electromyography

The recording of electrical activity of the human esophagus is still in an experimental phase. A recent modification of the recording technique provides for better tracings with less discomfort for the patient. Originally needle electrodes were used, which were built in a "suction capsule."[6] We have now replaced the needles by small electrodes incorporated into the rims of the suction orifices. The capsules are sufficiently small to allow recordings to be made at three different levels simultaneously, together with pressure recordings. Electrical recordings give more direct information on the type (striated or smooth) of muscle contraction, which is particularly important to the study of function and dysfunction of the zone of transition from striated to smooth muscle and to the study of phenomena such as deglutitive inhibition.

Twenty-four-hour pH and pressure monitoring

In many normal subjects and in patients with reflux disease, episodes of acid reflux occur intermittently as a result of "inappropriate," transient LES relaxations or as a result of a low basic LES tone.[7] This acid must be cleared from the esophagus in order to prevent damage to the esophageal mucosa. Measurement of pH with miniature glass or antimony electrodes, positioned 5 cm above the LES, is used to assess esophageal clearance. Short-term intraesophageal pH measurement is often insufficient to demonstrate the intermittent occurrence of gastroesophageal reflux. In fact, the same holds true for the manometric recording of motility disorders that occur intermittently and unpredictably. We recently developed a system that allows the recording in ambulatory patients of both pH changes and pressure changes at different levels of the esophagus for periods of 24 hours or more.[8,9] The intraluminal probe features one or two glass electrodes with an intraluminal reference electrode and three integrated pressure transducers. The pH and pressure changes are recorded on the tape of a portable cassette recorder. A computer program allows the plotting of the 24-hour pH measurements and the analysis of these data quantitatively. The main advantage of the system is that it allows the correlation of gastroesophageal reflux, esophageal motility disorders, and symptoms such as chest pain or heartburn.

MECHANISMS OF ESOPHAGEAL PERISTALSIS

Two main theories on the mechanism of esophageal peristalsis have been proposed. The first theory holds that the peristaltic progression is controlled by the deglutition center in the rhombencephalon, which emits sequential impulses to progressively more distal segments of the esophagus. The second theory attributes the peristaltic nature of the smooth-muscle contraction to an aborally increasing latency gradient in esophageal smooth-muscle contraction, an entirely peripheral mechanism. In favor of the second hypothesis is the fact that opossum and monkey esophagi do not need the deglutition center to produce peristaltic esophageal contractions. Christensen and Lund[10] showed that peristaltic contractions can be elicited in vitro in the smooth-muscle opossum esophagus by balloon distention. Moreover, we showed, many years ago, that in vivo stimulation of the distal cut end of the vagus may result in a peristaltic contraction in spite of the simultaneous activation of the entire gullet.[11] In a series of very elegant studies, Christensen[12] studied the source of the aborally increasing latency gradient of the esophageal smooth muscle contractions during peristalsis. A number of esophageal gradients were found: a gradient in intracellular potassium concentration, a gradient in passive permeability of the muscle cell membranes to potassium, a gradient in the resting membrane potential, and a gradient in rebound contraction following the period of hyperpolarization. However, the mechanism of the last gradient, the gradient in rebound contraction of circular muscle, is still unknown.

Other evidence in favor of the peripheral theory comes from the observation of Gidda et al.[13] that the progression characteristics of the peristaltic contraction can be changed by changing the stimulus parameters of vagal efferent stimulation. Suprathreshold stimuli produce peristaltic contractions; near-threshold stimuli resulted in simultaneous or even antiperistaltic contractions.

On the other hand, there is evidence that the smooth muscle esophagus is activated sequentially. Gidda and Goyal[14] made direct recordings of swallow-evoked action potentials in single vagal preganglionic fibers and found that two types of vagal fibers innervate the thoracic esophagus of the opossum: short-latency fibers, discharging within 1 second of swallowing, and long-latency fibers, showing a range of latencies from 1 to 5 seconds, which is similar to the range of latencies of peristaltic contractions. The type of esophageal muscle innervated by these fibers is not clearly established. The best candidate for the sequential cholinergic activation would seem to be the longitudinal layer. Sugarbaker et al.[15] measured the latencies of contractions at various levels of the opossum esophagus by means of strain gauges sutured onto the wall of the gullet. In the longitudinal muscle, the onset of contraction after swallowing occurred in an aboral sequence, whereas vagal stimulation resulted in simultaneous contractions. In the circular muscle, both swallowing and vagal stimulation resulted in latencies of contractions that were longer in distal parts as compared with the more proximal part of the esophagus. This observation indicates that the sequential activation of longitudinal muscle during peristalsis is centrally mediated.

On the basis of these recent and some older observations, the control of esophageal peristalsis can be schematically presented as follows. In the striated muscle part of the esophagus, peristalsis is under direct control of the rhombencephalic deglutition center. Via the nucleus ambiguus it provides sequential activation of progressively more distal esophageal segments. In the smooth muscle part of the esophagus the control is different. Not only are the motor neurons located in the nucleus dorsalis, but within 1 second of swallowing inhibitory neurons of the entire smooth muscle esophagus are centrally activated to produce almost simultaneous hyperpolarization of all circular muscle fibers. A still enigmatic peripheral mechanism then results in a latency gradient of the rebound circular muscle contraction. In contrast, the longitudinal muscle is activated sequentially by the central sequencing mechanism.

Obviously, in such a control system, the central control must be coordinated with the peripheral control: contraction of striated muscle must be coordinated with smooth muscle contraction, and longitudinal muscle contraction must be coordinated with circular muscle contraction. The mechanism of this coordination is unknown. It is tempting to speculate that the deglutition center plays a role in this coordination. Indeed, the deglutition center is directly responsible for the central sequencing, and, at the same time, it has control over the peripheral latencies of circular muscle contraction via modulation of the inhibitory stimulus parameters. And here, afferent information from the esophagus to the deglutition center comes into play to modulate the deglutition response via modulation of the central inhibitory activation.

DRINKING AND EATING

Most studies on esophageal transit and motility are performed with single swallows. In everyday life about one fifth of our daily 1000 swallows are taken in rapid succession during drinking and eating. When swallows are taken in rapid succession, two phenomena may change the stereotyped deglutitive response: first, the deglutitive inhibition and, second, the so-called refractory period following peristalsis. The deglutitive inhibition accompanying the second of two consecutive swallows may inhibit the first deglutitive response. Conversely, the second deglutitive response may be affected by the refractory period following the first swallow. Which of these phenomena will have a dominant effect depends upon the time interval between the two swallows and the esophageal level reached by the first deglutitive contraction at the time of the second swallow. On the basis of manometric, electromyographic, and radiocinematographic observations in our laboratory,[16,17] the following picture of deglutitive inhibition and deglutitive refractory periods in the human esophagus can be constructed:

1. Deglutitive inhibition. If a second swallow occurs when the peristaltic contraction elicited by the first deglutition is still in the striated muscle part of the esophagus (i.e., after an interval of less than 2, or perhaps 3, seconds), this contraction stops immediately. The pressure peak drops or (if the interval is very short) hardly develops, and the spike burst is cut off. Radiocinematography shows that the progress of the barium bolus is halted.

If the first deglutitive contraction had already reached the smooth muscle part of the esophagus at the time of the second deglutition (i.e., if the interval is more than 4 to 5 seconds), the spike burst is not immediately interrupted, though it is shortened. A pressure wave that had already begun can reach a normal amplitude, and a barium bolus is not halted at once. The distal progression of the contraction, however, is inhibited; spike activity and pressure peaks no longer appear at more distal recording sites.

2. Deglutitive refractory period. The contraction that follows the second of two deglutitions is often abnormal itself. When swallows are taken with an interval of less than 3 seconds, the first deglutitive contraction is wiped out by the deglutitive inhibition and replaced by a contraction wave that has an earlier onset but that is otherwise normal.

When the interval between two deglutitions is 4 seconds or more, the first contraction sequence already has passed down the upper 5 or 6 cm of the esophagus; the second deglutition often produces simultaneous pressure peaks in the upper part of the gullet.

With somewhat longer intervals the second contraction sequence tends to be peristaltic, but of low amplitude. When the two contractions join, the first is inhibited and the second proceeds in a normal peristaltic way. Even if the interval between two swallows is longer, the second deglutitive pressure complex may be simultaneous and of low amplitude. An interval of 20 to 30 seconds is required for consecutive swallows to produce normal deglutitive responses.

REFERENCES

1. Mei, N., Aubert, M., Crousillat, J., and Ranieri, F.: Sensory innervation of the lower esophagus of the cat: comparison with the other parts of the digestive system. In Daniel, E.E., editor: Proceedings of the Fourth International Symposium on Gastrointestinal Motility, Vancouver, 1974, Mitchell Press, pp. 585-591.
2. Christensen, J.: Origin of sensation in the esophagus, Am. J. Physiol. **246** (Gastrointest. Liver Physiol. 9):G221-G225, 1984.
3. Rodrigo, J., Fernandez, C.V., Vidal, M.A., and Pedrosa, J.A.: Vegetative innervation of the esophagus. II. Intraganglionic laminar endings, Acta Anat. **92**:79-100, 1975.
4. El-Ouazzani, T., and Mei, N.: Electrophysiological properties and role of the vagal thermoreceptors of lower esophagus and stomach of cat, Gastroenterology **83**:995-1001, 1982.
5. Rodrigo, J., Nava, B.E., and Pedrosa, J.: Study of vegetative innervation in the oesophagus. I. Perivascular endings, Trab. Inst. Cajal Invest. Biol. **62**:39-65, 1970.
6. Vantrappen, G: Measurement of electrical activity. In Postgraduate course of the American Gastroenterological Association: the esophagus, Bal Harbour, Fla., May 1971, p. 26.
7. Dent, J., Dodds, W.J., Friedmann, R.H., Sekiguchi, T., Hogan, W.J., Arndorfer, R.C., and Petrie, D.J.: Mechanism of gastroesophageal reflux in recumbent asymptomatic human subjects, J. Clin. Invest. **65**:256-267, 1980.
8. Vantrappen, G., Servaes, J., Janssens, J., and Peeters, T.: Twenty-four hour esophageal pH and pressure recording in outpatients. In Wienbeck, M., editor: Motility of the digestive tract, New York, 1982, Raven Press, pp. 293-297.
9. Janssens, J., Vantrappen, G., and Ghillebert, G.: 24-hour recording of esophageal pressure and pH in patients with noncardiac chest pain, Gastroenterology **90**:1978-1984, 1986.
10. Christensen, J., and Lund, G.F.: Esophageal responses to distension and electrical stimulation, J. Clin. Invest. **48**:408-419, 1969.
11. Vantrappen, G., and Hellemans, J.: Esophageal motility, Rendiconti Rom. Gastroenterol. **2**:7-19, 1970.
12. Christensen, J.: The oesophagus. In Christensen, J., and Wingate, D.L., editors: A guide to gastrointestinal motility, Bristol, England, 1983, John Wright & Sons, Ltd., pp. 75-100.
13. Gidda, J.S., Cobb, B.W., and Goyal, R.K.: Modulation of esophageal peristalsis by vagal efferent stimulation in opposum, J. Clin. Invest. **68**:1411-1419, 1981.
14. Gidda, J.S., and Goyal, R.K.: Swallow-evoked action potentials in vagal preganglionic efferents, J. Neurophysiol. **52**:1169-1180, 1984.
15. Sugarbaker, D.J., Rattan, S., and Goyal, R.K.: Swallowing induces sequential activation of esophageal longitudinal smooth muscle, Am. J. Physiol. **247** (Gastrointest. Liver Physiol. 10): G515-G519, 1984.
16. Hellemans, J., Vantrappen, G., and Janssens, J.: Electromyography of the esophagus. In, Vantrappen, G., and Hellemans, J., editors: Diseases of the esophagus, New York, 1974, Springer Verlag, pp. 270-285.
17. Janssens, J.: The peristaltic mechanism of the esophagus, Leuven, Belgium, 1978, Acco.

2 Gastroesophageal reflux: the role of delayed gastric emptying and duodenogastric reflux

Fernando Azpiroz

Prolonged studies using esophageal pH monitoring have clearly shown that gastroesophageal reflux (GER) is a normal event that occurs regularly in healthy persons.[1,2] The question then arises: why in some circumstances does GER produce only subjective symptoms, while in other circumstances it produces objective lesions? In normal circumstances noxious and protective mechanisms are in an equilibrium that results in the healthy state. However, when noxious factors overcome the compensatory mechanisms of defense, the equilibrium is disrupted and damage occurs. Pathologic reflux (producing symptoms or lesions) may be the consequence of (1) an excessive persistence of the refluxed material in contact with the esophgus (impaired esophageal clearance), (2) an especially noxious refluxed material, or (3) an excessive volume refluxed over time. The last case occurs when the factors inducing GER (intragastric volume and pressure) overcome the competence mechanisms of the gastroesophogeal junction, to which I will refer in a broad sense as the lower esophageal sphincter. Therefore, factors that modify intragastric content (e.g., delayed gastric emptying) may increase GER.

In this chapter I will review the integrative aspects of the gastroesophageal junction within the context of the upper digestive system. This information will provide the background for a discussion of the role of delayed gastric emptying and duodenogastric reflux in the pathogenesis of GER.

PHYSIOLOGY OF THE UPPER DIGESTIVE SYSTEM

The lower esophageal sphincter (LES) is anatomically and functionally associated with the proximal part of the stomach. The stomach, although an anatomic unit, is functionally divided into proximal and distal parts. The proximal part behaves as a reservoir and, like the LES, has the particular ability to generate a regulated tonic muscular contraction (gastric tone). The distal part and the pylorus interact as a functional unit. The proximal and distal regions partly overlap in an area where the electrophysiologic and mechanical properties are transitional.[3]

Fasting state

During fasting in humans and carnivorous animals the motor and secretory activities in the upper digestive system follow a pattern of cyclic variations.[4,5] This fasting pattern is a succession of interdigestive cycles. The motor correlate of an interdigestive cycle was first recognized in the dog as alternating periods of quiescence and bursts of intense electrical activity (reflecting contractions) migrating along the small intestine. In each region of the intestine, each cycle (about 100 minutes' duration in the dog) consists of a phase of quiescence (phase I), followed by a phase of increasing irregular activity (phase II), and culminating in a phase of intense activity (phase III). During phase III, the small bowel generates intense phasic contractions (50 to 100 mm Hg intraluminal pressure) at the maximum possible rate (13 to 19 contractions per minute). Each phase III propagates from the duodenum to the ileocolonic junction in about 100 minutes in the dog, so that, when a phase III is reaching the terminal ileum, the subsequent phase III appears in the duodenum.[4] This relationship is not exact, and each cycle may be considered an independent event. Furthermore, a high degree of interdigestive cycle variability exists in humans.

The stomach and the LES participate in this sequence of events, but with specific characteristics. The stomach and LES in the dog present a period of quiescence (about 80% of the duration of the interdigestive cycle), followed by a period of activity (20% of the cycle). During the period of activity, the LES and the proximal part of the stomach increase their tonic contraction (sphincter tone and gastric tone) and generate intense phasic contractions (50-100 mm Hg) at a maximum rate of 1 per minute.[4,6] A similar situation may prevail in humans, although some differences exist.[7,8] During the period of activity, the distal part of the stomach (antrum) generates peristaltic contractions at a rate of 3 (human) to 5 (dog) per minute. Antral contractions start in the gastric corpus and propagate to the pylorus. Phase III activity starts in the duodenum after the initiation of the period of activity in the stomach. Coinciding with the simultaneous phasic contractions in the LES and proximal stomach, antral contractions are markedly increased and duodenal phase III activity is temporarily interrupted, reflecting a close coordination of the LES, stomach, and duodenum.[6]

Gastric secretion, biliary secretion, and pancreatic secretion vary cyclically during fasting and are synchronized with the motor events in the stomach and duodenum. During the phase of quiescence (phase I) the secretory activity is low or absent, but a peak of secretion appears during late phase II.[5]

Gastric content during fasting also follows cyclic variations. During phase II, secretory activity starts and duodenogastric reflux occurs. The result is an accummulation of secretions, debris, and swallowed saliva. During phase III the propulsive contractions of the proximal stomach, coordinated with antral peristalsis and duodenal activity, clear the stomach and duodenum. Therefore, at the beginning of the period of quiescence (phase I), the stomach is empty. Nondigestible solids remaining in the stomach are emptied during the first phase III after the digestive period.[9]

GER occurs in healthy individuals during fasting, but the relationship of GER with the various phases of the interdigestive cycle has not been established.

Vagal discharge in abdominal fibers and blood levels of some gut hormones change in parallel to other events during the interdigestive cycle. However, the regulation of these orderly changes during fasting has not been elucidated.[4]

Fed state

After a meal a profound change occurs in the whole upper digestive system, involving also neural and humoral mechanisms.[9] Coinciding with each group of swallows, the basal tonic contraction of the LES (sphincter tone) and proximal stomach (gastric tone) decreases, allowing the passage (LES relaxation) and reception (gastric receptive relaxation) of the ingested material.[10,11]

After the acute receptive relaxation, the proximal stomach maintains a low level of gastric tone (lasting about 1 hour in the dog), which allows the accommodation process of the stomach to its content and prevents a major increase in intragastric pressure.[6,11] Phasic contractions of the LES and proximal stomach are abolished.[6,12] At the same time, LES pressure increases and regular antral peristalsis appears. The interdigestive cyclic activity is interrupted, and the small intestine presents a pattern of continuous irregular contractions, named the "fed pattern." The manometric configuration of this intestinal fed pattern is indistinguishable from the pattern of fasting phase II activity, although its functional significance may be different. Gastric secretion, biliary secretion, and pancreatic secretion also appear. Gastric liquid emptying starts immediately after ingestion, but intragastric volume remains constant during the first postcibal hour, because high rates of secretion compensate for the volume emptied.[9]

About 30 to 60 minutes after ingestion a series of changes occur in an ill-defined sequence. Ingested solids begin to be emptied from the stomach and follow subsequently a linear emptying pattern.[13] Gastric tone substantially increases from the low level maintained during the previous accommodation phase.[11] Gastric secretion decreases to a "plateau" phase, and intragastric content gradually decreases. This process continues for a variable period of time, depending on the size and composition of the meal (about 3 hours for a standard meal in humans). After the meal empties, a phase III clearly establishes the restoration of the interdigestive pattern.[9]

Regulatory mechanisms in the postcibal period

In healthy persons, GER is more frequent in the postcibal period.[2] This increase in GER is determined by the dynamic equilibrium between LES competence and intragastric content.

LES competence is modified after intestion of a meal. The postcibal increase in LES pressure is, at least in part, vagally mediated and depends on the size and composition of the meal.[10] Specific nutrient compositions have specific effects; protein meals increase LES pressure, while fat has the opposite effect. The intestine plays a role in this regulation; protein perfusion into the duodenum induces a tonic contractile response in the LES, and fat perfusion decreases it. Gastric alkalinization contributes to the postcibal increase in LES tone; a gastrin-mediated mechanism is in debate.[10,14] The effect of gastric distention on LES competence has not been clearly established. Large meals fail to increase LES pressure initially[15]; a contributing factor might be the decrease in LES pressure produced by increased intragastric pressure, even if the accommodation process of the stomach mitigates this effect.[16] Furthermore, the anatomic changes brought about by distention might reduce LES competence.

Intragastric volume in the postcibal period is determined by the rates of gastric secretion and emptying. Gastric distention and alkalinization stimulate gastric secretion by a combined vagus- and gastrin-mediated mechanism.[9] This stimulatory effect gradually decreases as gastric acidification and emptying take place. The intestinal phase of gastric secretion starts shortly after ingestion, triggered by the liquids delivered into the small bowel, and therefore overlaps the gastric stimulatory phase. Although nutrients in the proximal intestine have a net stimulatory effect, the responses to specific nutrients vary; proteins are stimulatory, while fat, and probably carbohydrate, are inhibitory. In the distal intestine, all three inhibit gastric secretion.[9]

Gastric emptying is a major determinant of intragastric volume during the postcibal period. The stomach liquifies the meal and delivers into the intestine a mixture of secretions, ingested liquids, and ingested solids reduced to a suspension of particles of less than 1 mm.[12] Therefore, although ingested liquids are ready to be delivered into the intestine, ingested solids require a preliminary grinding process. The antrum, in coordination with the pylorus, accomplishes this task, acting as a discriminatory barrier (sieve) and grinding pump.[17] The proximal stomach behaves as a reservoir; by modulating its tonic contraction (gastric tone), it allows the accommodation of ingested food and participates in regulating the emptying process. Tonic contraction of the proximal stomach squeezes liquids through the segment of regulated resistance generated by the antroduodenal area, while solids are trapped by the antropyloric barrier and ground by propulsive and retropulsive forces of the antral pump. Therefore, the proximal stomach is instrumental in emptying the liquid phase and feeding the antropyloric pump. Conversely, the finely tuned interaction between gastric tone and antroduodenal resistance to flow results in the regulated liquid emptying at a suitable rate for intestinal processing. Whether antral peristalsis has also a transport function and actively propels liquids and ground solids into the duodenum remains controversial. Some data suggest antral transport may contribute to liquid emptying.[13]

The rate of gastric emptying depends on the characteristics of the meal: size, consistency, caloric content, and nutrient composition.[9] The regulation of gastric emptying is achieved by specific modulation of the interacting mechanisms that determine emptying: gastric tone, antral grinding of solids, and antroduodenal resistance to flow.

1. Gastric tone during fasting is maintained by a vagal cholinergic input.[18] Receptive relaxation during swallowing is vagally mediated. Gastric distention induces a vagally mediated relaxation to allow the accommodation process. The intestine exerts a feed-back regulation, which is nutrient specific at different regions of the small bowel. For instance, fat in the proximal intestine decreases gastric tone (gastric relaxation), while carbohydrate has no effect. On the contrary, in the distal intestine, fat has no effect, while carbohydrate induces a marked gastric relaxation.[19] These effects are, at least in part, mediated by a nonadrenergic, noncholinergic vagal pathway.[20]

2. Gastric distention stimulates antral peristalsis,[6] thereby activating the grinding pump. This effect may be both vagus and gastrin mediated. Solid particles within the stomach may enhance this effect.[9] Fat and acid in the intestine inhibit antral peristalsis.[21]

3. Resistance to flow across the antroduodenal area has not been characterized during the postcibal period. During fasting, antroduodenal resistance is determined by the tonic activity of the pylorus, which is the predominant factor during motor quiescence, and by duodenal phasic contractions.[22] A similar situation may prevail in the fed state. Gastric distention induces irregular duodenal contractility.[6] Acid and nutrients, particularly fat, in the proximal intestine induce pyloric closure, stimulate duodenal motility, and, therefore, probably increase resistance.[23]

The digestive process markedly affects the secretion (stimulation or inhibition) of gut hormones.[9] Exogenous administration of pentagastrin, CCK, pancreatic polypeptide, or neurotensin, which increases during the digestive period, disrupts the cyclic interdigestive pattern and induces a motor activity that resembles the fed pattern. However, the physiologic relevance of these effects is not known. Other data suggest that the development of the digestive pattern is vagally mediated. Probably the concept of a "universal" fed pattern with a unique regulating mechanism is illusory. Specific functions are intimately regulated by interacting neurohumoral mechanisms, which achieve the integrated response adapted to each particular situation during the digestive process.

Conclusion

This sequence of events occurring during fasting and after a meal provides a picture of the functional integration of the LES within the broader context of the digestive system, in which specific functions are interrelated in a chain of causes and effects, involving neural and humoral mechanisms. In particular, in any given circumstance, an equilibrium of interacting factors will determine the occurrence and effects of GER.

ROLE OF DELAYED GASTRIC EMPTYING IN GASTROESOPHAGEAL REFLUX

Scintigraphic methods allow the selective study of the solid and liquid components of a meal. The definition and labeling of the solid component requires special attention. The stomach probably discriminates solids on the basis of the consistency and size (greater than 1 mm) of the particles mixed with the liquid phase.[17] These particles require a specific processing (grinding) before being emptied. Semisolid food may require a dilution and mixing process different from the processing of solids. As a matter of fact, gastric emptying for the spectrum of the semisolid type of food lies somewhere between the rates for solids and liquids, depending on the food's viscosity.[24] It is clinically meaningful to divide the solid emptying curve into a lag phase and an emptying phase.[13] The lag phase is the interval required for the initiation of solid emptying, which is determined by the appearance of marker outside the gastric area (defined as the scintigraphic region of interest). The emptying phase of solids thereafter follows a linear pattern, accurately defined by its slope. Emptying of a liquid marker follows an exponential pattern, because of the dilution of the ingested liquids (liquid marker) with gastric secretion.[13] However, the actual volume of liquids emptied (ingested plus secreted) is linear.[9]

Pathogenesis of delayed gastric emptying

Gastric emptying is determined by the interaction of (1) the tonic contraction of the proximal stomach (gastric tone), (2) antral peristalsis, and (3) antrointestinal resistance to flow.

Impairment of the *tonic contraction* of the proximal stomach has not been evidenced in humans, because of methodologic problems involved in measuring gastric tone "in vivo." However, experimental and clinical data suggest that impaired gastric tone causes delayed gastric emptying of both solids and liquids.

Antral hypomotility affects primarily the grinding process of solids required before emptying. In this case, a delayed solid emptying with a prolonged lag phase coexists with a normal liquid emptying. Antral dysmotility can be demonstrated by manometric techniques, provided multiple recording ports are closely spaced (1 cm apart) along the antroduodenal area, to identify, first, the pylorus and, consequently, the terminal antrum.[13]

The transport function of antral peristalsis remains controversial. In some patients, antral hypomotility and normal intestinal motility are associated with delayed gastric emptying of solids and liquids. Therefore, impaired antral transport caused by hypomotility has been postulated.[23] However, delayed liquid emptying in these patients might have been caused by a concomitant failure of the proximal stomach, which was not tested.

An increased *resistance to flow across the antroduodenal area* may produce delayed gastric emptying. This resistance factor has not been measured in relation to gastric emptying. Nor has the physiologic significance of intestinal manometric patterns been established. However, combined manometric and gastric emptying studies have identified a group of patients with normal antral motility, intestinal dysmotility, and delayed gastric emptying. Gastric emptying was prolonged for both solids and liquids, but the lag phase for solid emptying was normal. These data suggest that increased intestinal resistance may delay gastric emptying, even though a normal antral motor activity maintains the lag phase for solid emptying within the normal limits.[23] This concept is further supported by experimental studies that show accelerated gastric emptying after duodenal myotomy.[25]

Contribution of delayed gastric emptying to gastroesophageal reflux

The question of how delayed gastric emptying contributes to GER is open to speculation because only indirect data are available. In healthy subjects GER is more frequent postprandially than during fasting.[2] Therefore, when the postcibal period is prolonged by delayed gastric emptying, the reflux time over 24 hours will be increased. Some features observed in GER patients may aggravate the consequences of persistent postcibal gastric content. For instance, the increase in LES pressure in response to supine position or food ingestion does not occur in GER patients.[26] If delayed gastric emptying is also present, a synergism of factors will occur during night time: supine position, stomach not empty, and lack of LES response to both. GER patients with delayed gastric emptying are predominantly supine (or combined) refluxers and tend to have more severe esophagitis.[27]

In patients with delayed gastric emptying of both solids and liquids, cumulative gastric secretion with small losses through the pylorus may increase intragastric volume substantially. Gastric distention in this case may overcome the competence mechanisms of the gastroesophageal junction.[16]

In the hypothetic group of patients with increased outlet resistance as a cause of delayed gastric emptying, increased gastric tone (and consequently high intragastric pressure) may be required to achieve emptying. It has been speculated that increased intragastric pressure may contribute to GER.[27] Furthermore, increased intragastric pressure may produce a decrease in LES pressure.[16]

Clinical association between delayed gastric emptying and gastroesophageal reflux

Delayed solid emptying with normal liquid emptying has been demonstrated in about half of GER patients,[28,29] probably because of the association of impaired LES pressure and antral hypomotility.[30] In most instances, no symptoms related to delayed gastric emptying were present. When impaired LES function and delayed gastric emptying coexist, the latter aggravates the consequences of GER. GER patients with impaired LES pressure and delayed gastric emptying develop more severe esophagitis than patients with normal emptying.[27]

GER may be caused by a generalized disease (e.g., diabetes, scleroderma) affecting the digestive tract. Esophageal dysfunction, gastrointestinal manometric abnormalities, and delayed gastric emptying have been recognized in such conditions. Progressive systemic sclerosis (scleroderma) is frequently complicated by severe GER. In these patients, esophageal dysfunction is frequently associated with delayed gastric emptying of solids and liquids, suggesting a concomitant involvement of the proximal stomach (impaired gastric tone) and/or intestine (increased outlet resistance). Delayed gastric emptying may be a determining factor for the severe consequences of GER in these patients.[31]

Infants with GER constitute a particular subgroup in which delayed gastric emptying of liquids is frequent and coexists with normal or elevated LES pressure. In infants, altered esophageal body motility associated with fundic dysmotility (but normal LES) has been postulated as the underlying cause of GER.[32] Studies in adults suggest that delayed gastric emptying and/or motor abnormalities in the esophageal body are the major determinants of severe reflux esophagitis.[27] The association of both factors in infants explains the severe complications frequently produced by GER.

Interestingly, delayed gastric emptying and acid hypersecretion have been reported in a group of GER patients in which esophageal clearance tests and LES basal pressure were similar to those of a healthy control group.[33] It seems, therefore, that at least in some patients, delayed gastric emptying may be the principal factor determining pathologic GER.

On the basis of the frequent association of delayed gastric emptying and esophagitis, it has been speculated that delayed gastric emptying may be the consequence of vagal involvement by the panmural extension of the esophageal inflammatory process.[27] Delayed emptying in this case would aggravate the esophageal process, closing a pathogenetic vicious circle.

Management

A substantial proportion of patients with GER may present with delayed gastric emptying, generally subclinical. Furthermore, GER patients with delayed gastric emptying seem to be a heterogeneous group, in which the cause of delayed gastric emptying, the mechanisms by which delayed gastric emptying contributes to GER, and additional concurrent factors in the pathogenesis of GER (e.g., impaired esophageal clearance, impaired LES function) are variable. Therefore, a careful diagnostic evaluation is advisable before treatment, particularly if surgical therapy is indicated. Dyspeptic symptoms and manometric abnormalities have been reported after fundoplication. Although in this series preoperative manometric evaluation was not performed, postoperative vagal integrity was verified by the gastric secretory response to insulin hypoglycemia.[34] Thus, preexistent gastrointestinal motor dysfunction may produce a failure of antireflux surgical treatment.

Therapy should be directed at the etiopathogenic mechanisms involved in each case. General dietary measures will avoid factors that decrease LES pressure and delay gastric emptying (e.g., large meals, fat). Medical treatment with agents that improve esophageal motor function, LES competence, and gastric emptying has been helpful.[30,35]

ROLE OF DUODENOGASTRIC REFLUX IN GASTROESOPHAGEAL REFLUX

Like GER, duodenogastric reflux (DGR) is a normal event that occurs in healthy humans, as well as in other species.[5,36] In the fasting state, DGR occurs regularly during phase II of the interdigestive motor complex, but the stomach empties during phase III. Therefore, under normal conditions the presence of enteric content in the stomach during fasting is of limited duration. The occurrence of this event (and the limitation of its effects) is determined by the interaction of timed factors. During phase I, the circumstances are favorable for DGR to occur (gastroduodenal motor quiescence and low antroduodenal resistance to flow). However, the nonavailability of duodenopancreatic secretion in the duodenum precludes reflux. During phase II, although both aborally directed transport mechanisms and antroduodenal resistance increase, biliopancreatic secretion loads the duodenum and part of it refluxes into the stomach. During phase III the enteric refluxate is cleared from the stomach by the highly propulsive gastric motility and is propelled downstream by the intestinal migrating motor activity.[5]

DGR in the postcibal period has been well documented in normal individuals.[9] Passage of enteric content through the pylorus is bidirectional. Therefore, the amount of enteric refluxate within the stomach is determined by the dynamic equilibrium between reflux and clearance. The latter is closely related to gastric emptying.[36]

Mechanisms by which duodenogastric reflux contributes to the pathogenesis of gastroesophageal reflux (Table 2-1)

If DGR is a normal event (as is GER), a question at this point arises: why and how does DGR contribute to the pathogenesis of GER? The answer depends on (1) the excess availability of enteric refluxate within the stomach, (2) failure of protective mechanisms that prevent enteric refluxate from entering the esophagus, and (3) the physicochemical characteristics of the enteric refluxate within the esophagus.

The presence of *enteric refluxate within the stomach* depends on (1) the availability of biliopancreatic secretion in the duodenum, (2) the resistance to flow across the antroduodenal area, and (3) the gastric clearance mechanisms.

The availability of biliopancreatic secretion in the duodenum is determined by the rates of biliopancreatic secretion and the aborad duodenal transport. A most important point to consider in this context is the timing of factors. To this end the effect of cholecystectomy on DGR is controversial. However, the current physiologic understanding supports a possible pathogenic role of cholecystectomy in DGR. With a functioning gallbladder, DGR does not occur during phase I of the interdigestive motor cycle, because of the lack of biliary excretion into the duodenum at this time. However, with the reservoir and cyclic excretory function of the gallbladder lacking after cholecystectomy, bile will be continuously ex-

TABLE 2-1. Pathogenic role of duodenogastric reflux in gastroesophageal reflux

Availability of enteric refluxate in the stomach	Availability of enteric refluxate in the duodenum	Biliopancreatic secretion / Duodenal motility
	Antropyloric resistance	Pyloric activity
	Gastric clearance	Antral peristalsis / Gastric tone
Passage of enteric refluxate into the esophagus	Antireflux mechanisms	LES competence
Physiochemical characteristics of enteric components in the esophagus	Composition / Concentration / pH	Biliopancreatic secretion / Gastric dilution / Gastric acid secretion

creted and may reflux into the stomach during phase I.

Aborad duodenal propulsion is achieved by duodenal contractility. During motor quiescence (i.e., phase I) propulsion is absent and intraluminal content would accumulate in the duodenum and partly reflux into the stomach (i.e., after cholecystectomy). Conversely, intense motor activity (i.e., phase III) prevents GER by washing out duodenal content. During the postcibal period, both secretion and duodenal motor activity are closely regulated. Potent secretagogues (e.g., fat) also stimulate duodenal motility, favoring aborad propulsion.[21] A desynchronization of regulatory mechanisms may therefore cause DGR. Retrograde duodenal propulsion has also been postulated as a factor in DGR. However, this point remains unsettled because the intimate organization and functional significance of duodenal motility have not been completely elucidated.

Resistance to flow across the antroduodenal area opposes reflux. Resistance changes cyclically during the interdigestive motor cycle.[37] During phase I, resistance is low and predominantly generated by the tonic constriction of the pyloric sphincter. Resistance increases during phase II and peaks during phase III. During intense motor activity (i.e., phase III) duodenal phasic contractility is the major determinant of resistance.[22] Therefore, active transport is associated with high resistance, in analogy to a revolving door that transports in a closed system. Furthermore, resistance is similar for duodenogastric flow and gastroduodenal flow, which indicates lack of a valvular mechanism at the antroduodenal junction.[37]

Antroduodenal resistance during the postcibal period has not been evaluated. Continuous antral peristalsis may play a role in opposing reflux. Pyloric activity and motility in the first duodenal portion are regulated by the composition of intraluminal content (i.e., fat, acid) delivered into the intestine.[21] Failure of those mechanisms that increase resistance may increase DGR. Lack of pyloric response to duodenal acid infusion has been reported in a patient with alkaline reflux esophagitis.[38]

Gastric clearance of enteric refluxate is achieved by the motor activity of the stomach. During fasting, gastric clearance is produced by the phase III motor activity. In the dog, emptying at this point takes place in a stepwise fashion, when the propulsive phasic contractions of the proximal stomach coincide with increased antral peristalsis and interruption of duodenal activity.

In patients without cyclic interdigestive activity, gastric clearance will fail to occur during fasting and refluxed material will accumulate for prolonged periods of time in the stomach.

In the postcibal period, phasic activity of the proximal stomach is suppressed and clearance is closely associated with gastric emptying.[6,36] Gastric tone plays a major role in determining the direction of flow across the pylorus, by establishing a pressure gradient across the antroduodenal area. Antral peristalsis probably opposes enteric reflux into the reservoir cavity of the stomach (proximal stomach) and clears refluxed material within the antral canal.

The timing of the interaction of the preceding mechanisms determines the amount and duration of enteric refluxate within the stomach available for esophageal reflux. During fasting, the cyclic nature of events results in a limited presence of enteric refluxate in the stomach.

In the postcibal period, all the partial functions are finely orchestrated to achieve an integrated result. When gastric tone is high, emptying will occur, depending on the antroduodenal resistance. Conversely, when gastric tone is low, antoduodenal resistance will determine the occurrence of DGR. For instance, fat in the intestine stimulates biliopancreatic secretion and decreases gastric tone, but, on the other hand, it stimulates pyloric contraction and duodenal motility, thereby increasing antroduodenal resistance and aborad transport of duodenal content. The result allows adequate intestinal digestion, providing high enzymatic activity and slow gastric delivery, without DGR. A dissociation of these regulatory mechanisms will increase DGR. This is beautifully illustrated by the effects of atropine, which decreases gastric tone, antroduodenal resistance, and duodenal transport (inhibition of overall motor activity by cholinergic blockade). As a result, the preexisting duodenal content promptly refluxes into the stomach and gastric emptying is stopped.[36]

Increased DGR has been reported in a portion of GER patients, but because of the methodology used in these studies (duodenal barium infusion), conclusions are to be drawn with caution.[39] The association of alkaline GER and delayed gastric emptying suggests that a motor dysfunction involving the upper digestive tract may be present in some patients.[40]

Passage of enteric refluxate into the esophagus is especially noxious because of, first, the injurious potential of enteric content[41]; second, the longer esophageal clearance time required for alkaline reflux episodes[42]; and third, the fact that the increase in LES pressure induced by acid reflux into the esophagus (preventing further reflux episodes) will not be elicited by alkaline reflux.[43] However, specific protective mechanisms may operate under normal conditions, preventing the passage of enteric refluxate into the esophagus. Enteric reflux may buffer intragastric acid, elevating the pH. Gastric alkalinization in this case will induce an increase in LES pressure.[10,14] Furthermore, intragastric bile in experimental animals induces an increase in LES pressure without changing intragastric pH. In patients with alkaline esophageal reflux, LES pressure is below the normal range.[44] Thus, it seems that LES impairment is an important factor in the pathogenesis of enteric esophageal reflux.

The final noxious effect of enteric refluxate in the esophagus is determined by the *physicochemical characteristics* of the different constituents refluxed and the mucosal resistance. The deleterious effect of enteric content (bile salts, lisolecithin, pancreatic enzymes) on the esophageal mucosa has been well documented. Damage is determined by the concentration of each component and the pH.[41,45]

The concentration of enteric refluxate is determined by the amount refluxed into the stomach and by gastric dilution. The concentration of noxious components in the normal stomach is well below the injurious range.[45] Under normal conditions, fasting DGR occurs during phase II, when the stomach is not empty and refluxed material is diluted. However, if reflux occurs in an empty stomach (during phase I), the concentration of noxious components may achieve injurious levels. Alkaline reflux esophagitis has been reported in association with achlorhydria.[38] Lack of gastric dilution may be a pathogenic factor in the esophageal damage under this circumstance. Increased concentration of bile salts in gastric aspirate has been found in some GER patients.[46] Furthermore, abnormal bile composition has been found in patients with postsurgical reflux gastritis,[47] which suggests that alterations in bile composition may participate in the pathogenesis of reflux esophagitis.

Experimental studies have shown that the injurious potential of duodenal content (biliopancreatic secretion) increases at acid pH. In a group of patients with alkaline esophageal reflux, the degree of esophagitis was lower than in acid refluxers, suggesting that alkaline pH prevented damage.[48] However, the composition of the refluxate was not determined in this study. When enteric refluxate mixes with gastric content, two phenomena take place: dilution of noxious components and a reaction of neutralization between gastric acid and duodenal alkali. However, the relation between buffer capacity and injurious potential in duodena content has not been established. Therefore, esophageal pH determinations do not accurately reflect the presence of enteric components at noxious concentrations in the esophageal refluxate.

Clinical perspective

Patients with enteric reflux gastritis may present symptoms or objective findings of esophageal involvement. However, more intriguing is the possibility of pathologic GER produced by enteric refluxate in the absence of symptomatic reflux gastritis. In a manner similar to the case of asymptomatic delayed gastric emptying in GER patients, DGR may play a role in the pathogenesis of GER without producing a gastric syndrome.

Alkaline esophageal reflux in healthy volunteers, detected by prolonged esophageal pH monitoring, is infrequent.[1,42] Further studies on a population of GER patients have identified a small proportion of patients with alkaline esophageal reflux.[27,42,48] These patients presented with impaired LES function, suggesting that different factors interact to produce the final consequences (symptoms or lesions) of GER. Also supporting a multifactorial process is the simultaneous occurrence of delayed gastric emptying in some patients with alkaline esophageal reflux.[40] Probably the patients in whom DGR significantly contributes in the development of symptoms or lesions of GER constitute a very specific subgroup. However, the actual incidence may well be higher than reported to date. Indeed, it seems that abnormal DGR is present in a substantial proportion of GER patients,[39] although this observation needs to be verified with more reliable methods. Esophageal pH monitoring is limited in identifying an enteric contribution to esophageal reflux; acid esophageal reflux does not exclude the participation of enteric noxious components in the refluxate. On the other hand, esophageal reflux of enteric content may not produce a detectable change in pH and therefore some of the enteric reflux episodes may occur undetected, although simultaneous gastric pH monitoring in this case might identify the occurrence of DGR.[48]

Studies quantifying DGR and determining the concentration of enteric components in esophageal refluxate are needed to elucidate the contribution of DGR to GER. Effort should be directed toward the identification and comprehensive management of this subgroup of patients in whom a generalized or multifactorial process results in pathologic GER.

REFERENCES

1. DeMeester, T.R., Johnson, L.F., Joseph, G.J., Toscano, M.S., Hall, A.W., and Skinner, D.B.: Patterns of gastroesophageal reflux in health and disease, Ann. Surg. **184**(4):459-470, 1976.
2. Holscher, A.H., and Weiser, H.F.: Reflux characteristics in health and disease. In Roman, C., editor: Gastrointestinal motility, MTP Press Limited. Lancaster, England, 1984, MTP Press, Ltd., pp. 63-69.
3. Szurszewski, J.H.: Electrophysiological basis for gastrointestinal motility. In Johnson, L.R., editor: Physiology of the gastrointestinal tract, New York, 1981, Raven Press, pp. 1435-1466.
4. Itoh, Z., Aizawa, I., and Sekiguchi, T.: The interdigestive migrating complex and its significance in man, Clin. Gastroenterol. **11**(3):497-521, 1982.
5. Keane, F.B., DiMagno, E.P., and Malagelada, J.-R.: Duodenogastric reflux in humans: it relationship to fasting antroduodenal motility and gastric, pancreatic, and biliary secretion, Gastroenterology **81**:726-731, 1981.
6. Azpiroz, F., and Malagelada, J.-R.: Pressure activity patterns in the canine proximal stomach: response to distention, Am. J. Physiol. **247**(10):G265-G272, 1984.
7. Azpiroz, A., and Malagelada, J.-R.: Tonic activity of the human stomach during fasting: quantification by an electronic barostat (abstract), Gastroenterology **88**:1312, 1985.
8. Dent, J., Dodds, W.J., Sekiguchi, T., Hogan, W.J., and Arndorfer, R.C.: Interdigestive phasic contractions of the human lower esophageal sphincter, Gastroenterology **84**:453-460, 1983.
9. Malagelada, J.-R.: Gastric, pancreatic, and biliary responses to a meal. In Johnson, L.R., editor: Physiology of the gastrointestinal tract, New York, 1981, Raven Press, pp. 893-924.
10. Goyal, R.K., and Cobb, B.W.: Motility of the pharynx, esophagus, and the esophageal sphincters. In Johnson, L.R., editor: Physiology of the gastrointestinal tract, New York, 1981, Raven Press, pp. 359-391.
11. Azpiroz, A., and Malagelada, J.-R.: Physiological variations in canine gastric tone measured by an electronic barostat, Am. J. Physiol. **248**(11):G229-G237, 1985.
12. Holloway, R.H., Blank, E., Takahashi, I., Dodds, W.J., Hogan, W.J., and Dent, J.: Variability of lower esophageal sphincter pressure in the fasted unanesthetized oppossum, Am. J. Physiol. **248**(11):G398-G406, 1985.
13. Camilleri, M., Malagelada, J.-R., Brown, M.L., Becker, G., and Zinsmeister, A.R.: Relation between antral motility and gastric emptying of solids and liquids in humans, Am. J. Physiol. **249**:G580-G585, 1985.
14. Nebel, O.T., and Castell, D.O.: Lower esophageal sphincter pressure changes after food ingestion, Gastroenterology **63**(5):778-783, 1972.
15. Maher, J.W., Crandall, B.S., and Woodward, E.R.: Effects of meal size on postprandial lower esophageal sphincter pressure (LESP), Surg. Forum **28**:342-344, 1977.
16. Muller-Lissner, S.A., and Blum, A.L.: Fundic pressure rise lowers esophageal sphincter pressure in man, Hepatogastroenterology **29**:151-152, 1982.
17. Meyer, J.H., Ohashi, H., Jehn, D., and Thompson, J.B.: Size of liver particles emptied from the human stomach, Gastroenterology **80**:1489-1496, 1981.
18. Azpiroz, F., and Malagelada, J.-R.: The role of vagal input in the control of gastric tone (abstract), Gastroenterology **88**:1312, 1985.
19. Azpiroz, F., and Malagelada, J.-R.: Intestinal control of gastric tone, Am. J. Physiol. **249**:G501-G509, 1985.
20. Azpiroz, F., and Malagelada, J.-R.: Vagally mediated gastric relaxation induced by intestinal nutrients in the conscious dog (abstract), Clin. Res. **33**:318A, 1985.
21. Keinke, O., and Ehrlein, H.-J.: Effect of oleic acid on canine gastroduodenal motility, pyloric diameter and gastric emptying, Q. J. Exper. Physiol. **68**:675-686, 1983.
22. Mearin, T., Azpiroz, F., and Malagelada, J.-R.: Role of the pylorus in fasting antroduodenal resistance to flow (abstract), Dig. Dis. Sci. **30**:783, 1985.
23. Camilleri, M., Brown, M.L., and Malagelada, J.-R.: Relationship between impaired gastric emptying and abnormal gastrointestinal motility, Gastroenterology **91**(1):94-99, 1986.
24. Prove, J., and Ehrlein, H.-J.: Motor function of gastric antrum and pylorus for evacuation of low and high viscosity meals in dogs, Gut **23**:150-156, 1982.
25. Bortolotti, M., Pandolfo, N., Nebiacolombo, C., Labo, G., and Mattioli, F.: Gastroenterology **81**:910-914, 1981.
26. Funch-Jensen, P., and Oster, M.J.: Influence of food intake and postural changes on gastroesophageal sphincter pressure in patients with reflux esophagitis and in controls, Scand. J. Gastroenterol. **17**:279-281, 1982.
27. Little, A.G., DeMeester, T.R., Kirchner, P.T., O'Sullivan, G.C., and Skinner, D.B.: Pathogenesis of esophagitis in patients with gastroesophageal reflux, Surgery **88**(1):101-107, 1980.
28. McCalum, R.W., Mensh, R., and Lange, R.: Definition of the gastric emptying abnormality present in gastroesophageal reflux patients. In Wienbeck, M., editor: Motility of the digestive tract, New York, 1982, Raven Press, pp. 355-362.
29. Velasco, N., Hill, L.D., Gannan, R.M., and Pope, C.W., II: Gastric emptying and gastroesophageal reflux, Am. J. Surg. **44**:58-62, 1982.
30. Behar, J., and Ramsby, G.: Gastric emptying and antral motility in reflux esophagitis: effect of oral metoclopramide, Gastroenterology **74**:253-256, 1978.
31. Maddern, G.J., Horowitz, M., Jamieson, G.G., Chatterton, B.E., Collins, P.J., and Roberts-Thompson, P.: Abnormalities of esophageal and gastric emptying in progressive systemic sclerosis, Gastroenterology **87**:922-926, 1984.
32. Hillemeier, A.C., Grill, B.B., McCallum, R., and Gryboski, J.: Esophageal and gastric motor abnormalities in gastroesophageal reflux during infancy, Gastroenterology **84**:741-746, 1983.
33. Baldi, F., Corinaldesi, R., Ferrarini, F., Stanghellini, V.,

Miglioli, M., and Barbara, L.: Gastric secretion and emptying of liquids in reflux esophagitis, Dig. Dis. Sci. **26**(10):886-889, 1981.

34. Stanghellini, V., and Malagelada, J.-R.: Gastric manometric abnormalities in patients with dyspeptic symptoms after fundoplication, Gut **24**:790-797, 1983.

35. McCallum, R.W., Fink, S.M., Lerner, E., and Berkowitz, D.M.: Effects of metoclopramide and bethanechol on delayed gastric emptying present in gastroesophageal reflux patients, Gastroenterology **84**:1573-1577, 1983.

36. Sonnenberg, A., Muller-Lissner, S.A., Schattenmann, G., Siewert, J.R., and Blum, A.L.: Duodenogastric reflux in the dog, Am. J. Physiol. **242**(5):G603-G607, 1982.

37. Mearin, F., Azpiroz, F., and Malagelada, J.-R.: A new system for measuring "in vivo" the resistance to flow across the antroduodenal junction (abstract), Clin. Res. **32**:747A, 1984.

38. Orlando, R.C., and Bozymski, E.M.: Heartburn in pernicious anemia: a consequence of bile reflux, N. Engl. J. Med. **289**:522-523, 1973.

39. Donovan, J.A., Harding, L.K., Keighley, M.R.B., Griffin, D.W., and Collis, J.L.: Abnormalities of gastric emptying and pyloric reflux in uncomplicated hiatus hernia, Br. J. Surg. **64**:847-848, 1977.

40. Mattioli, F., and Pandolfo, N.: Gastric emptying and duodeno-gastric reflux in patients with gastro-esophageal reflux (abstract), Gut **24**:A361, 1983.

41. Safaie-Shirazi, S., DenBesten, L., and Zike, W.L.: Effect of bile salts on the ionic permeability of the esophageal mucosa and their role in the production of esophagitis, Gastroenterology **68**(68):728-733, 1975.

42. Pellegrini, C.A., DeMeester, T.R., Wernly, J.A., Johnson, L.W., and Skinner, D.B.: Alkaline gastroesophageal reflux, Am. J. Surg. **135**:177-184, 1978.

43. Ahtaridis, G., Snape, W.J., and Cohen, S.: Lower esophageal sphincter pressure as an index of gastroesophageal acid reflux, Dig. Dis. Sci. **26**(11):993-998, 1981.

44. Laitinen, S., Mokka, R.E.M., and Larmi, T.K.I.: Effect of intragastric bile on canine lower esophageal sphincter pressure, Scand. J. Gastroenterol. **13**:369-372, 1978.

45. Duane, W.C., Wiegand, D.M., and Gilberstadt, M.L.: Intragastric duodenal lipids in the absence of a pyloric sphincter: quantitation, physical state, and injurious potential in the fasting and postprandial states, Gastroenterology **78**:1480-1487, 1980.

46. Crumplin, M.K.H., Stol, D.W., Murphy, G.M., and Collis, J.L.: The pattern of bile salt reflux and acid secretion in sliding hiatal hernia, Br. J. Surg. **61**:611-616, 1974.

47. Gadacz, T.R., and Zuidema, G.D.: Bile acid composition in patients with and without symptoms of postoperative reflux gastritis, Am. J. Surg. **135**:48-52, 1978.

48. Little, A.G., Martinez, E.I., DeMeester, T.R., Blough, R.M., and Skinner, D.B.: Duodenogastric reflux and reflux esophagitis, Surgery **96**(2):447-454, 1984.

Gastroesophageal reflux: the role of delayed gastric emptying and duodenogastric reflux

DISCUSSION

Paolo Bechi

There has been a lot of research into GER in the last few years, which has greatly improved our knowledge of this problem. However, much remains to be done.

Although some time has passed since Pope stated in *Gastroenterology* that "the LES is not enough,"[1] too often GER has been considered an exclusively LES-dependent phenomenon. In the present chapter Dr. Azpiroz appropriately emphasizes the close relationship of GER and esophageal and LES function to what happens more distally (i.e., gastrointestinal motility and secretion and their possible alterations and consequent DGR). As widely demonstrated in the chapter, at least in some persons, GER must be considered the result of an impairment of foregut motility-absorptive-secreting function.

GER may be caused by transient inversions of pressure gradient between the proximal stomach and the LES. DGR may be caused by transient impairments of the dynamic equilibrium between gastric motility and emptying and antrointestinal resistance to flow. As opportunely pointed out in the chapter, impaired antrointestinal outlet resistance is a potential cause of DGR, delayed gastric emptying, increased gastric tone and, consequently, GER. However, for GER and DGR to occur, it is necessary that the stomach and duodenum are not empty when such reflux-favoring conditions take place.

In healthy subjects reflux, because of its quantity, quality, time, and persistence, is not able to induce mucosal injury and symptoms. This happens because of the correct synchronization of the functional pattern of the foregut. Any modification of the motility-absorptive-secreting pattern, as well as functional or organic modifications of the biliary tract, may result in abnormal reflux. Therefore, although some time ago a correct physiopathologic definition of reflux could be based on a standard esophageal manometric study and esophageal pH monitoring, certainly this would not be sufficient today. Esophageal pressure and pH studies should be combined at least with gastric and small intestinal manometry, study of the gastric emptying and secretion, gastric pH monitoring, and functional studies of the biliary tree. It is also probable that what seems to be enough for a correct physiopathologic interpretation today will not be sufficient in the near future. New questions will be raised by the continuous expansion of knowledge. Moreover, the problem is not purely speculative, since an appropriate diagnostic evaluation on clinical grounds is important for treatment, especially if surgery is indicated. Some reported unsatisfactory results of antireflux procedures[2] might be explained on the basis of findings of a more accurate physiopathologic approach to reflux.

Before a decision is made about how to study patients with suspected reflux, the following problem should be resolved: which patients should be suspected of having reflux and consequently studied? Obviously, the answer is patients with classical symptoms of GER (heartburn, regurgitation, and dysphagia) and those with chronic respiratory disorders of unknown origin and noncardiac chest pain. But DGR does not cause any typical symptom, and nonacid GER is often said to be asymptomatic.[3] Therefore, all the patients with a "dyspeptic" syndrome should be considered to have the potential for reflux and must be studied to exclude gastric, duodenal, biliary, or bowel disease.[4]

"If you're seeking reflux, then measure reflux."[1] The problem of measuring acid GER has been brilliantly solved with the use of esophageal pH monitoring. The duration of monitoring is now under discussion, but there is no doubt that 24-hour monitoring has made the most important contribution to knowledge of acid GER.[5] However, the problem of measuring nonacid GER and DGR has still to be completely solved.

All the tests devised to measure DGR involve the use of some form of gastric intubation to estimate bile acids, either in the fasting state or on overnight aspiration. Other tests consist of the passage of a tube through the pylorus and into the duodenum and the injection of radiopaque or radioactive substances. Technetium-labeled HIDA scintigraphy seems the least invasive and most physiologic of the tests for reflux assessment. However, the main problem with a scintiscan is the short duration of the study period. At present, therefore, combined esophageal and gastric pH monitoring seems to be the best method for studying nonacid GER and DGR, with DGR being indicated by a sudden rise in gastric pH and GER by a sudden drop or rise in esophageal pH (both unrelated to food intake) simultaneous with or immediately following a DGR episode. However, combined pH monitoring is not able to quantify reflux or to identify its composition but simply to assess the contact time of duodenal and gastric refluxate with gastric and esophageal mucosa, respectively. Therefore, a completely satisfactory method for measuring reflux and identifying its composition is not available. For this reason the real enteric contribution (which could also be present in acid GER) to GER is still hardly detectable, and the real effect on mucosa and the clinical relevance of nonacid GER and DGR are still to be determined and are the object of opposite opinions.[6,7] Moreover, while GER lesions are still under discussion and early markers of injury are to be defined, we are still unable to correlate DGR with a gastric histologic counterpart. This is so true that the postoperative "alkaline gastritis syndrome" is now under discussion and has even been rejected as "neither a useful concept nor a definable condition."[8]

The lack of a perfect method for assessing reflux and, to a lesser extent, the limited knowledge of its subjective and objective consequences certainly cause some confusion about reflux and its pathophysiology. However, as pointed out in the chapter, GER in some patients is a very complex phenomenon caused by a generalized or multifactorial process of the foregut, which needs complex diagnostic tools.

The chapter points out with precision the "state of the art" in the pathophysiology of upper gut motility, GER, and DGR. More information is to be expected from histochemical and ultrastructural studies of the foregut, which, guided by functional knowledge, could improve knowledge of function. Histochemical and ultrastructural findings on the LES seem to be of particular interest. On electron microscopy, an LES that functions well shows numerous intercellular contacts between morphologically and numerically normal nerve endings, interstitial cells of Cajal, and smooth muscle cells, making a muscular bundle that is considered the anatomic and functional unit of the human esophagus.[9] In achalasic patients, rare nerve endings and interstitial cells of Cajal are found together with damaged smooth-muscle cells with fewer intercellular contacts as compared with controls.[10] Histochemically, VIP, abundant in the normal human LES and considered an inhibitory neurotransmitter, has been found to be reduced or lacking in achalasic patients.[11] In contrast, in patients with hypertensive sphincters (which could be considered the opposite of the situation found in many patients with reflux) no damage of the muscle wall components is seen, but ultrastructural signs of enhanced activity of all interstitial cells of Cajal and of some smooth muscle cells (cytoplasms particularly rich in mitochondria and smooth endoplasmic reticulum) are found.[10] Little is known about LES, gastric, pyloric, and duodenal specimens of patients affected by GER and/or DGR, but it would certainly be interesting to study them, in view of the functional aspects highlighted in the chapter.

REFERENCES

1. Pope, C.E., II: Is LES enough? Gastroenterology **71**:328-329, 1976.
2. Bremner, C.G.: Gastric ulceration after fundoplication operation for gastroesophageal reflux, Surg. Gynecol. Obstet. **148**:62-64, 1979.
3. Pellegrini, C.A., DeMeester, T.R., Wernly, J.A., Johnson, L.F., and Skinner, D.B.: Alkaline gastroesophageal reflux, Am. J. Surg. **135**:177-184, 1978.
4. Alexander-Williams, J.: Alkaline reflux gastritis: a myth or a disease? Am. J. Surg. **143**:17-21, 1982.
5. Johnson, L.F., DeMeester, T.R.: Twenty-four-hour pH-monitoring of the distal esophagus, Am. J. Gastroenterol. **63**:325-332, 1974.
6. Gillison, E.W., Decastro, V.A.M., Nyhus, L.M., Kusakari, K., and Bombeck, C.T.: The significance of bile reflux esophagitis, Surg. Gynecol. Obstet. **134**:419-424, 1972.
7. Little, A.G., Martinez, E.I., DeMeester, T.R., Blough, R.M., and Skinner, D.B.: Duodenogastric reflux and reflux esophagitis, Surgery **96**:447-454, 1984.
8. Meyer, J.H.: Reflextions on reflux gastritis, Gastroenterology **77**:1143-1145, 1979.
9. Faussone-Pellegrini, M.S., and Cortesini, C.: Ultrastruc-

tural features and localization of the intestinal cells of
Cajal in the smooth muscle coat of human esophagus, J.
Submicrosc. Cytol. **17:**187-197, 1985.

10. Faussone-Pellegrini, M.S., and Cortesini, C.: The muscle coat of the lower esophageal sphincter in patients with achalasia and hypertensive sphincter: an electron micro-scopic study, J. Submicrosc. Cytol. **17:**673-685, 1985.

11. Aggestrup, S., Uddman, R., Sundler, F., Fahrenkrug, J., Håkanson, R., Sørensen, H.R., and Hambraeus, G.: Lack of vasoactive intestinal polypeptide nerves in esophageal achalasia, Gastroenterology **84:**924-927, 1983.

PART II DIAGNOSIS

CHAPTER 3 Update on esophageal pH monitoring

Hans-Fred Weiser, Elfriede Bollschweiler, Rüdiger Lange, and J. Rüdiger Siewert

Postulating a multifactorial etiology, Dodds et al.[1,2] identified reflux disease as a disorder whose development depends on one or more of the following factors:

1. Competency of the antireflux barrier
2. Volume of gastroesophageal reflux
3. Chemical composition of the regurgitate
4. Efficiency of gastroesophageal acid clearance
5. Protective factors of the esophageal mucosa

This view of a multifactorial etiology leads to a more accurate pathophysiologic understanding of reflux disease and avoids the isolated consideration of single aspects. However, at the same time, it requires a comprehensive approach toward the diagnosis of reflux disease.

Central to esophageal diagnosis is the direct visual examination of the esophageal mucosa by endoscopy. Only endoscopy allows the judgment of the severity of the morphologic alterations and the indirect estimation of the amount of gastroesophageal reflux.[3] The earliest grossly visible manifestation of reflux is a mucosal erythema of the terminal esophagus, classified by Siewert and Ottenjann as stage Ia of the disease, followed by solitary or multiple isolated mucosal lesions, which may be coated by fibrin after having reached the submucosa (stage Ib).[4] These mucosal lesions are typically located on the posterior esophageal wall on top of the mucosal folds, presumably because of the predominant exposure of this area to the regurgitate. With the progression of the disease, solitary lesions coalesce (stage IIa). These confluent lesions may cover a large area, but not yet the entire circumference. Frequently, the formation of fibrinous membranes is observed at the bottom of these lesions, which may become superinfected by *Candida* fungi (stage IIb).

Stage III is characterized by the above described lesions around the entire esophageal circumference. In this stage of the disease, adequate therapy may still lead to complete healing. Finally, complicated reflux disease (stage IV) is characterized by ulceration, by stenosis, and eventually by bleeding episodes from the inflamed mucosa or Barrett ulcers. In this stage of the disease, complete mucosal restoration is no longer seen. According to Siewert et al., the uncomplicated endobrachyesophagus, which Savary and Miller classified as stage IV of reflux esophagitis, should not be regarded as a symptomatic complication of reflux disease, but rather as a final end-stage condition of reflux esophagitis, identified histologically by a columnar-cell scar.[4] Finally, in addition to morphologic examination, endoscopy allows the sampling of tissue biopsies, a prerequisite for the identification of malignant transformation in the area of the inflamed mucosa.

Next to endoscopy, intraluminal manometry was used as an indirect method of identifying pathologic reflux by the assessment of the sufficiency of gastroesophageal closure. However, recent investigations have shown that routine manometry does not allow an exact discrimination between sufficient and insufficient esophageal closure mechanisms, since the pressure in the gastroesophageal segment is inconsistent, varying significantly from one minute to the next. Furthermore, inappropriate relaxations of the lower esophageal sphincter may also cause reflux.[5-9] Therefore the results of isolated manometric examinations, even if under ideal conditions, are hardly reproducible, are not representative, and are consequently of little meaning. The problem of pressure variability could be solved by long-term manometry, which requires total immobilization of the patient and an unphysiologic condition for the measuring period.[7,10,11]

Therefore, methods should be preferred that measure the consequence of an insufficient esophageal closure mechanism (i.e., gastro-esophageal reflux) directly in the terminal esophagus. A suitable method for the direct intraluminal determination of the hydrogen ion concentration in the regurgitate is long-term esophageal pH monitoring. However, according to the theory of the interionic interaction, pure aqueous electrolyte solutions are a prerequisite for pH determinations. In the clinical setting, pH is measured in mixed solutions and its results must be interpreted accordingly.[12]

Two types of electrodes are used nowadays for clinical pH monitoring—oxide electrodes, such as the antimony electrode, and diffusion electrodes, such as the silver-glass electrode. Both types used to have the disadvantage of needing an extracorporeal reference electrode. Therefore, so-called combined miniature glass electrodes have been developed, whose electrode chamber is filled with a reference electrolyte with an extremely low water-vapor pressure. The reference electrolyte (Friscolyt) in our pH probe (Ingold 440 M4) serves two purposes—first, to suppress the diffusion potential at the inner side of the ion-exchange membrane and, second, to provide a zero potential for the silver–silver chloride reference electrode in the lumen of the probe. Using highly integrated chips with low power absorption, miniaturized circuit arrangements, and miniaturized combined pH electrodes, De-Meester and Johnson reported their first experiences with pH monitoring in healthy subjects and in patients with known reflux disease.[13,14] Like Stanciu et al. and Wallin and Madsen, they assumed that pH 4 may be the best threshold value to discriminate between physiologic and pathologic reflux conditions. The rationale for this assumption was derived from the finding that only 2.4% of the examined volunteers exhibited values below pH 4. In contrast, when pH 5 had been used as a limit, 37.7% of the volunteers had to be included.[9,15]

However, these reports are not in conformity with similar investigations from our institution. We found that 19 out of 31 healthy volunteers (16 males, 15 females, average age 49.4 ± 3.7 years), or 60%, exhibited at least one episode of gastric pH below 1 during the 24-hour measuring period. Values below 3 were found in all volunteers at one time or another during the measuring period, and 30% showed values below 4, along with the occurrence of alkaline gastroesophageal reflux up to pH values of 8.5.[16] These results questioned the primary importance of pH as the sole discriminating parameter between physiologic and pathologic reflux and necessitated further analysis of the data.

The analyses of the relative duration (percent per hour) for the total measuring period from pH 1 to pH 9 in 115 patients with endoscopically identified reflux esophagitis (Fig. 3-1) showed the highest significance level ($p < 0.0005$) for the discrimination between healthy subjects and patients with mild reflux disease on the one hand and between patients with mild and severe reflux disease on the other hand (Fig. 3-2 and Table 3-1).

These results demonstrate that pH 4 may be used as a discriminator between physiologic and pathologic reflux only when the hydrogen ion concentration is evaluated together with the mucosal exposure time per measuring period. However, even then, pH 4 only distinguishes between the healthy and the diseased. Therefore, the determination of gastroesophageal reflux in relation to body position, the patient's state of consciousness, and food intake also needs to be determined, which requires other measuring parameters. As early as 1980, Dodds et al. introduced the duration of single reflux episodes as a discriminating criterion.[2] According to this report, each reflux episode of longer than 5 minutes should be considered pathologic. However, this criterion still did not allow a sufficient characterization of reflux disease. Only the evaluation of gastroesophageal reflux on the basis of the total duration of episodes with pH less than 4 and the number of single reflux episodes of longer than 5 minutes allowed a sufficient differentiation between healthy and severely reflux-diseased patients. However, parameters for further discrimination between different stages of the disease on the basis of pH data still needed to be found.

Computerized analysis of long-term reflux profiles finally allowed the identification and determination of the median number of reflux episodes per hour, of the median reflux duration per hour, and of the number of reflux episodes with a duration greater than 5 min in relation to different phases of the measuring period.[14,17-19]

For the statistical analysis, the median was used as a middle value, since the measurements belong to the metric system and are not normally distributed. Graphically the distributions are represented by curves with multiple peaks or with a shift to the left, respectively. The 95% confidence interval represents the limits within which the median of further measurements should be found. The nonparametric Wilcoxon-Mann-Whitney-test was used to determine whether the medians for the duration and the number of reflux episodes per hour are significantly different among the subgroups. The same applies for the frequency distribution of the pH values.

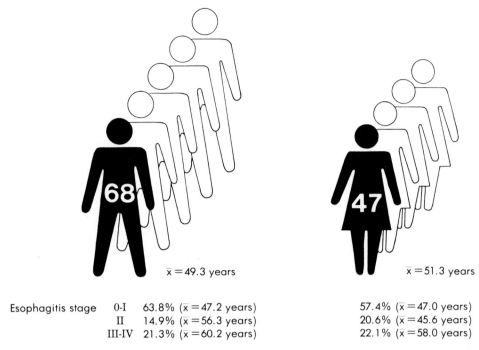

Esophagitis stage   0-I   63.8% ($\bar{x}$ = 47.2 years)   57.4% ($\bar{x}$ = 47.0 years)
               II   14.9% ($\bar{x}$ = 56.3 years)   20.6% ($\bar{x}$ = 45.6 years)
          III-IV   21.3% ($\bar{x}$ = 60.2 years)   22.1% ($\bar{x}$ = 58.0 years)

Fig. 3-1. Age distribution of 115 patients with esophagitis stage 0 to IV. The average age was 50 years. Data show relative duration of reflux (percent per hour).

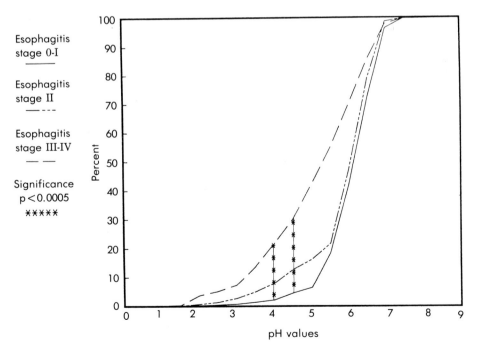

Fig. 3-2. Cumulative frequency of pH monitoring (medians). Largest distance between two curves occurs at pH 4, demonstrating optimal discrimination between stages at this value.

TABLE 3-1. Cumulative frequency of pH monitoring (median in percent)

pH steps	Esophagitis stage 0-I	Significance 0-1/2	Esophagitis stage II	Significance 2/3-4	Esophagitis stage III-IV
	(%)	p =	(%)	p =	(%)
0	0	0.94	0	0.16	0
0.5	0	0.93	0	0.08	0
1.0	0	0.56	0	0.13	0.01
1.5	0	0.12	0.02	0.03	0.19
2.0	0.12	0.005	0.55	0.06	3.62
2.5	0.32	0.0028	1.26	0.012	5.05
3.0	0.59	0.001	2.61	0.0063	7.23
3.5	1.25	0.0000	4.85	0.0013	13.45
4.0*	2.02	0.0000	7.85	0.0001	21.47
4.5	4.46	0.0002	12.65	0.0002	29.93
5.0	6.37	0.0089	16.13	0.0001	42.18
5.5	18.41	0.20	21.63	0.0004	54.79
6.0	42.05	0.45	47.41	0.0281	69.99
6.5	72.59	0.25	79.12	0.52	85.67
7.0	96.45	0.08	98.75	0.46	97.96
8.0	99.91	0.37	99.97	0.28	99.93
9.0	99.97	0.60	99.97	0.43	99.93

*Optimal discrimination between mild and severe forms of reflux disease at pH 4 ($p < 0.0005$).

On the basis of the above mentioned investigations in healthy volunteers, we have tried to determine threshold values to distinguish between healthy and barely pathologic gastroesophageal reflux.[27,28] This has led to the following characterization of physiologic reflux:

1. The pH value of the regurgitate is greater than 4 and less than 7.
2. Reflux episodes during the day occur primarily during the prandial and postprandial periods.
3. Nighttime reflux occurs during the first half of the night.

This definition is in accord with recent reports that showed that pH 4, with an exposure time of 6% to 7% of the total measuring period, allows a valuable discrimination between physiologic and pathologic reflux.[9,13-15,18,20-22] The importance of reflux during the fasting period and during the second half of the night, which had been emphasized by Dent and Euler, could also be confirmed by us.[1,7]

Dodds et al. assumed that the transnasally inserted pH electrode might cause hypersalivation by mechanical irritation of the pharyngeal mucosa. However, this contention is questioned by two facts. First, saliva, at a pH of approximately 7.8, possesses only negligible buffer capacity, so that large volumes of saliva would be required to dilute the regurgitate or wash off the electrode head. This effect would still not alter the reflux profiles, since it occurs in volunteers as much as in patients. Second, the production of saliva almost ceases during sleeping periods, so that night reflux, which is typical of pathologic reflux conditions, remains uninfluenced.[23-25]

Using the above described criteria, the analysis of long-term pH data from patients with endoscopically verified reflux disease revealed that reflux esophagitis stages II, III, and IV are associated with increased frequency and intensity of reflux and an increased number of reflux episodes of longer than 5 minutes during the awake phase, as compared either to healthy volunteers or to the groups (Figs. 3-3 to 3-5, Tables 3-2 and 3-3). Furthermore, 89% of physiologic reflux occurs during the prandial and postprandial periods. In patients with esophagitis stage II, we saw only 64.6% of prandial and postprandial reflux and in patients with esophagitis stage III or IV just 29.3%, meaning a significant shift in the occurrence of daytime reflux toward the fasting periods.

The analysis of the reflux profile during the sleeping phase yielded similar results. In patients with esophagitis stage II, we observed an average of 1.2 reflux episodes per hour, as opposed to patients with esophagitis stage III or IV, who exhibited 2.7 reflux episodes per hour ($p < 0.002$). The regurgitate exposure time was 4.9

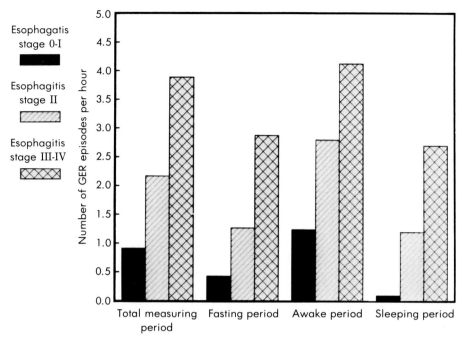

Fig. 3-3. Gastroesophageal reflux pattern in 115 patients with reflux disease of differing degrees of severity.

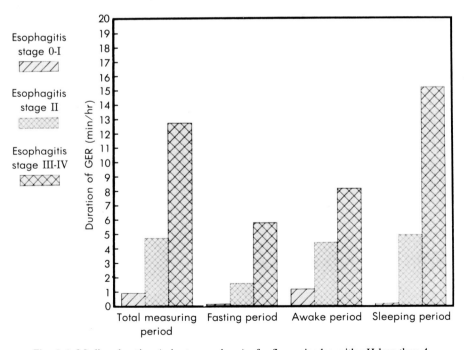

Fig. 3-4. Median duration (minutes per hour) of reflux episodes with pH less than 4.

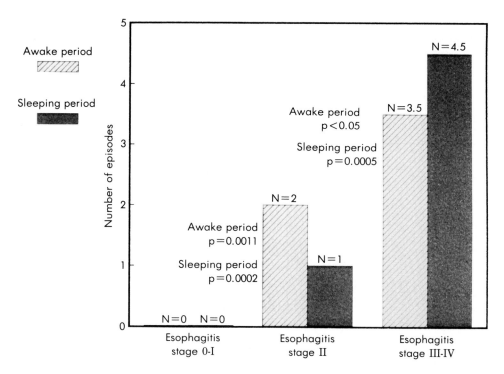

Fig. 3-5. Number of reflux episodes longer than 5 minutes in 115 patients with esophagitis stage 0 to I, stage II, or stage III to IV.

TABLE 3-2. Number of reflux episodes per hour with pH values less than 4

Esophagitis	Total measuring period	Fasting period	Awake period	Sleeping period
Stage 0-I (n = 69)				
Median (95% konf. I)	0.91	0.43	1.24	0.10
	(0.44, 1.34)	(0.16, 0.70)	(0.87, 1.59)	(0.00, 0.44)
Significance	.0018	.1150	.0200	.0005
Stage II (n = 21)				
Median (95% konf. I)	2.17	1.27	2.80	1.20
	(1.55, 2.60)	(0.26, 2.20)	(1.05, 3.42)	(0.33, 1.70)
Significance	.0113	.0112	.0215	.0019
Stage III-IV (n = 25)				
Median (95% konf. I)	3.89	2.88	4.13	2.70
	(2.63, 10.87)	(1.20, 7.10)	(2.56, 6.08)	(1.73, 4.60)

min/hr, as opposed to 15.2 min/hr ($p < 0.001$), respectively (Tables 3-2 and 3-3).

A second important factor for the development of symptomatic reflux is the occurrence of reflux during the second half of the night. In healthy subjects and patients with mild reflux esophagitis (stage 0 or I), the reflux during the night subsides within 2 to 3 hours. Patients with esophagitis stage II show persistent reflux during the second half of the night, albeit decreasing overall. In contrast, patients with esophagitis stage III or IV show continuously increased gastroesophageal re-

TABLE 3-3. Median duration (min/hr) of reflux episodes with pH values less than 4*

Esophagitis	Total measuring period	Fasting period	Awake period	Sleeping period
Stage 0-I (n = 69)				
Median (95% konf. I)	0.93 (0.48, 1.36)	0.13 (0.00, 0.61)	1.18 (0.71, 1.72)	0.18 (0.00, 0.60)
Significance	.0000	.0113	.0001	.0000
Stage II (n = 21)				
Median (95% konf. I)	4.73 (3.92, 5.86)	1.56 (0.05, 2.49)	4.40 (2.34, 6.39)	4.91 (2.13, 7.37)
Significance	.0000	.0072	.0399	.0001
Stage III-IV (n = 25)				
Median (95% konf. I)	12.75 (8.57, 14.32)	5.77 (0.88, 7.47)	8.16 (4.16, 13.69)	15.20 (10.26, 22.40)

*Results of 115 patients with reflux disease of differing severities.

flux during the entire sleeping phase (Fig. 3-6).

Hence, the discrimination between mild and severe forms of reflux disease may be based on the threshold value pH 4, the number of reflux episodes per hour, and the reflux duration per hour during various measuring periods. In our study, the number of reflux episodes lasting longer than 5 minutes varied from 0 to 4.5, with notable overlapping between the groups. In addition, the analysis of the number of reflux episodes per hour showed a low significance level. Therefore, we analyzed our data on the bases of the pH threshold value and the duration of reflux per hour. For sufficient discrimination among the groups, reflux parameters in the groups with lesser reflux should be lower than the 95% confidence interval of the next group (with more severe reflux). This leads to the following graduation:

Esophagitis stage 0 to I: less than 4 minutes of reflux per hour; equivalent to 7% of the measuring period

Esophagitis stage II: more than 4 minutes of reflex per hour, but less than 8 minutes; equivalent to 7% to 14% of the measuring period

Esophagitis stage III to IV: more than 8 minutes of reflux per hour; equivalent to more than 14% of the measuring period.

In addition, we classify gastroesophageal reflux as mild if the reflux episodes during the day occur mainly during the prandial and postprandial periods and if the reflux during the night is increased, albeit decreasing, toward morning. Similarly, severe gastroesophageal reflux is characterized not only by a median reflux duration of more than 14% per measuring period but also by persistent day reflux during fasting periods and by continous night reflux.

In regard to diagnosis of reflux disease and choice of treatment, the 24-hour long-term pH monitoring may be a valuable but not indispensible tool, in addition to endoscopy and the clinical history. Table 3-4 compares the sensitivity and specificity of pH monitoring and endoscopy. In cases in which the esophageal mucosa is morphologically unaltered, pH monitoring may provide substantial diagnostic data about pathologic reflux. Furthermore, pH monitoring reveals individual reflux profiles, which in turn allow the initiation of medical or surgical treatment, according to the stage and time course of the disease. Following the patient's reflux profile, medical treatment should be administered at times of maximal reflux—for example, only at night in mild cases or continuously in severe cases. If medical therapy does not prevent reflux sufficiently, surgical therapy should be initiated.[26,27]

In addition, the effect of drugs on pathologic reflux may be examined by pH monitoring. A study from our institution showed significant differences in all reflux parameters when Ranitidine was compared to placebo.[28]

Finally, the effectiveness of surgical antireflux therapy may also be assessed by pH monitoring. Recently, we reported the complete suppression of reflux following valvuloplasty or the implantation of the Angelchik antireflux prosthesis.[29]

In conclusion, pH monitoring may be con-

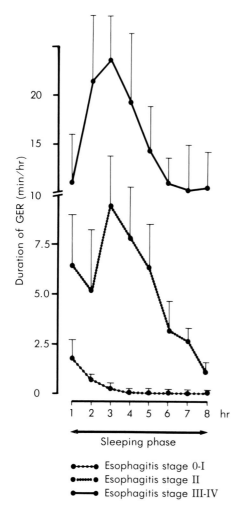

●····● Esophagitis stage 0-I
●┄┄● Esophagitis stage II
●━━━● Esophagitis stage III-IV

Fig. 3-6. Median reflux duration (minutes per hour) during the sleeping phase. Continuously decreasing reflux in healthy volunteers and patients with esophagitis stage I. Delayed decrease of reflux during the second half of the night in patients with esophagitis stage II. Persistent reflux in patients with esophagitis stage III to IV.

sidered an important adjuvant to endoscopy for the diagnosis and management of reflux disease.

SUMMARY

Because of the multifactorial etiology of reflux disease, a comprehensive approach to its diagnosis is required. Esophageal pH monitoring is an adjuvant diagnostic procedure to endoscopy, especially in cases in which symptomatic reflux is not associated with morphologic alterations of the esophageal mucosa. Furthermore, the evaluation of pH data allows a classification of the severity of reflux disease corresponding to the endoscopic findings. Medical or surgical treatment may be initiated, and its effectiveness may be assessed by examination of the individual reflux profile.

REFERENCES

1. Dodds, W.J., Hogan, W.J., and Miller, W.: Reflux esophagitis, Am. J. Dig. Dis. **21**:49-61, 1976.
2. Dodds, W.J., Hauser, R., Hogan, W.J., Dent, J., et al.: Gastroesophageal reflux (GER) and esophageal clearance in normal human volunteers and patients with reflux-esophagitis. In Christensen, J.M., editor: Gastrointestinal motility, New York, 1980, Raven Press, pp. 87-88.
3. Savary, M.: L'expression endoscopique de l'oesophagite par reflux, International bronchoesophagological society, XIII congrès, Lyon, 1971, SIMEP, 1971, Villeurbanne, pp. 101-118.
4. Siewert, J.R., Ottenjann, R., Heilmann, K., and Neis, A.: Therapie und Prophylaxe der Refluxösophagitis. I. Epidemiologie, Z. Gastroenterol. (In press.)
5. Ahtaridis, G., Snape, W.J., and Cohen, S.: Lower esophageal sphincter pressure as an index of gastroesophageal acid reflux, Dig. Dis. Sci. **26**:993-998, 1981.
6. Chattopadhyay, D.K., and Pope, C.E., II: Lower esophageal sphincter pressure's variability destroys its usefulness, Gastroenterology **76**:1111, 1979.

TABLE 3-4. Specificity and sensitivity of pH monitoring compared to endoscopy (percent)*

	Stage 0-I	Stage II	Stage III-IV
Sensitivity[†]	94%	52%	72%
Specificity[‡]	85%	88%	97%
Positive predictive value[§]	90%	50%	86%
Negative predictive value[‖]	91%	89%	93%
Validity[¶]	91%	82%	91%

*Definition: median duration of reflux episodes per hour during the entire measuring period: ≤ 4 min equivalent to esophagitis stage 0-I; > 4 min and ≤ 8 min equivalent to esophagitis stage II; > 8 min equivalent to esophagitis stage III-IV.
[†]Right pos./(r. pos. + f. neg.)
[‡]Right neg./(r. neg. + f. pos.)
[§]Right pos./(r. pos. + f. pos.)
[‖]Right neg./(r. neg. + f. neg.)
[¶](r. pos. + r. neg.)/(r. pos. + f. pos. + r. neg. + f. neg.)

7. Dent, J., Dodds, W.J., Friedman, R.H., et al.: Mechanism of gastroesophageal reflux in recumbent asymptomatic human subjects, J. Clin. Invest. **65:**256-267, 1980.

8. Euler, A.R., and Byrne, W.J.: Twenty-four-hour esophageal intraluminal pH probe testing: a comparative analysis, Gastroenterology **80:**957-961, 1981.

9. Stanciu, C., Hoare, R.C., and Bennett, J.R.: Correlation between manometric and pH tests for gastroesophageal reflux, Gut **18:**536-540, 1977.

10. Ask, P., Edwall, G., and Tibbling, L.: Combined pH and pressure measurement device for esophageal investigations, Med. Biol. Eng. **19:**443-446, 1981.

11. Clark, J., DeMeester, T.R., Johnson, L., and Skinner, D.B.: Twenty-four-hour lower esophageal pH monitoring and the lower esophageal sphincter, Surg. Forum **26:** 362-363, 1975.

12. Sörensen, S.P.L.: Enzyme, Z. Biochemie **21:**131-201, 1909.

13. DeMeester, T.R., and Johnson, L.F.: The evaluation of objective measurements of gastroesophageal reflux and their contribution to patient management, Surg. Clin. North Am. **56:**39-53, 1976.

14. Johnson, L.F.: 24-hour-pH monitoring in the study of gastroesophageal reflux, J. Clin. Gastroenterol. **2:**387-399, 1980.

15. Wallin, L., and Madsen, T.: 12-hour simultaneous registration of acid reflux and peristaltic activity in the esophagus, Scand. J. Gastroenterol. **14:**561-566, 1979.

16. Weiser, H.F., Pace, F., Lepsien, G., Müller-Lissner, S.A., Blum, A.L., and Siewert, J.R.: Gastroösophagealer Reflux: was ist physiologisch? Dtsch. Med. Wochenschr. **107:**366-370, 1982.

17. Branicki, F.J., Evans, D.F., et al.: A frequency-duration index (FDI) for the evaluation of ambulatory recordings of gastro-esophageal reflux, Br. J. Surg. **71:**425-430, 1984.

18. O'Sullivan, G.C., DeMeester, T.R., Smith, R.B., et al.: Twenty-four-hour pH monitoring of esophageal function, Arch. Surg. **116:**581-590, 1981.

19. Weiser, H.F.: Reflux characteristics of healthy volunteers examined by 24-hour-pH recording. In Wienbeck, M., editor: Motility of the digestive tract, New York, 1982, Raven Press, pp. 287-301.

20. Corazziari, E., Pozzessere, C., Dani, S., et al.: Intraluminal pH and esophageal motility, Gastroenterology **75:**275-277, 1978.

21. DeMeester, T.R., Johnson, L.F., Joseph, G.J., et al.: Patterns of gastroesophageal reflux in health and disease, Ann. Surg. **184:**459-470, 1976.

22. Kaye, M.D.: Postprandial gastroesophageal reflux in healthy people, Gut **18:**709-712, 1977.

23. Helm, J.F., Dodds, W.J., Hogan, W.J., Egide, M.S., and Wood, C.: Flow and acid neutralization capacity of human saliva, Gastroenterology **78:**1181, 1980.

24. Helm, J.F., Dodds, W.J., Hogan, W.J., et al.: Acid neutralizing capacity of human saliva, Gastroenterology **83:**69-74, 1982.

25. Kapila, Y.V., Dodds, W.J., Helm, J.F., et al.: Relationship between swallow rate and salivary flow, Dig. Dis. Sci. **29**(6):528-533, 1984.

26. Skinner, D.B.: Pathophysiology of gastroesophageal reflux, Ann. Surg. **202**(5):546-556, 1985.

27. Weiser, H.F., and Siewert, J.R.: Investigations with the 24-hour solid state pH-metry: correlation between gastroesophageal reflux extent and reflux sequelae, Surg. Gastroenterol. **1:**327-334, 1982.

28. Weiser, H.F., Gubernatis, G., and Siewert, J.R.: Einfluss von Oxmetidin und Ranitidin auf das Refluxverhalten von Patienten mit Ösophagitis, Gastroenterol. **21:** 580-584, 1983.

29. Weiser, H.F., Wu, Y.Q., and Siewert, J.R.: Supercontinence following antireflux surgery: evaluation by pH-metry, Dig. Surg. **1:**185-189, 1984.

Update on esophageal pH monitoring

DISCUSSION

Tom R. DeMeester

The essay by Dr. Weiser and associates on 24-hour esophageal pH monitoring reflects the difference between European and American definitions of gastroesophageal reflux disease. As spokesmen for the European position, they concur that symptoms are not a reliable guide to the presence of disease. This is particularly true for atypical symptoms, and even though typical symptoms have a higher relationship to the presence of disease, they also can be misleading. Consequently, Dr. Weiser and his co-workers use the presence of endoscopic esophagitis to define the disease. The problem with this approach is that esophagitis is a complication of the disease, and it is unwise to identify a disease by a complication, for not every patient with the disease will develop the complication. The authors agree that gastroesophageal reflux disease is multifactorial and that its presence cannot be identified simply by the existence of endoscopic esophagitis but contend that when endoscopic esophagitis is present, the diagnosis is reliable. We would concur, provided other causes of esophagitis, such as drug-induced injuries, radiation, or repetitive vomiting, are excluded.

We have defined gastroesophageal reflux disease as an increase in esophageal exposure to gastric juice. Instead of attempting to identify a population of patients with the disease by the presence of a complication, and measuring their esophageal exposure to acid gastric juice, we have measured the exposure in normal subjects who are free of symptomatic or objective evidence of a foregut abnormality. Our position is that in this situation it is easier to define normality than disease. Symptomatic patients whose esophageal acid exposure significantly exceeds that measured in normal subjects are considered to have gastroesophageal reflux disease. Typical symptoms or a complication of the disease is not essential. This approach is analogous to attempt-

ing to define dwarfism by first determining normal height distribution rather than finding and measuring those who appear to be dwarfs.

The difference in the definition of the disease has caused confusion on both sides of the Atlantic. For example, Dr. Weiser and associates have indicated that manometry of the lower esophageal sphincter is not helpful in determining the presence of disease. We have found that a severe manometric defect—that is, a sphincter pressure below the 2.5 percentile, overall length below the 2.5 percentile, or abdominal length below the 5th percentile of normal subjects—is associated with a high probability of increased esophageal exposure to gastric juice. As a consequence, manometry is helpful in identifying the sphincter as a cause of increased esophageal exposure to gastric juice. When manometry is normal, other causes of increased esophageal exposure to gastric juice must be considered. One such cause is decreased esophageal clearance after physiologic reflux episodes. This occurs in patients who have an esophageal motility disorder, decreased saliva production, or a hiatal hernia. Other causes of increased esophageal acid exposure in patients with normal sphincter manometrics are gastric in origin. Among them are increases in intragastric pressure, independent of intraabdominal pressure, to levels that exceed sphincter pressure. This can occur after eating in a patient who has lost the active relaxation of the stomach because of a previous vagotomy. Another factor is gastric dilatation. This is not synonymous with increased gastric pressure but rather simple dilatation of the stomach with shortening of the overall sphincter length, similar to the shortening of the neck of a balloon on inflation. This can occur with excessive aerophagia or simple gluttony. A persistent gastric reservoir secondary to delayed gastric emptying can increase the probability of gastroesophageal reflux and also result in increased esophageal exposure to gastric juice. This is similar to the hazard of aspiration when the stomach remains full. Gastric hypersecretion is another factor that can cause increased esophageal exposure to gastric juice. In this situation the quantity and concentration of gastric acid in each physiologic reflux episode overwhelm the buffering capacity of the saliva and result in an abnormal esophageal acid exposure. In Chapter 8 there is a more detailed discussion of these factors.

On both sides of the Atlantic a pH of 4 is accepted as the most critical cut-off level in the detection of acid reflux. The common occurrence of physiologic reflux during the postprandial period and its rarity at night are also accepted. Similarly, there is agreement that saliva causes little alteration in pH monitoring data, since it is stimulated by the pH probe in both patients and normal subjects.

Dr. Weiser and his associates use 24-hour esophageal pH monitoring to identify factors that differentiate patients with esophagitis from normal subjects. We agree that patients with esophagitis reflux more frequently and have an increase in the number of episodes that last longer than 5 minutes. We also agree that patients with esophagitis have an increase in the number of reflux episodes during the fasting periods between meals and during sleep. An observation made by Dr. Weiser and associates is that during the second half of the night reflux is particularly predominant in patients with esophagitis. This finding suggests that these patients may have lost the alkaline gastric tide because of gastric hypersecretion.

Dr. Weiser and co-workers encourage the use of 24-hour pH monitoring as a means to evaluate medical and surgical therapy. We strongly agree, but would emphasize that a reduction in the percent time the pH is less than 4 in patients receiving medical therapy can mean the cessation of reflux, or also a change in the hydrogen ion concentration of the refluxed gastric juice that can be misinterpreted as a cessation of reflux. In this situation, patients taking H_2 blockers can show improvement on 24-hour pH monitoring but reflux continues unabated. The change in the pH imposed by the H_2 blocker has removed the tag used to measure reflux but does not improve the antireflux barrier. Consequently, the improvement in 24-hour pH monitoring may not be reflected in healing of the esophageal mucosa, as pointed out in Chapter 8.

In contrast to Dr. Weiser and associates, we consider 24-hour pH monitoring an indispensable tool for the diagnosis of gastroesophageal reflux disease. Currently, it is the most reliable means by which one can measure increased esophageal exposure to acid gastric juice. Symptoms are the indication to perform the study but are an unreliable indicator of the presence of disease. Endoscopy is used to assess the presence of a complication of the disease, such as esophagitis, stricture, or Barrett's esophagus. We agree with Dr. Weiser and associates that 24-hour pH monitoring allows the physician to tailor the therapy to the patient; for example, patients who reflux only during the night need only nighttime therapy.

It is our opinion that 24-hour esophageal pH monitoring should be performed before starting H_2 antagonists in patients with reflux symptoms unresponsive to antacid, dietary, and postural therapy. If the results are normal, the diagnosis of gastroesophageal reflux should be questioned and a search initiated for another cause of the symptoms. If increased esophageal exposure to gastric juice is documented, then the reason should be determined; that is, is it due to an esophageal, a valvular, or a gastric abnormality? Patients who have a mechanically defective valve are likely to become drug dependent for relief of symptoms and are prone to developing complications of the disease. Consequently, they should be offered the benefits of antireflux surgery as an alternative form of therapy before the development of complications.

4 Recent advances in esophageal manometry

André Duranceau and Glyn G. Jamieson

The clinical evaluation of a patient will often lead the practitioner to suspect esophageal dysfunction. However, the subjectivity of esophageal symptoms and the lack of correlation with objective damage mean that clinical diagnosis in this area can be difficult. Radiologic evaluation of swallowing allows a brief evaluation of esophageal function when the contrast medium traverses the different regions of the esophagus. These observations cannot be prolonged, because of the risks of radiation. This lack of quantification by means of radiology led to nuclear medicine evaluation of esophageal function. Radionuclide techniques quantitate in a way that radiology does not. However, the tests lack specificity. Scintiscanning methods allow documentation of transit abnormalities but not documentation of the type of contractions, the peak pressures produced, or the duration of the contractions.[1] Scintiscanning can usefully demonstrate the presence of gastroesophageal reflux, but the presence of a hernia or poor esophageal emptying influences the results.[2] Despite the ease of these techniques, their role in the diagnosis and management of esophageal disease remains to be established.

Esophageal manometry records pressures simultaneously at several levels. This permits evaluation of the esophageal body as well as the proximal and distal esophageal sphincters. The advantage is the objective recording of pressures and swallowing wave patterns, which can be compared to the normal. However, there are still a large number of contraction abnormalities that are not easily classified as one of the major motor disorders.

In 1974 Pope described three areas in which esophageal manometry had a role in the clinical evaluation of patients: first, the preoperative documentation of abnormalities in patients with established gastroesophageal reflux disease; second, the evaluation of chest pain of undetermined origin, especially in patients with negative coronary arteriograms; and third, the evaluation of

patients with suspected motor disorders. He emphasized that good manometric recordings were dependent on careful attention to the many factors influencing the technique. Thus, esophageal manometry should be performed and interpreted by clinicians who have an interest in these disorders of the esophagus.[3]

TECHNICAL ADVANCES IN ESOPHAGEAL MANOMETRY

When Kronecker and Meltzer first measured intraesophageal pressures, they used small balloons.[4] This method remained in use until it was shown that the size of the balloon had a strong influence on the recordings of pressures.[5] This led to the introduction of small catheters, which were assembled with terminal openings separate from each other, allowing the recording of pressures at different points along the esophagus. These catheters were fluid filled and were intermittently flushed to ensure a constant column of liquid and less dampening.[6] The nonperfused catheters, however, showed marked variability from patient to patient, and the recorded pressures were not an accurate reflection of the true pressure events. The principle of constant infusion for catheter systems was demonstrated by Quigley and Brody.[7] Pope demonstrated that the infused catheter system was much more reliable in studying lower esophageal sphincter pressures.[8] The continuous infusion system was initially provided by a mechanical type of infusion pump (Harvard), with the infusion rate having a direct influence on the pressure values recorded. Although low flow rates did not affect baseline pressures and allowed better recordings of sphincter pressures, higher flow rates were necessary to prevent damping or pump artifacts.[9,10]

To record more accurately the changing pressures in time ($\Delta P/\Delta T$) the subsequent development that occurred in perfusion manometry was a different perfusion principle, whereby a constant and smaller volume of water was delivered through a noncompliant capillary system by a constant pressure.[11] Despite more accurate pressures being recorded, the constant movement of the esophagus following deglutition made sphincter recordings less accurate. This led Welch and Drake to compare a rapid pull-through method to the stationary pull-through recording, which was usually used.[12] However, the problem of variations in sphincter pressure values and whether they were real or merely due to movement of the sphincter proximal or distal to the recording orifice was solved by the introduction of a 5-cm-long perfused sleeve. This acts as a pressure sensor, recording the highest pressure at any point over its length. It thus provides a reliable measurement of lower esophageal sphincter pressure despite movement of the gastroesophageal junction.[13] Design modifications in the sleeve have made it the most accurate method of recording lower esophageal sphincter values as well as relaxation events.

Contraction pressures in the body of the esophagus are still best assessed by the noncompliant transducers or intraesophageal transducers that were used as early as 70 years ago but were too bulky to allow more than one to be swallowed at a time.[14] Gauer subsequently introduced a new generation of microtransducers.[15] The major advantages of these recording devices are the ease of the technique without a water-perfused system, and the more accurate recording of pharyngeal contractions.[16] The disadvantages are the cost of the multiple-transducer catheter and the expense involved in maintenance and repair.

Since esophageal motility is recorded most often with water-perfused systems, the effects of a number of variables have been assessed. Kaye and Showalter[17] and Lydon et al.[18] showed that increasing the size of the catheter assembly increased the pressure recorded in the lower esophageal sphincter. Stef et al.[19] showed that as the catheter internal diameter is increased, the recorded pressures will increase for given infusion rates. If the catheter length is increased, a "dragging" effect is imposed on the system and recorded pressures are diminished.

Swallowing in the absence of a bolus (dry swallow) may fail to initiate an esophageal contraction or may result in weaker contractions. Swallowing a liquid bolus causes stronger and longer contractions to appear. The quality of the bolus may also affect the recording, since a cold bolus may abolish contractions, while solid food will cause stronger and longer contractions.[20,21] The resting time between swallows can also affect peristalsis, with short periods leading to weak, frequently nonpropulsive waves. Longer resting periods between swallowing result in stronger and better organized contractions.

Despite the significant improvement in the various aspects of the manometric recording techniques, Pope suggested that the inaccuracies of these recordings, except for extremes, made the pressure measurements useless.[22] Meyer and Castell, on the other hand, saw these techniques as accurate and reproducible.[23] Esophageal motility studies remain indicated in the investigation of dysphagia or chest pain of undetermined origin, in the objective diagnosis of motor disorders, and in patients in whom surgery is contemplated for gastroesophageal reflux.

NORMAL ESOPHAGEAL MOTILITY
Pharyngeal function

Water-filled and infusion systems are the least accurate to measure pharyngeal function. Dodds et al. measured pharyngeal contractions in human subjects by means of intraluminal strain gauges and found average contraction pressures of 200 mm Hg, with recorded pressures up to 600 mm Hg.[16] The pharynx will contract during 0.2 to 0.5 seconds. It is the rapidity of the pharyngeal contraction wave (9 to 25 cm/sec) that is recorded in this fashion. Frequently, before the single pharyngeal peak an initial increase in pressure is observed: this is usually caused by the tongue thrust, the air column, or the advancing bolus.

Upper esophageal sphincter function

The upper esophageal sphincter (UES) is a high-pressure zone that separates the pharynx from the esophagus (see Fig. 4-1). This sphincter corresponds anatomically to the cricopharyngeus muscle, a muscle sling attached posteriorly to both laminae of the cricoid cartilage. The configuration and location of this muscle give it a role similar to the string tied to both ends of a bow, with a pressure exerted mostly in an anteroposterior direction. Winans documented this asymmetry within the sphincter, with 100 mm Hg pressures in the AP position and 30 mm Hg in the lateral orientation.[24] When swallowing occurs, the tonic contraction of the sphincter disappears and the pressure falls to ambient resting pressure. At this moment in time, pharynx and esophagus become a common cavity and the rapidly progressing wave from the pharynx traverses the sphincter area, pushing the bolus and closing the sphincter at the same time. The resulting pres-

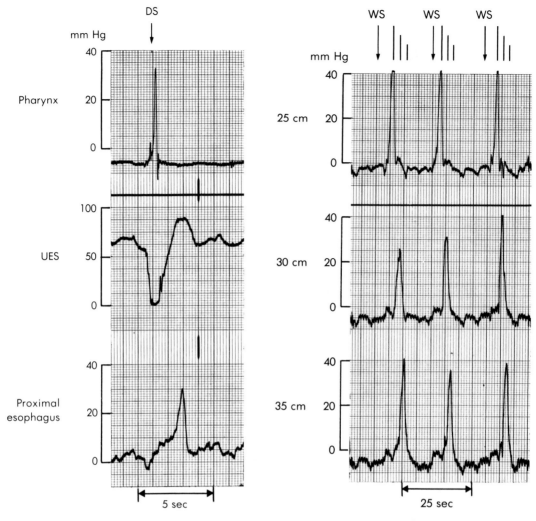

Fig. 4-1. Upper esophageal sphincter pressures compared with those of the pharynx and proximal esophagus. *DS,* Dry swallow.

Fig. 4-2. Esophageal body peristalsis. *WS,* Wet swallow.

TABLE 4-1. Comparison of results obtained with various methods of recording esophageal body motility

Author	Method	Proximal esophageal contractions (mm Hg)	Distal esophageal contractions (mm Hg)
Vantrappen and Hellemans (1967)[58]	Unperfused	28.6	37.5
Pope (1970)[9]	Perfused	20-50	35-100
Dodds et al. (1975)[16]	Perfused	55-70	60-70
Duranceau et al. (1983)[26]	Perfused	48-59	54-74
Nelson et al. (1983)[59]	Perfused	99-109	101-44
Humphries and Castell (1977)[28]	Microtransducers	35-55	58-65

sures during sphincter closure are frequently double the resting pressures. When the peak pharyngeal contraction and the duration of pharyngeal contraction meet a totally relaxed sphincter area, normal coordination is said to be present. With recording techniques used, normal coordination is seen in nearly 100% of swallows.[25,26] With the limitations of the side hole–perfused manometry system straddling a sphincter that shows considerable excursion during swallowing, newer methods of recording upper esophageal function are needed, especially in the assessment of oropharyngeal dysphagia. A model of the pressure sensor sleeve, modified for use in the upper sphincter, looks as though it may produce greater fidelity of recording in this area.[27]

Esophageal body function

After the closure of the upper esophageal sphincter, the esophageal contraction travels down the esophageal body at a speed of 2 to 5 cm/sec (Fig. 4-2). The contraction, which occurs in response to deglutition, progresses slower in the proximal striated muscle area and then becomes faster in the lower half—except just above the lower sphincter, where it is seen to slow again.[28] In a similar fashion, peak contraction pressures are weak in the striated esophagus and stronger in the distal esophagus. The values obtained in recording esophageal body motility vary from author to author, and the influence of differing recording techniques can be seen in Table 4-1.

It can be seen that rapidly perfused systems record pressures as accurately as strain gauges on the esophageal lumen. Hollis and Castell showed a decrease in the amplitude of esophageal contractions in older patients.[29] Primary peristalsis or a normal peristaltic contraction in response to swallowing is seen in 97% of all swallows in the normal population.[26] Secondary contractions occur more often in response to distention or irritation and represent an active defense mechanism of the esophagus. Tertiary contractions may be an abnormal response to swallowing or may appear spontaneously between swallowings. Rubin et al. suggested a relationship between esophageal motor disorders and the emotional states of the patients during recordings. Nonpropulsive contractions and repetitive spontaneous contractions were observed when motor function of the esophageal body was recorded during "affectively charged conversation."[30]

Spontaneous tertiary contractions occur in healthy individuals but are also observed in patients with a strongly anxious personality.[31] The resting pressure in the esophageal body

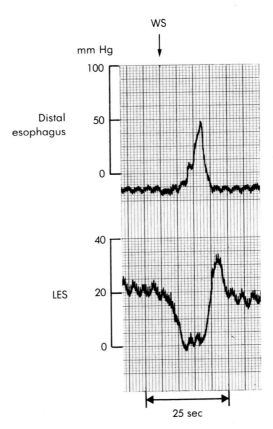

Fig. 4-3. Lower esophageal sphincter pressures compared with those of the distal esophagus. *WS,* Wet swallow.

reflects negative intrathoracic pressure except in the most proximal portion, where it tends to be close to atmospheric pressure. Obstruction, mechanical or functional, will result in increased resting pressures and abnormal body function.

Lower esophageal sphincter function

The lower esophageal sphincter (LES) is a zone of increased resting pressure, 2 to 4 cm long, located just proximal to the squamocolumnar junction in the distal esophagus (see Fig. 4-3). Its main function is to act as a barrier to the reflux of gastric and duodenal contents into the esophagus. The level of basal tone recorded in the lower esophageal sphincter is influenced by sphincter asymmetry, esophageal movement during contraction, the fed state of the patient, and the equipment used.[22,23] The introduction of the pressure sleeve by Dent allowed more accurate recording of the pressure events in the sphincter.[13] The normal resting lower esophageal sphincter pressure (LESP) ranges between 15 and 25 mm Hg.

During relaxation the pressure in the sphincter falls to ambient resting pressure. This relaxation usually occurs immediately following deglutition. The sphincter remains open during passage of the bolus from esophagus to stomach, and it closes with the passage of the peristaltic wave. This creates a closing pressure, following which the sphincter goes back to its normal resting pressure. The lower esophageal sphincter is affected by the same variables that affect all manometric recordings, as well as by physiologic, pharmacologic, and endocrine factors. These are summarized on Table 4-2.

OROPHARYNGEAL DYSPHAGIA

Oropharyngeal dysphagia is a symptom complex that include difficulty in swallowing solids or liquids, with pharyngo-oral and pharyngonasal regurgitations, food sticking in the throat, and repetitive aspirations. It is rare for pain symptoms to be associated with proximal-sphincter dysphagia.

Oropharyngeal dysphagia may be classified into five different areas of dysfunction:

A. Neurologic
  1. Central nervous system:

TABLE 4-2. Factors influencing lower esophageal sphincter function

Factors	Increased LESP	Decreased LESP	Unchanged LESP
Neural	Cholinergic drugs Anticholinesterases Alpha-adrenergic agents	Intravenous atropine Beta-adrenergic agents Vagotomy (in animals) Alpha-adrenergic antagonists	Oral atropine Vagotomy (humans)
Hormonal	Gastrin Prostaglandin F_2A Motilin Bombesin	Secretin Cholecystokinin Glucagon Progesterone Estrogen Prostaglandins E_1, E_2, and A_2	
Myogenic	Resting muscle tone	Possibly aging Possibly diabetes	
Mechanical	Surgical correction	Hiatal hernia Abnormal phrenoesophageal ligament insertion Absent intraabdominal esophageal segment Nasogastric tube	
Drugs	Caffeine Urecholine Methacholine hydrochloride Edrophonium Metoclopramide Betazole Metiamide	Theophylline Nicotine Alcohol Epinephrine Isoproterenol Phentolamine Nitroglycerine	Caffeine Cimetidine
Foods	Protein	Fats—Chocolate	
Other factors	Gastric alkalinization Gastric distention	Gastrectomy Smoking Hypoglycemia Gastric alkalinization Hypothyroidism Amyloidosis Pernicious anemia Epidermolysis Bullosa Gastric acidification	

a. Cerebrovascular accident
b. Amyotrophic lateral sclerosis
c. Brainstem tumors
d. Parkinson's disease
e. Degenerative disorders
2. Peripheral nervous system:
   a. Peripheral neuropathy (diabetic, alcoholic)
   b. Bulbar poliomyelitis
B. Neuromuscular
  1. Motor end plate disease: myasthenia gravis
  2. Skeletal muscle disease:
    a. Muscular dystrophy
    b. Inflammation
    c. Metabolic myopathy
C. Structural
  1. Intrinsic lesions of pharyngoesophageal junction:
    a. Zenker's diverticulum
    b. Webs
    c. Inflammatory disease
    d. Oropharyngeal and hypopharyngeal carcinoma
  2. Extrinsic compression of pharyngoesophageal junction:
    a. Thyroid disease
    b. Lymphadenopathy
    c. Abnormal vessels
    d. Hyperostosis of the cervical spine
D. Iatrogenic
  1. Radiotherapy
  2. Neck surgery (thyroidectomy, tracheostomy)
  3. Pharyngeal or laryngeal resection, recurrent laryngeal nerve palsy
E. Gastroesophageal reflux

Central nervous system and neuromuscular diseases are responsible for oropharyngeal symptoms in nearly 80% of all patients with oropharyngeal dysphagia.[32] When central neurologic disease is present, the formation of a solid or liquid bolus preparatory to the initiation of a swallow seems to be the main problem in these patients. Dysphagia secondary to poor propulsion from partial pharyngeal paralysis and "paradoxical" pharyngeal contraction may result from cerebrovascular accidents. Sphincter incoordination and secondary dysphagia are also seen after selective denervation, such as the paralysis of a recurrent laryngeal nerve.

In the neuromuscular disorders, myasthenia gravis may show progressive weakening of pharyngeal contractions with repetitive deglutitions. Pure muscular disease leads to poor pharyngeal contraction. The upper esophageal sphincter then acts as a functional obstruction against the powerless pharynx. Esophageal-body contraction abnormalities are seen usually with proximal dysfunction.

When no neurologic or neuromuscular disease is found and functional abnormalities are present at the pharyngoesophageal junction, oropharyngeal dysphagia is classified as structural. Zenker's diverticulum patients have been shown to have lower resting pressures in the sphincter, with incoordination abnormalities in approximately 25% of all swallows.[33,34] Entirely normal function of the upper esophageal sphincter area may be seen more often than the abnormal patterns described. Local intrinsic or extrinsic lesions cause mainly a mechanical obstruction to the bolus movement. (See Fig. 4-4.)

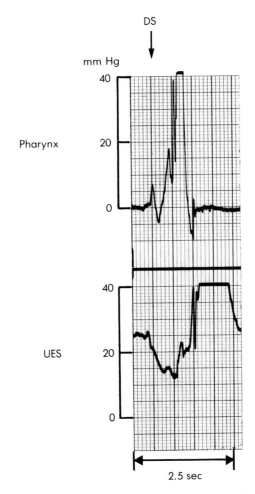

Fig. 4-4. Pressures measured during upper esophageal sphincter dysfunction resulting from Zenker's diverticulum. *DS*, Dry swallow.

Radiotherapy and laryngectomy can result in significant contraction abnormalities in the pharynx and in the upper esophageal sphincter.[32] Spastic contractions of the sphincter may be encountered in up to 25% of this category of patients. Coordination and relaxation abnormalities in the upper sphincter are also noted after laryngectomy. Even patients having a simple tracheostomy or patients who have undergone thyroid resection or parathyroid exploration may have difficulties in swallowing because of inhibition of the hypomandibular complex or because of simple inhibition of the laryngeal excursion by scarring.[35]

Since it has been shown that acid infusion causes an increase in upper sphincter pressure, gastroesophageal reflux has been implicated in upper sphincter dysfunction as well. However, confusing reports exist on the responses of the proximal sphincter to reflux. Distention of the esophagus with a balloon or with fluid causes a sustained increase in upper sphincter pressures.[36,37] Moreover, when acid is used to perfuse the esophagus, the upper sphincter shows a stronger increase in pressure. Hunt et al. observed an increase in upper sphincter resting pressure in the presence of reflux.[38] This has not been documented, however, by Sondheimer[39] in infants or by Gerhardt et al.[40] in adults. The presence of a lower resting pressure in the upper sphincter with a pharyngoesophageal diverticulum is confusing as well, since this condition is frequently associated with a hiatal hernia and reflux.

Despite all the reported observations in the experimental and clinical literature, the knowledge about two major factors, (1) the marked asymmetry of the sphincter and (2) the significant excursion of the larynx, pharynx, and proximal esophagus during deglutition, make all manometric interpretations of pharyngoesophageal function and dysfunction open to discussion. Until newer recording techniques are in general use, symptom evaluation, the presence or absence of normal voluntary deglutition with intact antepulsion and retropulsion of the tongue, and appropriate cineradiographic technique remain the best means to assess upper esophageal function abnormalities.

ESOPHAGEAL PERISTALTIC ABNORMALITIES

Abnormal esophageal contractions can be classified into hypomotility disorders, which include achalasia and scleroderma, and hypermotility disorders, which include the diffuse spasm abnormality and the hypertensive lower esophageal sphincter. This classification is not capable of covering a gray zone of esophageal motility studies, a zone that includes a wide spectrum of abnormal contractions not typical of any of the better recognized primary motor disorders.

The motility disturbances of achalasia are diagnostic. Complete absence of peristalsis is observed in response to all swallows, both in the proximal esophagus and in the distal esophagus. When the patient swallows, all contractions are simultaneous and of low amplitude, showing an identical pattern at all levels of recording. In the early stages of the disease the contractions may be more vigorous.[41] The resting pressure in the esophageal body is usually positive and is a sign of poor esophageal emptying. When bethanechol is given to a patient with achalasia, the esophageal body and the lower esophageal sphincter will react vigorously with an increase in spontaneous activity and more frequent and higher-pressure contractions both in the body and in the lower sphincter. Chest pain frequently accompanies this reaction. In achalasia the lower esophageal sphincter is usually hypertensive, with poor or absent relaxation. The pressure gradient may show an artificial fall in pressures when they are recorded with a side-hole perfused system. The sphincter abnormalities are better observed with the use of a Dent sleeve. Any obstructive lesion can be responsible for an achalasia-like recording, and abnormal motor function must always be correlated with clinical radiologic and endoscopic findings. (See Fig. 4-5.)

The major difference to be found in scleroderma as opposed to achalasia is the almost invariable loss of coordinated peristalsis, but only in the distal two thirds of the esophagus. Contractions are also significantly weaker. Lower esophageal sphincter tone is usually reduced or absent. These abnormalities may be found in patients investigated for reflux symptoms but with no symptoms or signs related to their collagen disease. The presence, duration, and severity of Raynaud's phenomenon, the single most frequent clinical finding with scleroderma, does not correlate with esophageal function.[42] A number of abnormal contraction patterns can be seen with the disease, ranging from simple loss of peristalsis to progressive loss of contractile strength by smooth muscle atrophy and submucosal collagen deposition. Some patients with scleroderma show intact esophageal waves, while others present weaker contractions and values of the lower sphincter. The extreme form of the disease, that is, progressive systemic sclerosis, is usually associated with total paralysis of the smooth

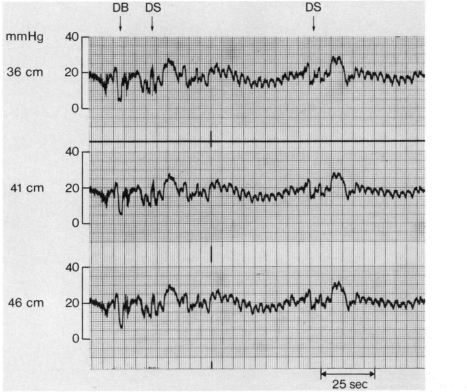

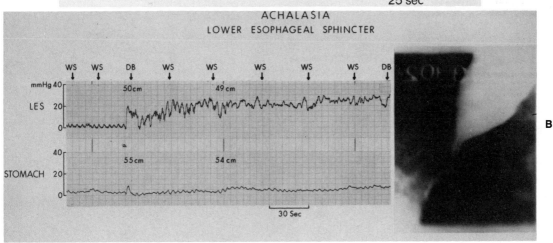

Fig. 4-5. A, Weak flat waves of achalasia with high resting pressure in the esophageal body. *DB,* Deep breath, *DS,* dry swallow. **B,** Poorly relaxing lower esophageal sphincter in achalasia.

muscle esophagus and absent lower esophageal sphincter. When diffuse esophageal infiltration is present with amotility, the same motor abnormalities can be identified in the distal digestive tract.[43,44] In this setting motility studies are particularly important, since a standard antireflux procedure built around an esophagus involved in such a process may produce poor results in esophageal emptying. (See Fig. 4-6.)

A hyperdynamic esophagus is seen in diffuse

spasm and with a hypertensive lower esophageal sphincter. The association of hypercontractions and premature closure of the lower sphincter with an epiphrenic diverticulum has led to the sobriquet of "supersqueeze esophagus." Esophageal motility studies in diffuse esophageal spasm of the idiopathic type reveal normal function of the proximal sphincter and of the striated muscle portion of the esophagus. The abnormal contractions in the lower two thirds of the esophagus are

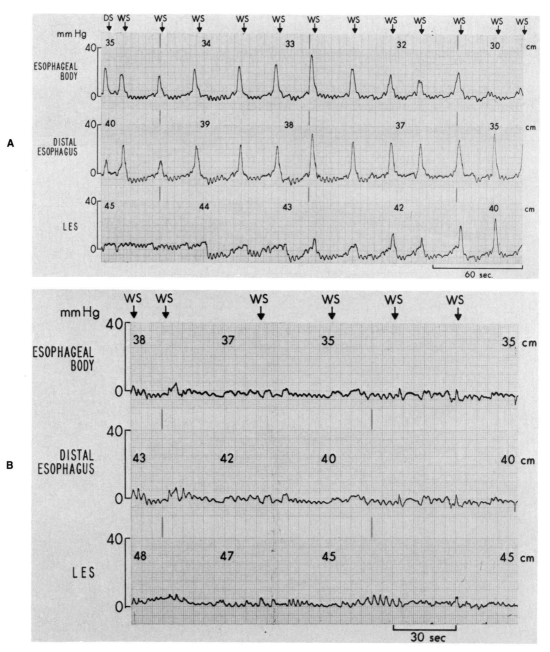

Fig. 4-6. A, Retained contraction force of the esophageal body in scleroderma. *DS,* Dry swallow; Wet swallow. **B,** Amotility with absent lower esophageal sphincter in scleroderma.

usually tertiary in type. The pressures following deglutition are exaggerated, of prolonged duration, and frequently repetitive.[45,46] Spontaneous tertiary contractions of similar character may be observed between swallows. The lower esophageal sphincter in diffuse spasm may show normal pressure and relaxation. A hypertensive sphincter with poor relaxation can also be observed.[47] A good correlation between clinical radiologic and manometric abnormalities should help to dif-

ferentiate the primary idiopathic form of spasm from the more frequent abnormal contraction observed in reflux disorders or in the highly tense patient. (See Fig. 4-7.)

The hypertensive lower esophageal sphincter has been described by Pederson and Alstrup[48] as well as by Berger and McCallum.[49] It is characterized by elevated sphincter pressures with normal relaxation of the sphincter and normal propulsion in the esophageal body. However,

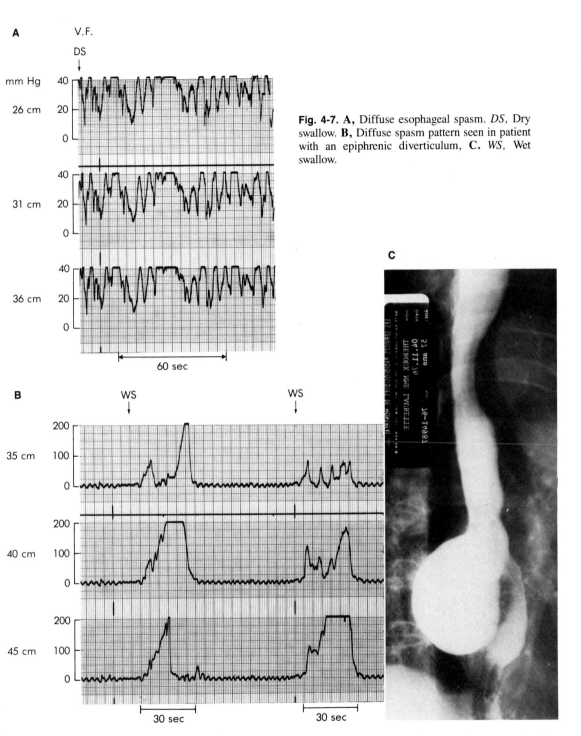

Fig. 4-7. A, Diffuse esophageal spasm. *DS,* Dry swallow. **B,** Diffuse spasm pattern seen in patient with an epiphrenic diverticulum, **C.** *WS,* Wet swallow.

basal pressures in the lower sphincter can reach high levels associated with phase III activity of the migrating motor complex, and this makes the diagnosis of hypertensive sphincter as a pathologic entity somewhat uncertain. Severe contraction abnormalities both in regard to pressures generated and in regard to coordination can also be seen with or without lower sphincter abnormalities.[50]

Despite the description of a progression from a state of diffuse esophageal spasm to achalasia[51] and of regression to normal peristalsis from achalasia,[52] it remains difficult to associate the various motor abnormalities considered as "primary" with each other. These abnormalities may all be part of a disease spectrum. Only continuous observations of these abnormalities with documentation of evolution and transformation over time will permit better classification of these disorders.

ESOPHAGEAL MOTOR ABNORMALITIES IN REFLUX DISEASE

Episodes of transient sphincter relaxation occur in normal individuals, resulting in the occurrence of gastroesophageal reflux.[53] These relaxations occur mainly after meals. Since the lower esophageal sphincter is asymmetric and the gastroesophageal junction mobile with respiration and swallowing, the resting pressure and the relaxation period of the lower esophageal sphincter must be studied using a long perfused sleeve.

Atkinson et al.[54] observed that the lower esophageal sphincter was low when reflux was present. This was further observed later with better recording techniques. Manometric evaluation of the lower esophageal sphincter by a low-compliance infusion system has become essential in the management of patients with gastroesophageal reflux disease. In addition to providing information on the actual values of the sphincter, this system allows assessment of changes produced by drug administration or surgical repair. Diminished lower esophageal sphincter pressures are usually associated with the presence of reflux as proved by pH recording[55]; and when pressures in a lower esophageal sphincter are found to remain persistently between 0 and 10 mm Hg, this observation shows good specificity (84%). Despite the fact that patients with no sphincter or poor sphincter function can be presumed to have gastroesophageal reflux, pH recording of reflux episodes over a 24-hour period remains the method of choice to document objectively the actuality of reflux. High values for lower esophageal pressures are not usually associated with reflux and the finding of normal esophageal mucosa; normal values in lower esophageal sphincter resting pressure mean that a diagnosis of reflux disease is most unlikely. Objective documentation of reflux events or of the pathologic consequences of reflux then becomes essential. A hypertensive sphincter reaction may be observed in a small number of patients with established reflux. Whether this represents an exaggerated defense reaction of the sphincter zone in response to reflux insult remains to be proved.

The effects of chronic gastroesophageal reflux on motor function of the esophageal body are less well documented. It seems logical to think that after the initial loss of sphincter function, the succeeding episodes of reflux eventually lead to dysmotility on a transient basis at first but with more permanent abnormalities on a long-term basis. The normal defense response of the esophagus when perfused with acid or when subjected to a reflux episode is to produce a secondary peristaltic wave, which will clear the reflux toward the stomach. Active swallowing with primary waves will also help to clear the esophagus of its contents.[56]

Early studies have shown that the simple infusion of acid produces little change in the motor function of the esophagus.[57] However, an acid bolus in the esophageal lumen results in more frequent secondary peristalsis. If the esophagus is exposed to both acid and alkaline contents, more contraction abnormalities result, leading to longer contact periods of the refluxate with the esophageal mucosa and to more damage. Progressive damage may result in weaker esophageal contractions with poorer emptying capacity. The lower esophageal sphincter zone is abolished at the same time by the production of esophagitis, but this hypotension is a reversible abnormality. If reflux esophagitis progresses to cause motor abnormalities in the esophagus comparable to those seen in scleroderma, it remains to be seen whether such changes are permanent or reversible. It is also not certain whether motor abnormalities are ever the initiating factor in primary gastroesophageal reflux disease.

Esophageal motility studies provide objective documentation of the abnormalities present in primary motor disorders and in reflux esophagitis. Similarly, objective documentation of results of medical or surgical therapy can be obtained.

REFERENCES

1. Blackwell, J.N., Hannan, W.J., Adams, R.D., and Heading R.C.: Radionuclide transit studies in the detection of esophageal dysmotility, Gut **24:**421-426, 1983.
2. Fisher, R.S., Malmud, L.S., Roberts, G.S., and Lobis, I.F.: Gastroesophageal scintiscanning to detect and quantitate GE reflux, Gastroenterology **70:**301-308, 1976.
3. Pope, C.E.: Esophageal motility: who needs it? Gastroenterology **74:**1337-1338, 1974.
4. Kronecker, H., and Meltzer, S.J.: Der Schulkmechanismus, seine Erregung und seine Hummung, Arch. P.F. Physiol. Leipz. [Suppl.], pp. 338-362, 1883.
5. Ingelfinger, F.J.: Esophageal motility, Physiol. Rev. **38:**533-584, 1958.
6. Code, C.F., Creamer, B., Schlegel, J.F., Olsen, A.M., Donoghue, F.E., and Andersen, H.A.: An atlas of esophageal motility in health and disease, Springfield, Ill., 1958, Charles C Thomas, Publisher.
7. Quigley, J.B., and Brody, D.A.: A physiologic and clinical consideration of the pressures developed in the digestive tract, Am. J. Med. **13:**397-406, 1959.
8. Pope, C.E.: A dynamic test of sphincter strength: its

application to the lower esophageal sphincter, Gastroenterology **52**:779-786, 1967.

9. Pope, C.E.: Effect of infusion on force of closure measurements in the esophagus, Gastroenterology **58**:616-624, 1970.

10. Hollis, J.B., and Castell, D.O.: Amplitude of esophageal peristalsis as determined by rapid infusion, Gastroenterology **63**:417-422, 1972.

11. Arndorfer, R.C., Stef, J.J., Dodds, W.J., Linehan, J.H., and Hogan, W.J.: Improved infusion system for intraluminal esophageal manometry, Gastroenterology **73**:23-37, 1977.

12. Welch, R.W., and Drake, S.T.: Normal lower esophageal sphincter pressure: a comparison of rapid vs slow pull-through technique, Gastroenterology **78**:1446-1451, 1980.

13. Dent, J.: A new technique for continuous sphincter pressure measurement, Gastroenterology **71**:263-267, 1976.

14. Hurwitz, A.L., Duranceau, A., and Haddad, J.K.: Disorders of esophageal motility, vol. 16 in the series Major problems in internal medicine, Philadelphia, 1979, W. B. Saunders Co.

15. Gauer, O.H., and Gienapp, E.: A miniature pressure recording device, Science **112**:404-405, 1950.

16. Dodds, W.J., Hogan, W.J., Lydon, S.B., Stewart, E.T., Stef, J.J., and Arndorfer, R.C.: Quantitation of pharyngeal motor function in normal human subjects, J. Appl. Physiol. **39**:692-696, 1975.

17. Kaye, M.D., and Showalter, J.P.: Measurement of pressure in the lower esophageal sphincter: the influence of catheter diameter, Am. J. Dig. Dis. **19**:860-863, 1974.

18. Lydon, S.B., Dodds, W.J., Hogan, W.J., and Arndorfer, R.C: The effect of manometric assembly diameter on intraluminal esophageal pressure recording, Am. J. Dig. Dis. **20**:968-970, 1975.

19. Stef, J.J., Dodds, W.J., Hogan, W.J., Linehan, J.H., and Stewart, E.T.: Intraluminal esophageal manometry: an analysis of variables affecting recorded fidelity of peristaltic pressures, Gastroenterology **67**:221-230, 1974.

20. Winship, D.H., Viegas De Andrade, S.R., and Zboralske, F.F.: Influence of bolus temperature on human esophageal motor function, Clin. Invest. **49**:243-250, 1970.

21. Funch-Jensen, P., and Jacobsen, E.: Esophageal peristalsis before, during and after food intake in healthy people, Scand. J. Gastroenterol. **16**:209-212, 1981.

22. Pope, C.E.: Is measurement of lower esophageal sphincter pressure clinically useful? Dig. Dis. Sci. **26**:1025-1027, 1981.

23. Meyer, G.W., and Castell D.O.: In support of the clinical usefulness of lower esophageal sphincter pressure determination. Dig. Dis. Sci. **26**:1028-1031, 1981.

24. Winans, C.S.: Manometric asymmetry of the lower esophageal high pressure zone, Am. J. Dig. Dis. **22**:348-354, 1977.

25. Hurwitz, A.L., Nelson, J.A., and Haddad, J.K.: Oropharyngeal dysphagia: manometric and cineesophagraphic findings, Am. J. Dig. Dis. **20**:313-324, 1975.

26. Duranceau, A.C., DeVroede, G., Lafontaine, E., and Jamieson, G.G.: Esophageal motility in asymptomatic volunteers, Surg. Clin. North Am. **63**:777-786, 1983.

27. Dent, J.: Personnal communication, 1985.

28. Humphries, T.J., and Castell, D.O.: Pressure profile of esophageal peristalsis in normal humans as measured by direct intraesophageal transducers, Am. J. Dig. Dis. **22**:641-645, 1977.

29. Hollis, J.B., and Castell, D.O.: Esophageal function in elderly men: a new look at "presbyesophagus," Ann. Int. Med. **80**:371-374, 1974.

30. Rubin, J., Nagler, R., Spiro, H.M., and Pilot, M.L.: Measuring the effect of emotions on esophageal motility, Psychosom. Med. **24**:170-176, 1962.

31. Watier, A., DeVroede, G., Duranceau, A., et al.: Constipation with colonic intertia: a manifestation of systematic disease? Dig. Dis. Sci. **28**:1025-1033, 1983.

32. Hurwitz, A.L., and Duranceau, A.: Upper esophageal sphincter dysfunction: pathogenesis and treatment, Dig. Dis. Sci. **23**:275-281, 1978.

33. Ellis, F.H., Jr., Schlegel, J.F., Lynch, V.P., and Payne, W.S.: Cricopharyngeal myotomy for pharyngo-esophageal diverticulum, Ann. Surg. **170**:340-349, 1969.

34. Duranceau, A., Rheault, M.J., and Jamieson, G.G.: Physiological response to cricopharyngeal myotomy and diverticulum suspension, Surgery **94**:655-662, 1983.

35. Bonanno, P.C.: Swallowing dysfunction after tracheostomy, Ann. Surg. **174**:29-33, 1971.

36. Enzmann, D.R., Harell, G.S., and Zboralske, F.F.: Upper esophageal responses to intraluminal distention in man, Gastroenterology **72**:1292-1298, 1977.

37. Gerhardt, D.C., Schuck, T.J., Bordeaux, R.A., and Winship, D.H.: Human upper esophageal sphincter: response to volume, osmotic and acid stimuli, Gastroenterology **75**:268-274, 1978.

38. Hunt, P.S., Connell, A.M., and Smiley, T.B.: The cricopharyngeal sphincter in gastric reflux, Gut **11**:303-306, 1970.

39. Sondheimer, J.M.: Upper esophageal sphincter and pharyngo-esophageal motor function in infants with and without gastroesophageal reflux, Gastroenterology **85**:301-305, 1983.

40. Gerhardt, D.C., Castell, D.O., Winship, D.H., and Shuck, T.: Esophageal dysfunction in esophagopharyngeal regurgitation, Gastroenterology **78**:893-897, 1980.

41. Sanderson, D.R., Ellis, F.H., Schlegel, J.F., and Olsen, A.M.: Syndrome of vigorous achalasia: clinical and physiologic observations, Dis. Chest **52**:508-517, 1967.

42. Hurwitz, A.L., Duranceau, A., and Postlethwait, R.W.: Esophageal dysfunction and Raynaud's phenomenon in patients with scleroderma, Am. J. Dig. Dis. **21**:601-606, 1976.

43. Maddern, G.J., Horowitz, M., Jamieson, G.G., Chatterton, B.E., Collins, P.J., and Roberts-Thomson, P.: Abnormalities of esophageal and gastric emptying in progressive systemic sclerosis, Gastroenterology **87**:922-926, 1984.

44. Hamel-Roy, J., DeVroede, G., Arhan, P., Tetreault, L., Duranceau, A., and Ménard, H.: Comparative esophageal and anorectal motility in scleroderma, Gastroenterology **88**:1-7, 1985.

45. Kramer, P.: Diffuse esophageal spasm, Mod. Treatment **7**:1151-1162, 1970.

46. Bennett, J.R., and Hendrix, T.R.: Diffuse esophageal spasm: a disorder with more than one cause, Gastroenterology **59**:273-279, 1970.

47. Ritcher, J.E., and Castell, D.O.: Diffuse esophageal spasm: a reappraisal, Ann. Intern. Med. **100:**242-245, 1984.

48. Pederson, S.A., and Alstrup, P.: The hypertensive gastroesophageal sphincter: a manometric and clinical study, Scand. J. Gastroenterol. **7:**531-534, 1972.

49. Berger, K., and McCallum, T.W.: The hypertensive lower esophageal sphincter, Gastroenterology **80:**1109, 1981.

50. Hurwitz, A.L., Way, L.W., and Haddad, J.K.: Epiphrenic diverticulum in association with an unusual motility disturbance: report of surgical correction, Gastroenterology **68:**795-798, 1975.

51. Kramer, P., Harris, L.D., and Donaldson, R.M.: Transition form symptomatic diffuse spasm to cardiospasm, Gut **8:**115-119, 1967.

52. Mellow, M.M.: Symptomatic diffuse esophageal spasm: manometric follow-up and response to cholinergic stimulation and cholinesterase inhibition, Gastroenterology **73:**237-240, 1977.

53. Dent, J., Dodds, W.J., Friedman, R.H., Sekiguchi, T., Hogan, W.J., Arndorfer, R.C., and Petrie, D.J.: Mechanisms of gastroesophageal reflux in recumbent asymptomatic human subjects, J. Clin. Invest. **65:**256-267, 1980.

54. Atkinson, M., Edwards, D.A.W., Honour, A.J., and Rowlands, E.N.: The esophagogastric sphincter in hiatus hernia, Lancet **2:**1138-1142, 1957.

55. Haddad, J.K.: Relation of gastroesophageal reflux to yield sphincter pressures, Gastroenterology **58:**175-184, 1970.

56. Dodds, W.J., Dent, J., Hogan, W.J., Helm, J.F., Hauser, R., Patel, G.K., and Egide, M.S.: Mechanisms of gastroesophageal reflux in patients with reflux esophagitis, N. Engl. J. Med. **307:**1547-1552, 1982.

57. Siegel, C.I., and Hendrix, T.R.: Esophageal motor abnormalities induced by acid perfusion in patients with heartburn, J. Clin. Invest. **42:**686-695, 1963.

58. Vantrappen, G., and Hellemans, J.: Studies on the normal deglutition complex, Am. J. Dig. Dis. **12:**255-266, 1967.

59. Nelson, J.L., Richter, G.E., Gohns, D.N., Castell, D.O., and Centola, G.M.: Esophageal contraction pressures are not affected by normal menstrual cycles, Gastroenterology **87:**867-871, 1984.

Recent advances in esophageal manometry

DISCUSSION

J.E. Dussek

Professors Duranceau and Jamieson have given a comprehensive description of conventional manometric investigation of the esophagus, but they have been reticent about including some recent advances that indicate the direction in which esophageal manometry might proceed.

Radiologic evaluation of the esophagus is dismissed somewhat cursorily. The esophagus is analogous to the heart. It is a pumping chamber with an inlet valve (cricopharyngeus) and an outlet valve (lower esophageal sphincter). Its muscular architecture is similar (long inner and outer spirals), and it is affected by similar drugs (e.g., the calcium antagonists and nitrates). Likewise, the esophagus is investigated in a way similar to the way in which the heart is investigated, with contrast radiology and pressure studies. Each gives different but complementary information. Perhaps one should bear in mind that in cardiology more emphasis is now being placed on the radiologic studies than on pressure and saturation data.

A properly conducted barium meal will supply a great deal of information. Liquid barium is ideal for showing anatomic and structural details. Solid barium (e.g., bread coated in barium) will give excellent information about function at all levels. Recordings on videotape or cineradiographic film allow the information to be played back repeatedly at any speed required (as with coronary angiograms). Acid barium studies may reveal reflux-induced motility disorders. One might even ask whether there is any place for esophageal manometry in the face of an entirely normal solid barium swallow.

TECHNICAL ADVANCES IN ESOPHAGEAL MANOMETRY

The progression from intraesophageal balloon catheter open-tipped catheters, culminating in the Arndorfer system, is well described, but microtransducer or strain gauges unfortunately receive scant mention. I consider solid-state manometry to be *the* recent advance.

It has been traditional to use a catheter with three sensors 5 cm apart, whether they be fluid filled or solid state. By gradually withdrawing the catheter through the esophagus it has been possible to evaluate all regions of it, but *not* synchronously. The usual way of recording the data is on moving paper, using either pens and ink or light-sensitive paper. Multichannel pen writers are becoming increasingly expensive. Being mechanical, they are prone to mechanical problems and wear. We are now in the computer age, and it seems sensible to use a solid-state computerized system.

At Guy's Hospital, and also at the South East Regional Cardiothoracic Unit, both in London, England, the following system is used.

The esophageal catheter contains six microtransducers, each 5 cm apart (Fig. 4-8). The proximal sensor is thus 25 cm from the distal one. Under most circumstances, this means that when the proximal sensor is in the cricopharyngeus, the lower one is at the lower esophageal sphincter. The other four sensors are thus at 5-cm intervals along the whole length of the esophagus. It is therefore possible on one swallow to see cricopharyngeal action, esophageal peristalsis, and LES relaxation, all on the same tracing (Fig. 4-9). The diameter of the catheter is only 32 mm, and where acid infusion is required, a fine-bore catheter can be fixed to it. It has the disadvantage that the addition of a pH sensor makes it rather bulky.

The microtransducers relay through an interface to a desk-top computer, and the tracings are shown on a video display unit. Hard copies may be printed (Figs. 4-10 and 4-11), and the whole

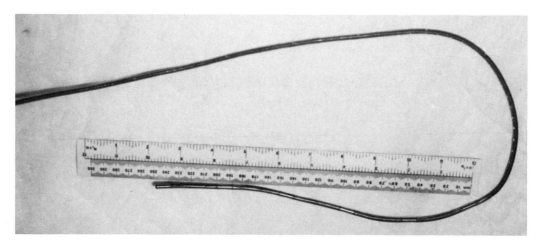

Fig. 4-8. Six-transducer pressure probe.

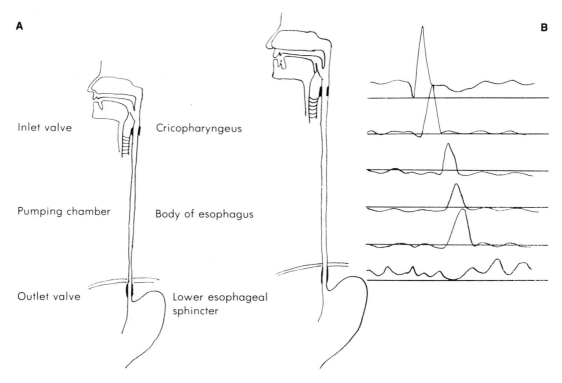

Fig. 4-9. A, The esophagus has an inlet valve, a pumping chamber, and an outlet valve. **B,** Measurements of esophageal pressure may be made at several levels in the esophagus simultaneously.

examination recorded on a floppy disk for subsequent reanalysis.

The system has many advantages:
1. The whole of the esophagus may be seen at once.
2. The response is rapid, enabling pharyngeal and cricopharyngeal activity to be studied more easily.
3. The tracings produced may be expanded electronically, allowing more detailed analysis.
4. Electronic analysis is simple and free of observer error.
5. The apparatus is very simple to use and, being devoid of mechanical parts, needs almost no maintenance.
6. The storage of data on floppy disks means that should one want to look at different parameters at a later date, it is a relatively simple matter to write another program to analyze the data.
7. A solid-state system is now as cheap as, if

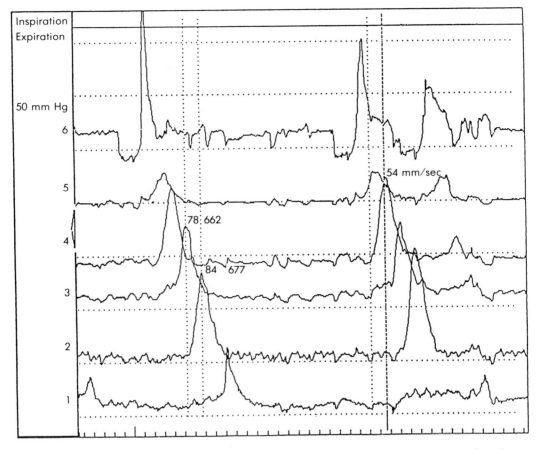

Fig. 4-10. Typical tracing of a normal swallow. Transducer no. 6 is in the cricopharyngeus, and no. 1 is just proximal to the LES. The numbers alongside the pressure waves of the first swallow represent the amplitude in millimeters of mercury (first number) and time of the measurement in tenths of a second after the start of the recording (second number). The figure of 54 mm/sec beside tracing 4 of the second swallow is the rate of change of pressure against time ($\Delta P/\Delta T$)—that is, a rise in pressure of 54 mm Hg per second. The inspiration/expiration channel (top) is not in use.

not cheaper than, multiple pen writers.

There are disadvantages; the catheter is slightly bulky and stiff. Repairs to it, though very infrequent, require specialist expertise, take time, and are relatively expensive compared with fluid-filled catheters. However, the disadvantages are small compared with the considerable advantages mentioned.

Although we use a six-sensor probe at present, there is no reason why more or fewer sensors should not be used, and the next logical step should be to have at least two sensors facing in different directions for studying the cricopharyngeus. We have not used a sleeve for looking at the LES and cannot comment on its efficacy, although it looks to be a sensible way of assessing this difficult region—if, however, the necessary bulk of the sleeve does not in itself alter LES tone.

Although the system described demonstrates

the whole of the esophagus, we also use a pull-through technique to assess the LES. The distal transducer is withdrawn 1 cm at a time, from stomach to esophagus, and the program is designed so that the mean pressure over 5 seconds is recorded at each point (Fig. 4-12).

It seems logical that the next step forward will be 24-hour ambulatory manometry, using a simplified technique. Allied to 24-hour electrocardiographic monitoring, it may be helpful in differentiating between cardiac and esophageal pain.

USES OF MANOMETRY
Acid clearance

Some laboratories perform acid clearance studies in which a bolus of 0.1N hydrochloric acid is instilled into the esophagus and the

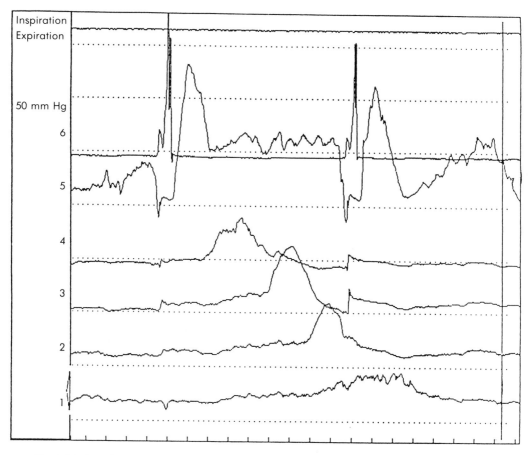

Fig. 4-11. A tracing that is similar to Fig. 4-10, except that the time base is expanded (each vertical line at the bottom is 1 second) and transducer no. 6 is in the pharynx and no. 5 is in cricopharyngeus.

number of swallows taken to clear the acid is noted. Patients with macroscopic esophagitis tend to have prolonged acid clearance as compared with patients with reflux but no esophagitis.[1] Unfortunately, at present no therapeutic benefit has resulted from this finding.

Intraoperative manometry

The essence of an effective antireflux operation would appear to be the creation of an adequate high-pressure zone at the lower esophageal sphincter. It thus seems sensible to monitor the pressure in this region on the operating table while an antireflux operation is being performed. Hill has been an enthusiastic advocate of this technique,[2] and Cooper et al. have similarly found it helpful.[3]

Manometry and atypical chest pain

Both angina and esophageal pain are common, and occasionally it may be difficult to differentiate between the two.[4] Indeed, they may coexist, or angina may even be linked to esophageal

disorders, particularly gastroesophageal reflux. A significant number of patients investigated by coronary angiography for angina have normal coronary arteries, and a diagnosis of coronary spasm is frequently invoked. However, esophageal spasm is far more common than coronary spasm. Esophageal manometry is being used increasingly to help differentiate between esophageal and coronary artery pain.

Two tests appear to be useful:
1. Acid instillation. The classic Bernstein test may provoke pain. The pain may be similar to that which was thought to be angina, or it may be different. Unfortunately, acid instillation into the esophagus may trigger myocardial ischemia with diagnostic electrocardiographic changes.[5] If, however, diffuse esophageal spasm ensues with accompanying pain, it may be assumed that this is responsible for the symptoms.
2. Edrophonium provocation test.[6] Diffuse esophageal spasm or disordered motility may be produced by the injection of 10 mg

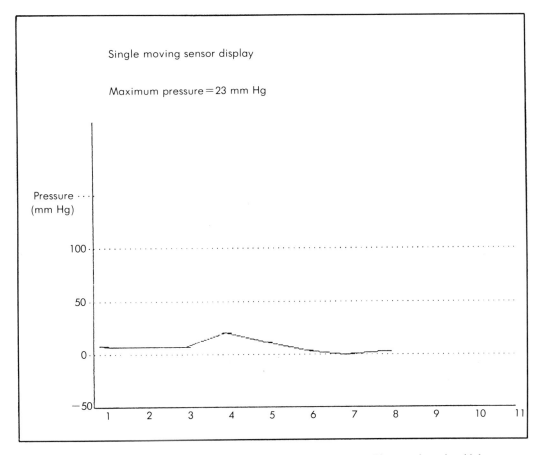

Single moving sensor display

Maximum pressure = 23 mm Hg

Fig. 4-12. Tracing demonstrating lower esophageal sphincter pressure. The transducer is withdrawn across the LES from the stomach, with measurements being made at 1-cm intervals. The resting intragastric pressure is slightly positive, with a rise to 23 mm Hg in the LES and a fall of zero in the thorax.

of edrophonium IV. If this disordered motility coincides with the pain being investigated, it is reasonable to infer that the esophagus is responsible for the pain.

Unfortunately, despite the elegant methods available for investigating both coronary artery disease and esophageal function, one cannot always reach a clear-cut and unequivocal conclusion.

Manometry in monitoring anesthesia

The lower esophagus consists of smooth muscle and is therefore not affected by the conventional muscle relaxants used during anesthesia. It is thought that secondary and tertiary peristaltic waves may be abolished by sufficient depth of anesthesia. It is suggested that the manometric profile should be monitored under general anesthesia following the rapid inflation of an intraesophageal balloon. The abolition of secondary and tertiary peristalsis implies adequate depth of anesthesia.[7]

THE FUTURE

It is probable that intraesophageal probes will become smaller and more sensitive. Telemetry (at present still in its infancy) should enable more meaningful measurements to be made. The combination of ambulatory pH monitoring, manometry, and electrocardiography, once miniaturization of the hardware is accomplished, should enable us to understand the symptomatology and pathogenesis of esophageal disorders more easily.

REFERENCES

1. Skinner, D.B., and Booth, D.J.: Assessment of distal esophageal function in patients with hiatal hernias and/or gastro esophageal reflux, Ann. Surg. **172:**627-637, 1970.
2. Hill, L.D.: Intraoperative measurement of lower esophageal sphincter pressure, J. Thorac. Cardiovasc. Surg. **75:** 378-382, 1978.
3. Cooper, J.D., Gill, S.S., Nelems, J.M., and Pearson, F.G.: Intraoperative and post operative esophageal

manometric findings with Collis gastroplasty and Belsey hiatal hernia repair for gastro-esophageal reflux, J. Thorac. Cardiovasc. Surg. **74:**744-751, 1977.

4. Anon.: Angina and esophageal disease, Lancet **1:**191-192, 1986.

5. Mellow, M.H., Simpson, A.G., et al.: Esophageal acid perfusion in coronary artery disease: induction of myocardial ischemia, Gastroenterology **85:**306-312, 1983.

6. London, R.L., Ouyang, A., et al.: Provocation of esophageal pain by ergonovine or edrephonium, Gastroenterology **81:**10-14, 1981.

7. Evans, J.M., Davies, W.L., and Wise, C.C.: Lower esophageal contractility: a new monitor of anaesthesia, Lancet **1:**1151-1154, 1984.

CHAPTER 5 New endoscopic techniques

Philippe Monnier and Marcel Savary

In the study of the esophagus, we have come to distinguish two types of endoscopies: medical endoscopies, whose aim is diagnostic, and surgical endoscopies, whose aim is therapeutic.

DIAGNOSTIC ENDOSCOPY
Optical and technical possibilities

Paradoxically, the new gastrofibroscopes of the Olympus OES series have not been responsible for the diagnostic and therapeutic advances made recently in esophageal pathology. Even though their optical quality is much superior to that of the previous models, their instrumental possibilities remain distinctly inferior to those obtained with the rigid esophagoscopes. The same is true of the Olympus or Welch Allyn types of videoendoscopes, whose high-quality video imagery is definitely an improvement in lesion assessment but whose instrumental possibilities equal those of traditional fibroscopes.

Those who use both fibroscopes and rigid endoscopic systems daily often find that they must perform rigid endoscopy after initial fibroscopy, especially when they are confronted with complex pathologies located at the pharyngoesophageal junction or the gastroesophageal junction.

The difficulties encountered in diagnostic endoscopy generally concern early stages and complicated late stages of esophageal pathology. For example, it is impossible to differentiate between benign and malignant pathologies in their early stages. Early-stage reflux esophagitis, columnar epithelialization of the lower esophagus, and squamous cell carcinoma can all present the same endoscopic morphology (Plate 1).

The role of the endoscopist is a particularly difficult one; he or she should be able to diagnose the pathology based on the macroscopic aspect of the lesion, and confirm the diagnosis histologically with a precise and selective biopsy. This necessitates high-quality optical equipment and great stability in macroscopic observation and endoscopic technical ability (in biopsying as well as in possible endoscopic treatments).[1]

The drive for precise, meticulous technique has given renewed favor to rigid endoscopy, which ensures better stability of the instruments, and also to the practice of general anesthesia, which allows greater stability of the lesion to be observed, biopsied, or treated (Plate 2).

If we add the optical performances, the ease of handling provided by the rigid system, and the surgical possibilities offered by the different-sized open tubes, it is clear that the open Storz or Wolf type of optical esophagoscope gives the best results in terms of high-quality observation and intervention, and this is true for all age groups. Of course, the endoscopist must have sufficient experience to enable him or her to use this potential to the fullest.

Early-stage reflux esophagitis and early squamous cell carcinoma provide two striking examples of the optical and instrumental advantages of the rigid system.

Early-stage reflux esophagitis

Even though reflux esophagitis is the most frequently encountered illness of the upper digestive tract, the study of early histologic lesions by peptic erosion had advanced solely as a result of the findings of rigid endoscopy.[2]

The technical problems inherent in supravestibular selective biopsy proved insurmountable with the gastrofibroscope. The instability between the biopsy forceps and the target (because of peristaltic waves or the flexibility of the fibroscopes) and the tangential approach to the mucosa (the biopsy forceps being parallel to the axis of the fibroscope) do not allow precise manipulation (see Plate 2). This explains why histopathologic criteria of early-stage reflux esophagitis are so vague and often completely different from one author to another.[3-5]

Our study, based on 50 cases (with 10 additional cases recently included), proves that in stage I reflux esophagitis, the supravestibular lesion exists as an epithelial erosion associated with a neutrophilic infiltration of the lamina propria.[2] There is no diffuse infiltration (histologically seen as papillary elongation or inflammatory lymphocytic or plasmocytic infiltration) without endoscopic signs of epithelial erosions.

Endoscopically and histologically, stage I reflux esophagitis is a topographically asymmetric lesion, often macular or linear. None of the reference biopsy specimens taken at *the same level* as the supravestibular erosive lesion but in a normal-looking squamous epithelium showed any histologic signs of inflammation (Plate 3).

Our study was performed using a rigid endoscope, taking first a selective biopsy of the lesion, followed by epinephrine swabbing to stop any bleeding, then a second biopsy taken at the same level but in a normal mucosa, and finally a third biopsy taken 5 cm proximally in the esophagus (Plate 4). With the gastrofibroscope, positive correlations were much rarer, because of the poorer optical quality, the difficulties mentioned before concerning hyperselective biopsy, and also the problems involved in obtaining good hemostasis and visualization for the second and third biopsies.[2]

Early forms of squamous cell carcinoma

According to the recent statistics published by Froelicher and Miller concerning over 900,000 upper digestive tract endoscopies performed in Europe, positive diagnosis of early-stage carcinoma was 10 times less frequent for the esophagus than for the stomach (correction being made for the respective incidences of the two lesions).[6] The most common form of intraepithelial or microinvasive carcinoma of the esophagus often presents as a slight discoloration of the mucosa (leukoplakia, erythroplakia or leukoerythroplakia), sometimes associated with a surface irregularity (slightly elevated or depressed), and with no alteration of the esophageal wall.[7] When the lesion is of the elevated leukoplakia type, endoscopic diagnosis is easy, no matter what optical system is used. Unfortunately, this is the least common form of early carcinoma. The flat erythroplakia type of lesion requires a high-performance optical system to be diagnosed, especially since this form can easily be mistaken for other benign lesions (Plate 5) (see also Plate 1).

Vital staining using Lugol's solution or toluidine blue is very helpful in endoscopic diagnosis, and application of stain by rigid endoscope is much easier than by a fibroscope (Plate 6).[8]

When the lesion is located in the hypopharynx or the esophageal os or cervical esophagus, diagnosis with a fibroscope becomes extremely difficult. Open rigid tubes allow the endoscopist to remove secretions by suction, and to explore mucosal folds and expose the lesion completely, to perform selective vital staining, to visualize the lesion perfectly, and to photograph and biopsy selectively in the best possible conditions. During exploration of the hypopharynx and the esophageal os, a surgical microscope or a laparoscope can also be used to further enhance the quality of the observation (Plate 7).

Vital staining

Vital staining has made a great contribution to endoscopic diagnosis, showing tumor limits in a multicentric pattern, directing biopsies, revealing satellite lesions in dysplasia or intraepithelial carcinoma, diagnosing second primary tumors, and, above all, detecting the "occult" form of dysplasia and intraepithelial carcinoma of the esophagus, whose existence is now firmly established.

Three percent Lugol's solution is a negative tumor marker; that is, normal esophageal mucosa and regions of glycogenic acanthosis are colored brown, whereas pathologic mucosa (esophagitis, columnar metaplasia, or early carcinoma) do not stain (Plate 8).[9-11]

Practically speaking, staining via the rigid endoscope is done simply by swabbing through the open tube. With the gastrofibroscope, it is done using a spray via a catheter passed into the biopsy forceps canal of the endoscope.

Toluidine blue (aqueous solution, 1%) is a metachromatic stain having great affinity for cell nuclei. Its cellular penetration is approximately five to seven layers. Tissues having high cellular density and high nucleus/plasma ratios take up the stain rapidly and retain it for at least an hour.[12,13]

Practically, the staining is done in three steps:
1. Mucolysis: abundant washing with 1% acetic acid to eliminate excess mucus and food particles
2. Staining: washing with 1% toluidine blue for 1 minute
3. Stain removal: abundant washing with 1% acetic acid

Swabbing with acetic acid (the mechanical effect of swabbing helps clean the mucosa) improves the quality of endoscopic visualization (see Plate 6).

Toluidine blue is particularly suitable for the smooth mucosa of the esophagus. False positives are frequent (mucus, food particles, erosions, and so on), but false negatives are rare in the esophagus and are always due to intraepithelial carcinoma of the hyperkeratotic type. This elevated white form of "in situ" cancer does not escape endoscopic detection, because of its striking macroscopic appearance. The contribution of toluidine blue is that it detects the less obvious form of early carcinoma (depressed erythroplastic type, occult type).[14]

Thanks to the recent advances in rigid endoscopy of the upper digestive tract (micropharyngoscopy, rigid esophagoscopy), diagnostic possibilities for early-stage hypopharyngeal and esophageal cancer have been developed. This type of instrumentation must be used in screening programs such as those introduced in the pretherapy workup of patients having an ear, nose, or throat carcinoma, who have a 20% risk of simultaneous second primary carcinoma of the upper digestive tract.[15,16]

Advanced-stage esophageal pathology

In the study of advanced-stage esophageal pathology, which is often complex, the use of endoscopic instrumentation has, we feel, allowed considerable progress to be made.

In stage IV reflux esophagitis, one can find stenosis, ulcer formation, and metaplastic columnar epithelialization, which can produce benign or malignant lesions.[1] Endoscopic investigation is often made difficult by salivary and food-particle stagnation, bleeding, and the presence of the stenosis. The most interesting part of the esophagus is that part located distal to the stenosis, and this is why we always complete the pretherapy workup of a stenotic reflux lesion discovered by fibroscopy with a rigid-type surgical endoscope.[17]

After inspection of the suprastenotic region, the character, location, and size of the stenosis are precisely defined. Then its "dilatability" is explored, and we consider dilatation as an integral part of all esophageal stenosis investigation. The stricture is explored carefully to detect any suspicious lesions (ulcers, erosions, columnar metaplasia, adenocarcinoma). After measurement of the length of the stenosis, the exploration is continued down to the diaphragmatic hiatus. If columnar epithelialization is present, the type and length of endobrachyesophagus are determined (after Lugol's staining where necessary). Biopsies are taken of all macroscopic lesions observed, and finally nonselective biopsy specimens at different levels all along the endobrachyesophagus are taken for histologic confirmation and screening for dysplasia (Plate 9).

It is our experience that all these maneuvers (dilatation, hemostasis, swabbing, selective and nonselective biopsies) necessitate the modern rigid endoscope (stability, optical quality, open-tube exploration, and precision).

In regard to diagnosis, as paradoxical as it may seem, high-quality rigid esophagoscopes represent distinct progress in oncologic exploration as well as in investigation of complex benign lesions such as stenosis.

If the endoscopist hopes to solve the multiple problems presented by esophageal pathology at all ages of life, he or she must use *diversified instruments* (rigid and flexible endoscopes of all sizes, dilatation systems that are efficient and safe, lasers of different types, and so on). Neither the gastrofibroscope nor the rigid esophagoscope can meet all these requirements by themselves.

Endoscopic ultrasonography

The pretherapy work-up of benign and malignant esophageal lesions has been made even more precise by the introduction of endoscopic ultrasonography. This technique gives more useful information concerning the esophageal wall and the mediastinum than does the CT scan.[18]

Endoscopic ultrasonography is becoming more and more important as a complement to radiologic (barium swallow, CT scan) and endoscopic investigation of the esophagus. It plays an important role in three sectors.

Analysis and staging of benign tumors[19-21]

The most common benign esophageal tumor is the leiomyoma, seen as a distinct mass of low echodensity. Sometimes, ultrasonography shows the origin of the tumor as being the muscularis mucosae or the muscularis propria of the esophagus (Fig. 5-1). A differential diagnosis should be made between leiomyoma and metastatic carcinoma of the extrinsic lymph nodes, often of bronchial origin. The value of bronchoscopy in such cases is obvious.

Staging of esophageal carcinoma[18,21,22]

Here is where endoscopic ultrasonography plays its most interesting role. Esophageal carcinoma presents as a nondistinct echo-poor lesion. Tio and Tytgat[22] believe that staging must allow (screening for metastatic lymph nodes aside) distinction between:

1. Tumors involving only the esophageal wall without metastatic nodes: permitting in toto exeresis and possible cure
2. Tumors involving only the esophageal wall,

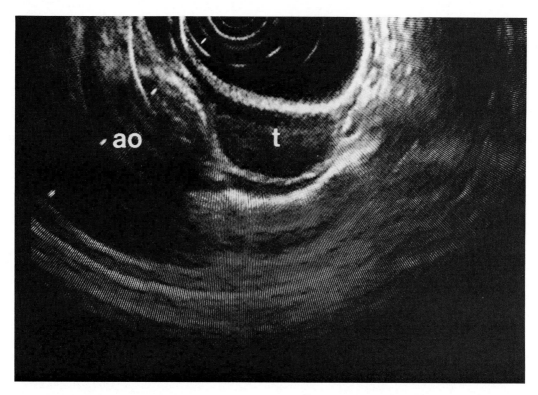

Fig. 5-1. Endoscopic ultrasonographic image compatible with a leiomyoma. Endoscopic ultrasonography shows an ellipsoid hypoechogenic homogenous echo pattern with sharply demarcated borders (*t*) beyond normal mucosa adjacent to the descending aorta (*ao*). (From Tio T.L., and Tytgat, G.N.J.: Atlas of transintestinal endosonography, Aalsmeer, The Netherlands, 1986, Drukkerij Mur-Kostverloren.)

with mediastinal lymph node metastasis, or well-circumscribed tumors extending beyond the esophageal wall: exeresis possible but only palliative surgery

3. Tumors penetrating into the mediastinum with local organ invasion (aorta, pericardium, bronchi, diaphragm): surgical exeresis impossible (Fig. 5-2).

Endoscopic ultrasonography using fourth-generation instruments (Olympus GF-UM 2) is more efficient in determining the operability of an esophageal carcinoma than is the CT scan. However, it is not yet able to distinguish between an "early" intramucosal carcinoma and an "early" submucosal carcinoma. In some cases, a submucosal carcinoma can be distinguished from a carcinoma that has already infiltrated the muscular layer of the esophagus. In inoperable cases, this distinction should help in choosing cases to be treated by photodynamic therapy ("early" carcinoma infiltrating maximally to the submucosa). Even though the esophageal wall is seen ultrasonographically as five layers, practically speaking it is difficult to visualize them because of the direct contact between the transducer and the esophageal wall. The use of a balloon filled with water surrounding the transducer does alleviate somewhat this problem, but it also flattens the esophageal wall by distention. Analysis of the histologic layers of the wall becomes problematic even if the balloon is only slightly filled.

Detection and staging of esophageal varices

In transverse section, varices appear as round echo-poor structures. Endoscopic ultrasonography diagnoses not only submucosal varices, but deep intramural and periesophageal varices as well (Fig. 5-3).[23] Excessive inflation of the balloon must be avoided, since this causes collapse of the veins by compression. Endoscopic ultrasonography is very useful in following up patients after sclerotherapy.

Videoendoscopy

Videoendoscopy is another recent breakthrough in upper digestive tract endoscopy, not because of its instrumental qualities, which are comparable to those found in other gastrofibroscopes, but rather because of the new analytic

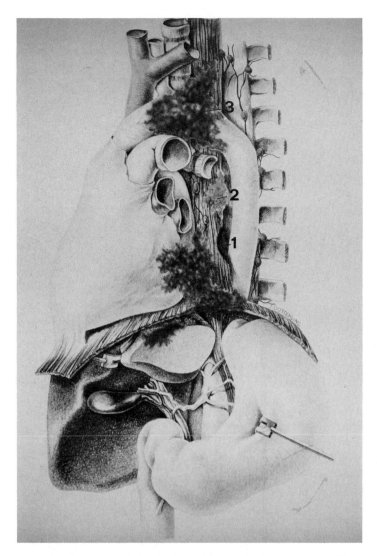

Fig. 5-2. Left lateral oblique view of the distal esophagus and midesophagus. *1*, Clearly demarcated malignancy without penetration through the organ boundaries (muscularis propria) and with no evidence of lymph node involvement; indicative of local resectability with intention of curability. *2*, Clearly demarcated malignancy with penetration through the organ boundaries (muscularis propria) and with lymph node involvement, suggesting the palliative nature of the resection. *3*, Malignancy deeply penetrating into the surrounding tissues (aorta, pericardium, bronchus, diaphragm) and/or organ (adjacent liver) or liver metastasis, strongly suggesting nonresectability. (From Tio, T.L., and Tytgat, G.N.J.: Atlas of transintestinal endosonography, Aalsmeer, The Netherlands, 1986, Drukkerij Mur-Kostverloren.)

process it brings to the endoscopic images recorded.

The image obtained by a videoendoscope is produced by a microchip camera placed at the tip of the flexible endoscope. Resolution quality is excellent, and distinctly superior to that obtained by conventional fibroscopes.[24]

Above all, videoendoscopy offers the possibility of "freezing" the sequence on the television screen when needed. For the first time, mor-

phologic analysis on a stable model is possible, and not only by one endoscopist, but, if desired, by a panel of experts seated anywhere a television monitor can be installed.

Since the observer's attention is not captured by the dynamic aspect of the esophagus and its peristaltic waves or by the movements of the endoscope, it can be fully concentrated on the analysis of the lesions. In addition, this "frozen" document allows consultation and discussion of

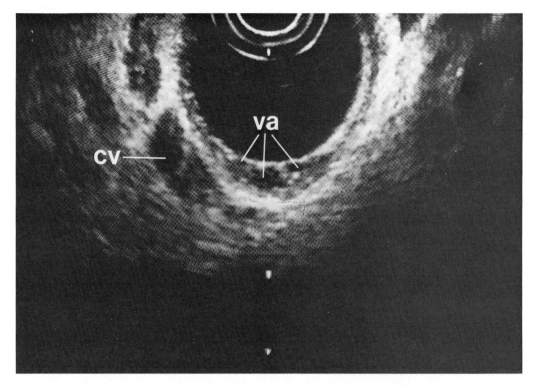

Fig. 5-3. Endoscopic ultrasonographic image of esophageal varices. Endoscopic ultrasonography shows anechoic ellipsoid structures (*va*) in the submucosal layer, compatible with esophageal varices. Collateral veins (*cv*) adjacent to the esophageal wall are also clearly visible.

the pathology, thereby providing a wider potential for diagnosis. The ideal site for a biopsy, for example, can be decided upon calmly after discussion.

Moreover, this system provides an unequalled potential for stocking of endoscopic sequences for teaching and for the follow-up of patients. It represents, in fact, the first step toward teleconferences on endoscopic documents.

THERAPEUTIC ENDOSCOPY

Some endoscopic maneuvers considered to be therapeutic are actually part of diagnostic investigation. Such is the case in regard to dilatation of benign esophageal stenosis. Other therapeutic sectors now being developed include use of the Nd-YAG and carbon dioxide lasers and phototherapy.

Endoscopic dilatation

In spite of their efficiency, endoscopic dilatations of esophageal stenoses were associated until recently with an unacceptably high incidence of iatrogenic perforation.[25-27]

Use of the Savary-Gilliard bougies has solved this problem.[17] In over 1000 dilatations performed in three medical centers for benign stenosis (peptic, postoperative, postactinic, caustic, web, Schatzki, and so on), not one case of perforation was reported. During the same period, the operation-related mortality rate associated with endoscopic intubation using this same system dropped to below 2% in a series of over 200 cases.[28]

The technical improvements involve three main elements:

1. The bougies. Made of polyvinylchloride, they measure 100 cm long and have a central lumen 1.8 mm in diameter, which allows them to slide on a metallic guide wire. They are smooth and noncompressible but flexible in the longitudinal axis. The proximal tip is formed by a straight 8-cm-long segment followed by a dilator cone (Fig. 5-4).

2. The metallic guide wire. The tip is made of a spring with variable coil whose turns are progressively wider apart toward the distal extremity. This system ensures a progressive flexibility that prevents acute angulation at the rigid junction with the metallic guide wire. Even when placed perpendic-

A   B

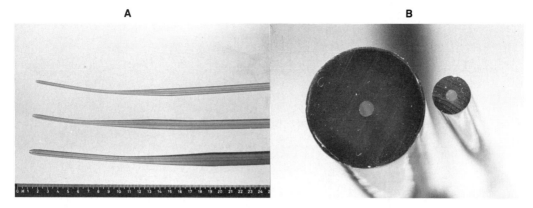

Fig. 5-4. Savary-Gilliard dilatation bougies. **A,** The dilatation cone is extremely profiled. It follows a 4-cm straight segment and stays in a constant 4- or 5-degree angle, depending upon the caliber of the bougie. Because of this construction, dilatation is very gentle and progressive, causing minimal mucosal trauma. **B,** The bougies have a hollow core, 1.8 mm in diameter, allowing them to be advanced on a guide wire.

ular to the mucosal surface, the tip curves around progressively and pulls the rigid segment along with it without risk of perforation (Fig. 5-5).

3. The prosthesis introducer. This system consists of a bougie 10.5 mm in diameter and 100 cm long and a graduated prosthesis introducer made of semirigid polyvinyl chloride, which is slipped over the bougie and introduced into the cuff of the prosthesis, and then fixed securely at its proximal tip by a conical ring (Fig. 5-6).

Only the combined use of the metallic guide wire, Savary-Gilliard bougies, and the Dumon-Gilliard prosthesis introducer can provide maximum safety under all conditions. However, high-quality material is not enough to lower the complication rate; rigorous, systematic technique is necessary.

Esophageal dilatation and adequate medical treatment can be sufficient in cases of peptic stenosis. A few dilatations often suffice to relieve dysphagia symptoms, which recur with successive flare-ups of the illness.

Nd-YAG laser

The introduction of lasers in medicine has given therapeutic endoscopy a new wind. In the esophagus, the most commonly used laser is the Nd-YAG (neodymium : yttrium-aluminum-garnet). Thanks to its wavelength, it has interesting hemostatic qualities, and at high power can be used to vaporize tissue.

In esophagology, the main application is the lumen repermeabilization of inoperable obstructive carcinomas.[29] No author has yet presented a

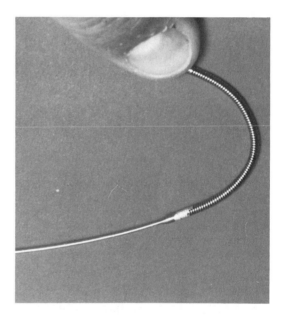

Fig. 5-5. Flexible guide wire. Compared to the metallic guide used in the Eder-Puestow system, the head of this guide wire is formed by a spring with coils that become longer spirals as they approach the distal end. This provides progressive rigidity, which avoids sudden angulation between the nonflexible part of the metallic guide and the head.

randomized study comparing the morbidity, mortality, and swallowing possibilities following treatment by endoscopic intubation, surgical bypass, and Nd-YAG laser repermeabilization. One must admit that the indications for each of these palliative treatments are different. In an inoperable patient, an exophytic tumor is a good indica-

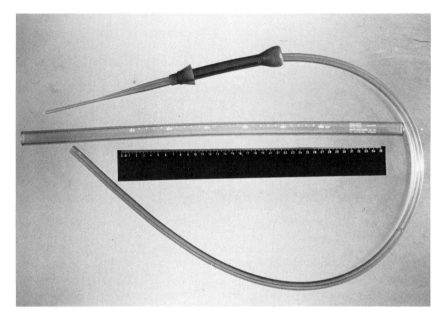

Fig. 5-6. Dumon-Gilliard prosthesis introducer. This system is composed of a Savary bougie measuring 10.5 mm in diameter and 100 cm long. The prosthesis introducer is passed through the cuff of the prosthesis, and attached to the proximal end by means of a conical ring. The bougie/prosthesis/prosthesis introducer system is a single unit, allowing easy introduction.

tion for laser repermeabilization, whereas an esophagobronchial fistula can be treated properly only by endoscopic intubation. In all cases in which bypass surgery can be performed without excessive mortality risk, it must be the preferred treatment, since it offers the best quality of swallowing and survival.

Among benign esophageal pathologic conditions, indications to perform endoscopic Nd-YAG laser therapy are rare and apply nearly always to exceptional cases.

Heterotopic secreting gastric mucosa

After submitting to complete workups (radiocinema, esophageal manometry, esophagoscopy) for pharyngeal paresthesia associated with intermittent dysphagia, several patients were found to have only heterotopic secreting gastric mucosa located just below the esophageal os. Endoscopic treatment by vaporization using the Nd-YAG laser completely relieved symptoms in three cases treated thus far (Plate 10). This little-known cause of pharyngeal paresthesia is a good indication for this type of endoscopic treatment. In the future, the same technique may be applied to noncircular supravestibular columnar metaplasia, lesions we know risk degeneration into adenocarcinoma (Plate 11).

Benign tumors

Unless there is an absolute contraindication to surgery, benign tumors (mostly leiomyomas) should not be treated endoscopically. Traditional exeresis should always be the preferred treatment, since the result is more reliable. Thanks to endoscopic ultrasonography, it is now possible to show the degree of wall involvement (tumors in the submucosa or coming from the muscularis propria). In small submucosal lesions, endoscopic Nd-YAG laser treatment can be done *occasionally,* only if the risk of surgery is inordinately high (Plate 12).

Dysplasia and in situ carcinoma

Dysplasia and in situ carcinoma, which are forerunners of invasive carcinoma, can be treated by laser under the following conditions only:

1. As part of a multiple-site carcinoma of the upper digestive tract (mouth, pharynx, esophagus)
2. As a small, distinct lesion (after toluidine blue or Lugol's staining) and not as a part of a field cancerization (Plate 13).

The justification for this treatment lies in the excessive morbidity or mortality related to thoracotomy or esophageal stripping in debilitated alcoholic smokers.

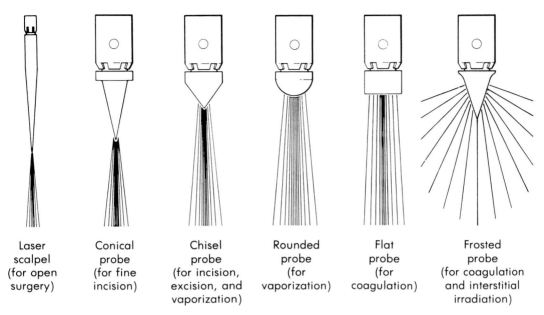

| Laser scalpel (for open surgery) | Conical probe (for fine incision) | Chisel probe (for incision, excision, and vaporization) | Rounded probe (for vaporization) | Flat probe (for coagulation) | Frosted probe (for coagulation and interstitial irradiation) |

Fig. 5-7. Contact laser probes and their energy distribution patterns. Contact laser probes offer a completely new method of delivering Nd-YAG energy to tissue, and overcome many of the limitations encountered with the conventional noncontact medical laser systems. The optical properties and geometric designs of the different contact laser probes shape the laser energy to suit the requirements of various endoscopic techniques. (Courtesy Surgical Laser Technologies, Medicor Nederland B.V.)

The recent development of contact laser probes should allow more precise endoscopic exeresis, with less coagulation necrosis and therefore less risk of hollow-organ perforation (Figs. 5-7 and 5-8). Clinical experimentation tends to show that tissue vaporization allows more precise control of the power densities delivered.[30,31]

Carbon dioxide laser

In regard to the hypopharynx and esophageal os, the possibility of direct inspection under general anesthesia permits use of endoscopy coupled with the surgical microscope (suspended micropharyngoscopy), along with all the therapeutic possibilities offered by the Nd-YAG and carbon dioxide lasers.

Benign lesions

All benign lesions located on the laryngeal margins or on the posterior hypopharyngeal wall are accessible to carbon dioxide laser therapy. Thanks to the qualities of the carbon dioxide laser (minimum coagulation necrosis), these endoscopic maneuvers never require intubation or a nasogastric tube. It is the era of endoscopic microsurgery.

Malignant lesions

The same degree of security can be obtained for "early" carcinomas, as long as the following conditions are fulfilled:

1. Perform exeresis after vital staining (Lugol's or toluidine blue).
2. Expose the lesion completely.
3. Obtain a surgical specimen for histologic analysis of the surgical cuts.
4. Refrain from endoscopic treatment if the "early" carcinoma is too diffuse (field cancerization) (Plate 14).

Palliative repermeabilization of esophageal carcinoma at the hypopharynx or at the level of Killian's sphincter must be done after dilatation so as to avoid accidental perforation. Micropharyngoscopy using the surgical microscope allows good exposure of the esophageal os and safe use of the carbon dioxide laser. The repermeabilization can be done with less risk of perforation than with the Nd-YAG laser, since there is less edema and inflammatory reaction. Moreover, patient comfort is improved (Plate 15). This is also a good indication for use of contact laser probes using the Nd-YAG laser.[30,31]

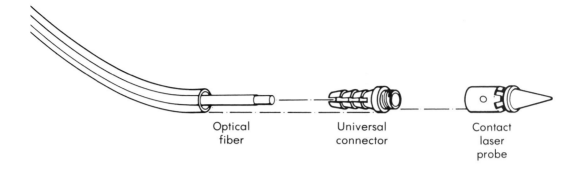

Fig. 5-8. Endoscopic contact laser probe. The contact laser probe (neutral synthetic sapphire crystal) can be affixed to a standard optical fiber and passed through any rigid or flexible endoscope for use in an ever-increasing range of endoscopic applications. (Courtesy Surgical Laser Technologies, Medicor Nederland B.V.)

Photodetection and photodynamic therapy

Though still experimental, photodetection and phototherapy of early carcinomas after injection of a photosensitizing agent seem to hold promise for the future.[32-34]

The principal is based on exploiting the preferential accumulation properties of cancerous tissue for hematoporphyrin (HPD), which renders the cells photosensitive:

1. When accumulated in a malignant tumor, HPD emits red fluorescent light when exposed to ultraviolet (405-nm) rays. This property is used to locate "early" cancers, which are invisible by conventional methods.
2. When exposed to another wavelength (630-nm for HPD), the HPD induces a photochemical reaction that theoretically destroys carcinoma cells selectively (high concentration of HPD in tumor cells compared to normal cells). This phototoxicity is caused by the production of the free radical O^-, which is highly toxic to cells (Plate 16).

Experimentally the process is much more complex, since it involves several parameters in cell necrosis. It seems that the interruption of the microcirculation by destruction of capillary endothelium plays a major role in determining the tumor necrosis.[35]

In any case, this "treatment of the future" can only be used for "early" carcinomas (in situ, microinvasive, or submucosal), since a transmural destruction of a tumor could cause organ perforation.

For the esophagus, the advantages of photodetection and phototherapy for "early" cancers are obvious:

1. Detection of "early" carcinomas, especially the occult or erythroplastic type, which is very difficult using conventional methods.
2. The morbidity and mortality of esophagectomy remain high in spite of surgical and anesthesiologic advances (poor general condition of alcoholic and cigarette-smoking patients, who constitute the main candidates for esophageal cancer in Western countries).

However, these techniques are far from being applicable in everyday clinical endoscopy. The numerous problems involved in the chemistry of the photosensitive agents (complex mixture of HPD, for example) and in the comprehension of tumoral necrosis, and the technical problems involved in irradiation of a hollow organ, are not yet solved.

The future techniques will probably be based on the discovery of more stable molecules for sensitization and on the development of optimal irradiation systems for different geometric configurations.

CONCLUSIONS

In esophageal endoscopy, recent diagnostic and therapeutic progress has come from the following developments:

1. Use of diversified rigid and flexible endoscopes, with a "comeback" of rigid endoscopes (Hopkins-type telescope optical systems) for complex pathologies (workup for stenosis with endobrachyesophagus) and for pretherapy investigations of some early-stage pathologies ("early" carcinomas, reflux esophagitis lesions, lesions of the hypopharyngeal and gastroesophageal junction, and so on)
2. Endoscopic ultrasonography, by far more helpful in staging esophageal lesions (benign tumors, varices, and carcinomas) than is the CT scan
3. Videoendoscopy (Welch Allyn type), which represents a new approach to the study of lesion morphology, follow-up of patients, and documentation and teaching of endoscopic semiology
4. Endoscopic dilatation, with development of safer, efficient equipment, which greatly contributed to lowering the morbidity and mortality rates involved in dilatation
5. Carbon dioxide, Nd-YAG, and dye lasers, which are extremely useful when used judiciously in the diagnosis and treatment of "early" carcinomas (especially in situ and intramucosal carcinomas) as well as in the treatment of certain benign pathologic conditions

At the present time, the diagnostic and therapeutic possibilities for endoscopy are so impressive that they may tempt the endoscopist to go beyond the strict indications that we know should be respected. When the choice of several therapeutic modalities is open to discussion (endoscopic laser therapy, endoscopic dilatations, or other treatment), a multidisciplinary team approach must be used. The final decision must be, whenever possible, the consensus of several specialists (surgeon, gastroenterologist or ear, nose, and throat endoscopist, radiotherapist, oncologist, and so on) and must be adapted to the special aspects of the individual patient (type and location of lesion, age, general health condition, patient's desire for treatment, concomitant illness, and so on). The problem is multifactorial, and so must be its assessment; otherwise we may see a seemingly paradoxical drop in the cure rate and quality of patient survival in spite of technologic progress.

REFERENCES

1. Savary, M., and Miller, G.: The esophagus. In Gassman, S.A., editor: Handbook and atlas of Endoscopy, Solothurn, Switzerland, 1978.
2. Monnier, P., and Savary, M.: Contribution of endoscopy to gastro-oesophageal reflux disease, Scand. J. Gastroenterol. 19(106):26-44, 1984.
3. Ismail-Beigi, F., and Pope, C.E.: Histological consequences of gastro-oesophageal reflux in man, Gastroenterology 58:163-174, 1970.
4. Kobayashi, S., and Kasugai, T.: Endoscopic and biopsy criteria for the diagnosis of oesophagitis with the fiberoptic oesophagoscope, Am. J. Dig. Dis. 19:345-352, 1974.
5. Seefeld, U., Krejs, G.J., Siebenmann, R.E., and Blum, A.L.: Esophageal histology in gastroesophageal reflux, Am. J. Dig. Dis. 22:956-964, 1977.
6. Froelicher, P., and Miller, G.: Esophageal cancer limited to the mucosa and submucosa in Europe. In DeMeester, T.R., and Skinner, D.B., editors: Esophageal disorders: pathophysiology and therapy, New York, 1985, Raven Press, pp. 355-357.
7. Monnier, P., Savary, M., and Anani, P.: Endoscopic morphology of "early" esophageal carcinoma. In DeMeester, T.R., and Skinner, D.B., editors: Esophageal disorders: pathophysiology and therapy, New York, 1985, Raven Press, pp. 333-345.
8. Papazian, A., Descombes, P., Capran, J.P., and Lorriaux, A.: Fréquence du cancer de l'oesophage synchrone des cancers des voies aéro-digestives supérieures (100 cas): Intérêt des colorations vitales au Lugol et au bleu de toluidine, Gastroenterol. Clin. Biol. 9:16-22, 1985.
9. Mandard, A.M., Tourneux, J., Gignaux, M., Blanc, L., Segol, P., and Mandard, J.C.: In situ carcinoma of the esophagus: macroscopic study with particular reference to the Lugol test, Endoscopy 12:51-57, 1980.
10. Voegeli, R.: Die Schillersche Iodprobe im Rahmen der Oesophagusdiagnostik, Pract. Oto-rhino-laryngol. 28:230-239, 1966.
11. Toriie, S., Kohli, Y., Akasaka, Y., and Kawai, K.: New trial for endoscopical observation of esophagus by dye scattering method, Endoscopy 7:75-79, 1975.
12. Monnier, P., Savary, M., Pasche, R., and Anani, P.: Intraepithelial carcinoma of the oesophagus: endoscopic morphology, Endoscopy 13:185-191, 1981.
13. Mashberg, A.: Final evaluation of tolonium chloride rinse for screening of high-risk patients with asymptomatic squamous carcinoma, J. Am. Dent. Assoc. 106:319-323, 1983.
14. Monnier, P., Savary, M., and Pasche, R.: Contribution of toluidine blue to bucco-pharyngo-oesophageal cancerology, Acta Endoscopica 11(4-5):299-315, 1981.
15. Pasche, R., Savary, M., and Monnier, P.: Multifocalité du carcinome épidermoïde sur les voies digestive supérieure et respiratoire distale: technicité du diagnostic endoscopique, Acta Endoscopica 11:277-291, 1981.
16. Savary, M., Crausaz, P.H., and Monnier, P.: La place de l'endoscopie totale aéro-digestive supérieure en cancérologie, Schweiz. Med. Wochenschr. 109:838-840, 1979.

17. Monnier, P., Hsieh, V., and Savary, M.: Endoscopic treatment of esophageal stenosis using Savary-Gilliard bougies: technical innovations, Acta Endoscopica **15**(2): 119-129, 1985.

18. Tio, T.L., Den Hartog Jager, F.C.A., and Tytgat, G.N.J.: The role of endoscopic ultrasonography in assessing local resectability of oesophagogastric malignancies, Scand. J. Gastroenterol. **21**(123):78-86, 1986.

19. Strohm, W.D., and Classen, M.: Benign lesions of the upper GI tract by means of endoscopic ultrasonography, Scand. J. Gastroenterol. **21**(suppl. 123):41-46, 1986.

20. Yasuda, K., Nakajima, M., and Kawai, K.: Endoscopic ultrasonography in the diagnosis of submucosal tumor of the upper digestive tract, Scand. J. Gastroenterol. **21**(suppl. 123):59-67, 1986.

21. Tio, T.L., and Tytgat, G.N.J.: Atlas of transintestinal ultrasonography, ed. Smith Kline & French, Drukkerij Mur-Kostverloren B.V., Aalsmeer, The Netherlands, 1986.

22. Tio, T.L., and Tytgat, G.N.J.: Endoscopic ultrasonography in the assessment of intra- and transmural infiltration of tumours in the oesophagus, stomach and papilla of Vater and in the detection of extra-oesophageal lesions, Endoscopy **16**:203-210, 1984.

23. Caletti, G.C., Bolondi, L., Zani, L., Brocchi, E., Guizzardi, G., and Labo, G.: Detection of portal hypertension and esophageal varices by means of endoscopic ultrasonography, Scand. J. Gastroenterol. **21**(suppl. 123):74-77, 1986.

24. Classen, M., and Phillip, J.: Electronic endoscopy of the gastrointestinal tract: initial experience with a new type of endoscope that has no fiberoptic bundle for imaging, Endoscopy **16**(1):16-19, 1984.

25. Luna, L.L.: Endoscopic treatment of esophageal strictures, Endoscopy **15**(1):203-206, 1983.

26. Earlam, R., and Cunha-Melo, J.R.: Benign esophageal strictures: historical and technical aspects of dilatation, Br. J. Surg. **68**(12):829-836, 1981.

27. Tulman, A.B., and Boyce, H.W.: Complications of esophageal dilatation and guidelines for their prevention, Gastrointest. Endosc. **27**(4):229-234, 1981.

28. Dumon, J.F., Castro, R., Merrick, B., Hancy, A., and Dupin, B.: Experience of 1100 esophageal dilatations: In Book of abstracts, 4e Symposium international d'endoscopie digestive, Paris, May 1984.

29. Fleischer, D., and Sivak, M.U., Jr.: Endoscopic Nd-YAG laser therapy as palliation for esophagogastric cancer: parameters affecting initial outcome, Gastroenterology **89**(4):827-831, 1985.

30. Joffe, S.N.: Contact neodymium-YAG laser surgery in gastroenterology: a preliminary report, Lasers Surg. Med. **6**(2):155-157, 1986.

31. Ohyama, M.: Treatment of head and neck tumors by contact Nd-YAG laser surgery, Auris Nasus Larynx **12**(2):138-142, 1985.

32. Dougherty, T.J.: Photodynamic therapy (PDT) of malignant tumors, CRC Crit. Rev. Oncol. Hematol. **2**:83-116, 1984.

33. Kessel, D.: Hematoporphyrin and HPD: photophysics, photochemistry and phototherapy, Photochem. Photobiol. **39**:851-859, 1984.

34. Hayata, Y., Kato, H. Okitsu, H., Kawaguchi, M., and Konaka, C.: Photodynamic therapy with hematoporphyrin derivative in cancer of the upper gastro-intestinal tract, Semin. Surg. Oncol. **1**:1-11, 1985.

35. Star, W.M., Marijnissen, J.P.A., Van Berg–Blok, A.E., Versteeg, A.A.C., and Reinhold, H.S.: In vivo observation of the effects of HPD-photosensitization on the microcirculation of rat mammary tumor and normal tissues growing in transparent chambers. In Jori, G., and Perria, C., editors: Photodynamic therapy of tumors and other diseases, Libreria Progetto Padova, pp. 239-242, 1985.

PLATE 1. Difficulties encountered in endoscopic diagnosis of some esophageal pathologies.

A. **Stage I reflux esophagitis.** The erosive erythroplastic form closely resembles the erythroplastic-type "early" squamous cell carcinoma in **B.**

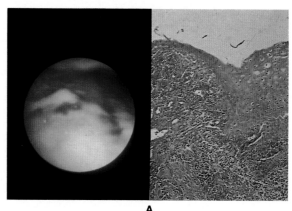

A

B. **In situ carcinoma.** Selective biopsy is necessary to distinguish this lesion from stage I reflux esophagitis.

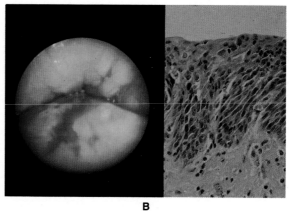

B

C. *Left,* endobrachyesophagus; *right,* diffuse erythroplastic-type microinvasive squamous cell carcinoma. Vital staining and selective biopsy alone can distinguish the two conditions.

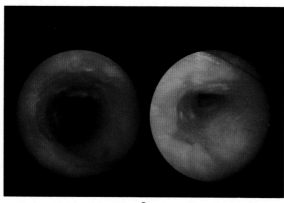

C

PLATE 2. Examples illustrating the need for multiple supravestibular biopsies.

A. Combination of linear erosive lesions and islands of columnar epithelium. Only a high-quality optical instrument allows endoscopic differential diagnosis between these two lesions. The slightly foveolar aspect of the columnar epithelium can be recognized at high resolution.

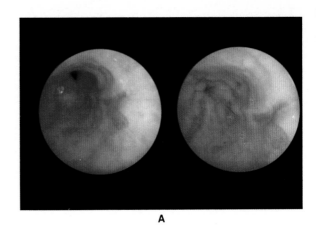

A

B. Thanks to its stability and to the angulation of the biopsy forceps, rigid esophagoscopies allow selective biopsy of the supravestibular linear erosion and of the island of columnar epithelium and finally a reference biopsy of normal squamous epithelium, thus confirming the asymmetric topography of reflux esophagitis lesions. These biopsies require stability of the regions to be biopsied (general anesthesia), instrument stability (rigid esophagoscope), and meticulous hemostasis (epinephrine applied locally). These criteria are not fulfilled with a fibroscope.

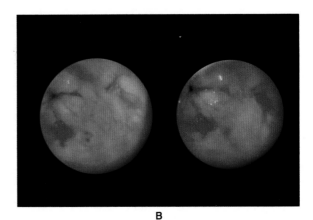

B

PLATE 3. Histologic study of stage I reflux esophagitis.

A. Fibrin-covered supravestibular linear erosion.

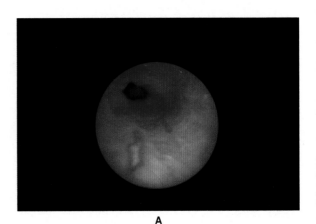

A

B. Histologic view: abrasion of the squámous epithelium and neutrophilic inflammatory infiltration of the lamina propria.

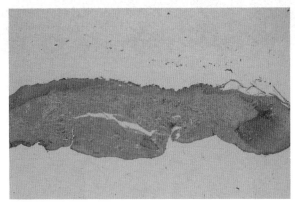

B

C. Reference biopsy specimen taken in endoscopically normal region shows no histologic sign of inflammation.

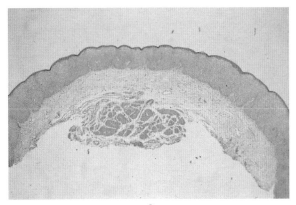

C

PLATE 4. Biopsy mapping for histologic study of stage I reflux esophagitis.

In all cases of supravestibular lesions suspected of being stage I or II reflux esophagitis, the first biopsy was taken on the erythroplastic zone (covered with fibrin or not). Two reference biopsy specimens were taken from endoscopically normal mucosa at the same level as the first biopsy and 5 cm proximally. These biopsies were always free of inflammatory infiltration, which shows again the asymmetric topography of supravestibular reflux esophagitis lesions.

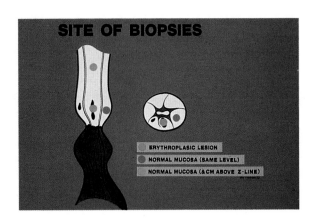

SITE OF BIOPSIES

ERYTHROPLASIC LESION
NORMAL MUCOSA (SAME LEVEL)
NORMAL MUCOSA (&CM ABOVE Z-LINE)

PLATE 5. In situ carcinoma (multicentric erythroplastic type) of the posterior esophageal wall.

A. Photo taken using rigid esophagoscope: the erythroplastic reticulate pattern is well visible and distinct. The whitish yellow spot is exudate 5 days after a biopsy.

B. Same lesion photographed with a fibroscope: only the spot (postbiopsy exudate) is visible; the erythroplastic region does not show up at all. The difference in optical resolution of endoscopes probably explains why the diagnostic efficiency of routine esophagogastroduodenoscopies is so low for "early" carcinoma of the esophagus.

C. Same lesion after vital staining with toluidine blue: multicentric aspect becomes obvious.

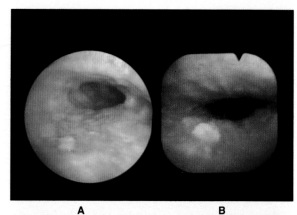
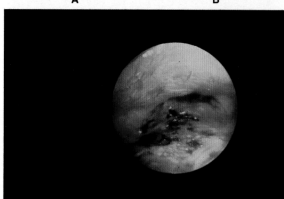

A   B

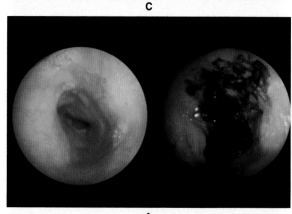

C

PLATE 6. Comparison of toluidine blue vital staining using rigid esophagoscope or gastrofibroscope.

A. Erythroplastic-type microinvasive carcinoma of the esophagus, clearly shown after vital staining with toluidine blue.

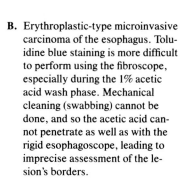

A

B. Erythroplastic-type microinvasive carcinoma of the esophagus. Toluidine blue staining is more difficult to perform using the fibroscope, especially during the 1% acetic acid wash phase. Mechanical cleaning (swabbing) cannot be done, and so the acetic acid cannot penetrate as well as with the rigid esophagoscope, leading to imprecise assessment of the lesion's borders.

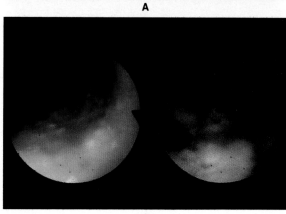

B

PLATE 7. Microinvasive carcinoma of the right piriform sinus (laparoscopic examination using suspended microscope blade).

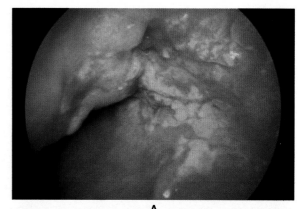

A

A. Thanks to the laparoscope and the suspended blade of the microlaryngoscope, a panoramic visualization of the piriform sinus can be obtained. Here is a leukoerythroplastic multicentric lesion. It is a horseshoe-shaped lesion involving the medial and lateral borders of the right piriform sinus.

B. Same lesion after toluidine blue staining: leopard-skin aspect characteristic of multicentric lesions is apparent.

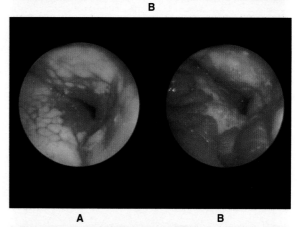

B

PLATE 8. Endobrachyesophagus before and after staining with Lugol's solution.

A. The squamous cell–columnar junction is clear even without vital staining.
B. Lugol's solution colors the glycogen-rich squamous cells brown; the glycogen-free columnar epithelium does not stain at all. In more difficult cases, staining with Lugol's solution can be useful in showing the upper limits of columnar metaplasia or spots of "early" squamous cell carcinoma.

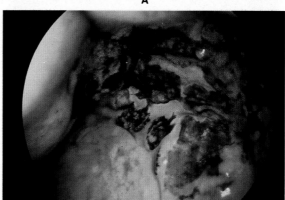

A   B

PLATE 9. Stenosis in an endobrachyesophagus.

Not only must the suprastenotic columnar cell epithelium be biopsied, but the infrastenotic region must be biopsied as well. The stenosis in the middle of an endobrachyesophagus is due to a residual strip of squamous cell epithelium. After dilatation, serial biopsy specimens of the type II endobrachyesophagus are taken systematically.

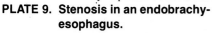
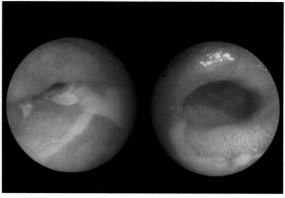

PLATE 10. Proximal heterotopic gastric mucosa, located directly below the esophageal os.

A. Round 3- to 4-mm-diameter disk located at the 3-o'clock position.

B. Status after Nd-YAG laser superficial vaporization. Disappearance of symptoms (over 1-year follow-up).

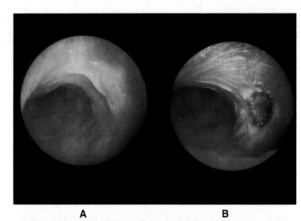

A   B

PLATE 11. Asymmetric columnar metaplasia of the supravestibular region.

On the strip of columnar metaplasia, slightly exophytic mucosa can be seen. Selective biopsy confirmed diagnosis of simple columnar hyperplasia. In other cases, we have seen adenocarcinomas develop on these noncircular areas of columnar metaplasia. It would appear advisable to vaporize these strips of metaplasia using an Nd-YAG laser so as to avoid degeneration into adenocarcinoma.

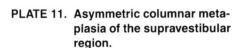

PLATE 12. Granular cell myoblastoma of the right anterolateral wall of the middle third of the esophagus.

A. Small whitish yellow submucosal elevated lesion measuring 3 to 4 mm at its largest diameter. Patient inoperable because of cardiopulmonary risk.

B. Status after Nd-YAG laser vaporization. No relapse as of last follow-up (3 years after treatment).

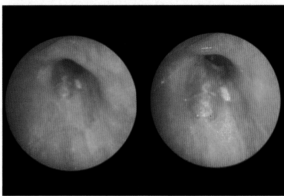

A   B

PLATE 13. Solitary and multicentric forms of "early" carcinoma of the esophagus.

A. Microinvasive carcinoma seen as a solitary spot 3 mm in diameter. Clear limits apparent after toluidine blue vital staining. With the rigid esophagoscope, biopsy–subtotal exeresis is performed and complementary Nd-YAG laser vaporization is done. This type of early carcinoma can be treated by endoscopy alone as long as the conditions are optimal and the follow-up strict.

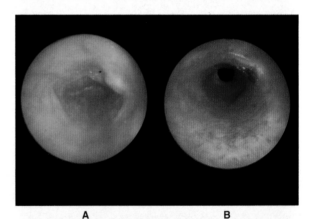

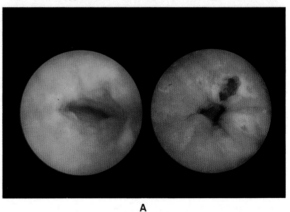

A

B. Example of a carcinoma less advanced histologically than that shown in **A.** It is an occult multicentric-type in situ carcinoma, seen only after vital staining with toluidine blue. The surgical specimen confirmed the noninvasive character of the lesion. The wide spread (5.3 cm) of the lesion precludes Nd-YAG laser treatment. In the future, this type of lesion could be treated by phototherapy after preliminary injection of a photosensitivization solution.

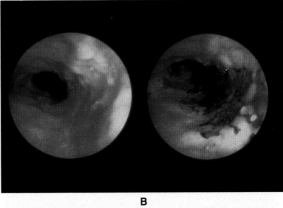

B

PLATE 14. Microinvasive carcinoma of the pharynx treated by endoscopic methods.

A. Perfect visualization of the tumor after vital staining with toluidine blue makes endoscopic exeresis with the carbon dioxide laser possible.

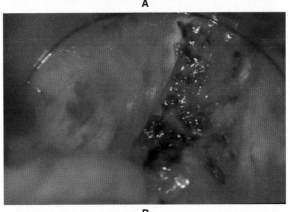

A

B. Status after treatment with the carbon dioxide laser. The raw surface is left to reepithelialize.

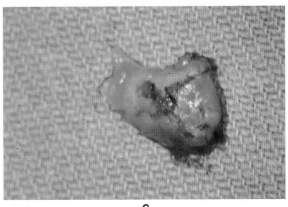

B

C. The specimen can be examined histologically and its borders inspected to confirm complete exeresis.

C

PLATE 15. Carcinoma of the cervical esophagus infiltrating the submucosa of the esophageal os.

A. Visualization of tumor obtained using micropharyngoscope (photo with laparoscope). After catheterization of the stenosis, the endoscopic repermeabilization can be done using the carbon dioxide laser and the surgical microscope.

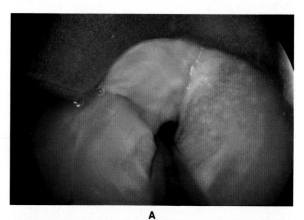

A

B. Status after repermeabilization with the carbon dioxide laser. Coagulation necrosis is less than with the Nd-YAG laser, and this diminishes postoperative edema and inflammatory reaction that lead to dysphagia. This is particularly true in the hypopharyngeal region.

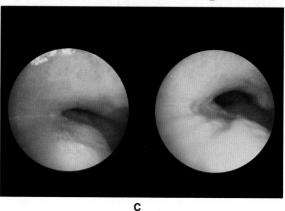

B

PLATE 16. Photodynamic therapy of a microinvasive carcinoma of the esophagus (ENT cancer patient with multiple synchronous primary tumors).

A. Endoscopic view before treatment: the "early carcinoma," located on the left lateral wall of the esophagus, is of the depressed erythroplastic type.

B. Endoscopic view 10 days after treatment: localized necrosis at the site of the lesion.

C. Endoscopic view 6 months after treatment: endoscopically, total disappearance of the lesion. The control biopsy showed a dense scarring of the lamina propria and a normal squamous epithelium. Follow-up: 1 year without evidence of recurrence.

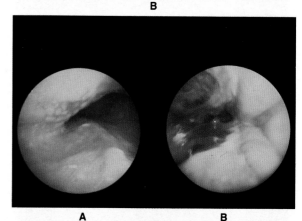

A   B

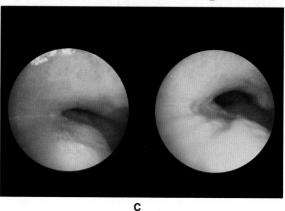

C

CHAPTER 6 Esophageal scintigraphy and tests of duodenogastric function

Mark K. Ferguson and James W. Ryan

The current tests of esophageal function include barium contrast esophagram with or without cinefluoroscopy, manometry, the acid clearance test,[1] and the standard acid reflux test.[2] This broad range of testing provides useful information about the anatomy and function of the esophagus. However, frequently more than one test is required to evaluate esophageal function for clinical decisions, and each individual test has its own inherent limitations. Both the imaging and the nonimaging techniques alter the normal physiology of the esophagus, and the contrast agents employed do not satisfactorily equate with either the liquid or the solid phase of foods normally ingested. These tests are poorly reproducible because they are performed for short periods that are isolated in time, and they may not measure the usual activity of the esophagus. In addition, the nonimaging techniques are invasive, requiring the presence within the esophagus of a catheter recording system that can cause significant discomfort to the patient during testing and alter the normal response of the esophagus to acid or foods. Finally, the imaging techniques are at best semiquantitative, and their accurate interpretation relies heavily on the experience of the radiologist performing the test.

PRINCIPLES OF ESOPHAGEAL SCINTIGRAPHY

Radionuclide techniques for measuring esophageal transit were introduced by Kazem in 1972 and have subsequently undergone modifications to improve accuracy and versatility.[3-7] There are several advantages to esophageal scintigraphy. It reflects the physiology of swallowing and esophageal clearance much more closely than do the other tests currently used. A variety of liquids and solids can be labeled for measurement by scintigraphy. The results can be quantified with the use of a dedicated computer or microprocessor and do not rely extensively on the experience of the operator performing the test, as is the case with barium swallows. Invasive recording systems are not required, providing a more accurate measure of the response of the upper gastrointestinal system to swallowing and making the procedure much more acceptable to patients. Multiple isotope swallows can be performed over an extended period of time, to increase the reliability of the data. Finally, because the isotopes are given in very small or "tracer" quantities, the radiation exposure is significantly less than that involved in a standard gastrointestinal radiographic examination.

The techniques used for esophageal scintigraphy are straightforward. Patients are examined in the upright or supine position in front of a large-field-of-view gamma scintillation camera with a parallel hole collimator. Anterior views have been frequently used, but we prefer the posterior view since the attenuation of the photons from the esophageal activity is relatively uniform in this view, making the data more reliable for quantitation. After an overnight fast, 5 to 15 ml of water at room temperature containing 150 to 300 μCi of technetium 99m sulfur colloid is instilled into the patient's mouth with a syringe, and a swallow is performed on command. Dry swallows are performed subsequently at 15- to 30-second intervals, and data are acquired for 1 to 20 minutes on a computer or microprocessor. Either serial (list) mode or rapid frame rate (0.15 to 0.40 seconds) is used with swallows that transit rapidly through the esophagus, but longer intervals (up to 15 seconds) may be used in patients with markedly delayed bolus transit, such as those with achalasia.

After completion of the acquisition phase of the study, the data are replayed by the computer

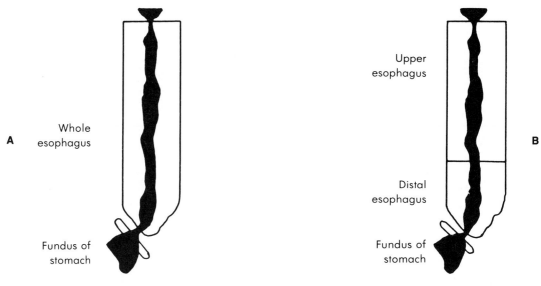

Fig. 6-1. ROIs used to generate time-activity curves of radioactive water bolus transit. **A,** On the summed image of the water swallow the whole esophagus extends from the upper esophageal sphincter to the lower esophageal sphincter. The small ROI over the proximal stomach is used for timing purposes only. **B,** The whole esophageal ROI is subdivided into two smaller regions— proximal two thirds and distal one third. (From Ryan, J.W., O'Sullivan, G.C., Brunsden, B.S., VanDaalen, J., and DeMeester, T.R.: Digital scintigraphy in achalasia. In DeMeester, T.R., and Skinner, D.B., editors: Esophageal disorders: pathophysiology and therapy, New York, 1985, Raven Press.)

in cine format for viewing and for quantitation. A summed image of the swallow is formed so that regions of interest (ROIs) can be drawn (Fig. 6-1). The site of the lower esophageal sphincter is easily identified on this image in most patients, so that the esophagus is readily separated from the stomach, and ROIs representing the whole esophagus, the upper two thirds and the lower one third of the esophagus, and the proximal stomach are constructed. The esophagus can be subdivided further, but the main distinction in the esophageal transit is between the lower region, corresponding to the esophagus posterior to the heart, and the remaining proximal esophagus. Time-activity curves are generated for each region, and the curves are smoothed once (Fig. 6-2). The percent of activity cleared in one swallow and the time for maximum clearance are determined. Clearance is defined as follows:

$$C_t = \frac{E_{max} - E_t}{E_{max}} \times 100$$

where C_t represents percent of esophageal clearance at time t; E_{max} is the maximum count rate in the esophagus; and E_t is the esophageal count rate at time t. The transit time is taken as the interval from the initial entry of the bolus into the esophagus until the maximal clearance from the esophagus in one swallow.[6] In normal subjects who swallow in the upright position, esophageal

transit of a water bolus is rapid, being completed in less than 10 seconds; in the supine position there is a slower bolus transit, but it is still complete within 15 seconds after the swallow (Table 6-1). In subjects with delayed clearance the transit time measurements usually indicate the time to achieve 90% or greater clearance of activity from the esophagus, and multiple dry swallows may be performed during this interval. Substances other than water, including pudding, egg salad, gelatin cubes, and marshmallows, can also be radiolabeled for scintigraphic studies of esophageal motor function.

MOTILITY DISORDERS

Scintigraphic measurements are useful in quantitating abnormalities in esophageal function in patients with scleroderma or achalasia. In one study with patients supine, esophageal clearance of a water bolus was only 5% to 40% following multiple swallows, compared with clearance of greater than 90% after one swallow in normal subjects.[5] Although some believe there is an adynamic pattern in both achalasia and scleroderma, we have found that esophageal scintigraphy using rapid frame rates does not always demonstrate an adynamic pattern in achalasia, since occasional patients have significant clear-

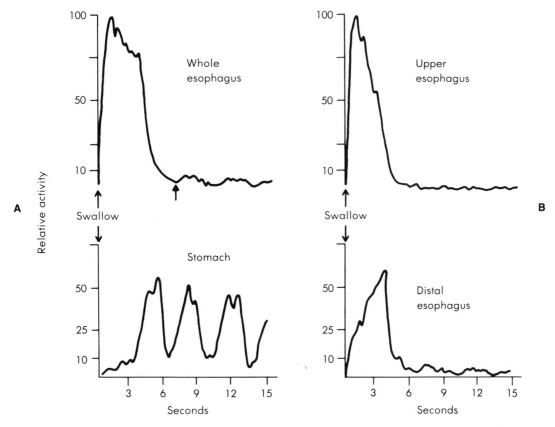

Fig. 6-2. Time-activity curves of a swallow in a normal subject sitting upright. **A,** The bolus rapidly enters the esophagus, and a small portion is cleared by 1 second; 90% clearance occurs before 6 seconds; and clearance is complete between 6 and 9 seconds. Arrow in the whole esophageal ROI indicates the time used to calculate maximum clearance of activity from the whole esophagus. The small amount of detectable activity after this time is attributable to a scatter effect from tracer in the fundus of the stomach. Activity levels in the stomach ROI fluctuate because of gastric peristalsis. **B,** The bolus rapidly enters the upper esophagus and transits quickly to the lower esophagus, where there is a delay before a rapid clearance event into the stomach. The lower esophageal curve is a reflection of the combined entrance and exit events of the liquid bolus in the distal esophagus. (From Ryan, J.W., O'Sullivan, G.C., Brunsden, B.S., VanDaalen, J., and DeMeester, T.R.: Digital scintigraphy in achalasia. In DeMeester, T.R., and Skinner, D.B., editors: Esophageal disorders: pathophysiology and therapy, New York, 1985, Raven Press.)

ance from the esophagus after a single upright swallow, and other patients demonstrate spontaneous intraesophageal "shuttling," or displacement of activity from one esophageal region to another without significant clearance from the esophagus.[6] (See Fig. 6-3.)

Esophageal scintigraphy is also of value in the diagnosis of other dynamic motility disorders, including diffuse esophageal spasm and a large variety of nonspecific motor disorders of the esophagus. Both can have delayed clearance and abnormal intraesophageal movements of tracer, although occasional swallows are normal.[7,8] Similar findings are also present in patients with esophageal peristaltic waves of increased amplitude, or "nutcracker" esophagus.[9] Possibly the greatest value of esophageal scintigraphy is its

TABLE 6-1. Water swallows in normal subjects

	Position	
Parameter	**Upright** (n = 10)	**Supine** (n = 10)
Sex (M/F)	4/6	5/5
Age (years) (x ± SD)	31 ± 12	33 ± 13
Transit time (sec) (x ± SD)	6.6 ± 1.1	10.3 ± 1.7
Clearance (%) (x ± SD)	93.7 ± 2.0	92.0 ± 4.0

From Ryan, J.W., O'Sullivan, G.C., Brunsden, B.S., VanDaalen, J., and DeMeester, T.R.: Digital scintigraphy in achalasia. In DeMeester, T.R., and Skinner, D.B., editors: Esophageal disorders: pathophysiology and therapy, New York, 1985, Raven Press.

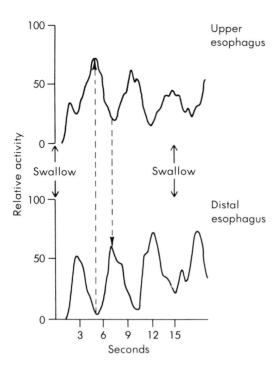

Fig. 6-3. Spontaneous shuttling in achalasia. Time-activity curves from the proximal and distal esophagus were generated at a frame rate of 0.15 seconds. Water swallowed by the patient sitting upright rapidly reaches the distal esophagus, but no clearance into the stomach occurs. Shuttling begins with the spontaneous retrograde movement of water from the distal to the proximal esophagus *(left arrow)* and continues with return of the bolus to the distal esophagus *(right arrow)*. Periodicity is approximately 4.9 seconds. (From Ryan, J.W., O'Sullivan, G.C., Brunsden, B.S., VanDaalen, J., and DeMeester, T.R.: Digital scintigraphy in achalasia. In DeMeester, T.R., and Skinner, D.B., editors: Esophageal disorders: pathophysiology and therapy, New York, 1985, Raven Press.)

potential to quantitate esophageal clearance. This is the best way to assess the effectiveness of therapy for esophageal motility disorders such as achalasia after dilatation or myotomy[10-12] or diffuse esophageal spasm following therapy with nitrates or calcium antagonists.[13]

Disorders of esophageal transit and emptying are also found in patients with dysphagia who have normal findings on manometry and upper gastrointestinal (UGI) radiography; and when dysphagia is a prominent symptom, one half to two thirds of these patients have abnormalities on esophageal scintigraphy.[14,15] These abnormalities occur whether the scintigraphic examination is performed with a liquid or a solid bolus and are manifested as delayed transit with retention of tracer proximally at times. Thus, esophageal scintigraphy is more sensitive than radiography or manometry for the detection of nonspecific motor disorders.

GASTROESOPHAGEAL ACID REFLUX

Esophageal scintigraphy is frequently abnormal in the presence of esophagitis or gastroesophageal reflux (GER) as determined by using 24-hour pH monitoring. Experimentally, esophagitis chemically induced with acid instillation results in doubling of esophageal transit time.[16] In patients with abnormal results of extended esophageal pH monitoring but with normal UGI radiographic results and no primary esophageal motor abnormality on manometry, abnormalities of esophageal emptying are discovered on esophageal scintigraphy in over 80%.[17] The results of esophageal scintigraphy in patients with acid reflux with or without esophagitis are not entirely uniform, however, and less striking correlations have been obtained by other investigators.[18]

Until the development of prolonged esophageal monitoring, there was no way to quantitate GER. Although esophageal pH monitoring is of benefit in the diagnosis and management of patients with suspected reflux, the test is somewhat cumbersome, time consuming, and invasive.[19] For these reasons, alternatives are sought that are more accessible to physicians and patients and that also provide quantitative estimates of GER. Gastroesophageal scintigraphy is the only other current technique that satisfies these requirements. In one technique the patient ingests 300 μCi, of technetium 99m sulfur colloid in 300 ml of acidified orange juice and after 10 to 15 minutes is positioned supine under a gamma camera for acquisition of anterior views.[20] A special abdominal binder is placed around the upper abdomen in beltlike fashion. With the use of a sphygmomanometer, the pressure on the binder is increased sequentially in 20 mm Hg increments from 0 to 100 mm Hg, with 30-second images, being acquired at each level. A pressure increment of 20 mm Hg on the abdominal binder corresponds to approximately a 5 mm Hg increase in pressure gradient across the lower esophageal sphincter. Gastroesophageal reflux is calculated by using the formula

$$R = \frac{E_t - E_b}{G_0} \times 100$$

where R equals percent gastroesophageal reflux; E_t equals esophageal counts at time t; E_b equals esophageal background counts; and G_0 equals gastric counts at the beginning of the study. If 4% or more of reflux activity is considered abnormal, the reflux scintiscan is positive in up to 90% of symptomatic patients, a considerably higher positive rate than is found in other diagnostic tests, including gastroesophageal fluoroscopy, manometry, endoscopy, and endoscopic biopsy.[20,21] Unfortunately, this means of assessing GER quantitatively has not been compared directly with results of extended pH monitoring, our most reliable method for the diagnosis of pathologic reflux. We believe that with modification and refinement, gastroesophageal scintigraphy will one day serve as an excellent screening examination for patients with symptoms of gastroesophageal reflux, particularly those patients whose symptoms are not classic and may represent motility problems.[17]

In the pediatric group the diagnosis and treatment of gastroesophageal reflux presents a special problem. Since reflux is very common in infants and children, the differentiation between benign and pathologic reflux is difficult except when symptoms are present, and pathologic GER can be much more life threatening than in the adult. Because of the invasive nature of some of the standard tests for GER and the difficulty of performing them in pediatric patients, other, less quantitative, measurements are frequently used to diagnose reflux. When extended esophageal pH monitoring is used, however, the results correlate well with severity of symptoms.[22] Gastroesophageal scintigraphy is available as a screening test for gastroesophageal reflux in children and has a sensitivity of 75% when compared with the standard acid reflux test.[23] When gastroesophageal scintigraphy is compared with extended esophageal pH monitoring in infants and children with suspected GER, the accuracy of scintigraphy is 79% with a specificity of 93%, considerably higher than the specificity of 21% that is offered by upper gastrointestinal radiography.[24] Abdominal binders are not used in reflux studies in children, as a safety precaution, but hand pressure on the abdomen has been suggested by some.

GASTRIC EMPTYING

Motility disorders that accompany gastroesophageal reflux are not confined only to the esophagus but are also associated with delayed gastric emptying in patients with pathologic GER. We frequently obtain scintigraphic gastric emptying studies in patients with reflux to delineate the possible contribution of abnormal gastric motility or gastric outlet obstruction to this problem. Gastric emptying studies can be performed with the use of tracers that reflect either the solid or the liquid phases of a meal. A simple liquid phase study uses oatmeal intermixed with technetium 99m sulfur colloid as the test meal. Gamma camera images of the abdomen are acquired on a computer or microprocessor serially at intervals of every 5 to 15 minutes for 1½ to 2 hours or until the stomach activity has been substantially reduced. After correction for physical decay of the isotope, the percentage of activity remaining in the stomach ROI is calculated for each recorded time interval and plotted semilogarithmically. A line that best fits the percent of regained activity versus time is generated, with the slope of the line expressing the rate of emptying. Normal subjects and patients with reflux but without esophagitis have a normal gastric emptying half-time of about 70 minutes; in patients with reflux and esophagitis, gastric emptying half-time is frequently delayed beyond 100 minutes.[25,26]

Similar findings are present in patients in the pediatric group with symptomatic GER confirmed by prolonged esophageal pH monitoring. In these patients the rate of gastric emptying correlates with the severity of reflux symptoms and complications.[22,27] Because of the significant percentage of reflux patients with delayed gastric emptying, greater than 40% in two studies,[28,29] the use of pharmacologic agents that enhance gastric emptying is popular in the treatment of gastroesophageal reflux, and their effectiveness can be monitored in part with the gastric emptying scan. Scans from a patient with prolonged gastric emptying that responded to metaclopromide are shown in Fig. 6-4.

Dual-isotope gastric scintigraphy, for simultaneous assessment of liquid- and solid-phase gastric emptying, has been reported and can be accomplished with gamma cameras available in most institutions.[30] One advantage of solid-phase studies is that they can detect more subtle abnormalities than the liquid-phase studies, but they also require longer acquisition times. Examples of solid-phase markers include scrambled eggs mixed with technetium 99m sulfur colloid and chicken liver labeled in vivo with the same agent. Indium 111 DTPA is currently used to label the liquid phase and is now approved for routine use by the Food and Drug Administration for this purpose. These studies can also be repeated serially to assess therapeutic interventions.

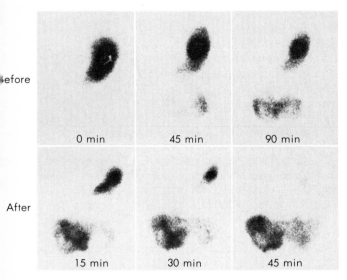

Before

After

0 min   45 min   90 min

15 min   30 min   45 min

Fig. 6-4. Gastric emptying before and after intravenous metoclopramide. This patient had prolonged gastric emptying (half-time of 114 minutes) during the initial 90 minutes of the study. Shortly thereafter, 10 mg of metoclopramide was given intravenously over 5 minutes and the stomach emptied rapidly, with a half-time of 20 minutes.

ALKALINE REFLUX

Substances other than gastric acid, including bile salts, pancreatic enzymes, and alkali, are involved in the pathogenesis of esophagitis both experimentally and clinically. Reflux of duodenal contents into the stomach is associated with esophagitis, particularly in the presence of alkaline reflux gastritis. However, reflux of duodenal contents into the esophagus in patients with an intact stomach and pylorus is not a common clinical problem. In fact, periods of duodenogastric alkaline reflux appear to protect the esophagus from inflammation.[31] The origin of alkaline contents in the esophagus is important to determine, for the source may be either saliva or duodenal contents. Saliva is an important contributor to alterations in esophageal pH and can influence results of invasive studies of acid clearance.[17,32,33] An effective means of determining whether duodenogastric reflux of alkaline material contributes to alkaline GER is extended gastroesophageal pH monitoring. In this method, in addition to standard pH monitoring of the distal esophagus, a pH probe is placed in the stomach 5 cm distal to the lower esophageal sphincter and pH is monitored during an identical 24-hour period. Esophageal alkaline reflux occurs during the periods in which esophageal pH is greater than 7. Gastric alkaline reflux is less well defined, but since the intragastric pH is usually quite low, it is assumed to occur when the pH recorded by the distal probe rises above 4 or 5. This technique enables the detection of misdiagnosed cases of alkaline reflux.[34]

In patients who have had partial or total gastrectomies, the problem of alkaline reflux esophagitis is more apparent clinically. In such patients, alkaline reflux esophagitis is normally accompanied by alkaline gastritis, evident on endoscopic examination. Confirmation of duodenogastric reflux in these patients can be accomplished by means of hepatobiliary scintigraphy (HBS) using technetium 99m iminodiacetic acid (IDA) derivatives such as disofenin with simultaneous imaging of the stomach and gallbladder. After an overnight fast the study is initiated with an intravenous injection of 5 mCi of technetium 99m IDA. Anterior images of the upper abdomen that include the gallbladder and stomach in the field of view are acquired until the gallbladder fills well (usually after 30 minutes). The patient then ingests a 300-ml liquid meal (240 ml Ensure, 30 ml Lipomul, 30 ml water), which will initiate a gallbladder contraction within a few minutes in normal subjects, and imaging is continued for 1 hour or until the gallbladder contracts maximally (Fig. 6-5). The data are fed into an on-line computer or microprocessor. Separate regions of interest can be drawn to encompass the gallbladder and the stomach, respectively. The rate and amount of gallbladder emptying and also a gastric reflux index can be calculated. The duodenogastric reflux index is a measure of the bile reflux from the duodenum into the stomach over a specified time period and is defined as the increase in technetium 99m activity in the stomach ROI divided by the decrease in activity in the gallbladder during this interval.[35] In the initial description of the technique, a second isotope, Indium 111 DTPA (250 μCi), was added to the liquid meal, and dual-isotope scintigraphy was performed. The rate of gastric emptying can also be calculated with this technique. In the original study, the normal subjects had a peak reflux index of 8.2% ± 6.0% at 15 minutes after ingesting the meal, while the asymptomatic patients with Billroth II gastroenterostomies had a peak reflux index of 24.6% ± 4.7% at 30 minutes. In symptomatic postsurgical patients the reflux indices were considerably higher at 30 minutes, with the maximal index of 86.3% ± 7.1%.

An alternate method of quantitating the duodenogastric reflux employs an intravenous injection of synthetic cholecystokinin (Kinevac) to contract the gallbladder at a predetermined

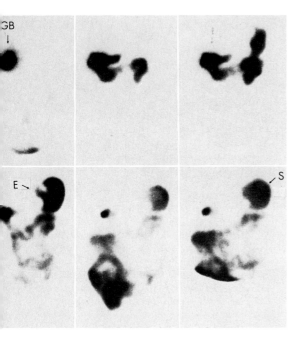

Fig. 6-5. Duodenogastric reflux. This patient had a hemigastrectomy with a Billroth I and subsequently a Billroth II gastroenterostomy. **A,** The gallbladder *(GB)* is well filled after 5 mCi techetium 99m disofenin intravenously. Following this image a liquid meal was given and imaging resumed. **B** to **E,** The gallbladder contracts in response to the meal, and tracer enters the small intestine. Stomach activity is seen in **C** to **E,** and reflux into the distal esophagus *(E, arrow)* occurs in **D.** This degree of gastric reflux is markedly abnormal. **F,** The stomach region *(S)* is confirmed following ingestion of a small dose of technetium 99m sulfur colloid in water.

time in the HBS study. After an appropriate interval to allow for bile activity to reflux into the stomach, the quantities reaching the stomach are measured by imaging the patient after a small capsule containing a known amount of technetium 99m pertechnetate is swallowed. The stomach ROI can be accurately outlined after a small dose of technetium 99m sulfur colloid in water is ingested. The lower limit of reflux detected by this method is about 0.5% of the injected dose of the technetium 99m hepatobiliary radionuclide.[36]

SUMMARY

In summary, many tests are currently available for assessing upper gastrointestinal functions, and quantitation can be accomplished with either invasive or noninvasive modalities. Of the latter, scintigraphic techniques that have evolved over the past two decades can be readily performed in

most clinical nuclear medicine facilities. These techniques use minute amounts of radioactivity to measure physiologic functions in health and disease by external monitoring without disturbing the functions (tracer principle). The radiation burdens are low, most patients accept them favorably, and serial studies can be performed to evaluate various medical and surgical therapeutic modalities. Future developments in nuclear medicine should expand the usefulness of these techniques.

REFERENCES

1. Booth, D.J., Kemmerer, W.T., and Skinner, D.B.: Acid clearing from the distal esophagus, Arch. Surg. **76:** 731-734, 1968.
2. Skinner, D.B., and Booth, D.J.: Assessment of distal esophageal function in patients with hiatal hernia and/or gastroesophageal reflux, Ann. Surg. **172:**627-637, 1970.
3. Kazem, I.: A new scintigraphic technique for the study of the esophagus, Am. J. Roentgenol. Radium Ther. Nucl. Med. **115:**681-688, 1972.
4. Bosch, A., Dietrich, R., Lanero, A., et al.: Modified scintigraphic technique for the dynamic study of the esophagus, Int. J. Nucl. Med. Biol. **4:**195-199, 1977.
5. Tolin, R.D., Malmud, L.S., Reilley, J., and Fisher, R.S.: Esophageal scintigraphy to quantitate esophageal transit (quantitation of esophageal transit), Gastroenterology **76:**1402-1408, 1979.
6. Ryan, J.W., O'Sullivan, G.C., Brunsden, B.S., Van-Daalen, J., and DeMeester T.R.: Digital scintigraphy in achalasia. In DeMeester, T.R., and Skinner, D.B., editors: *Esophageal disorders: pathophysiology and therapy,* New York, 1985, Raven Press, pp. 439-446.
7. Russell, C.O.H., Hill, L.D., Holmes, E.R., III, Hull, D.A., Gannon, R., and Pope, C.E., II: Radionuclide transit: a sensitive screening test for esophageal dysfunction, Gastroenterology **80:**887-892, 1981.
8. Blackwell, J.N., Hannan, W.J., Adam, R.D., and Heading, R.C.: Radionuclide transit studies in the detection of esophageal dysmotility, Gut **24:**421-426, 1983.
9. Benjamin, S.B., O'Donnell, J.K., Hancock, J., Nielsen, P., and Castell, D.O.: Prolonged radionuclide transit in "nutcracker esophagus," Dig. Dis. Sci. **28:**775-779, 1983.
10. Rozen, P., Gelfond, M., Salzman, S., et al.: Radionuclide confirmation of the therapeutic value of isosorbide, dinitrate in relieving the dysphagia in achalasia, J. Clin. Gastroenterol. **4:**17-22, 1982.
11. Rozen, P., Gelfond, M., Salzman, S., et al.: Dynamic, diagnostic, and pharmacological radionuclide studies of the esophagus in achalasia, Radiology **144:**587-590, 1982.
12. Holloway, R.H., Krosin, G., Lange, R.C., Baue, A.E., and McCallum, R.W.: Radionuclide esophageal emptying of a solid meal to quantitate results of therapy in achalasia, Gastroenterology **84:**771-776, 1983.
13. McCallum, R.W.: Radionuclide scanning in esophageal

disease, J. Clin. Gastroenterol. **4:**67-70, 1982.

14. Russel, C.O.H., Pope, C.E., II, Gannan, R.M., Allen, F.D., Velasco, N., and Hill, L.D.: Does surgery correct esophageal motor dysfunction in gastroesophageal reflux? Ann. Surg. **194:**290-296, 1981.

15. Kjellen, G., Svedberg, J.B., and Tibbling, L.: Solid bolus transit by esophageal scintigraphy in patients with dysphagia and normal manometry and radiography, Dig. Dis. Sci. **29:**1-5, 1984.

16. Beauchamp, G., Taillefer, R., Devito, M., Levasseur, A., and Lamoureux, C.: Radionuclide esophagogram in the evaluation of experimental esophagitis: manometric and histopathologic correlations. In DeMeester, T.R., and Skinner, D.B., editors: *Esophageal disorders: pathophysiology and therapy,* New York, 1985, Raven Press, pp. 77-81.

17. Ferguson, M.K., Ryan, J.W., Little, A.G., and Skinner, D.B.: Esophageal emptying and acid neutralization in patients with symptoms of esophageal reflux, Ann. Surg. **201:**728-735, 1985.

18. van Heukelem, H.A., Blom, H., Camps, J.A.J., Gooszen, H.G., Pauwels, E.K.J., and Biemond, I.: Assessment of esophageal motility by radionuclide transit studies in patients with reflux esophagitis and a pathologic 24-hour pH study. In DeMeester, T.R., and Skinner, D.B., editors: *Esophageal disorders: pathophysiology and therapy,* New York, 1985, Raven Press, pp. 83-86.

19. DeMeester, T.R., Wang, C.I., Wernly, J.A., Pellegrini, C.A., Little, A.G., Klementschitsch, P., Bermudez, G., Johnson, L.F., and Skinner, D.B.: Technique, indications, and clinical use of 24-hour esophageal pH monitoring, J. Thorac. Cardiovasc. Surg. **79:**656-670, 1980.

20. Fisher, R.S., Malmud, L.S., Roberts, G.S., et al.: Gastroesophageal (GE) scintiscanning to detect and quantitate GE reflux, Gastroenterology **70:**301-308, 1976.

21. Menin, R.A., Malmud, L.S., Petersen, R.P., Maier, W.P., and Fisher, R.S.: Gastroesophageal scintigraphy to assess the severity of gastroesophageal reflux disease, Ann. Surg. **191:**66-71, 1980.

22. Hillemeier, A.C., Grill, B.B., McCallum, R., and Gryboski, J.: Esophageal and gastric motor abnormalities in gastroesophageal reflux during infancy, Gastroenterology **84:**741-746, 1983.

23. Blumhagen, J.D., Rudd, T.G., and Christie, D.L.: Gastroesophageal reflux in children: radionuclide gastroesophagography, AJR **135:**1001-1004, 1980.

24. Seibert, J.J., Byrne, W.J., Euler, A.R., Latture, T., Leach, M., and Campbell, M: Gastroesophageal reflux—the acid test: scintigraphy or the pH probe? AJR **140:**1087-1090, 1983.

25. Little, A.G., DeMeester, T.R., Rezai-Zadeh, K., and Skinner, D.B.: Abnormal gastric emptying in patients with gastroesophageal reflux, Surg. Forum **28:**347-348, 1977.

26. Little, A.G., DeMeester, T.R., Kirchner, P.T., O'Sullivan, G.C., and Skinner, D.B.: Pathogenesis of esophagitis in patients with gastroesophageal reflux, Surgery **88:**101-107, 1980.

27. McCallum, R.W., Berkowitz, D.M., and Lerner, E.: Gastric emptying in patients with gastroesophageal reflux, Gastroenterology **80:**285-291, 1981.

28. Hillemeier, A.C., Lange, R., McCallum, R., Seashore, J., and Gryboski, J.: Delayed gastric emptying in infants with gastroesophageal reflux, J. Pediatr. **98:**190-193, 1981.

29. Little, A.G., DeMeester, T.R., and Skinner, D.B.: Combined gastric and esophageal 24-hour pH monitoring in patients with gastroesophageal reflux, Surg. Forum **30:**351-353, 1979.

30. Moore, J.G., Christian, P.E., and Coleman, R.E.: Gastric emptying of varying meal weights and composition in man: evaluation by dual liquid and solid phase isotopic method, Dig. Dis. Sci. **26:**16-22, 1981.

31. Little, A.G., Martinez, E.I., DeMeester, T.R., Blough, R.M., and Skinner, D.B.: Duodenogastric reflux and reflux esophagitis, Surgery **96:**447-454, 1984.

32. Helm, J.F., Dodds, W.J., Hogan, W.J., Soergel, K.H., Egide, M.S., and Wood, C.M.: Acid neutralizing capacity of human saliva, Gastroenterology **83:**69-74, 1982.

33. Helm, J.F., Dodds, W.J., Pelc, L.R., Palmer, D.W., Hogan, W.J., and Teeter, B.C.: Effect of esophageal emptying and saliva on clearance of acid from the esophagus, N. Engl. J. Med. **310:**284-288, 1984.

34. Pellegrini, C.A., DeMeester, T.R., Wernly, J.A., Johnson, L.F., and Skinner, D.B.: Alkaline gastroesophageal reflux, Am. J. Surg. **135:**177-184, 1978.

35. Tolin, R.D., Malmud, L.S., Stelzer, F., et al.: Enterogastric reflux in normal subjects and patients with Billroth II gastroenterostomy, Gastroenterology **77:**1027-1033, 1979.

36. Svedberg, J.B., Karlquist, P.A., Lindstrom, E., and Sjodahl, R.: New scintigraphic method for the quantitative measurement of enterogastric reflux, Scand. J. Gastroenterol. **19:**947-952, 1984.

Esophageal scintigraphy and tests of duodenogastric function

DISCUSSION

Gilles Beauchamp and Raymond Taillefer

It is now more than 10 years since the description by Kazem of esophageal scintigraphy.[1] Nuclear medicine using computer data processing has now added another dimension to the evaluation of esophagogastric problems. Since it is relatively easy to perform a safe and noninvasive test, the use of isotopes has spread as a method to provide quantitative parameters of esophageal and gastric motor disorders.

Ferguson and Ryan have discussed the currently available techniques for the assessment of the esophagogastroduodenal unit. Among those techniques, some will help in identifying the motor and transit problems of the pharynx, esophagus, and stomach, using solid or liquid. Other techniques will delineate the presence of reflux of acid from the stomach into the esophagus and alkaline secretion from the duodenum into the stomach.

Ferguson and Ryan have written an excellent review of all these tests. We will add some of our personal thoughts and methodology in regard to this topic.

EVALUATION OF MOTOR DISORDERS OF THE ESOPHAGUS AND STOMACH
Radionuclide esophageal transit study

The radionuclide esophageal transit study (RETS) is a relatively recent technique. However, since its introduction there have been many variations and improvements to the initial technique.

Concerning the methodology of this test, one must insist on the necessity of performing this study in the upright as well as in the supine position. Solids and liquids are used, to have a more complete evaluation of the function of the esophagus. The study needs to be conducted under the supervision of someone who has knowledge of esophageal physiology. The duration of the data acquisition can vary from 2 to 15 minutes, with a digital recording from 0.1- to 5-second intervals, depending on the symptoms or the esophageal disorders under investigation.

Standardization of the technique and evaluation of a normal population are necessary before the results can be relied on for clinical decisions. One must also stress the importance of communication between the laboratory and the clinician in order to make the results interpretable.

Evaluation of esophageal clearance

Esophageal clearance can be evaluated by radiology or by prolonged pH monitoring. RETS, because it uses physiologic markers and provides quantitative data, is one of the most reliable techniques for evaluating esophageal clearance. With the time-activity curves derived from the digitalized data, it provides the clinician unique information unavailable by other means. This quantitation of clearance is important in evaluating disease itself and in its treatment.

In achalasia, RETS provides a physiologic quantitative evaluation of esophageal emptying.[2-5] When the study is performed in the upright position with a solid meal, one can appreciate the time taken to evacuate the esophagus. When the examination is performed in a supine position with a liquid meal, it provides an opportunity to evaluate regurgitation and tracheal aspiration.

We have had some experience with patients complaining of dysphagia but in whom gastroesophageal reflux has been excluded by endoscopy and manometry. In such patients an abnormal RETS finding has been the factor persuading us to perform prolonged pH monitoring to exclude gastroesophageal reflux.

RETS can also evaluate the esophageal transit time prior to antireflux surgery. Some patients with gastroesophageal reflux disease have clearance problems related to an underlying disease, which needs to be considered before an antireflux operation is performed. Dysphagia and motor disorders can occur after any antireflux surgery.[6] In this situation, RETS can define the severity of the motor dysfunction, as well as its disappearance or persistence after surgery.

Atypical chest pain is a frequent diagnostic problem, for which an extensive cardiac workup, including thallium 201 myocardial imaging and coronary angiography, is carried out. A large percentage of these patients are found to have normal test results. RETS should be performed to complete the investigation and to eliminate the possibility of an esophageal motor dysfunction.

In patients with normal manometric and radiologic findings who complain of dysphagia, RETS can detect esophageal clearance disorders.[7-9]

Evaluation of swallowing and pharyngeal clearance

By means of the hypopharyngeal time derived from the time-activity curve clearance, pharyngeal emptying can be evaluated. RETS can also demonstrate pharyngonasal or pharyngooral regurgitations. It can also detect tracheal aspiration.[2] We think that RETS is a useful tool in the evaluation of pharyngeal disorders and will help to quantitate hypopharyngeal emptying time in patients with muscular dystrophy or other causes of oropharyngeal dysphagia.[2] If these patients undergo cricopharyngeal myotomy, the results of the surgery can be assessed and compared.

Evaluation of esophageal replacement surgery

Using a longer period of scanning, one can study the gastric interposition emptying time and assess the transit of the esophageal remnant as well as the clearance of the intrathoracic stomach. Tracheal aspiration and reflux can then be properly identified at the same time. This type of study can also be carried out to evaluate colonic interposition.

• • •

We must recognize that RETS is a test that has been performed for only a short period of time. It has not and will not replace conventional investigation in esophageal disorders. However, it can help in screening. Ferguson and Ryan have reported their experience with the use of isotope swallows as a valuable screening method for gastroesophageal reflux.[10] More is to be developed in the field of screening.

Radionuclide gastric emptying study

Gastric physiology is complex, and gastric emptying is regulated by a combination of factors. Among those factors are meal composition, stomach motility, and pyloric and duodenal motor activity, which all need to be considered in measuring gastric emptying.[11]

The gastric emptying of liquids is determined by contractions of the fundus and proximal stomach. Solids are emptied by contraction of the distal stomach and relaxation of the pylorus. Liquids empty from the stomach faster than solids, with an exponential emptying curve. Solids empty more slowly, following a linear curve. Delayed gastric emptying can be secondary to a mechanical obstruction at the gastric outlet or to a functional obstruction resulting from a pump failure.

During the last decade, new diagnostic techniques have contributed to our knowledge of gastric emptying pathophysiology.

The myoelectric gastrography, ultrasonography, and radionuclide studies are important technical advances in evaluating gastric motility disorders.[12,13] Many variables affect gastric emptying, and we find in the literature many different ways of conducting the examination.[13-15] Although there are common basic technical aspects to the evaluation of gastric emptying, the different variations introduced have led to discordant conclusions. We must recognize several potential inaccuracies that can reduce the sensitivity and specificity of the radionuclide gastric emptying evaluation. Among the many factors affecting the test are the type of camera used, the distribution of radionuclide in the stomach, and the way in which the data are analyzed.[14]

We think that every laboratory has to standardize the technique and establish its own normal values with the liquid and solid meals.

In clinical practice, the physician will use the radionuclide gastric emptying study for two purposes: first, to provide quantitative measurements of gastric emptying rate for solids and liquids in patients with symptoms of gastric emptying disorders and, second, to provide an accurate method of evaluating treatment effectiveness.

Since radionuclide tests are usually performed after radiologic and endoscopic studies, mechanical obstruction is rarely evaluated by scintigraphy. Pump failures, which are recognized by an abnormal gastric emptying curve, are numerous. In clinical practice what we see more often are the gastric emptying problems related to esophageal and gastric surgery when the vagus has been injured or deliberately cut.

There is also gastroparesis secondary to medication, metabolic disease such as diabetes, neurologic disorders, gastric disease, anorexia nervosa, and idiopathic problems.

Gastroesophageal reflux also can be secondary to gastric stasis. This is why every patient with severe gastroesophageal reflux should have an evaluation of the stomach capability of emptying. It is even more important for someone contemplating an antireflux operation to make sure the gastric emptying is normal. Performing a very effective antireflux procedure in a patient with a severe gastric emptying disorder might relieve the gastroesophageal reflux but leave the patient with a severe, incapacitating gas bloating. This is the reason why we now perform a gastric emptying study on every patient undergoing an antireflux procedure, trying to predict which patients have the potential for developing such a problem after surgery.

Some patients develop diarrhea after antireflux surgery. It can be secondary to a rapid emptying of liquids from the stomach or to trauma to the vagus nerve. It can also be due to gas bloating. The performance of preoperative and postoperative liquid gastric emptying studies can help in understanding such a problem if it appears. Ideally one should also evaluate the gas emptying of the stomach before and after surgery. We could probably recognize those patients who could potentially develop postoperative gas bloating difficulties.

EVALUATION OF ACID AND ALKALINE REFLUX WITH RADIONUCLIDE
Gastroesophageal acid reflux study

Measurement of gastroesophageal reflux with radionuclides offers a noninvasive and physiologic alternative to other procedures performed in clinical practice. Nonscintigraphic modalities have a common limitation: none of them provide quantitation of gastroesophageal reflux. Gastroesophageal scintigraphy has been introduced as a technique designed to quantitate gastroesophageal reflux in terms of the following parameters: the number of reflux episodes, their frequency, relative degree (reflux index), and extension of reflux (esophageal level); it can also evaluate the time required by the esophageal defense mechanisms to clear the refluxed fluid.

As for other radionuclide techniques used in the evaluation of gastroesophageal function, different acquisition protocols are described in the literature.[14,16,17] Many variables are involved in this type of study: patient's position, composition and volume of the radiolabeled liquid, amount of

radioactivity, use of maneuvers to induce reflux, acquisition protocol (including the total duration of the study and the number of seconds per image), data analysis and display, and criteria for a positive result. All these factors render the comparison between different techniques very difficult. This can explain the wide range of diagnostic accuracy found in different reports.[18-21] Furthermore, one must admit that very few good studies are found in the literature on why this wide range exists.

In our institution, we address an adult population. A radionuclide esophageal transit study is always performed concomitantly with a gastroesophageal reflux study. This may allow the detection of an esophageal motor dysfunction. Gastroesophageal activity is recorded at 5-second intervals for 30 or 60 minutes. An external inflatable abdominal binder is not used to increase the gastroesophageal pressure gradient. It may be uncomfortable for the patient and it does not appear to be physiologic. We prefer to induce reflux by using Valsalva maneuvers performed for 15 seconds at 30-second intervals for the last 5 minutes of the study.

There are two ways to quantify and express the results. The first is the gastroesophageal reflux index computed according to the formula of Fisher et al.[16] According to these authors, an index of 4% or greater is considered an evidence of gastroesophageal reflux. One limitation of this method however, is that ideally the radionuclide has to be introduced into the stomach through a nasogastric tube in order to avoid radiocolloid esophageal stasis, which can result in a false-positive test. Taking this drawback into consideration, Velasco et al.[17] introduced another method to express the results of a gastroesophageal reflux study. Instead of using static counts over the esophageal area, they measured transient peaks of esophageal radioactivity on a time-activity curve. A gastroesophageal reflux episode is then defined as a peak of activity with a value exceeding at least twice the baseline count value.

Mucosal adherence of the radiotracer is then of no significance, and this technique allows one to perform a RETS study concomitantly.

In our experience, the sensitivity of radionuclide studies in adult patients is more in the range of 70% rather than the previously reported sensitivity of 90%[16] for the detection of gastroesophageal reflux.

Radionuclide detection of gastroesophageal reflux is particularly well suited to pediatric and geriatric patients. It does not require intubation, has a low radiation burden, and can document pulmonary aspiration and gastric emptying, and esophageal function can be assessed simultaneously as well. Radionuclide studies are a reliable way to identify suspected gastroesophageal reflux and to assess the results of medical or surgical treatment.

In a recent study by Shay et al. of postprandial gastroesophageal reflux events, frequency and clearance were both evaluated simultaneously by scintigraphy and pH monitoring.[22] It was found that scintigraphy discerned postprandial reflux events and their clearance better than the pH probe. However, in this study, gastric emptying was a limiting factor in the use of scintigraphy for prolonged monitoring. In daily practice, if the radionuclide study does not detect significant gastroesophageal reflux despite strongly suggestive symptoms, 24-hour pH monitoring is recommended.

Duodenogastric alkaline reflux study

The advent of flexible endoscopy has helped the clinician to recognize the occurrence of bile in the stomach, especially in the postoperative period. The antropyloroduodenal unit can be disturbed by any surgery on the vagus, stomach, or duodenum. Excessive duodenogastric reflux may also occur in other circumstances.

Primary duodenogastric reflux is probably a very rare disease but can happen and needs to be recognized.

The problem with alkaline reflux is accuracy in diagnosis. Because of the nonspecificity of the endoscopic and histologic findings, we need a better test to identify bile reflux. A number of tests have been used to identify bile in the stomach and esophagus, but none is completely satisfactory.[23] However, a nice study was concluded by Houghton et al., in which duodenogastric reflux was assessed using ^{99m}Tc-labeled butyliminodiacetic acid (BIDA) scintigraphy and intragastric bile acid levels. There was a significant correlation between both free and total intragastric bile acid levels and the degree of isotopic bile reflux, except when reflux was mild.[24]

Because of the difficulties in diagnosing and treating such a disease, some have questioned whether the disease really exists at all.[25,26] We have faced difficulties in determining which of our patients have the disease and would benefit from a Roux-en-Y procedure.

We have not been impressed with the quantification of bile reflux by scintigraphy. We have had to base our diagnoses on severity and duration of symptoms along with the lack of psychiatric disorders. We have waited at least 6 months to see the effect of medical treatment before considering

surgery. We have not tried the intragastric alkali infusion described by Warshaw.[27] With this test, alkali is placed in the stomach and will reproduce the symptoms in patients with alkaline reflux gastritis, with a 90% accuracy in diagnosis. There is certainly a place for clinical research in that particular aspect of gastroesophageal reflux.

CONCLUSION

Ferguson and Ryan have well described and discussed the current esophageal, gastric, and duodenal scintigraphic tests. Although these tests have not revolutionized our approach to esophageal problems, they have given us more quantitation of the esophagogastric physiology. The use of radionuclide studies in the investigation of digestive problems is in its beginning. More basic research and clinical trials need to be conducted in that field to help the surgeon in understanding the pathophysiology of such complex diseases.

REFERENCES

1. Kazem, I.: A new scintigraphic technique for the study of the esophagus, Am. J. Roentgenol. Radium Ther. Nucl. Med. 115:681-688, 1972.
2. Taillefer, R., and Beauchamp, G.: Radionuclide esophagogram, Clin. Nucl. Med. 9:465-483, 1984.
3. Taillefer, R., Beauchamp, G., Duranceau, A.C., and Lafontaine, E.: Nuclear medicine and esophageal surgery, Clin. Nucl. Med. 11:445-460, 1986.
4. Rozen, P., Gelfond, M., Zaltman, S., et al.: Dynamic, diagnostic and pharmacological radionuclide studies of the esophagus in achalasia: correlation with manometric measurements, Radiology 144:587-590, 1982.
5. Rozen, P., Gelfond, M., Zaltman, S., et al.: Radionuclide confirmation of the therapeutic value of isosorbide dinitrate in relieving the dysphagia in achalasia, J. Clin. Gastroenterol. 4:17-22, 1982.
6. Kjellen, G., Fransson, S.G., Johansson, K.E., et al.: Scintigraphy, radiography, and acid clearing in dysphagia patients after anti-reflux surgery, Scand. J. Gastroenterol. 19:1022-1026, 1984.
7. Kjellen, G., Swedberg, J.B., and Tibbling, L.: Solid bolus transit by esophageal scintigraphy in patients with dysphagia and normal manometry and radiography, Dig. Dis. Sci. 29:1-5, 1984.
8. Russell, C.O.H., Hill, L.D., Holmes, E.R., et al.: Radionuclide transit: a sensitive screening test for esophageal dysfunction, Gastroenterology 80:887-892, 1981.
9. De Caestecker, J.S., Blackwell, J.N., Adam, R.D., Hannan, W., Brown, J., and Heading, R.C.: Clinical value of radionuclide esophageal transit measurement, Gut 27:659-666, 1986.
10. Ferguson, M.K., Ryan, J.W., Little, A.G., and Skinner, D.B.: Esophageal emptying and acid neutralization in patients with symptoms of esophageal reflux, Ann. Surg. 201:728-735, 1985.

11. Akkermans, L.M.A., Johnson, A.G., and Read, N.W.: Gastric and gastroduodenal motility, Surgical Science Series 4, New York, 1984, Praeger Publishers, p. 332.
12. Bolondi, L., Bortolotti, M., Santi, V., Galletti, T., Gaiani, S., and Labo, G.: Measurement of gastric emptying time by real-time ultrasonography, Gastroenterology **89:**752-759, 1985.
13. Minami, H., and McCallum, R.W.: The physiology and pathophysiology of gastric emptying in humans, Gastroenterology **86:**1592-1610, 1984.
14. Christian, P.E., Datz, F.L., Sorenson, J.A., et al.: Technical factors in gastric emptying studies, J. Nucl. Med. **24:**264-268, 1983.
15. Horowitz, M., Collins, P.J., and Shearman, D.J.C.: Disorders of gastric emptying in humans and the use of radionuclide techniques, Arch. Intern. Med. **145:**1467-1472, 1985.
16. Fisher, R.S., Malmud, L.S., Roberts, G.S., et al.: Gastroesophageal scintiscanning to detect and quantitate G.E. reflux, Gastroenterology **70:**307-308, 1976.
17. Velasco, N., Pope, C.E., II, Gannan, R.M., Roberts, P., and Hill, L.D.: Measurement of esophageal reflux by scintigraphy, Dig. Dis. Sci. **29:**977-982, 1984.
18. Seibert, J.J., Byrne, W.J., Evler, A.R., et al.: Gastroesophageal reflux—the acid test: scintigraphy or the pH probe? AJR **140:**1087, 1983.
19. Fung, W.P., Van der Scharf, A., and Grieve, J.C.: Gastroesophageal scintigraphy and endoscopy in the diagnosis of esophageal reflux and esophagitis, Am. J. Gastroenterol. **80:**245, 1985.
20. Paton, J.Y., Cosgriff, P.S., and Nanayakkara, C.S.: The analytical sensitivity of Tc-99m radionuclide "milk" scanning in the detection of gastroesophageal reflux, Pediatr. Radiol. **15:**381, 1985.
21. Hoffman, G.C., and Vansant, J.H.: The gastroesophageal scintiscan, Arch. Surg. **114:**727-728, 1979.
22. Shay, S., Eggli, D., Maydonovitch, C., and Johnson, L.: Postprandial gastroesophageal reflux event frequency and clearance: a simultaneous comparison of scintigraphy vs pH monitoring, Gastroenterology **90:**1630, 1986.
23. Earlam, R.: Bile reflux and the Roux en Y anastomosis, Br. J. Surg. **70:**393-397, 1983.
24. Houghton, P.W.J., McC.Mortensen, N.J., Thomas, W.E.G., Cooper, M.J., Morgan, A.P., and Davies, E.R.: Intragastric bile acids and scintigraphy in the assessment of duodenogastric reflux, Br. J. Surg. **73:**292-294, 1986.
25. Alexander-Williams, J.: Alkaline reflux gastritis: a myth or disease? Am. J. Surg. **143:**17, 1982.
26. Meyer, J.H.: Reflections on reflux gastritis, Gastroenterology **77:**1143, 1979.
27. Warshaw, A.L., Johnson, H., and Welch, C.E.: The alkaline reflux gastritis problem, Surg. Gastroenterol. **1:**175-178, 1982.

CHAPTER 7 The laboratory in the diagnosis of esophageal disease

Hugoe R. Matthews and Ian P. Adams

In the preceding chapters attention has been focused on recent developments in esophageal diagnosis, with particular reference to individual diagnostic techniques. It is also important, however, to consider the way in which these different tests are integrated in the diagnosis of the individual patient. This chapter, therefore, is concerned principally with an analysis of all the cases referred to our laboratory for clinical studies during 1983, in order to examine the general role of the esophageal laboratory in a surgical department.

HISTORY

In Birmingham a part-time esophageal laboratory was first established by Professor J.L. Collis in 1968 at the Queen Elizabeth Hospital. Manometric and pH studies were performed, but the quality of data recording tended to be inconsistent, since the tests were conducted by research fellows of varying degrees of ability and enthusiasm. In 1980, therefore, a qualified physiologist (I.P.A.) was appointed full time to perform all studies, and the laboratory was integrated with the Regional Department of Thoracic Surgery at East Birmingham Hospital, under the direction of the present author (H.R.M.). We were then able to provide a reliable and continuous diagnostic service, both to the thoracic surgical unit and to patients referred from any other source. Since that time the workload has increased steadily, and a second member of staff (also trained in physiologic measurement) was appointed in 1985. In that year a total of 208 patients received clinical studies, of whom 126 were from the author's practice and 82 were from other clinicians.

WORKLOAD

In the year chosen for analysis (1983) a total of 235 manometric, pH, or Bernstein tests were performed on 137 patients, of whom 101 were from the author's practice and 36 were from other clinicians (see Table 7-1). Excluded from this analysis are three patients in whom studies were attempted but could not be completed—because of anxiety in two and inability to pass the lower esophageal sphincter in one (with achalasia). They, however, indicate a very low "failure rate," which we attribute to the fact that all tests were performed by a permanent member of staff with 4 years' experience of the appropriate techniques. Also excluded are all patients in whom studies were performed purely for research purposes.

TESTS PERFORMED

Most patients were referred for investigation of possible reflux disease, motility disorders, unexplained chest pain, or recurrent attacks of vomiting; the tests used in each of these diagnostic categories are shown in Table 7-2. The miscellaneous group comprised five patients with systemic diseases and possible esophageal involvement, four who had undergone esophageal surgery elsewhere, two infants with possible esophageal symptoms, one patient with odynophagia, one with a previous bolus obstruction, and one with a columnar-lined esophagus and carcinoma.

PROPORTION OF PATIENTS TESTED

One of the important questions concerning the role of the laboratory is what proportion of

TABLE 7-1. Cases referred to the laboratory for clinical studies in 1983

Source	No. of patients	Tests performed			
		Manometry	pH	Bernstein	
Author (H.R.M.)	101	76	78	13	
Other thoracic surgeons	18 ⎫				
General surgeons	2 ⎬	30	27	11	
Physicians	16 ⎭				
Totals	137	106	105	24	(235)

TABLE 7-2. Use of tests in relation to provisional diagnosis

Diagnosis	No. of patients	Manometry No. (%)	pH No. (%)	Bernstein No. (%)
Reflux disorders	69	44 (64)	69 (100)	10 (15)
Motility disorders	39	39 (100)	14 (36)	1 (3)
Unexplained chest pain	8	7 (88)	7 (88)	6 (75)
Vomiting	7	5 (71)	6 (86)	2 (29)
Miscellaneous	14	11 (79)	9 (64)	5 (36)

patients require laboratory studies, but this cannot be answered when the population from which the patients were referred is not known. For this purpose, therefore, we have analyzed our own practice, in which that population is known and the proportion of patients referred to the laboratory can be calculated. In 1983 a total of 304 new inpatients with esophageal disease were seen by the author, of whom 101 had laboratory studies for clinical reasons. This represents 33% of all the patients and 51% of patients with nonmalignant disease. The eventual diagnoses in these patients and the tests used are shown in Table 7-3.

In this table we have separated the patients with sliding hiatal hernia into those with or without reflux esophagitis in order to emphasize an important difference in our policy for the two groups. As part of the diagnosis, one needs to know whether patients are having reflux, but if this is already established by the presence of reflux ulceration or stricture, then we believe that pH studies are not routinely required for clinical purposes. Also if a reflux stricture is very tight, then reflux may actually be prevented and this is one of the few circumstances in which pH studies may be misleading. They were performed, therefore, in only 9 of the 58 patients in this category, but they are essential whenever it is necessary to distinguish chemical esophagitis (i.e., alcohol or drug induced) from reflux inflammation. In our view it is in the group without esophagitis that

TABLE 7-3. Use of the laboratory within a known population of 304 new esophageal patients

Diagnosis	No. of patients	No. (%) referred to laboratory
Carcinoma	107	1 (1)
Sliding hiatal hernia		
With esophagitis	58	9 (16)
Without esophagitis	57	47 (83)
Paraesophageal hernia	11	0
Achalasia	19	15 (79)
Primary esophageal		
spasm	12	12 (100)
Miscellaneous	40	17 (43)

pH studies are particularly important, and measurements were made on 47 of the 57 patients in this category (the remainder had symptoms that were insufficient to require investigation at that time). In these patients the results are frequently crucial in determining what therapy is required; severe constant reflux may require operation, while mild reflux should be controllable by medical measures. If no reflux is identified, then irrelevant treatment is avoided and the clinician is prompted to search for an alternative source of the symptoms.

Table 7-3 also shows that laboratory studies were performed in all patients with esophageal spasm, in most of those with achalasia (the four exceptions having gross classical disease), but in none of the patients with paraesophageal hernia. The one patient with carcinoma was referred from another hospital with a suspected motility disorder, and it was only when manometry and pH studies were normal that endoscopy was repeated in our unit and a very small tumor discovered.

TWENTY-FOUR HOUR pH MONITORING

Twenty-four-hour pH monitoring was performed on all 69 patients referred to the laboratory with possible reflux (Table 7-2), and its importance is indicated in Table 7-4, in which the results are correlated with the radiologic evidence of reflux and the eventual selection for surgery. In 36 patients (groups 1 and 2) no reflux was detected by barium swallow, yet 26 of these had pathologic reflux on pH testing, of whom 15 subsequently required an antireflux repair. There was thus a "false-negative" rate of 72% for the radiologic assessment of reflux. In the 30 patients (groups 3 and 4) in whom reflux was identified radiologically, the correlation was better; 25 had reflux confirmed by pH studies, and 16 of these had an antireflux repair. However, five of the patients in groups 3 and 4 did not have pathologic reflux on pH testing, giving a "false-positive" rate of 17% for the radiologic assessment.

It is for these reasons that we would agree with Johnson and DeMeester[1] that 24-hour pH monitoring is the most accurate index of reflux that is currently available, and we never rely on the radiologic findings alone for this part of the diagnosis. Clearly, many factors determine whether a patient with a sliding hernia requires repair, but in patients without esophagitis we will not consider operation unless pathologic reflux

has been confirmed by pH testing. In this series there was only one exception to this rule (see Table 7-4), and that was in an unusual patient with a strongly positive Bernstein test and anatomic recurrence of a hernia following repair at another hospital, whose symptoms were relieved by a second repair.

Monitoring of pH was of course also used in other groups of patients, as shown in Table 7-2. In patients with motility disorders it was used to help unravel the functional consequences of previous operations (e.g., Heller's myotomy), to assess reflux in patients with scleroderma, or to distinguish primary esophageal spasm from reflux-induced secondary spasm. This distinction is particularly important with regard to therapy, since primary spasm requires an extended esophageal myotomy (if symptoms are sufficiently severe), while secondary spasm is satisfactorily treated by antireflux repair. Reflux was demonstrated in five of the seven patients investigated for angina-type chest pain and led to alterations in their medical therapy, but in this year none of this group required surgery. In the six patients with recurrent attacks of vomiting, pH studies helped to exclude an esophageal cause for their symptoms.

MANOMETRY

Manometric studies were performed in all 39 patients referred with suspected motility disorders (see Table 7-2), and the correlation with the radiologic results and the eventual therapy is shown in Table 7-5. In 11 patients with suspected achalasia (group 1) the diagnosis was confirmed in 10, all of whom were treated by operation, but one patient was found to have only an inert esophagus and thereby avoided an operation that

TABLE 7-4. Radiologic and pH results in 69 patients with suspected reflux

Radiologic findings	No. of patients (%)	pH findings	Treated by antireflux repair
No hernia, no reflux (group 1)	17 (25)	Reflux, 11	5
		No reflux, 6	0
Hernia, no reflux (group 2)	19 (28)	Reflux, 15	10
		No reflux, 4	0
Hernia with reflux (group 3)	16 (23)	Reflux, 13	10
		No reflux, 3	1*
Reflux, no hernia (group 4)	14 (20)	Reflux, 12	6
		No reflux, 2	0
Hernia and narrowing (group 5)	3 (4)	Reflux, 3	3
		No reflux, 0	0

*Patient with a recurrent hernia and strongly positive Bernstein test result (see text).

would have been at best useless and at worst damaging. In combination with pH testing, manometry was particularly valuable in the evaluation of the eight patients in group 2 with symptoms following a previous myotomy for achalasia (only one of whom was from our own practice); three of these had residual lower esophageal obstruction, but five did not and were suffering from an inert esophagus, with or without reflux. All patients except one required further surgery, and the choice of operation was determined by a combination of the laboratory, endoscopic, and operative findings.

In the 13 patients in group 3, manometry distinguished between those with diffuse esophageal spasm and those with hyperperistalsis, or a "nutcracker" esophagus. The treatment of these was broadly the same, but one patient was found to have a segmental loss of contractility which would not have responded to myotomy and required a colon interposition. Seven patients (groups 4 and 5) had no motility disorder identified at routine radiologic examination; five of these had manometric abnormalities, though none was severe enough to require operation.

Manometry was also performed in 44 patients with suspected reflux (see Table 7-2), principally to assess lower esophageal sphincter function and to look for associated motility disorders, but the results were rarely of importance in therapeutic decisions. Reflux was always measured independently by pH studies, and the use of the Belsey Mark IV repair means that there is no particular

concern if motility disorders are present. None of the patients with angina-type chest pain had significant manometric abnormalities (though we do not use provocative tests). Three of the patients with vomiting had minor disorders of motility, but these were judged to be unrelated to their symptoms.

BERNSTEIN TEST

Along with other workers we have found that results of the Bernstein test[2] do not correlate well with the presence or absence of esophagitis. When correctly performed, however, this test can show a dramatic connection between the patient's symptoms and the infusion of acid. Of the 24 patients studied (Table 7-2) only four had an unequivocally positive result and only one of these (with a recurrent hernia, previously mentioned) required surgery. Of the 20 patients with a negative result, 12 (60%) had reflux on pH testing and two had esophagitis.

MUCOSAL POTENTIAL DIFFERENCE

In our laboratory mucosal potential difference (PD) is measured routinely during manometric studies. An abrupt drop in the mucosal PD provides accurate localization of the squamocolumnar junction, which occasionally helps in the detection of a hiatal hernia, or of a columnar-

TABLE 7-5. Radiologic and manometric results in 39 patients with suspected motility disorders

Radiologic findings	No. of patients	Manometry results (with or without pH tests)	Treatment
Suspected achalasia (group 1)	11	Achalasia confirmed, 10	Heller's myotomy, 10
		Inert esophagus, 1	Dilated
Hold-up after previous myotomy (group 2)	8	Distal obstruction, 3	Repeat myotomy, 2; colon graft, 1
		Inert esophagus, 1	Dilated
		Inert esophagus and reflux, 4	Antireflux repair, 3; colon graft, 1
Spasm with or without diverticulum (group 3)	13	Diffuse spasm, 7	Long myotomy, 4; dilated, 2; nifedipine, 1
		Nutcracker esophagus, 5	Long myotomy, 4; dilated, 1
		Immotile segment, 1	Colon graft
Reflux only (group 4)	2	Spasm, no reflux, 1	Dilated
		Inert, no reflux, 1	Dilated
No abnormality (group 5)	5	No abnormality, 2	—
		Nutcracker esophagus, 1	Dilated
		Diffuse spasm, 1	Nifedipine
		Inert esophagus, 1	Dilated

lined esophagus (when there is a marked discrepancy between the level of the squamocolumnar junction and the position of the lower esophageal sphincter). We have not, however, found a good correlation between an irregular tracing and the presence or absence of esophagitis. The results therefore are rarely important in clinical management and have not been analyzed separately in this survey.

CASE REPORT

To illustrate how these various tests are integrated in the management of the individual patient, it may be helpful to cite a single example from our own practice:

In 1979 a 57-year-old Caucasian male was referred to our unit with severe pain during eating and with episodic regurgitation. At the first esophageal investigation a barium swallow was obtained (Fig. 7-1), which showed two obvious

anatomic abnormalities, a lower esophageal diverticulum and a moderately large paraesophageal hernia. The existence of the diverticulum implied the presence of distal esophageal obstruction, but the radiologic examination did not indicate whether this was due to distortion or pressure from the hernia, a reflux stenosis, a motility disorder in the distal esophagus, or a carcinoma. To investigate some of these possibilities, endoscopy was performed, but it demonstrated no mucosal ulceration, inflammation, stricture, or tumor, and these were effectively excluded as the cause of the diverticulum.

Further elucidation required the use of the laboratory, and esophageal manometry was next performed. This showed grossly disordered motility (i.e., esophageal spasm) in the segment between the diverticulum and the gastroesophageal junction. It was still uncertain, however, whether this spasm was "primary" or "secondary" to reflux resulting from the hernia. Twenty-four hour pH studies were therefore obtained, but

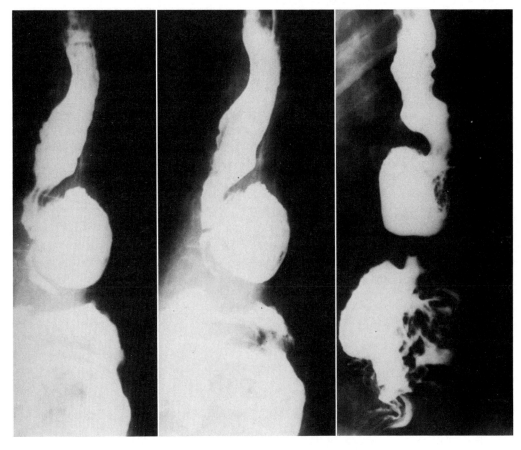

Fig. 7-1. Preoperative barium swallow showing esophageal diverticulum, a narrowed lower esophageal sphincter, and a paraesophageal hernia.

no gastroesophageal reflux was demonstrated, and whether the spasm was primary or secondary could not be determined. Unfortunately, at present there is no test (other than a trial of hernia repair) that will distinguish between these two alternatives. Hiatal hernia repair alone, however, would obviously be insufficient if primary spasm were present, so the patient was treated by lower esophageal myotomy, suspension of the diverticulum, and hiatal hernia repair, using a Belsey partial fundoplication (Fig. 7-2). In the 7 years since operation, he has been free of symptoms and has required no further esophageal treatment.

CONCLUSION

This chapter demonstrates clearly that esophageal diagnosis is not necessarily a simple matter —and it certainly means more than just being able to attach a label to any given patient. It may

be quite easy, for instance, to determine that a patient has a hiatal hernia simply from a lateral chest radiograph, but that does not tell us if the condition is serious or whether anything needs to be done about it. In its fullest sense, therefore, diagnosis means obtaining all the information that is necessary for a complete understanding of the pathologic processes that are at work in a particular patient, so that a decision can be made as to whether treatment is required and what form it should take.

This process is also illustrated in the case report. Laboratory studies should not be used indiscriminately but should be selected in order to answer specific questions that are relevant to the management of the individual patient. The results must then be interpreted correctly and integrated with the data from all the other investigations, including the history and examination, radiography, endoscopy, and any other special investigations that may be required. Clearly, for

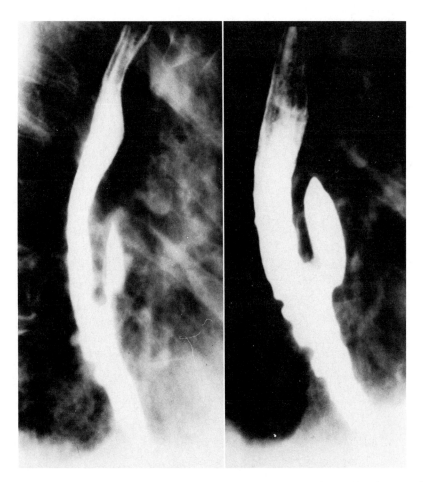

Fig. 7-2. Appearances on barium swallow following suspension of the diverticulum, lower esophageal myotomy, and Belsey partial fundoplication.

the correct conclusions to be drawn the laboratory results must be absolutely reliable, and we therefore take the view that studies should be performed by persons trained in physiologic measurement, and not by transient fellows (whose priorities lie elsewhere) or nurses (who generally do not have a full understanding of esophageal pathophysiology).

When esophageal laboratories first developed they were regarded primarily as research departments, but this is no longer the case. While the research function is still important, the laboratory is now also essential for the proper clinical management of many esophageal patients. As this survey has shown, it can help to determine which patients require operation, what procedure is appropriate, and, of equal importance, which patients will not benefit from surgery. Esophageal surgery is difficult enough without the added burden of an inaccurate diagnosis, and no operation, however brilliantly executed, will be benefi-

cial if it is performed for a nonexistent condition (e.g., an antireflux repair in a patient who does not have reflux). It is therefore ultimately the responsibility of the surgeon to ensure that a full assessment has been made before he or she undertakes any procedure on the esophagus. There are some areas of surgery in which the surgeon is no longer involved in diagnosis, but the esophagus, happily, is not one of them, and gratifyingly good results can be achieved provided that the surgeon has a thorough grasp of the investigative techniques and their application in clinical practice.

REFERENCES

1. Johnson, L.F., and DeMeester, T.R.: Twenty-four-hour pH monitoring of the distal esophagus, Am. J. Gastroenterol. **62:**325-332, 1974.
2. Bernstein, L.M., and Baker, L.A.: A clinical test for esophagitis, Gastroenterology **34:**760-781, 1958.

The laboratory in the diagnosis of esophageal disease

DISCUSSION

Lawrence F. Johnson

In the preceding chapter the authors describe their use of esophageal function testing in a clinical surgical practice. Although the majority of their experience was confined to the evaluation of patients with gastroesophageal reflux, other esophageal disorders were examined. Thus, this report consists of a well-balanced one-year experience. In choosing me as a commentator for this series, the editors met the criteria not only of selecting an individual from across the Atlantic, but indeed of choosing a person from a cross discipline (i.e., an internist gastroentrologist). Since I cannot judge the criteria the authors used to select their patients for surgery, I would like to confine my comments concerning their experience to areas in which we agree or disagree, as well as to those areas in which their data may have limited usefulness to the reader. The only limitation in their data that I identified was that they did not give definitions for esophageal diagnoses and/or disorders seen in their laboratory. Therefore, it will be difficult for the reader to interpret their percentages or compare their experience with that of others. Hence, rather than comment on their percentages, I would like to take this opportunity to address certain aspects of their experience.

That the authors noted early on the need for a qualified physiologist to run their esophageal function laboratory is a valuable observation. Although the initial purpose of esophageal function laboratories was research, their clinical contribution has also been recognized. Unfortunately, this recognition has not always coincided with a clinical commitment to quality control consistent with that seen in a research laboratory. In the

The opinions or assertions contained herein are the private views of the author and are not to be construed as official or as reflecting the views of the Department of the Army or the Department of Defense.

clinical laboratory these tests are often administered by uninterested residents or busy clinicians who may delegate these tests to unsupervised technicians. Without attention to quality control by committed, permanent laboratory personnel, such as a clinical physiologist or a physician interested in esophageal disorders or disease, the information gained from these tests is meaningless. Although residents need to rotate through these laboratories in order to learn the nature, limitations, and proper use of these tests, they still need to be supervised by knowledgeable professionals committed to the minute details necessary to properly conduct these tests in order to achieve a meaningful result. The authors, in pointing this out, make a significant contribution to those interested in establishing an esophageal function laboratory.

Although it is often stated that "reflux" is established in patients with distal esophageal ulceration and/or stricture, and that pH tests are not required for clinical diagnosis as stated by the authors, this axiom may not be true. This results because of the problem, "you don't know what you don't know"; that is, pathologic degrees of gastroesophageal reflux are often diagnosed by "reflex" when one sees distal esophagitis, yet only recently have we become aware that erosive esophagitis and/or strictures can be caused by excessive cigarette smoking,[1] pill-induced esophageal injury,[2] herpesvirus, cytomegalogvirus, and streptococcal disease.[3] Thus, in these instances, esophagitis may obviously exist without an incompetent lower esophageal sphincter and pathologic degrees of gastroesophageal reflux. Although an incorrect diagnosis may not severely harm the patient if he were treated medically, this would not be the case if he were treated surgically. In this instance, an antireflux procedure would be performed for a dysfunction that did not exist. In my opinion, any patient who has an antireflux procedure should have esophageal function tests to demonstrate LES incompetence and pathologic degrees of gastroesophageal reflux.

I was intrigued by the authors' observation concerning the influence of a hiatal hernia and/or radiographic reflux on intraesophageal pH monitoring results. When they examined the four possible combinations between the presence or absence of a hiatal hernia and radiographic reflux for the total population (n = 69, Table 7-4), each of the four possible combinations represented approximately one-fourth of the individuals. The lowest risk for a positive pH reflux occurred in the group with no hiatal hernia and radiographic reflux (64%). In contrast, the highest scores occurred in those with radiographic reflux (85%) or a hernia with (81%) or without (78%) radiographic reflux. Despite the fact that hiatal hernias have been deemphasized in the pathophysiology of gastroesophageal reflux disease for the last two decades, recent clinical investigation with pH monitoring[4] and/or isotopes[5,6] has shown that the presence of a hernia delays esophageal acid clearance. This occurs when the patient assumes the recumbent posture. This delay in esophageal clearance provides prolonged acid mucosal contact, a risk factor for reflux esophagitis.[4,7,8] Although we should not return to qualitatively diagnosing gastroesophageal reflux in our patients on the basis of the presence or absence of a hiatal hernia, we need to acknowledge the contribution this finding makes to the pathophysiology of gastroesophageal reflux.

Although I agree with the authors that LES pressure is rarely important in making therapeutic decisions regarding patients with gastroesophageal reflux, there are some exceptions. First, the extremes of LES pressure can be used to manage patients. Virtually 100% of patients with an LES pressure less than 6 mm Hg have a positive pH reflux test (standard acid reflux test).[9] Moreover, an LES pressure less than 6 has recently been shown to help denote a population of symptomatic patients that respond well to antireflux surgery.[10] Symptomatic patients found to have an LES pressure greater than 20 mm Hg generally do not have a positive pH test, so one should question the diagnosis of gastroesophageal reflux in these patients.[9] Hence, extremely low or high LES pressures can be used as a screening test. Second, the determinants of the sphincter pressure and location can be used to precisely place pH probes for intraesophageal pH monitoring so that quality control concerning this test can be assured.

That the authors had a varied experience with the manometric demonstration of different esophageal disorders such as those shown in Table 7-2 indicates they were using manometry to precisely define all esophageal diseases and disorders seen in their practice. Primary peristaltic contraction waves in the body of the esophagus and normal LES relaxation are both important manometric events to demonstrate in all patients evaluated in an esophageal function laboratory. This is because patients with achalasia are often mistaken for those with gastroesophageal reflux, especially since the patients with achalasia may complain of a heartburn like-symptom.[11] In this situation, a fundoplication, effectively used in the surgical treatment of gastroesophageal reflux in patients with normal esophageal peristalsis and low LES pressure, would adversely affect patients with achalasia, who have no esophageal peristaltic contraction waves, along with high LES pressure, and poor to absent LES relaxation. In a similar manner, esophageal manometry also helps to identify other motor disorders that are sometimes confused with gastroesophageal reflux.[12]

I agree with the authors' observation and that of others[13] that results of the Bernstein test do not correlate with the presence or absence of esophagitis. Years ago, when esophagitis could only be detected by rigid endoscopy, such a positive correlation would have been clinically important. Today, however, the ease of fiberoptic endoscopy in detecting the presence or absence of esophagitis has made this lack of correlation irrelevant. At present, the Bernstein test is best employed to detect the presence of an acid-sensitive esophagus. Used in this manner, the Bernstein test has excellent results because almost 100% of patients with heartburn have a positive test.[14] Thus, the demonstration of an acid-sensitive esophagus, along with a low LES pressure (i.e., ≤ 6 mm Hg), excessive acid gastroesophageal reflux demonstrated by pH monitoring (especially at night), and slow acid clearance times will assure the surgeon that an antireflux procedure that augments LES pressure and in turn diminishes acid gastroesophageal reflux should improve the patient's symptoms. It is reasonable to ask the question, why do all these other tests if the Bernstein test is positive? These other tests are necessary because of the high incidence of false-positive Bernstein tests results; 14% of control subjects will have an acid-sensitive esophagus demonstrated during the Bernstein test, including those with no reflux symptoms, a normal LES pressure, and no reflux on pH testing.[14] The Bernstein test determines that the burning substernal chest pain is esophageal in origin and is induced by an acid pH. However, this test provides no information about the state of LES competence, the degree of reflux, or the ability of the esophagus to clear acid.

That the authors experienced a low percentage of patients with a positive Bernstein test (4 of 24) I believe attests, in part, to the limited number of patients with gastroesophageal reflux in whom they performed the test (10 of 69), as well as to the number of patients with nonreflux disorders in whom they used the test (Table 7-1). I was impressed, however, with the authors' observation that 60% of their patients with a negative Bernstein test had "reflux on pH testing and two had esophagitis." This suggests there are patients with severe gastroesophageal reflux who have little or no esophageal acid sensitivity. I feel this observation is valid because diminished esophageal acid sensitivity has been observed in patients with esophageal strictures,[15] Barrett's esophagus,[16] and alkaline gastroesophageal reflux.[17] Thus, a negative Bernstein test result, as the authors pointed out, does not obviate a diagnosis of gastroesophageal reflux disease.

The authors' preference for selectively intensifying the medical treatment of angina in patients with coronary artery disease and gastroesophageal reflux deserves comment. Although this is a standard of practice consistent with good clinical judgment on either side of the Atlantic, recent clinical investigation has elucidated a new relationship between angina and gastroesophageal reflux that deserves review. It has been found that acid perfusion of the esophagus in a patient with an acid-sensitive esophagus from reflux, as well as angina from coronary artery disease, will significantly increase the rate-pressure product.[18] This increase can reach the angina threshold just as if the patient had exercised. This phenomenon does not occur in patients who do not have an acid-sensitive esophagus during the Bernstein test, but have angina from coronary artery disease. Hence, one might intensify the treatment of reflux to lessen the angina, just the opposite of our current standard of practice.

The authors' clinical experience in their esophageal function laboratory for one year also reflects the broad range of disorders these units are now being asked to evaluate. For instance, seven patients were seen for unexplained vomiting. Although gastric and/or duodenal outlet obstruction can account for reflux symptoms and esophagitis,[12] most patients with either reflux esophagitis or Barrett's esophagus have no delay in their gastric emptying[19,20] Upright refluxers who may present with "vomiting" and/or severe regurgitation along with heartburn and aerophagia are of interest to surgeons, to whom such patients are often referred with a reflux diathasis recalcitrant

to medical management.[21] Surgeons should be reluctant to operate, because although a fundoplication can return their daytime gastroesophageal reflux to normal, these patients are left virtually incapacitated with a resultant gas bloating syndrome.[22] Fortunately, biofeedback has been objectively shown to diminish their daytime acid gastroesophageal reflux and improve their symptoms.[21] Hence, these motility units will evaluate a broad range of patients with various esophageal diseases or disorders.

Because esophageal surgery for benign conditions is rarely extirpative, surgeons need to direct their attention and plan their procedures to correct specific dysfunctions in accordance with physiologic principles. An esophageal function laboratory such as that described and used by the authors offers patients and surgeons the best chance to attain good results.

REFERENCES

1. Johnson, L.F., DeMeester, T.R., and Haggitt, R.C.: Endoscopic signs for gastroesophageal reflux objectively evaluated, Gastrointest. Endosc. **22**:151-155, 1976.
2. Kikendall, J.W., Friedman, A.C., Oyewole, M.A., Fleisher, D., and Johnson, L.F.: Pill-induced esophageal injury: case reports and review of the medical literature, Dig. Dis. Sci. **28**:174-182, 1983.
3. Johnson, L.F., and Moses, F.M.: Endoscopic evaluation of esophageal disease. In Castell, D.O., and Johnson, L.F., editors: Esophageal function in health and disease, New York, 1983, Elsevier North-Holland, Inc., pp. 237-254.
4. Johnson, L.F., DeMeester, T.R., and Haggitt, R.C.: Esophageal epithelial response to gastroesophageal reflux, a quantitative study, Am. J. Dig. Dis. **23**:498-509, 1978.
5. DeMeester, T.R., Lafontaine, E., Joelsson, B.E., et al.: The relationship of a hiatal hernia to the function of the body of the esophagus and the gastroesophageal junction, J. Thorac. Cardiovasc. Surg. **82**:547-558, 1981.
6. Mittal, R.K., Lange, R.C., and McCallum, R.W.: Identification and mechanism of delayed esophageal acid clearance in subjects with hiatal hernia, Gastroenterology **92**:130-135, 1987.
7. DeMeester, T.R., Johnson, L.F., Guy, G.J., Toscano, M.S., and Skinner, D.B.: Pattern of gastroesophageal reflux in health and disease, Ann. Surg. **184**:459-470, 1976.
8. Atkinson, M., and Van Gelder, A.: Esophageal intraluminal pH recording in the assessment of gastroesophageal reflux and its consequences, Am. J. Dig. Dis. **22**:265-370, 1978.
9. Thurer, R.L., DeMeester, T.R., and Johnson, L.F.: The distal esophageal sphincter and its relationship to gastroesophageal reflux, J. Surg. Res. **16**:418-423, 1974.
10. DeMeester, T.R., Bonavina, L., and Albertucci, M.: Nissen fundoplication for gastroesophageal reflux disease, Ann. Surg. **204**:9-20, 1986.

11. Wong, R.K.H., and Johnson, L.F.: Achalasia. In Castell, D.O., and Johnson, L.F., editors: Esophageal function in health and disease, New York, 1983, Elsevier Science Publishing Co., pp. 99-123.

12. Johnson, L.F.: Gastroesophageal reflux disease. In Spittell, J.A., Jr., editor: Clinical medicine, Hagerstown, Md., 1982, Harper & Row, Publishers, Inc., pp. 1-39.

13. Siegel, C.L., and Hendrix, T.R.: Esophageal motor abnormalities induced by acid perfusion in patients with heartburn, J. Clin. Invest. **42:**686-695. 1963.

14. Benz, L.J., Hootkin, L.A., Margulies, S., Donner, M.W., et al.: A comparison of clinical measurements of gastroesophageal reflux, Gastroenterology **62:**1-5, 1972.

15. Volpicelli, N.A., Yardley, J.H., and Hendrix, T.R.: A histopathologic demonstration of the association between gastritis and reflux esophagitis, Gastroenteroloy **68:**1007, 1975.

16. Johnson, D.A., Winters, C., Spurling, T.J., Cattaue, E.L., Chobanian, S.J., Hacker, J.F., and Hirszel, R.T.: Esophageal acid sensitivity in Barrett's esophagus, Gastroenterology **88:**1434, 1985.

17. Pellegrini, C.A., DeMeester, T.R., Johnson, L.F., and Skinner, D.B.: Alkaline gastroesophageal reflux, Am. J. Surg. **125:**177-183, 1978.

18. Mellow, M.H., Simpson, A.G., Watt, L., Schoolmeester, L., and Haye, O.L.: Esophageal acid perfusion in coronary artery disease: induction of myocardial ischemia, Gastroenterology, **85:**306-312, 1983.

19. Shay, S.S., Eggli, D., McDonald, C., and Johnson, L.F.: Gastric emptying of solid food in patients with gastroesophageal reflux, Gastroenterology **92:**459-465, 1987.

20. Johnson, D.A., Winters, C., Drane, W.E., Cattau, E.L., et al.: Solid phase gastric emptying in patients with Barrett's esophagus, Dig. Dis. Sci. **31:**1217-1220, 1986.

21. Shay, S.S., Johnson, L.F., Wong, R.K.H., Curtis, D.J., Rosenthal, R., Lamott, J.R., and Owensby, L.C.: Rumination, heartburn and daytime gastroesophageal reflux: a case study with mechanism defined and successfully treated with biofeedback therapy, J. Clin. Gastroenterol. **8:**115-126, 1986.

22. DeMeester, T.R., Johnson, L.F., Guy, J.J., Toscano, M.S., et al.: Patterns of gastroesophageal reflux in health and disease, Ann. Surg. **184:**459-470, 1976.

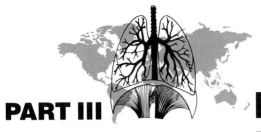

PART III   REFLUX PROBLEMS

CHAPTER 8

Definition, detection, and pathophysiology of gastroesophageal reflux disease

Tom R. DeMeester

DEFINITION

Gastroesophageal reflux disease accounts for approximately 75% of esophageal pathology and is among the most challenging diagnostic and therapeutic problems in benign esophageal disease. A major factor contributing to this challenge is the lack of a universally accepted definition of the disease.

Some have defined the disease as the presence of symptoms indicative of gastroesophageal reflux, such as heartburn and acid regurgitation.[1] There are at least three problems associated with defining the disease on symptomatic grounds. First, ascribing the cause of such typical symptoms as heartburn and acid regurgitation, in the absence of endoscopic esophagitis, to gastroesophageal reflux can be deceiving in that there are other disorders that can cause similar symptoms, such as achalasia, diffuse spasm, esophageal carcinoma, pyloric stenosis, cholelithiasis, gastritis, gastric or duodenal ulcer, and coronary artery disease.

Second, a symptomatic definition fails to incorporate the whole clinical spectrum of the disease. Gastroesophageal reflux is often associated with other disorders of the foregut, such as duodenogastric reflux[2] and esophagopharyngeal reflux.[3] The symptoms of the former are more gastric in character: epigastric pain, nausea, vomiting, postprandial fullness, and belching; symptoms of the latter are more respiratory in character: choking, chronic cough, wheezing, and hoarseness. When present, these symptoms can be of sufficient severity to override the typical symptoms of heartburn and regurgitation that are necessary to diagnose gastroesophageal reflux disease when defined on the basis of typical symptoms.

Third, a symptomatic definition of the disease does not provide the incentive to evaluate further the complaints of the patient. Foregut symptoms, like those previously mentioned, are among the most common complaints encountered by physicians. Because gastroesophageal reflux can have such a varied symptomatic presentation, no one symptom complex can be used to indicate its presence. Patients with poorly understood symptoms should be evaluated for the presence of gastroesophageal reflux disease. A symptomatic definition of the disease excludes this possibility, destroys diagnostic initiative, and encourages the use of nonspecific or shotgun therapy.

An alternative definition of gastroesophageal reflux disease is the presence of esophagitis on endoscopy. On the basis of this definition, only those symptomatic patients who have endoscopic esophagitis have the disease known as gastroesophageal reflux. There are problems with this definition as well. First, it assumes that all patients who have esophagitis have excessive regurgitation of gastric juice into the esophagus. Data indicate that this is true in 90% of patients, but in 10% the esophagitis results from other etiologies, the most common being unrecognized chemical injury from drug ingestion.[4,5] Second, the definition leaves undiagnosed those patients who have typical symptoms of gastroesophageal reflux—that is, heartburn or regurgitation—but do not have endoscopic esophagitis. Data indicate that this occurs in 40% of patients with typical symptoms of gastroesophageal reflux.[4] Obtaining an esophageal biopsy specimen is of little help, since the sensitivity and specificity of an epithelial biopsy specimen in the absence of endoscopic esophagitis are 0.75 and 0.9, respectively,[1] and depend on an interested pathologist for proper reading. Consequently, a large number of patients with complaints of sufficient severity to seek medical advice are treated expectantly. Third, the definition characterizes the disease on the basis of a complication of the disease. Esophagitis is a tissue injury that can occur as a consequence of the disease, but is not synonymous with the presence of the disease. Defining the disease by its complication is not a workable solution.

A third approach to defining gastroesophageal reflux disease is to measure the basic patho-physiologic abnormality accountable for the disease—the presence of more than normal esophageal exposure to gastric juice. In the past this was inferred by the presence of a hiatal hernia, later by endoscopic esophagitis, and more recently by a hypotensive lower esophageal sphincter pressure. Although these findings can occur with gastroesophageal reflux, it was difficult to always associate their presence with increased esophageal exposure to gastric juice. To measure the latter required the development of technology that allowed prolonged monitoring of the esophageal pH.[6] To use 24-hour esophageal pH monitoring to document the presence of increased esophageal exposure to gastric juice required the solution of three problems. First, initial monitoring studies showed that the esophagi of normal subjects were exposed to small amounts of gastric juice, usually after meals.[7] This became known as physiologic reflux, and in order to identify pathologic reflux it was necessary to measure what was normal physiologic reflux. Second, if measurement was necessary, what constituted a reflux episode and how should the data generated by 24-hour pH monitoring be expressed? Third, if several parameters, such as percent time of exposure, number of reflux episodes, and number of episodes lasting longer than 5 minutes, are used, how can they be assimilated into a single expression of normality or abnormality? Each of these questions is so important to the understanding of the pathophysiology of gastroesophageal reflux disease that it deserves separate discussion.

DETECTION

As already mentioned, it is difficult to define gastroesophageal reflux disease on the basis of symptoms or the presence of endoscopic esophagitis. Thus, to collect a group of patients who are representative of the disease is difficult, if not impossible. Consequently, to monitor the esophageal pH for 24 hours in a group of patients thought to have the disease, in order to determine characteristics of the 24-hour pH record that are

associated with disease, would be unlikely to result in a universally acceptable criterion. The approach used to solve this problem was to monitor a group of normal subjects, of appropriate age distribution, who had never had foregut symptoms, did not understand what the symptom of heartburn meant, had never taken any antacid therapy, had never had a reason to visit a physician regarding an upper gastrointestinal complaint, and had never had an upper gastrointestinal roentgenographic contrast study.[8] From the analysis of these records, it was noted that normal subjects rarely refluxed during sleep, but commonly did during and after eating. When reflux occurred, normal subjects rapidly cleared the gastric juice from their esophagi, regardless of position. A single reflux episode rarely caused a drop in esophageal pH below 4 for longer than 9 minutes, and over a 24-hour period, no more than three reflux episodes lasted longer than 5 minutes. In most situations, this exposure was without symptoms; however, a burning discomfort or a bitter taste occasionally occurred, which was annoying for a moment but rapidly cleared and was soon forgotten.

The observation in normal subjects that the cardia was significantly more competent during sleep in the supine position than while they were up and about in the upright position, seems paradoxical.[7] Why should it be easier for gastric juice to flow upward into the esophagus against gravity when the subject was upright than to spill into the esophagus when the subject was supine? There are four explanations for this. First, in the upright position there is a 12-mm pressure gradient between the resting positive intraabdominal pressure measured in the stomach and the most negative intrathoracic pressure measured at midesophageal level.[9] This gradient favors the flow of gastric juice up into the thoracic esophagus when a person is upright. The gradient diminishes when a person is supine, because of the elevation in the resting midesophageal pressure in this position.[10] Second, reflux episodes can occur in normal subjects when the lower esophageal sphincter relaxes on swallowing and the expected peristaltic sequences in the body of the esophagus fail to occur. This results in an unguarded moment when the relaxed sphincter is not protected by an oncoming peristaltic wave.[11] The average swallowing frequency in normal subjects is 72 times per hour while they are awake and in the upright position, and only seven times per hour while they are asleep and in the supine position.[12] Consequently, there are fewer opportunities for reflux to occur secondary to swallowing while a person is supine. Third, during the waking hours each pharyngeal swallow results in the ingestion of air, which collects in the stomach and causes gastric dilatation. When dilatation becomes excessive, a belch occurs.[13] Associated with the belch can be a reflux episode. Swallowing is less common in the supine position while a person is asleep. Consequently, there is less gastric dilatation and less tendency for belching to occur. Fourth, the lower esophageal sphincter pressure in normal subjects is significantly higher in the supine position than in the upright position.[14] This is due to the apposition of the hydrostatic pressure of the abdomen to the abdominal portion of the sphincter when a person is supine. In the upright position, the abdominal pressure surrounding the sphincter (that is, under the diaphragm) is negative compared to the atmospheric pressure and gradually increases the lower in the abdomen it is measured (see Table 8-1).[15] This pressure gradient tends to push gastric contents toward the cardia and encourages reflux into the esophagus when an individual is upright. In contrast, in the supine position, this pressure gradient diminishes and the abdominal hydrostatic pressure under the diaphragm increases, causing an increase in sphincter pressure and a more competent cardia.

Although 24-hour esophageal pH monitoring provided an objective means of detecting the occurrence of a pH change in the esophagus, there was no universal agreement as to what constituted a reflux episode and how the data collected by 24-hour pH monitoring should be expressed. At an international conference in Zurich, in April of 1986, on the technical aspects of intraluminal pH monitoring in humans,[16] the definition of a reflux episode was discussed and the majority of attendants agreed that for clinical diagnostic purposes, a reflux episode was a change in esophageal pH outside the range of 4 to 7 caused by the regurgitation of gastric contents into the esophagus. The range of 4 to 7 was used because 96% of the time, normal individuals maintained the esophageal pH within this range. Although it was recognized that changes in pH above 7 were less dependable than changes below 4, the former may indicate that alkaline gastric contents have been regurgitated into the esophagus and would encourage further investigation of that possibility. Using a pH of 4 as a cutoff point had considerable historical support as well. It was established as a reference point by Tuttle et al., who had shown that the onset of heartburn occurred when intraesophageal pH dropped to a value of less than 4.[17] Wallin and Madsen have shown that a pH value of less than 4, as opposed to less than 3 or 5, was the best discriminator in symptomatic volunteers,[18] and Vitale, et al. have shown that a pH value less than 4 best discriminates between symptomatic patients and controls.[19] In addition, animal data have strongly indicated that the proteolytic enzyme pepsin is a significant injurious agent in hemorrhagic erosive esophagitis.[20] This enzyme has a peak activity between the pH of 1.7 and the pH of 2.7 and is only 20% active at the pH of 4.

At the same Zurich conference a definition was constructed for the duration of a reflux episode: the time the esophageal pH is below 4 or above 7, or alternatively, the time the esophageal pH is at a pH interval below 4 (4 to 3, 3 to 2, 2 to 1, 1 to 0) or above 7 (7 to 8, 8 to 9). This definition, although very precise, posed a problem in determining when a reflux episode was over. This problem emerges when the esophageal pH at the end of a reflux episode fluctuates just above and below 4 before rising definitively above 4 and remaining above 4. Fig. 8-1 illustrates the problem and shows how a reflux episode could be recorded as a single episode or as one long episode followed by three short episodes.

Another area discussed at the Zurich conference was what constitutes an adequate length of test for intraesophageal pH monitoring—6, 18, or 24 hours. It was felt that patient tolerance permits a time period of 24 hours and that this

TABLE 8-1. Intraabdominal pressure (cm H_2O)

| Position of animal | Under diaphragm | | In lower part of abdomen |
	On inspiration	On expiration	
Supine	3.0	3.5	5.5
Erect	−3.5	−3.0	10.0
Head down	11.0	16.0	0.5
Head up (45 degrees)	−2.5	−2.0	8.0
Head down (45 degrees)	6.0	5.5	2.0
Supine (second reading)	3.0	3.5	5.5

From Lam, C.R.: Arch. Surg. **39**:1006, 1939. Copyright 1939, American Medical Association.

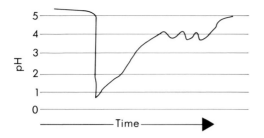

Fig. 8-1. Illustration of the difficulty of measuring the duration of a reflux episode. The problem is in determining the completion of an episode—that is, when the pH rises above 4 for the first time or when it stays above 4 for a period of time. The most precise definition is the former and allows for data collection without judgment.

would allow observation of gastroesophageal reflux patterns during one complete human circadian cycle. In addition, this period would allow physiologic activities such as eating in the upright position and sleeping in the recumbent position to be monitored. More important, it would obviate the common practice during short tests of having the patient assume a recumbent posture without falling asleep. Monitoring a patient in the supine position while he is awake is different from monitoring him while he is asleep. Although monitoring for a full 24-hour circadian cycle can be divided into a day segment and night segment, how should daytime and nighttime be defined for the patient being monitored: when does his day end and night begin? Should the determining factor be solar lighting with its seasonal change, an electric switch controlled by hospital policy, or observation of the patient's activity? Expecting personnel to record when the patient fell asleep or to define sleep polygraphically was deemed impractical. We subsequently found that forcing patients to lie recumbent for a period of time without sleeping results in increasing the supine reflux time over that measured during actual sleeping hours. In essence, it puts daytime reflux time into the night segment and makes the latter component less sensitive in detecting an abnormality. Consequently, we settled on having the patient define the two segments of the circadian cycle. He should be instructed to remain in the upright or sitting position while awake and to ingest three meals at the appropriate times. At night, bedtime should be signaled by having the patient turn a switch when he assumed a recumbent posture in preparation for sleep. Hence, the influence of both segments of the circadian cycle on the reflux pattern could be evaluated separately—that is, while the patient is awake in the

upright posture (before, during, and after meals) and while he is sleeping in the recumbent position at night.

In addition to the duration and division of the monitored period, there has not been universal agreement about how to express the pH data collected by the monitor. In 1974, we chose to express the 24-hour pH monitoring data as follows: (1) cumulative reflux time, expressed as percent of the monitored time, percent of the time monitored upright, and percent of the time monitored supine; (2) frequency of reflux episodes, expressed as number of reflux episodes per 24 hours; and (3) duration of reflux episodes, expressed as number of episodes longer than 5 minutes and the number of minutes in the longest episode.[6] This decision was based on clinical findings made in patients who were monitored and on the experience of other authors. Miller[21] had shown that control subjects seldom had reflux episodes lasting longer than 5 minutes, and we observed that patients who had disease often had profoundly long reflux episodes, which were not seen in normal subjects. Although we considered reporting these two duration parameters for both the upright time and the supine time, we felt that reporting them for the total 24-hour period would suffice. This is because the longest reflux episode usually occurred during the supine period and because episodes of more than 5 minutes had a similar detrimental effect whether they occurred in the upright position or the supine position. Hence, we felt that six parameters—that is, the cumulative acid exposure time for the upright, recumbent, and total 24-hour periods, expressed as percent time the pH was less than 4, along with the frequency of reflux episodes per 24 hours and the duration of reflux episodes during the 24 hours, expressed as the number of episodes lasting longer than 5 minutes and the length of the longest single episode, in minutes—would adequately quantitate all conceivable abnormal reflux patterns observed in patients with symptoms of gastroesophageal reflux disease.

To establish normal values, 49 asymptomatic control subjects were monitored, and the median and mean esophageal exposures to gastric juice were determined. From these reference points, upper limits of normal were established at the 90th percentile (see Table 8-2). If a symptomatic patient had an esophageal acid exposure outside the limits set for a normal subject, he was considered abnormal for the components measured. No effort was made to define a symptomatic population with the disease, since, as stated before, this was impossible. When normal values for the six components obtained from various

TABLE 8-2. Normal values* for 24-hour esophageal pH monitoring (n = 49)

Percent total time	<3.5
Percent upright time	<5.4
Percent supine time	<2.17
No. of episodes	<47
No. > 5 min	<3
Longest episode (min)	<16

Copyright Gastrosoft, Inc., Milwaukee, Wisc., 1985.
*90th percentile

centers throughout the world were compared at the Zurich conference, there was unexpected uniformity in their values.[16] This would indicate that esophageal acid exposure can be quantitated, and that in normal individuals it is similar despite nationality or dietary habits.

Today, ambulatory pH recorders allow patients to be monitored for 24 hours in the outpatient environment. This has raised the question of whether outpatient monitoring would result in greater esophageal exposure to gastric juice because of increased physical activity. Our experience in monitoring normal individuals in the hospital and in an outpatient environment has shown that the values obtained are similar. This would indicate that when the cardia is competent, the level of activity has no effect on esophageal exposure to gastric juice. Patients, on the other hand, tend to increase their esophageal exposure to gastric juice with activity. Restraining their activity in the hospital, however, does not return esophageal acid exposure to normal.

During the initial analysis of 24-hour esophageal pH records obtained from patients with typical symptoms of gastroesophageal reflux, it was noted that not all of the six parameters measured were uniformly abnormal. For instance, the component most commonly abnormal was acid exposure during the recumbent period, while the total number of reflux episodes per 24 hours had the lowest incidence of abnormality. This observation indicated a need to define when the 24-hour record was abnormal; in other words, even though the six components that were measured provided a means for identifying a variety of combinations, some of which were normal and others abnormal at the same time, it was unclear as to when an individual became abnormal.[8] To solve this problem, the standard deviation of the mean for each of the six components measured in 50 normal subjects was used as a weighting factor. The weighting factor for a component was divided into the value measured for that component in the patient. This gave a weight for each component according to the dependability and reliability of the measurement. For example, in normal subjects, the number of reflux episodes per 24 hours had a very wide standard deviation, resulting in a large number being used to weight the measured value in patients. This rewards few points for that particular component (points = measured value ÷ standard deviation). In contrast, normal individuals rarely reflux at night; therefore, the standard deviation for supine acid exposure is small. Consequently, an increase in nocturnal acid exposure is given greater weight and therefore more points. Hence, using the standard deviation as a weighting unit allows the data from normal individuals to be used to score the pH record of symptomatic patients in a manner that appropriately weights their departure from the physiologic reflux measured in normal subjects.

In order to use the standard deviation in this manner, it was necessary to deal with the data as though they were parametric data.[22] To do so, a zero point had to be established 2 standard deviations below the mean value measured for each particular component.[8] This technique allowed a scoring system to be built around the standard deviation as a weighting unit while treating the data as though they had a normal distribution. Thus, any measured value could be referenced to this zero point and in turn be awarded points whether it was below or above the normal mean value for that component (see Fig. 8-2). A 24-hour pH composite score was obtained by adding the weighted points calculated for each of the six components. The composite score was considered abnormal when it exceeded the mean plus 2 standard deviations of the score calculated from the 50 control subjects.

Recently, we have computerized this process and applied it to measure the amount of esophageal acid exposure at each whole-number pH threshold. The data are expressed as the percent time the esophageal pH is below 1, 2, 3, or 4, or above 7 or 8. The number of reflux episodes, the number of reflux episodes lasting longer than 5 minutes, and the longest reflux episode are also measured for each pH threshold. The data are shown graphically in Fig. 8-3, *A*. A score can be calculated for each pH threshold and also expressed graphically (Fig. 8-3, *B*). An IBM-compatible program to perform this function is available from Gastrosoft.*

At the present time 24-hour esophageal pH

---

*Copyright 1986, Gastrosoft, 611 N. Broadway, Milwaukee, Wisc. 53202.

Fig. 8-2. Concept of using the standard deviation as the scoring unit. Note the establishment of an abstract zero point 2 standard deviations below the mean value for total-period acid exposure. Theoretically, that allows scoring the measurement as though the normal values were parametric.

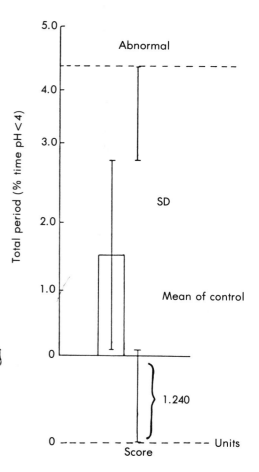

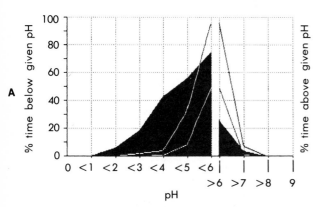

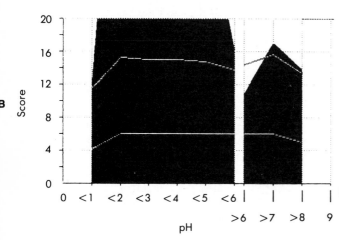

Fig. 8-3. A, Graphic display of ESOpHOGRAM showing the median and 90th percentile levels in 50 normal individuals, using whole pH values above and below 6 as thresholds. The black area represents measurements made in a patient with acid reflux; it shows increased exposure over that seen in normals below the pH of 5, 4, 3, and 2. **B,** The composite score used to express the overall pH result. The clear line represents the median score and 97.5 percentile of 50 normal subjects. The black area represents the score of the patient in **A** with increased esophageal acid and alkaline exposure measured at pH of <1, <2, <3, <4, <5, >7, and >8.

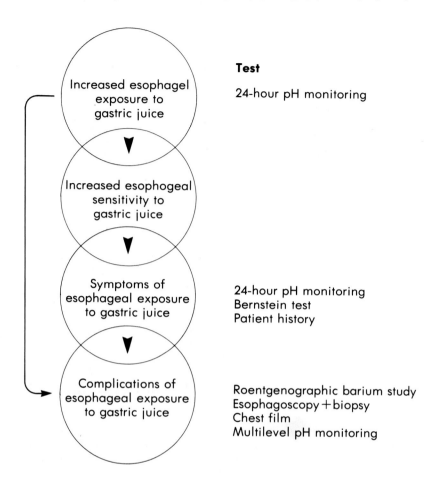

Test

24-hour pH monitoring

24-hour pH monitoring
Bernstein test
Patient history

Roentgenographic barium study
Esophagoscopy + biopsy
Chest film
Multilevel pH monitoring

Fig. 8-4. Pathophysiologic sequence of gastroesophageal reflux disease.

monitoring, when analyzed according to the above method, is the most accurate means of detecting increased esophageal exposure to gastric juice. It does not, however, determine the cause of the increased exposure.

PATHOPHYSIOLOGY

The pathophysiology of gastroesophageal reflux disease is illustrated in Fig. 8-4. The basic abnormality is increased esophageal exposure to gastric juice. This leads to an increased sensitivity of the esophagus to gastric juice, which in turn gives rise to symptoms of increased esophageal exposure to gastric juice. The latter is suggested by the patient's clinical history, supported by inducing the symptoms with the infusion of acid into the esophagus, and documented by relating the patient's symptoms to reflux episodes recorded during 24-hour esophageal pH monitoring. If the increased exposure to gastric juice persists, complications can occur, such as esophagitis, stricture, the development of

Barrett's esophagus, and progressive pulmonary fibrosis or recurrent pneumonia from repetitive pulmonary aspiration. Usually, but not always, the development of esophagitis or a luminal stricture is preceded by symptoms from an esophagus that has become sensitive to acid. A few patients, however, can develop these complications without going through the sensitivity and symptom stages. This is probably due to the reflux of gastric juice with a pH between 4 and 7 resulting in an increased esophageal exposure to gastric juice without the symptoms associated with acid reflux. Gastric juice of this pH can occur from duodenogastric reflux (see Fig. 8-5) or medical therapy with H_2 blockers. Consequently, the absence of classical symptoms cannot be used to exclude the presence of the disease, and monitoring the symptom of heartburn cannot be used to indicate control of the disease. On the other hand, visual confirmation of the presence of a complication is not an absolute indicator of the presence of gastroesophageal reflux disease. The detection of the disease requires, as previously discussed, the documenta-

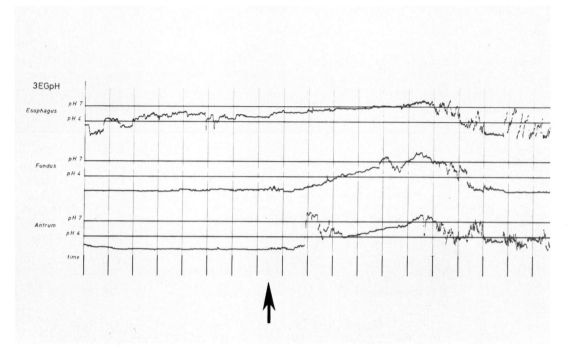

Fig. 8-5. Duodenogastric reflux in a patient with pH probes positioned in the antrum, fundus, and esophagus. Duodenogastric regurgitation occurs at arrow and alters the pH in the antrum, fundus, and esophagus. The esophageal pH rises within its normal band of 4 to 7 and does not move out of the normal pH band into <7 or >4 until late in the reflux episode. Vertical lines represent 1-hour intervals. (Courtesy S. Mattioli.)

tion of increased exposure of the esophagus to gastric juice, but this does not indicate the cause of the increased exposure.

Causes of increased esophageal exposure to gastric juice

There are three known causes of increased esophageal exposure to gastric juice in patients with gastroesophageal reflux disease. The first is a mechanically incompetent lower esophageal sphincter. The identification of this cause is important, since it is the one etiology that antireflux surgery is designed to correct. The other two causes are inefficient esophageal clearance of reflux gastric juice and abnormalities of the gastric reservoir that augment physiologic reflux, such as increased gastric pressure, excessive gastric dilatation, delayed gastric emptying, and/or increased gastric acid secretion.

Competence of lower esophageal sphincter

Sphincter pressure. The introduction of esophageal manometry demonstrated that the mean lower esophageal sphincter pressure measured in a population of patients with symptoms

associated with increased esophageal acid exposure was lower than that measured in a population of normal subjects.[23] This finding focused attention on sphincter pressure as the main factor by which competence of the cardia was maintained. Subsequent studies documented this clinical observation by showing that patients with a sphincter pressure of 5 mm Hg or less had a 75% incidence of increased esophageal exposure to gastric juice (see Fig. 8-6).[24] There was, however, no explanation why the amplitude of the lower esophageal sphincter pressure was lower in some individuals than in others. Various factors have been suggested, including neural, humeral, positional, and myogenic influences. A neuroexcitatory mechanism for the maintenance of basal sphincter tone has been questioned, since truncal vagotomy has no effect on the resting lower esophageal sphincter pressure.[25] Similarly, a pharmacologic mechanism has been proposed, since doses of cholinergic agents can cause an increase in sphincter pressure, and anticholinergic agents reduce it. However, the relevance of these observations to explain a low sphincter pressure has not been shown.[26] The influence of many hormones on the lower esophageal sphincter has

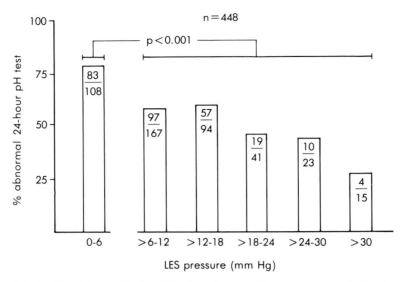

Fig. 8-6. Relationship of the amplitude of distal esophageal sphincter pressure to the incidence of an abnormal result of a 24-hour esophageal pH monitoring test. The incidence of an abnormal test result was significantly higher in patients with a pressure of 6 mm Hg or less.

been investigated, but the effects noted are associated with pharmacologic doses and probably do not represent the true physiologic situation.[26] The environmental location of the lower esophageal sphincter, either in the abdomen or in the chest, does not seem to be a major factor in the genesis of the pressure, since it can be measured when the chest and the abdomen are surgically opened and the distal esophagus is being held freely in the hand of the surgeon.[27]

It appears that under normal circumstances, neither neural, humeral, nor positional factors are responsible for maintaining an adequate resting sphincter pressure, and the explanation for a decreased sphincter pressure in some individuals is most probably an abnormality of myogenic function. Biancani and co-workers have shown that the lower esophageal sphincter's muscles' response to stretch is reduced in patients with incompetent cardias.[28] This suggested that the sphincter pressure depends on the length and tension properties of the sphincter's smooth muscle. Indeed, a reduction in sphincter pressure is associated with measured abnormalities in length-tension characteristics (see Fig. 8-7). Furthermore, a surgical fundoplication that restores sphincter pressure to normal also corrects the abnormal length-tension characteristics.[28]

Sphincter abdominal length. Despite the statistical correlations between the sphincter pressure and the presence of gastroesophageal reflux on a population basis, it became evident that the magnitude of the sphincter pressure was not always related to competence of the cardia in the

individual patient.[29] Some patients with low pressure had competent cardias, whereas others with high pressure had incompetent cardias. As further experience was gained, it became evident that there was a marked overlap between the sphincter pressure of normal subjects and that of patients who refluxed, and that the administration of atropine, which reduces the sphincter pressure, did not increase the incidence of gastroesophageal reflux in normal subjects.[30,31] This suggested that other factors besides the pressure of the sphincter were important in maintaining competence.

Further analysis of the data obtained from patients who underwent both esophageal manometry and 24-hour esophageal pH monitoring showed that the competence of the cardia was also related to the length of the sphincter exposed to the positive pressure environment of the abdomen (see Fig. 8-8).[24] The latter is measured manometrically as the length of sphincter below the respiratory inversion point. This finding drew attention to the intraabdominal position of the sphincter as an additional factor contributing to competence of the cardia. These manometric findings supported the anatomic measurement of Bombeck and co-workers, who showed a high correlation between the level of insertion of the phrenoesophageal membrane on the esophagus and the presence of esophagitis.[32] Even when a hiatal hernia was present, a portion of the sphincter was exposed to abdominal pressure because of the presence of the hernia sac, which acts as a conduit to transmit changes in intraab-

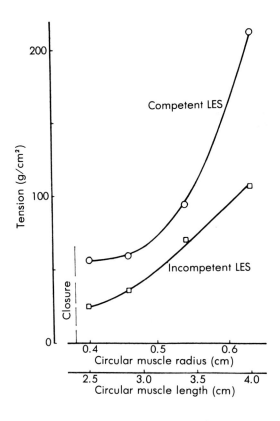

Fig. 8-7. Length-tension characteristics of competent and incompetent lower esophageal sphincters. The tension was calculated from pressure measurements according to the equation $Tm = Prm/tm$, where Tm is the average circular muscle tension, P the intraluminal pressure, rm the inner radius of the circular muscle layer, and tm its thickness. The radius of the circular muscle was calculated from the probe used. Circular muscle length equals muscle radius times 2. At closure the radius of the circular muscle is 0.38 cm, as indicated by the broken line. (From DeMeester, T.R.: Experimental and clinical evidence for mechanical factors in the competency of the cardia. In Van Heukelem, H.A., Gooszen, H.G., Terpstra, J.B., and Belsey, R.H.R., editors: Pathological gastroesophageal reflux, Amsterdam, 1982, Zuid-Nederlandse Uitgevers-Maatschappij B.V., pp. 17-34.)

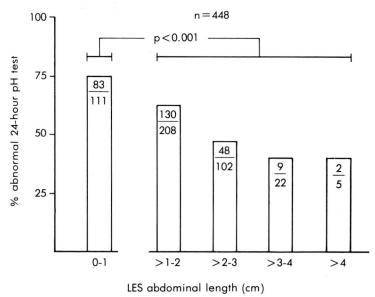

Fig. 8-8. Relationship of the abdominal length of the distal esophageal sphincter to the incidence of an abnormal result of a 24-hour esophageal pH monitoring test. The incidence of an abnormal test result was significantly higher in patients with an abdominal length of 1 cm or less.

dominal pressure through the diaphragm and around the distal esophagus contained within the sac. This structural arrangement allows for compression of the segment of the sphincter that is within the sac and that is exposed to abdominal pressure, to prevent reflux from occurring secondary to changes in intraabdominal pressure. Shortening the abdominal segment, whether it is in the hernia sac or not, results in a sphincter that mechanically is unable to be affected by

TABLE 8-3. Pressures (mm Hg) induced by respiratory and positional maneuvers in 10 patients

Maneuver	Thoracic esophagus	Lower esophageal sphincter		Gastric fundus
		Thoracic part	Abdominal part	
Valsalva	30.2 (± 3.6)	24.9 (± 4.6)*	30.7 (± 2.3)*	36.4 (± 1.3)
Leg raising	0.38 (± 0.1)	3.7 (± 3.5)†	16.3 (± 2.8)	17.2 (± 3.3)
Muller	< − 22	− 14.9(± 3.8)	16.1 (± 4.7)	7.3 (± 1.9)

Differences between thoracic and abdominal portions of the lower esophageal sphincter are all significant (p<.05) except for *. All measurements differ significantly from resting pressure (p<.05) except for †.

TABLE 8-4. Normal manometric values for the lower esophageal sphincter (n = 50)

	Mean	Mean − 2 SD	Mean ± 2 SD	Median	Percentile	
					2.5	97.5
Pressure (mm Hg)	13.8 ± 4.6	4.6	23.0	13	5.8	27.7
Overall length (cm)	3.7 ± 0.8	2.1	5.3	3.6	2.1	5.6
Abdominal length (cm)	2.2 ± 0.8	0.6	3.8	2	0.9	4.7

changes in abdominal pressure and consequently is incompetent.[33]

These findings suggested that the ability of the intraabdominal portion of the sphincter to increase its pressure following increases in intraabdominal pressure was an important component of a competent sphincter. Whether intrinsic pressure on the intraabdominal segment of the sphincter or an adaptive reflux response intrinsic to the cardia and the distal esophagus was responsible for the increase in pressure still needs to be discerned. With the first explanation, the behavior of the sphincter could be accounted for simply on the basis of intrinsic mechanical factors, whereas the second mechanism implicates complex neural reflexes, with less emphasis on a mechanical function of the cardia. To differentiate between these two possibilities, we challenged the lower esophageal sphincter with various intraabdominal and intrathoracic pressures and determined their effects on its thoracic and abdominal segments in patients whose reflux status was defined by 24-hour esophageal pH monitoring.[34] Table 8-3 shows changes in pressure induced by respiratory and positional maneuvers in 10 such patients. The results showed that each portion of the sphincter, abdominal or thoracic, was markedly affected by changes in its environment and that each was affected independently. An increase in abdominal pressure caused an increase in the luminal pressure of the abdominal portion of the sphincter and the stomach, while the thoracic portion and the esophagus remained unaffected, and vice versa. This behavior suggests that changes in sphincter pressure occurring with changes in environmental pressures are due sim-

ply to extrinsic mechanical factors rather than to complex neural reflexes. The esophagus is a soft muscular tube, and, as such, the intraluminal pressure of the sphincter results both from applied extrinsic environmental pressures and from the intrinsic myogenic tone. To prevent reflux, the tiny portion of intragastric pressure that is due to gastric muscle tone is all that must be controlled by the muscle of the lower esophageal sphincter, as long as both the abdominal portion of the sphincter and the stomach are able to respond similarly to environmental pressure changes. This study further showed that at least 1 cm of the sphincter must be exposed to the positive pressure environment of the abdomen in order for it to respond adequately to changes in environmental pressures. Lesser amounts result in a mechanical disadvantage, which allows reflux to occur with increases in intraabdominal pressure secondary to straining or to changes in body position. Of interest is that an abdominal length of sphincter measuring 1 cm or less is outside of the 97.5 percentile range measured in normal subjects (see Table 8-4). This, plus the above experimental findings, are independent observations that support the importance of the abdominal sphincter length as a factor in the ability of a sphincter to maintain competence.

Although these findings have focused on the mechanical components of the cardia in preventing reflux from spontaneous rises in intraabdominal pressure, the role of intraabdominal pressure as an etiological factor in reflux was based only on suggestive clinical histories. Therefore, we investigated whether spontaneous changes in intraabdominal pressure could cause gastroesophageal reflux and what percentage of reflux episodes are due to this mechanism.[35] This study was done in 19 patients with incompetent sphincters who had simultaneous 24-hour monitoring of esophageal pH and intraabdominal pressure. During the monitoring period there was an average of 2.7 reflux episodes per hour, with a similar number occurring during the day and night. Thirty-nine percent of the reflux episodes occurred either simultaneously with or within 30 seconds of an increase in intraabdominal pressure. The remaining 61% of the reflux episodes were unrelated to an increase in intraabdominal pressure.

We performed a clinical study that confirms the important role of sphincter pressure and abdominal length in the competence of the cardia.[36] Three hundred and ninety-one consecutive patients with symptoms suggestive of gastroesophageal reflux had both esophageal manometry and 24-hour pH monitoring. Table 8-5 was constructed by classifying the patients as to the length of the sphincter exposed to the positive pressure environment of the abdomen and the amplitude of its pressure. The competence of the cardia was evaluated with 24-hour pH monitoring of the distal esophagus, and the incidence of an incompetent cardia was calculated for each of the groups. The table shows that competence of the cardia is related to the level of pressure in the lower esophageal sphincter, the length of sphincter exposed to the positive pressure environment in the abdomen, and an interaction between both. It further shows that a minimum pressure and a minimum length of sphincter in the abdomen are simultaneously required for competence. For example, when the sphincter pressure is 5 mm Hg or less, the prevalence of gastroesophageal reflux approaches 90% irrespective of the length of the abdominal segment. Similarly, when the length of the abdominal segment is less than 1 cm, the prevalence of gastroesophageal reflux approaches 90% irrespective of the length of the abdominal segment. Similarly, when the length of the abdominal segment is less than 1 cm, the prevalence of gastroesophageal reflux approaches 90% irrespective of the amplitude of the pressure in the sphincter. The table further shows that a hypotensive sphincter can occur in the presence of an adequate length of sphincter in the abdomen and that normal sphincter pressure can occur in the presence of a short abdominal segment. This indicates that basal sphincter pressure is not caused by the positive pressure of the abdomen acting on the abdominal segment, but rather is due to an intrinsic myogenic factor. Further analysis of Table 8-5 shows that progressive

TABLE 8-5. Incidence of increased esophageal acid exposure in patients classified according to abdominal length* and pressure measurements of lower esophageal sphincter

Pressure (mm Hg)	Abdominal length (cm)		
	0-1	> 1-2	> 2
0-5			
%	92%	88%	87.5%
n	34/37	22/25	7/8
> 5-10			
%	90%	58%	68%
n	19/21	29/50	17/25
> 10-15			
%	86%	77%	76%
n	14/16	34/44	26/34
> 15-20			
%	67%	60%	71%
n	4/6	15/25	20/28
> 20			
%	90%	40%	19%
n	9/10	10/25	7/37

*Length (cm) of sphincter below respiratory inversion point.

increases in both lower esophageal sphincter pressure and the length of sphincter in the abdomen result in a decrease in the incidence of a positive 24-hour pH test. Thus, the relationship between abdominal length and sphincter pressure in reflux control is not strictly additive but includes an interaction effect. This indicates that changes in sphincter pressure or abdominal length also influence the relative contributions of each to the competence mechanism.

To understand this functional relationship, we developed an in vitro model in which we are able to study the functions of sphincter pressure and the length exposed to abdominal pressure individually and together.[24] On the basis of this study, we concluded that the competence of the cardia to challenges of intraabdominal pressure was solely the function of the length of the lower esophageal sphincter exposed to the positive pressure environment of the abdomen. Fig. 8-9 shows that in the absence of any sphincter pressure, an abdominal length of 4 cm is necessary to prevent reflux resulting from changes in intraabdominal pressure and that shorter lengths necessitate the addition of intrinsic sphincter pressure in order to maintain competence. Fig. 8-9 also shows that a minimum length of 1 cm of sphincter exposed to abdominal pressure is required to protect against challenges of increased intraabdominal pressure, since the amplitude of pressure necessary to achieve competence with

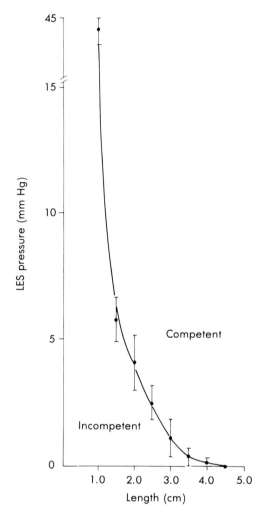

Fig. 8-9. Relationship of lower esophageal sphincter pressure and abdominal length to competence of the cardia. The plotted line represents the pressure necessary for a given abdominal sphincter length to maintain competence of the cardia against challenges of intraabdominal pressure. Lengths less than 1 cm cannot be compensated for by an increase in pressure, and incompetence is predictable.

less than this amount becomes infinite. Between these two extremes, the shorter the intraabdominal sphincter length, the greater the intrinsic sphincter pressure necessary to maintain competence. From this study, and studies in normal individuals, it became evident that patients who have a lower esophageal sphincter pressure of 6 mm Hg or less, or less than 1 cm of the sphincter below the respiratory inversion point, have a severe mechanical defect of the cardia. These values are in the 2.5 percentile of normal individuals (see Table 8-4).

Table 8-5 also indicates that other factors besides sphincter pressure and the length of

sphincter exposed to the positive pressure of the abdomen are important in maintaining the competence of the cardia; a number of patients who have adequate sphincter pressure and abdominal length continue to reflux, although the incidence of reflux in such patients is low.

Sphincter overall length. It was noteworthy that several of these patients had very short overall sphincter lengths. It was hypothesized that under these conditions reflux could occur, despite a normal lower esophageal sphincter pressure and abdominal length, because the length over which the pressure was exerted was insufficient to provide enough resistance to the flow of gastric contents into the esophagus. To test this hypothesis, the relationship of the lower esophageal sphincter pressure and overall length to the resistance to flow through the cardia was studied using an electrolytic transducer in an in vitro model.[13] This transducer was designed to measure the changes in resistance to the flow of electrons through an electrolyte fluid column caused by variations in the length and degree of compression of the column. The transducer was positioned across the sphincter portion of the model, and measurements were made after incremental increases in distal esophageal sphincter pressure and length. An independent linear increase in electrical resistance occurred with incremental increases in either lower esophageal sphincter pressure or length (see Fig. 8-10). These findings showed that resistance to the flow of electrons varies with changes in the cross-sectional area of the electrolyte column caused by changes in both sphincter pressure and the length over which the pressure is exerted. Thus, the resistance to flow through the cardia is related to the integrated effects of lower esophageal sphincter pressure and length.

This hypothesis was tested in the clinical situation.[13] Studies in asymptomatic subjects showed that the lower limit of normal for the length of the lower esophageal sphincter, based on the 2.5 percentile or 2 standard deviations below the mean, was less than 2 cm (see Table 8-4). Fig. 8-11 shows the incidence of an abnormal 24-hour pH test in patients with symptoms suggestive of gastroesophageal reflux who were classified according to overall sphincter length. Patients with an overall sphincter length less than 2 cm had a statistically increased incidence of an abnormal 24-hour test when compared with those with greater lengths. In Table 8-6 the patients in Fig. 8-11 were grouped according to lower esophageal sphincter pressure and overall length, and the incidence of an abnormal 24-hour pH test was calculated for each of the groups. As in Table

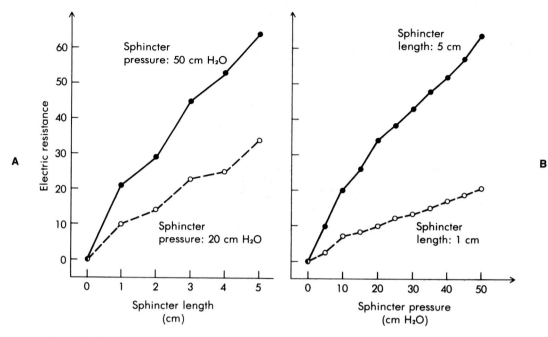

Fig. 8-10. The influence of overall sphincter length (**A**) and sphincter pressure (**B**) on resistance to flow of electrons through the cardia as measured by the electrolytic transducer. Resistance is expressed in relative units of deflection from the baseline on the strip recording.

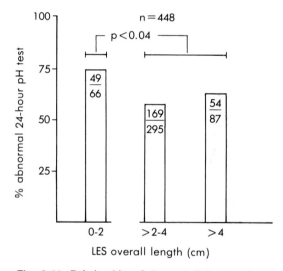

Fig. 8-11. Relationship of the overall length of the lower esophageal sphincter to the incidence of an abnormal 24-hour esophageal pH monitoring test. The incidence of an abnormal test was significantly higher in patients with a length of 2 cm or less.

TABLE 8-6. Incidence of increased esophageal acid exposure in patients classified according to overall length and pressure measurements of lower esophageal sphincter

Pressure (mm Hg)	Overall length (cm)		
	0-2	> 2-4	> 4
0-6			
%	74%	79%	81%
n	14/19	46/58	25/31
> 6-12			
%	82%	51%	69%
n	18/22	59/116	20/29
> 12-18			
%	65%	63%	40%
n	11/17	42/67	4/10
> 18-24			
%	80%	46%	30%
n	4/5	12/26	3/10
> 24			
%	67%	36%	29%
n	2/3	10/28	2/7

8-5, the importance of the lower esophageal sphincter pressure in maintaining competence of the cardia was shown, in that patients with a pressure of 6 mm Hg or less had a high incidence of an abnormal 24-hour test. This occurred regardless of the overall length of the lower esophageal sphincter. Table 8-6 also shows that patients with an overall sphincter length of less than 2 cm had a high incidence of an abnormal 24-hour test regardless of the resting lower esoph-

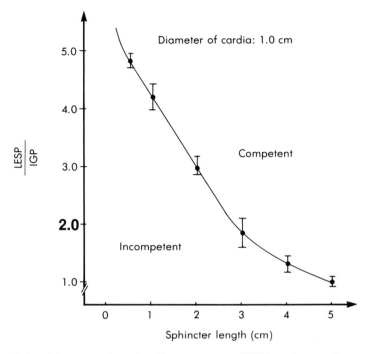

Fig. 8-12. Ratio of lower esophageal sphincter pressure (*LESP*) to intragastric pressure (*IGP*) necessary to maintain competence for a given overall sphincter length. The plotted line represents the ratio of pressure necessary for a given overall sphincter length to maintain competence of the cardia against challenges of intragastric pressure that rises above intraabdominal pressure.

ageal sphincter pressure. Progressive increases in lower esophageal sphincter pressure and in the overall length of the sphincter resulted in decreases in the prevalence of gastroesophageal reflux, but as was true in regard to abdominal sphincter length and pressure in Table 8-5, the relationship between overall length and sphincter pressure in reflux control was not strictly additive but included an interaction effect; changes in either influenced the contribution of each to the competence of the sphincter. The importance of the abdominal length of the sphincter is to resist reflux secondary to increases in intraabdominal pressure. The importance of the overall length of the sphincter is to retard reflux resulting from changes in intragastric pressure independent of intraabdominal pressure.

To understand this functional relationship, we again made overall use of our in vitro model, in which we could study the function of the sphincter's pressure and length individually and together.[13] Fig. 8-12 shows that the ratio of lower esophageal sphincter pressure to intragastric pressure necessary to maintain competence is inversely related to the overall length of the sphincter. When the sphincter length is 2 cm or less, a pressure in excess of two to three times the resting intragastric pressure, or 16 to 24 mm Hg

above an intragastric pressure of 8 mm Hg, is necessary to prevent reflux. Since this represents a high normal sphincter pressure, most patients with lower esophageal sphincters of only 2 cm in length will be prone to reflux with small increases in intragastric pressure.

Of importance is the fact that the overall sphincter length is affected by the degree of gastric dilatation[13]; that is, as the stomach dilates the sphincter becomes shorter, in a manner similar to the neck of a balloon becoming shorter on inflation. The relationship among overall sphincter length, gastric dilatation, and competence of the cardia is shown in Fig. 8-13. Dilatation of the stomach adversely affects the degree of competence achieved by a given length of sphincter. A cardia of 1 cm (30F) in diameter requires a sphincter of 3 cm in length to remain competent. A cardia of 3 cm (90F) in diameter requires a length of 5 cm for competence. Therefore, increasing the diameter of the cardia results in decreasing the competence of the cardia by reducing the overall length of the sphincter.

Summary. The resistance to gastroesophageal reflux provided by the cardia depends on the lower esophageal sphincter pressure, the length of the sphincter exposed to the positive pressure environment of the abdomen, and the overall

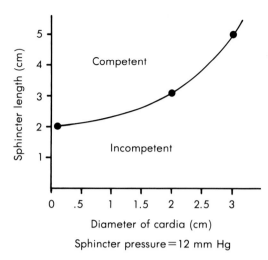

Sphincter pressure = 12 mm Hg

Fig. 8-13. Overall sphincter length necessary to maintain competence for a given diameter of the cardia. The plotted line represents the overall length of sphincter necessary to maintain competence of the cardia for a given degree of gastric dilatation as measured by the diameter of the cardia at the lower border of the sphincter.

length of the sphincter. From a clinical perspective, mechanical failure of the cardia is diagnosed by identifying with esophageal manometry inadequate mechanical characteristics. On the basis of the manometric measurements obtained from 50 control subjects (see Table 8-4), we have defined a mechanically inadequate cardia as one having any of the following: an average lower esophageal sphincter pressure of 6 mm Hg or less, an average lower esophageal sphincter length exposed to the positive pressure environment in the abdomen of 1 cm or less, and an average overall sphincter length of 2 cm or less. These values are in the 2.5 percentile, or 2 standard deviations below the mean measurements obtained from the normal subjects.

The most common cause of an incompetent cardia is an inadequate lower esophageal sphincter pressure, but the efficiency of a sphincter with normal pressure can be nullified by an inadequate abdominal length or an abnormally short overall length (see Fig. 8-14). Patients with low lower esophageal sphincter pressure, or those with normal pressure but short abdominal length, are

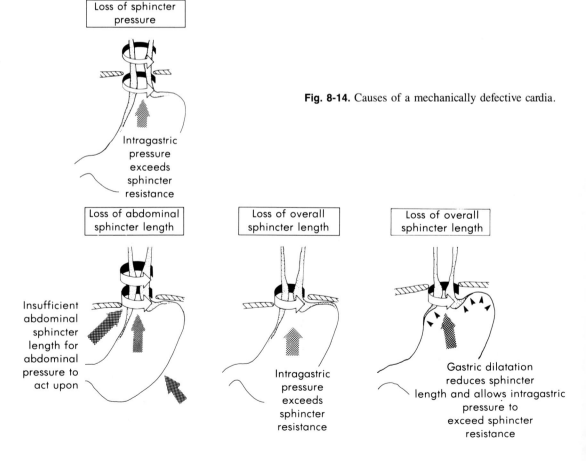

Fig. 8-14. Causes of a mechanically defective cardia.

unable to cope with reflux caused by fluctuations in intraabdominal pressure that occur with daily activities or changes in body position. Patients with low lower esophageal sphincter pressure, or those with normal pressure but short overall length, are unable to cope with reflux caused by increases in intragastric pressure in excess of intraabdominal pressure. In this situation, reflux can occur whenever the ratio of lower esophageal sphincter pressure to intragastric pressure is less than that necessary to provide competence for the overall length of sphincter present. Also, patients who have short overall sphincter length on a resting esophageal motility study are less able to protect against reflux caused by progressive gastric dilatation.

Surgery is a symptom-driven mechanical approach to the treatment of gastroesophageal reflux caused by a mechanically defective sphincter. Consequently, an antireflux procedure should be considered only for patients who have (1) uncontrolled symptoms of increased esophageal exposure to gastric juice (i.e., heartburn and regurgitation); (2) a documented increase in esophageal exposure to gastric juice as shown by 24-hour esophageal pH monitoring; and (3) a documented mechanical deficiency of the cardia on manometry. If the cardia is manometrically normal, the patient should be evaluated for other causes of abnormal esophageal exposure to gastric juice.

Esophageal clearance of reflux material

The second cause of increased esophageal exposure to gastric juice is inefficient esophageal clearance of reflux material. This is a relatively rare, isolated abnormality and is apt to occur in association with a mechanically defective cardia, which augments the esophageal exposure to gastric juice by prolonging the duration of each reflux episode.

Four factors important in esophageal clearance are gravity, esophageal motor activity, salivation, and the presence of a hiatal hernia.[7,33,37,38] The upright position enhances esophageal emptying as compared with the supine position, which explains the occurrence of severe reflux disease in patients who are nocturnal refluxers.[7] Normally, the esophagus is cleared by a peristaltic pressure wave initiated with a pharyngeal swallow—that is, primary peristalsis—or by local esophageal irritation or distention—that is, secondary peristalsis. The former is voluntary and is the major esophageal motor activity that clears the esophagus of reflux material in normal subjects. Secondary peristalsis can occur after the regurgitation of a large volume of gastric juice or after a sudden drop in esophageal pH.[39] The esophageal

activity initiated can be peristaltic or nonperistaltic—that is, simultaneous or repetitive contractions. When the latter occurs, it rarely causes dysphagia, but reduces the efficiency of esophageal clearance, and encourages the regurgitation of reflux material into the pharynx, which predisposes the patient to aspiration.[40]

Salivation contributes to esophageal clearance by neutralizing the minute amount of acid that is left following a peristaltic wave. Esophageal clearance time is increased significantly when saliva is removed by suction and, conversely, decreased when salivation is stimulated by oral lozenges.[38] Thus, esophageal acid clearance normally occurs as a two-step process and is aided by gravity when a person is in the upright position. First, virtually all of the gastric juice that is refluxed is evacuated from the esophagus by one or two peristaltic sequences, leaving a minimal residual amount that sustains a low pH. Second, the residual acid is neutralized by the swallowed saliva. The effectiveness of saliva in neutralizing the residual acid may contribute to a habit of repetitive pharyngeal swallowing and gum chewing in patients who have gastroesophageal reflux disease. This excessive pharyngeal swallowing activity can result in a cyclic process of gastric distention, belching, reflux, and more pharyngeal swallowing to clear the refluxed gastric juice.

A hiatal hernia can reduce esophageal propulsion efficiency, causing inadequate esophageal clearance.[33] Recent studies have shown that the presence of a hernia is unrelated to the competence of the cardia, but does contribute to a longer esophageal transit time. The decrease in transit time is not due to a motility disorder, but is secondary to the loss of esophageal anchorage in the abdomen. This significantly interferes with the mechanics of esophageal contractions in the distal third of the esophagus, with reduced efficiency in the clearing of refluxed gastric contents. Reduction of the hernia and effective anchoring of the esophagus in the abdomen improve the mechanics and esophageal clearance. In this regard, a patient with a mechanically defective cardia and a large hiatal hernia has a severely compromised antireflux mechanism. He lacks a mechanically effective lower esophageal sphincter to protect against the regurgitation of gastric juice into the esophagus and an effective clearance mechanism to evacuate the refluxed gastric juice back into the stomach.

In some patients, a hiatal hernia not only interferes with the mechanics of esophageal clearance but also restricts the forward propulsion of a swallowed bolus by what Edwards has termed "abnormal hiatal flow."[41] If the diaphragmatic hiatus forms a narrow slit, there can be an accumulation of swallowed material within the herniated stomach above the diaphragm, resulting in delayed passage of the bolus into the subdiaphragmatic stomach and symptoms of dysphagia. When the resistance to flow through the diaphragmatic hiatus is excessive, the herniated portion of the stomach becomes distended and the intragastric pressure within the hernia overcomes the sphincter pressure, and its contents regurgitate into the esophagus. As expected, these patients complain of regurgitation and dysphagia. Heartburn may or may not be present, depending on the competence of the sphincter and the presence of gastric juice in the herniated portion of the stomach.

Gastric function abnormalities

The third reason for increased esophageal exposure to gastric juice is abnormalities of gastric function. In this situation, the reflux of gastric contents occurs through a mechanically normal lower esophageal sphincter. There are four gastric abnormalities known to cause this: gastric dilatation,[13] increased intragastric pressure,[13] persistent gastric reservoir,[42] and increased gastric acid secretion.[43] As pointed out before, excessive gastric dilatation can shorten the overall length of a normal sphincter, resulting in incompetence of the sphincter and reflux of gastric contents into the esophagus. Excessive gastric dilatation can occur from aerophagia in patients who reflux and habitually swallow to clear the esophagus. Each pharyngeal swallow results in the propulsion of approximately 1 to 2 ml of air into the stomach. When the amount of air entering the stomach exceeds the capacity to evacuate it, gastric dilatation occurs, causing shortening of the sphincter and belching with further reflux. Patients who reflux tend also to be chronic gum chewers because the swallowed saliva helps to neutralize the acid in the esophagus. The repetitive swallowing, however, results in aerophagia, gastric distention, and reflux. Similarly, patients who have decreased saliva formation, as occurs with Sjögren's syndrome or after radiation therapy to the head and neck, swallow excessively and consequently also have aerophagia. Gastric dilatation can also occur from a loss of secondary peristalsis, usually as a result of a collagen vascular disease or diabetes. In these patients, distention of the esophagus does not initiate a secondary peristalsis, and repetitive pharyngeal swallows are needed in order to propel food into the stomach. This again leads to aerophagia. Simple gluttony is another mechanism of gastric dilatation, which

results in shortening of the sphincter and significant postprandial reflux.[7]

Increases in intragastric pressure can occur with or without gastric dilatation and result in reflux of gastric contents into the esophagus through a normal manometric sphincter. One cause of this is outlet obstruction of the stomach. Normally, this occurs during the physiologic act of vomiting, when the outlet of the stomach is obstructed by a strong antral contraction.[44] Another cause is a previous vagotomy that interrupts the normal active relaxation of the stomach.[44] The fundus and body of the stomach constitute a reservoir that is able to accommodate a large volume with minimal increases in pressure, because of active relaxation of the musculature. Interruption of the vagi interferes with active relaxation, resulting in greater gastric pressures with lower volumes.

A persistent gastric reservoir is another cause of reflux through a mechanically normal sphincter and is due to delayed gastric emptying.[45] This can be caused by myogenic abnormalities, such as gastric atony from advanced diabetes, diffuse neuromuscular disorders, idiopathic gastric paresis following a viral infection, or vagotomy. Nongastric causes are pyloric dysfunction and duodenal dysmotility. The latter would not only reduce gastric emptying but also cause an inefficient flow of duodenal contents in the aboral direction. Consequently, bile can regurgitate into the stomach, resulting in bile gastritis and gastroparesis secondary to inflammation.[2] Any factor that increases the volume and persistence of a gastric reservoir increases the probability of regurgitation through a mechanically normal sphincter, simply because the gastric reservoir remains full for a longer period and accentuates physiologic reflux. In such situations, the application of an antireflux procedure to a normal cardia would indeed stop the gastroesophageal reflux but also would potentiate the deleterious effects of existing gastric and duodenal pathology.

When the cardia is mechanically incompetent, increases in gastric volume secondary to delayed emptying can potentiate the abnormality by increasing the severity of reflux.[45] Augmentation of esophageal exposure to gastric juice secondary to delayed gastric emptying is a commonly unrecognized ingredient of gastroesophageal reflux disease. It is estimated that 40% of patients with gastroesophageal reflux disease have delayed gastric emptying.[46] This delay is most pronounced in patients who have endoscopic esophagitis and is probably due to transmural inflammation causing vagal paresis.[47] In this situation, the delayed gastric emptying is a consequence rather than a cause of gastroesophageal reflux disease.

Excessive gastric acid secretion can cause increased esophageal exposure to gastric juice in the presence of a manometrically normal sphincter. This is probably due to both increased gastric volume and the high acidity of that volume, both of which augment physiologic acid reflux.[43]

Dodds and associates suggest transient spontaneous relaxation of the distal esophageal sphincter as a cause of increased esophageal exposure to gastric juice.[48] In this situation, a normal sphincter relaxes spontaneously, unrelated to swallowing, to gastric baseline pressure, allowing reflux of gastric contents into the esophagus. The cause of the spontaneous relaxation is unknown, but may be of gastric origin and represent a physiologic belch. If this were so, the cause of the reflux would be a gastric phenomenon rather than an esophageal phenomenon. To diagnose this condition requires continuous pressure monitoring of the sphincter and the esophageal body along with pH monitoring of the esophagus over a 24-hour period, since episodes of spontaneous relaxation are unlikely to be captured during a short recording session. As a consequence, a large population of patients with the disease have not been able to be monitored and this hypothesis for increased esophageal acid exposure needs further substantiation.

Increased esophageal sensitivity to gastric juice and the development of reflux symptoms

There are two primary symptoms resulting from esophageal dysfunction—dysphagia and chest pain. Heartburn is considered part of the latter and is a form of chest pain that is typically esophageal in origin. Because we evaluate patients more frequently than normal subjects, physicians become programmed into thinking that the experience of heartburn indicates that acid has come into contact with the esophageal mucosa. The studies of Jones showed that the symptom of heartburn can arise from a variety of esophageal stimuli and are not always unrelated to

the presence of gastric acid in the esophagus.[49] He recorded the sensations experienced by normal subjects during the distention of a balloon at different levels in the esophagus (see Table 8-7). The majority of the subjects felt a sensation of choking or fullness when the balloon was inflated in the upper portion of the esophagus; a small percentage experienced a burning sensation. As the point of stimulation descended, the sensation of choking or fullness diminished and burning increased. More than half of the subjects examined felt definite burning the moment the balloon was inflated in the region of the cardia. Of interest was that a few subjects, in addition to the sensation of burning, felt as if something hot or sour was being carried up toward the mouth when a balloon was inflated near the cardia. Such findings explain why heartburn can be experienced by patients when the cause is other than irritation of the lower esophagus by regurgitated gastric juice.

In a second study, Jones placed a nasogastric tube just above the cardia in normal subjects and made observations on the effects of introducing various amounts of warm water, cold water, 0.1N sodium hydroxide, 0.1N hydrochloric acid, and gastric juice into the esophagus.[49] From this simple experiment, several observations were noteworthy. First, there was a wide variation in the amount of fluid that could be introduced into the esophagus before heartburn or any other sensation was experienced. Discomfort of one sort or another, usually burning, could be produced with as little as 5 ml of fluid or could require as much as 35 ml. The speed of introduction of the fluid was also an important factor. When it was allowed to run in slowly, frequently no sensation was produced. On the other hand, the rapid introduction of 10 to 15 ml of fluid with a syringe produced an almost instantaneous sense of discomfort or pain. It was further noted that the more frequently the injections of fluid were made, the more readily the discomfort was produced and the longer it persisted. When warm water was introduced, five of eight subjects noted a cool sensation, and three had a feeling of

TABLE 8-7. Predominant symptom experienced with balloon distention of the esophagus

Symptoms	Upper esophagus	Midesophagus	Lower esophagus
Choking or fullness	62% (18/29)	20% (5/25)	10% (3/29)
Heartburn	14% (4/29)	44% (11/25)	59% (17/29)*
Chest pain	10% (3/29)	8% (2/25)	10% (3/29)
Uncomfortable	14% (4/29)	20% (7/25)	21% (6/29)

Data from Jones, C.M.: Digestive tract pain, New York, 1938, Macmillan, Inc.

*Seven patients also complained of chest pain.

heartburn. When ice water was injected, all eight subjects had a distinct sensation of heartburn. The introduction of 0.1N hydrochloric acid had no effect in two subjects, produced a sensation of coolness in one, and in five caused a definite burning feeling, described as heartburn. In six of seven subjects, 01.N sodium hydroxide caused the same burning feeling but to a greater degree. Three subjects had their own gastric contents introduced into the lower end of the esophagus, and in two of these, heartburn was produced. In the third, only a sensation of coolness resulted.

From a clinical point of view, these studies indicate that the experience of heartburn by a normal subject is more dependent on the speed and repetition of the injection than on the chemical composition of the fluid placed in the lower esophagus. Consequently, in patients who complain of heartburn, chemical neutralization cannot be expected to bring universal relief of the discomfort. Although increased exposure of the esophagus to gastric juice is central to the pathophysiology of gastroesophageal reflux disease, the symptoms that it elicits can be variable. The development of an acid-sensitive esophagus appears to depend largely on the degree of esophageal distention that occurs with each reflux episode and on the frequency of the reflux event.

The mechanism by which acid provokes pain has been a matter of controversy. Some investigators have suggested that the pain associated with reflux is due to acid-induced muscle spasms.[50] Others have believed that induced motility changes are not an integral part of the pain mechanism.[17] The work of Atkinson and Bennett[51] suggests that the presence of acid in the esophagus has two independent effects: to produce pain and to increase nonpropulsive muscular activity. According to this view, the motility changes are not an essential part of the pain mechanism since in the presence of acid, pain or nonperistaltic contractions may occur in isolation, and when pain and a change in motility occur together, sodium bicarbonate infusion will relieve the pain without affecting the motility, and propantheline will abolish motility without relieving the pain.

Other studies have shown that the symptoms of heartburn and regurgitation are not a reliable guide to the presence of gastroesophageal reflux disease in patients who seek medical attention.[1] When the symptoms of heartburn and regurgitation were scored according to their degree of severity in symptomatic patients, only patients who had heartburn sufficiently severe to interfere with daily activities and regurgitation sufficient to cause symptoms of pulmonary aspiration could be reliably predicted to have a positive 24-hour test. Patients with less severe symptoms were unpredictable. This indicates that only in the most severely affected patients can the symptoms of heartburn and regurgitation be a reliable guide to the presence of disease. When symptoms are less severe or atypical, recognition is more difficult and the diagnosis depends on the objective measurement of increased esophageal exposure to gastric juice.

Complications of increased esophageal exposure to gastric juice

Chronic irritation of the esophageal mucosa by gastric juice has been implicated as the cause of the loss of surface epithelial cells seen in esophageal biopsy specimens from patients with gastroesophageal reflux disease (see Fig. 8-15).[52] This is reflected by a closer approximation of the apex of the papillae to the luminal surface and hyperplasia in the basal zone layer. This hypothesis has been supported in a study using 24-hour pH monitoring to correlate esophageal mucosa exposure to acid gastric juice with the epithelial papillary length and the thickness of the basal zone hyperplasia in esophageal mucosal biopsy specimens.[53] In patients with positive 24-hour pH records, the papillae extended for a significantly greater mean percentage length across the width of the epithelium (representing a loss of surface epithelial cells) than in patients with normal tests, and a regression analysis showed a significant direct correlation between the percent of papillary extension and the degree of distal esophageal acid exposure. This reactive epithelial change was reversible in that it significantly decreased in patients after antireflux surgery had returned the distal esophageal acid exposure to normal.

The relationship between esophageal acid exposure time and the epithelial reaction was also shown by studies on the pattern of reflux in patients with gastroesophageal reflux disease—that is, upright, supine, or bipositional.[4] When categorized, the mean papillary extension was found to exceed 60% of the width of the epithelium only in the supine and bipositional refluxers—that is, acid exposure that resulted from few reflux episodes but ones of long duration. In contrast, the mean papillary length was found to be normal in those patients who had only upright reflux—that is, acid exposure that resulted from frequent reflux episodes of short duration. Of importance was that although the total duration of the upright reflux episodes significantly exceeded the total duration of recumbent reflux episodes,

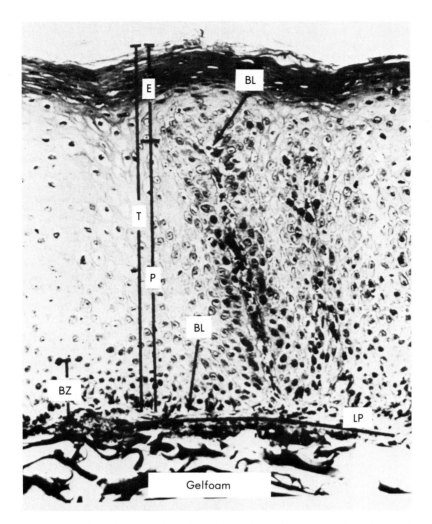

Fig. 8-15. Cross section of the esophageal epithelium from a biopsy specimen in a patient with increased esophageal exposure to gastric juice. *BZ,* Basal zone; *BL,* basal layer; *T,* total epithelial width; *P,* papillary length; *E,* protective epithelium above top of papillae; *LP,* lamina propria.

the upright acid exposure was less damaging to the esophageal mucosa because of rapid clearance. Thus, esophageal acid clearance time is more important in determining the epithelial reaction than the total magnitude of esophageal acid exposure. The concept appears to be that low-frequency, long-duration gastric juice exposure is more deleterious to the esophageal mucosa than high-frequency, short-duration exposure.

A similar effect is observed when the patterns of reflux are related to the incidence and severity of endoscopic esophagitis.[7] Fig. 8-16 shows that isolated supine gastric juice exposure is associated with a higher incidence of esophagitis and more severe esophagitis than is isolated upright exposure. Bipositional refluxers have the highest incidence of, and most severe, endoscopic esophagitis, which probably represents a severe form of

gastroesophageal reflux disease that started as isolated supine reflux. Thus, supine reflux appears to be the most critical factor in the development of esophagitis.

Considerable differences of opinion exist in regard to what ingredient in reflux gastric juice produces esophagitis. Ingredients in both gastric and duodenal secretions have been implicated. Twenty-four hour esophageal pH monitoring has shown that when pH records from patients with symptoms of gastroesophageal reflux disease are compared with records from asymptomatic controls, the patients have excessive esophageal exposure to acid (pH less than 4), alkaline (pH greater than 7), or acid and alkaline gastric contents (see Fig. 8-17).[54] Interestingly, the three types of pH exposure patterns are associated with comparable incidences and severities of esophagi-

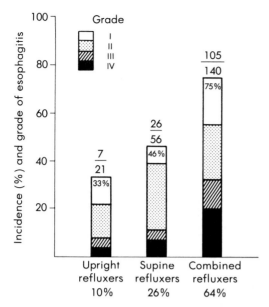

Fig. 8-16. Percent incidence and grade of esophagitis related to the pattern of reflux as detected by 24-hour pH monitoring in patients with increased esophageal exposure to gastric juice.

tis (see Fig. 8-18). These findings suggest that gastric contents as a whole, rather than hydrochloric acid in particular, are injurious to the squamous esophageal mucosa.

Quincke,[55] in 1879, was the first to draw the correlation between esophagitis and the digestive action of acid gastric juice. Subsequently, several studies were designed to identify the offensive agent in the gastric juice. These consisted of infusion experiments in which the substance under question was dripped continuously into the esophagus of an anesthetized animal,[55a] or experiments in which the lower esophageal sphincter was destroyed so that the reflux of gastric juice could occur.[55b] In the latter type of study, it was difficult to determine the exact composition of refluxed juice. This led to surgical experiments in which the esophagus was exposed to intestinal juices in such a manner that their composition could be controlled.[55c] The results of these studies seemed to show that a combination of acid and pepsin had a damaging effect on the esophageal mucosa of the species tested. However, in all of the experiments, a prolonged

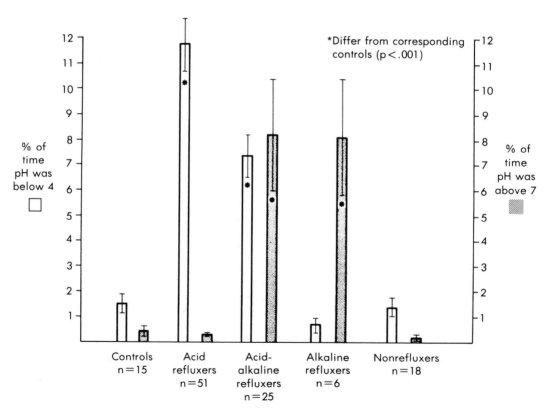

Fig. 8-17. Results of 24-hour pH monitoring of the distal esophagus in 15 asymptomatic patients and 100 symptomatic patients.

continuous exposure of the esophageal mucosa to the substance studied was necessary to produce a deleterious effect. The time required was in excess of that measured in patients with severe reflux esophagitis. In these patients, esophageal pH was below 4 for only 20% to 30% of the 24-hour period, and the exposure was not continuous but broken up into several episodes. These findings suggested that factors in addition to hydrochloric acid and pepsin were involved in the development of esophagitis in humans.

The occurrence of esophagitis in patients with achlorhydria[56] or after total gastrectomy[57] is a well-established clinical observation, and indicates that an offensive agent must be in the duodenal juice as well. In support of this, several authors have demonstrated a concomitant increase in duodenal gastric reflux in patients with symptomatic gastroesophageal reflux disease.[58-61] Bile, pancreatic secretions, and duodenal secretions are all potentially injurious ingredients in duodenal juice. Bile salts are considered to be the corrosive component of bile, and their presence in the esophagus has been correlated with symptomatic heartburn.[62] The corrosive components of pancreatic juice are activated enzymes such as trypsin, lipase, and carboxypeptidase, all of which have been shown to produce epithelial

changes when incubated with strips of esophageal mucosa.[63] These proteolytic enzymes are generally thought to be rapidly inactivated in the stomach. Experiments have demonstrated that the inactivation of trypsin by pepsin takes place at a pH below 3.5.[64] In the absence of pepsin, trypsin is stable in acid solution and present in an active form.[65] Active trypsin has been demonstrated in the human stomach at pH values between 3.5 and 7 for as long as 90 minutes after a test meal.[66]

The elegant experiments of Johnson and Harmon on in vivo perfusion of rabbit esophagi have shed considerable light on the pathogenesis of the mucosal injury and have explained the seemingly conflicting clinical observations regarding the reflux of gastric and duodenal juice.[67] These studies have shown that the esophageal squamous mucosa is resistant to hydrogen ion injury at a pH of 2 or above, and damaged when the pH drops below this level. Bile salts at concentrations found in gastric juice are potentially damaging to the esophageal mucosa, depending on the pH of the solution. When the pH of the gastric juice is less than the pK_a of the bile acid, the bile acid will precipitate out of solution and is no longer damaging to the mucosa. For example, at a pH of 2, the taurine-conjugated bile salts with pK_a values slightly less than 2 remain in solution and

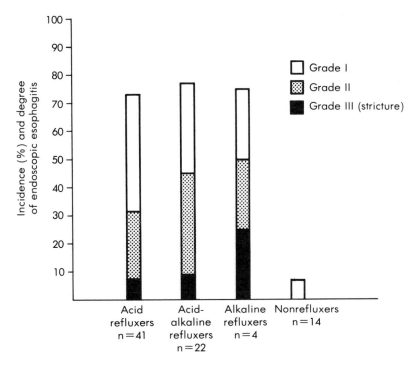

Fig. 8-18. Endoscopic results in symptomatic patients with different kinds of gastroesophageal reflux.

are damaging to the mucosa, while the unconjugated bile salts with pK_a values much greater than 2 are precipitated and noninjurious. When the pH of the gastric juice rises to 7, the unconjugated bile salts go into solution and injure the mucosa while the taurine-conjugated bile salts precipitate out and are noninjurious.

An important observation made from their experiments was that acid or bile could produce esophageal mucosal barrier abnormalities, such as changes in potential difference, hydrogen ion reflux, and permeability defects, yet neither alone nor combined could they produce morphologic lesions consistent with clinical reflux esophagitis. When the enzyme pepsin or trypsin was present in physiologic concentrations, significant gross and microscopic esophagitis resulted, depending on the pH of the perfusate. These observations appear to be applicable to the human, in that increased concentrations of pepsin have been found in the esophageal aspirates of patients with severe ulcerative esophagitis as opposed to those without esophagitis,[68] and erosive esophagitis comparable to that observed with excessive acid reflux has been seen following total gastrectomy.[57]

Johnson and Harmon's studies[67] suggested that trypsin may be a major injurious agent in an alkaline refluxate, and pepsin in an acid refluxate. It appears that the pH of the refluxed juice dictates which enzyme, if present, would be the injurious agent by providing the optimal pH range for its activity—that is, a pH of 2 to 5 for pepsin

and 5 to 8 for trypsin. These proteolytic enzymes appear to cause their mucosal damage by digesting surface tissue protein, since no injury occurs at nonoptimal pH values.

Johnson and Harmon's studies also pointed out an interaction between bile salts and pepsin or trypsin activity. The bile salt taurodeoxycholate significantly diminished, in a dose-dependent manner, the degree of esophagitis caused by pepsin in an acid environment. In contrast, soluble unconjugated bile salts significantly potentiate the degree of esophagitis caused by trypsin in an alkaline environment. Fig. 8-19 attempts to graphically illustrate these interactions.

Our current understanding is that the reflux of bile and pancreatic enzymes into the stomach could either increase or decrease the degree of esophagitis in a patient with gastroesophageal reflux. For instance, the reflux of duodenal contents into the stomach may prevent the development of peptic esophagitis in a patient whose gastric acid secretion maintained an acid environment, because the bile salts would attenuate the injurious effect of pepsin and the acid would inactivate the trypsin. Such a patient would have bile-containing acid gastric juice that when refluxed would irritate the esophageal mucosa, but cause less esophagitis than if it were acid gastric juice containing pepsin. In contrast, the reflux of duodenal contents into the stomach of a patient with limited gastric acid secretion can result in esophagitis, because the alkaline intragastric environment would support optimal

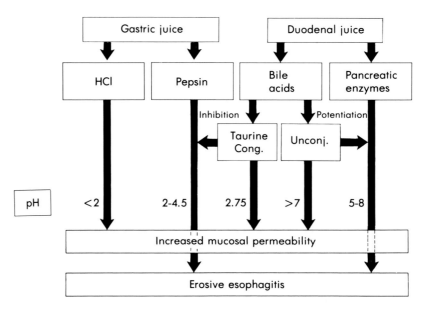

Fig. 8-19. Schematic diagram of the interaction of injurious agents refluxed into the esophagi of patients with gastroesophageal reflux disease.

trypsin activity and the soluble bile salts with a high pk_a would potentiate the effect. Hence, duodenal gastric reflux and the acid secretory capacity of the stomach interrelate to modulate the injurious effects of trypsin and pepsin on the esophageal mucosa by altering the pH and enzymatic contents of the reflux gastric juice. Fig. 8-5 shows how duodenal gastric reflux alters the pH of the gastric juice refluxed into the esophagus. As expected, this patient had symptoms of heartburn and severe esophagitis. If the duodenal gastric reflux was excessive so that alkaline gastric juice was predominantly refluxed, the patient would have esophagitis with minimal symptoms of heartburn. This explains why symptoms are not a reliable guide to the presence of the disease.

Similarly, the disparity in injury—that is, mucosal barrier abnormalities caused by acid and bile alone as opposed to gross esophagitis caused by pepsin and trypsin—provides an explanation for the poor correlation between the symptom of heartburn and endoscopic esophagitis. The reflux of acid gastric juice contaminated with duodenal contents could break the esophageal mucosal barrier, irritate nerve endings in the papillae close to the luminal surface, and cause severe heartburn. Despite the presence of intense heartburn, the bile salts present would destroy pepsin, the acid pH would inactivate trypsin, and the patient would have little or no gross evidence of esophagitis. In contrast, the patient who refluxed alkaline gastric juice may have minimal heartburn because of the absence of hydrogen ions in the refluxate, but severe endoscopic esophagitis because of bile salt potentiation of trypsin activity on the esophageal mucosa. Consequently, changing the pH of refluxed gastric juice from acid to alkaline, by the administration of H_2 blockers, may intensify the mucosal injury, while at the same time giving the patient a sense of security by alleviating the symptom of heartburn. Fig. 8-20 shows that the results of clinical studies with H_2 blockers suggest that this may occur, in that their administration markedly reduces symptoms but has a lesser effect in improving the endoscopic grade of esophagitis.[69]

When the composition of the refluxed gastric juice is such that sustained or repetitive esophageal injury occurs, two sequelae can result. First, a luminal stricture can develop from submucosal and eventually intramural fibrosis. Second, a Barrett's esophagus can develop by replacement of repetitively destroyed squamous mucosa with columnar epithelium. The columnar epithelium, although resistant to acid and therefore associated with the alleviation of the complaint of heartburn,

is subjected to severe forms of dysplasia, most likely because of continuous irritation from the refluxed gastric juice. This can lead to adenocarcinoma with an incidence that is yet to be determined but that is predicted to be between 0.5% and 10%.[70] Although this appears to be a small risk, it can be placed in better perspective when compared to the risk of lung cancer in a population of men between the ages of 55 and 64 who have smoked one pack of cigarettes per day for 20 years. The incidence of lung cancer in such a population is 227 per 100,000 individuals. In a similar-sized population of individuals with Barrett's esophagus, the incidence of adenocarcinoma is between 500 and 1000 per 100,000. When placed in this perspective, the risk of adenocarcinoma resulting from reflux emerges as a serious problem but one that may be completely solvable by the earlier recognition of severe reflux disease and proper therapy.

The development of extensive esophageal damage, such as a luminal stricture or Barrett's esophagus, is usually associated with a profound mechanical defect of the cardia and decreased acid clearance by the body of the esophagus. Studies have shown that patients with reflux-induced strictures or Barrett's esophagus have a more profound defect in sphincter pressure than patients with simple esophagitis, and, as expected, this results in a greater exposure of the distal esophagus to gastric juice.[71] Of interest is that the extent of the Barrett's involvement is related to the level of lower esophageal sphincter pressure, and that the number of reflux episodes 5 minutes or longer in duration is related to the severity of the valvular deficiency and the clearance function of the esophageal body.[71]

An esophageal stricture can be associated with severe esophagitis or Barrett's esophagus. In the latter situation it occurs at the columnar-squamous epithelial interface; this is the site of maximal inflammatory injury. As the columnar epithelium advances into the area of inflammation, the inflammation extends higher into the proximal esophagus and the site of the stricture moves progressively up the esophagus. Patients who have a stricture in the absence of Barrett's esophagus should have the presence of gastroesophageal reflux documented before the etiology of the stricture is ascribed to reflux esophagitis. In such patients the stricture may be due to a primary esophageal motility defect or a drug-induced chemical injury resulting from the lodgment of a capsule or tablet in the distal esophagus.[5] In such patients, dilatation usually corrects the problem of dysphagia and heartburn, which may have occurred only because of the chemical

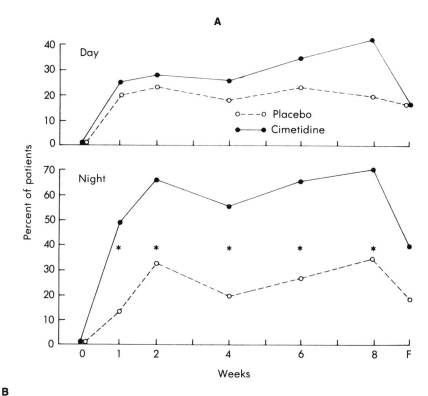

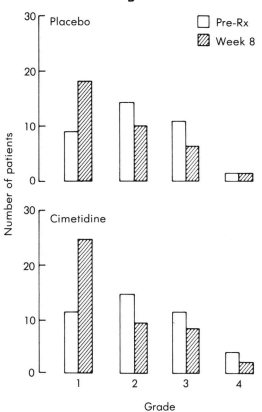

Fig. 8-20. A, Percentage of patients with gastroesophageal reflux disease who became pain free during the study period while receiving the H_2 blocker cimetidine or a placebo. Altering the pH of the refluxed gastric juice with H_2 blockers resulted in a significant decrease in symptoms ($p<0.05$). **B,** Endoscopic assessment of severity of esophagitis, from normal (grade 1) to severe (grade 4), in placebo and cimetidine patients. Altering the pH of the refluxed gastric juice with an H_2 blocker had little effect on the degree of endothelial damage, indicating that other ingredients in the gastric juice are injurious to the epithelium.

injury and does not need treatment. It is also possible for drug-induced injuries to occur in patients who have underlying esophagitis and a distal esophageal stricture secondary to gastroesophageal reflux. In this situation, a long string-like stricture progressively develops as a result of repetitive caustic injury from capsule or tablet lodgment on top of an initial reflux stricture. These strictures are often resistant to dilatation.[5]

When the refluxed gastric juice is of sufficient quantity, it can reach the pharynx with the potential for pharyngeal tracheal aspiration, causing symptoms of repetitive cough, choking, hoarseness, and recurrent pneumonia.[3] This is often an unrecognized complication of gastroesophageal reflux disease, since either the pulmonary or the gastrointestinal symptoms may predominate in the clinical situation and focus the physician's attention on one to the exclusion of the other. The presence of an esophageal motility disorder is observed in 75% of patients with reflux-induced aspiration and is believed to promote the aboral movement of the refluxate toward the pharynx.[40]

A complication of increased esophageal exposure to gastric juice, such as persistent endoscopic esophagitis, esophageal stricture, Barrett's columnar-lined esophagus, or radiographic evidence of repetitive aspiration pneumonia, in the presence of a mechanically defective sphincter should encourage early operative therapy. The probability that medical therapy can correct or successfully manage these complications in patients with a mechanically defective sphincter is low.[72] Persistence of medical therapy in this situation is likely to cause more functional damage until the only alternative becomes esophageal resection and colon interposition.[73]

REFERENCES

1. DeMeester, T.R., and Johnson, L.F.: The evaluation of objective measurements of gastroesophageal reflux and their contribution to patient management, Surg. Clin. North. Am. **56:**39-53, 1976.
2. Kaye, M.D., and Showalter, J.P.: Pyloric incompetence in patients with symptomatic gastroesophageal reflux, J. Lab. Clin. Med. **83:**198-206, 1974.
3. Pellegrini, C.A., DeMeester, T.R., and Johnson, L.F.: Gastroesophageal reflux and pulmonary aspiration: incidence, functional abnormality and results of surgical therapy, Surgery **86:**110-119, 1979.
4. DeMeester, T.R., Wang, C.I., Wernly, J.A., et al.: Technique, indications and clinical use of 24-hour esophageal pH monitoring, J. Thorac. Cardiovasc. Surg. **79:**656-667, 1980.
5. Bonavina, L., DeMeester, T.R., McChesney, L., et al.: Drug induced esophageal strictures, Ann. Surg. **206:**173-183, 1987.
6. Johnson, L.F., and DeMeester, T.R.: 24-Hour pH monitoring of the distal esophagus: a quantitative measure of gastroesophageal reflux, Am. J. Gastroenterol. **62:**325-332, 1974.
7. DeMeester, T.R., Johnson, L.F., et al.: Patterns of gastroesophageal reflux in health and disease, Ann. Surg. **184:**459-470, 1976.
8. Johnson, L.F., and DeMeester, T.R.: Development of the 24-hour intraesophageal pH monitoring composite scoring system, J. Clin. Gastroenterol. **8:**52-58, 1986.
9. Johnson, L.F., Lin, T.C., and Hong, S.K.: Gastroesophageal dynamics during immersion in water to the neck, J. Appl. Physiol. **38:**449-454, 1975.
10. Banchero, N., Schwartz, P.E., and Wood, E.H.: Intraesophageal pressure gradient in man, J. Appl. Physiol. **22:**1066-1074, 1967.
11. Dent, J., Dodds, W.J., Friedman, R.H., et al.: Mechanism of gastroesophageal reflux in recumbent asymptomatic human subjects, J. Clin. Invest. **65:**256-267, 1980.
12. Leon, C.S.C., Flanagan, J.B., Jr., and Moorrees, C.F.A.: The frequency of deglutition in man, Arch. Oral Biol. **10:**83-96, 1965.
13. Bonavina, L., Evander, A., DeMeester, T.R., et al.: Length of the distal esophageal sphincter and competency of the cardia, Am. J. Surg. **151:**25-34, 1986.
14. Babka, J.C., Hagar, G.W., and Castell, D.O.: The effect of body position on lower esophageal sphincter pressure, Am. J. Dig. Dis. **18:**441-442, 1973.
15. Lam. C.R.: Intra-abdominal pressure: a critical review and an experimental study, Arch. Surg. **39:**1006-1015, 1939.
16. Emde, C., Garner, A., and Blum, A.: Technical aspects of intraluminal pH-metry in man: current status and recommendations, Gut. (In Press.)
17. Tuttle, S.G., Rufin, F., and Battaneloo, A.: The physiology of heartburn, Ann. Intern. Med. **55:**292-300, 1961.
18. Wallin, L., and Madsen, T.: Twelve-hour simultaneous registration of acid reflux and peristaltic activity in the oesophagus: a study in normal subjects, Scand. J. Gastroenterol. **14:**561-566, 1979.
19. Vitale, G.C., Cheadle, W.G., Sarvi, S., et al.: Computerized 24-hour ambulatory esophageal pH monitoring and esophagogastroduodenoscopy in the reflux patient: a comparative study, Ann. Surg. **200:**724-729, 1984.
20. Lillemoe, K.D., Johnson, L.F., and Marmon, J.W.: Role of the components of the gastroduodenal contents in experimental acid esophagitis, Surgery **92:**276-284, 1982.
21. Miller, F.A.: Utilization of inlying pH probe for evaluation of acid-peptic diathesis, Arch. Surg. **89:**199-203, 1964.
22. Herrera, B.S.: The precision of percentiles in establishing normal limits in medicine, J. Lab. Clin. Med. **52**(1):34-42, 1958.
23. Haddad, J.K.: Relation of gastroesophageal reflux to yield sphincter pressures, Gastroenterology **58:**175-184, 1970.
24. DeMeester, T.R., Wernly, J.A., Bryant, G.H., et al.: Clinical and in vitro analysis of gastroesophageal competence: a study of the principles of antireflux surgery, Am. J. Surg. **137:**39-46, 1979.

25. Mann, C.V., and Hardcastle, J.D.: The effect of vagotomy of the human gastroesophageal sphincter, Gut **9**:688-695, 1968.

26. Castell, D.O.: The lower esophageal sphincter: physiologic and clinical aspects, Ann. Intern. Med. **83**: 390-401, 1975.

27. DeMeester, T.R.: What is the role of intraoperative manometry? Ann. Thorac. Surg. **30**:1-4, 1980.

28. Biancani, P., Zabinsky, M.P., and Behar, J.: Pressure, tension, and force of closure of the human lower esophageal sphincter and esophagus, J. Clin. Invest. **56**:476-483, 1975.

29. Thurer, R. L., DeMeester, T.R., and Johnson, L.F.: The distal esophageal sphincter and its relationship to gastroesophageal reflux, J. Surg. Res. **16**:418-423, 1974.

30. DeMeester, T.R., and Johnson, L.F.: The evaluation of objective measurements of gastroesophageal reflux and their contribution to patient management, Surg. Clin. North. Am. **56**:39-53, 1976.

31. Skinner, D.B., and Camp, T.R., Jr.: Relation of esophageal reflux to lower esophageal sphincter pressures decreased by atropine, Gastroenterology **54**: 543-551, 1968.

32. Bombeck, C.T., Dillard, D.H., and Nyhus, L.M.: Muscular anatomy of the gastroesophageal junction and role of phreno-esophageal ligament: autopsy study of sphincter mechanism, Ann. Surg. **164**:643-654, 1966.

33. DeMeester, T.R., Lafontaine, E., Joelsson, B.E., et al.: The relationship of a hiatal hernia to the function of the body of the esophagus and the gastroesophageal junction, J. Thorac. Cardiovasc. Surg. **82**:547-558, 1981.

34. Pellegrini, C.A., DeMeester, T.R., and Skinner, D.B.: Response of the distal esophageal spincter to respiratory and positional maneuvers in humans, Surg. Forum **27**: 380-382, 1976.

35. Wernly, J.A., DeMeester, T.R., Bryant, G.H., et al.: Intra-abdominal pressure and manometric data of the distal esophageal sphincter, Arch. Surg. **115**:534-539, 1980.

36. O'Sullivan, G.C., DeMeester, T.R., Joelsson, B.E., et al.: The interaction of the lower esophageal sphincter pressure and length of sphincter in the abdomen as determinants of gastroesophgeal competence, Am. J. Surg. **143**:40-47, 1982.

37. Helm, J.F., Riedel, D.R., Dodds, W.J., et al.: Determinants of esophageal acid clearance in normal subjects, Gastroenterology **85**:607-612, 1983.

38. Helm, J.F., Dodds, W.J., Hogan, W.J., et al.: Acid neutralizing capacity of human saliva, Gastroenterology **83**:69-74, 1982.

39. Madsen, T., Wallin, L., Boesby, S., et al.: Oesophageal peristalsis in normal subjects: influence of pH and volume during imitated gastroesophageal reflux, Scand. J. Gastroenterol. **18**:13-18, 1983.

40. DeMeester, T.R., Iascone, C., and Courtney, J.V.: The presence of occult esophageal disease in patients with chronic unexplained respiratory complaints: a prospective study. (In preparation.)

41. Edwards, D.A.W.: Radiological examination and quantitation of reflux in the hiatal hernia-reflux syndrome. In Van Heukelem, H.A., Gooszen, H.G., Terpstra, J.B., et al., editors: Pathological gastroesophageal reflux,

Amsterdam, 1982, Zuid Nederlandse Uitgevers Maatschappij BV, pp. 47-53.

42. Malagelada, J.R.: Physiologic basis and clinical significance of gastric emptying disorders, Dig. Dis. Sci. **24**: 657-661, 1979.

43. Boesby, S.: Relationship between gastroesophageal acid reflux, basal gastroesophageal sphincter pressure and gastric acid secretion, Scand. J. Gastroenterol. **12**: 547-551, 1977.

44. Davenport, H.W.: Physiology of the digestive tract, ed. 5, Chicago, 1982, Year Book Medical Publishers, Inc., pp. 52-69.

45. Ahtaridis, G., Snape, W.J., and Cohen, S.: Lower esophageal sphincter pressure as an index of gastroesophageal acid reflux, Dig. Dis. Sci. **26**:993-998, 1981.

46. McCallum, R.W., Berkowitz, D.M., and Lerner, E.: Gastric emptying in patients with gastroesophageal reflux, Gastroenterology **80**:285-291, 1981.

47. Little, A.G., DeMeester, T.R., Kirchner, P.T., et al.: Pathogenesis of esophagitis in patients with gastroesophageal reflux, Surgery **88**:101-107, 1980.

48. Dodds, W.J., Dent, J., Hogan, W.J., et al.: Mechanisms of gastroesophageal reflux in patients with reflux esophagitis, N. Engl. J. Med. **307**:1547-1552, 1982.

49. Jones, C.M.: Digestive tract pain, New York, 1938, Macmillan, Inc.

50. Siegel, C.I., and Hendrix, T.R.: Esophageal motor abnormalities induced by acid perfusion in patients with heartburn, J. Clin. Invest. **42**:686-695, 1963.

51. Atkinson, M., and Bennett, J.R.: Relationship between motor changes and pain during esophageal acid perfusion, Am. J. Dig. Dis. **13**:346-350, 1968.

52. Ismail-Beigi, F., and Pope, C.E.: Distribution of histological changes of gastroesophageal reflux in the distal esophagus of man, Gastroenterology **66**:1109-1113, 1975.

53. Johnson, L.F., DeMeester, T.R., and Haggitt, R.C.: Esophageal epithelial response to gastroesophagela reflux: a quantitative study, Am. J. Dig. Dis. **23**:498-509, 1978.

54. Pellegrini, C.A., DeMeester, T.R., Wernly, J.A., et al.: Alkaline gastroesophageal reflux, Am. J. Surg. **135**: 177-184, 1978.

55. Quincke, H.: Ulcus oesophagi ex digestione, Deutsch Arch. Klin. Med. **24**:72-78, 1879.

55a. Henderson, R.D., Mugashe, F., Jeejeebhoy, K.N., et al.: The role of bile and acid in the production of esophagitis and the motor defect of esophagitis, Ann. Thorac. Surg. **14**:465-473, 1972.

55b. Gillison, E.W., de Castro, V.A.M., Nyhus, L.M., et al.: The significance of bile in reflux esophagitis, Surg. Gynecol. Obstet. **134**:419-424, 1972.

55c. Kranendonk, S.E.: Reflux oesophagitis: an experimental study in rats, thesis, Rotterdam, 1980, Erasmus University.

56. Palmer, E.D.: Subacute erosive ("peptic") esophagitis associated with achlorhydria, N. Engl. J. Med. **262**: 927-929, 1960.

57. Helsingen, N.: Oesophagitis following total gastrectomy, Acta. Chir. Scand. [Suppl.] **273**:5-21, 1961.

58. Donovan, I.A., Harding, L.K., Keighley, M.R.B., et al.: Abnormalities of gastric emptying and pyloric

reflux in uncomplicated hiatus hernia, Br. J. Surg. **64:** 847-848, 1977.

59. Stol, D.W., Murphy, G.M., and Collis, J.L.: Duodeno-gastric reflux and acid secretion in patients with symptomatic hiatal hernia, Scand. J. Gastroenterol. **9:**97-101, 1974.

60. Crumplin, M.K.H., Stol, D.W., Murphy, G.M., et al.: The pattern of bile salt reflux and acid secretion in sliding hiatal hernia, Br. J. Surg. **61:**611-616, 1974.

61. Clemencon, G.: Nocturnal intragastric pH measurements, Scand. J. Gastroenterol. **7:**293-298, 1972.

62. Gillison, E.W., and Nyhus, L.M.: Bile reflux, gastric secretion and heartburn (abstract), Br. J. Surg. **58:**864, 1971.

63. Bateson, M.C., Hopwood, D., Milne, G., et al.: Oesophageal epithelial ultrastructure after incubation with gastrointestinal fluids and their components, J. Pathol. **133:**33-58, 1981.

64. Heizer, W.D., Cleveland, C.R., and Iber, F.L.: Gastric inactivation of pancreatic supplements, Johns Hopkins Med. J. **116:**261-270, 1965.

65. Northrop, J.H., Nunitz, M., and Herriott, R.M.: Crystalline enzymes, ed. 2, New York, 1948, Columbia University Press.

66. Wenger, J., and Trowbridge, C.G.: Bile and trypsin in the stomach following a test meal, South. Med. J. **64:** 1063-1064, 1971.

67. Johnson, L.F., and Harmon, J.W.: Experimental esophagitis in a rabbit model, J. Clin. Gastroenterol. **8**(suppl. 1):26-44, 1986.

68. Alwin, J.A.: The physiological basis of reflux oesophagitis in sliding hiatal diaphragmatic hernia, Thorax. **8:**38-45, 1952.

69. Behar, J., Brand, D.L., Brown, F.C., et al.: Cimetidine in the treatment of symptomatic gastroesophageal reflux, Gastroenterology **74:**441-448, 1978.

70. Spechler, S.J.: Endoscopic surveillance for patients with Barrett's esophagus: does the cancer risk justify the practice? Ann. Intern. Med. **106:**902-904, 1987.

71. Iascone, C., DeMeester, T.R., Little, A.G., et al.: Barrett's esophagus: functional assessment, proposed pathogenesis and surgical therapy, Arch. Surg. **118:** 543-549, 1983.

72. Lieberman, D.A., and Keeffe, E.B.: Treatment of severe reflux esophagitis with cimetidine and metoclopramide, Ann. Intern. Med. **104:**21-26, 1986.

73. Lieberman, D.A.: Chronic reflux esophagitis: is intensive long-term treatment necessary? (Abstract) Dig. Dis. Sci. **31**(suppl.):26S, 1986.

Definition, detection, and pathophysiology of gastroesophageal reflux disease
DISCUSSION

D.F. Evans

In recent years scientists and clinicians have increasingly studied all aspects of the gastrointestinal tract in order to increase their understanding of its physiology and to begin to understand the fundamental mechanisms responsible for disorders of this essential organ. Only by learning more of the physiology of a body system can the pathology be understood and hence methods of treatment be determined scientifically rather than empirically, as has often been the case in this particular area of medicine.

The esophagus has received wide attention among medical researchers for a number of reasons. First, because it constitutes the most proximal part of the gastrointestinal tract it is subjected to a considerable amount of abuse from ingestion of toxic and unsuitable foodstuffs. Second, it is the pathway through which all ingested nutrients pass, and without this constant input life cannot be sustained. Third, disorders of esophagus are common throughout the world; symptoms are very variable and in many cases do not relate to the severity or the nature of the disease.

Professor Tom DeMeester has for many years had a particular interest in esophageal disorders. As a surgeon his primary concern in treatment of the esophagus would be in the identification of patients for esophageal surgery, these being only a small proportion of the total number of patients with esophageal symptoms. Many disorders of the esophagus can obviously be effectively resolved without the need for surgery, so Dr. DeMeester not only has developed his skills in the operating theater but also has a wider knowledge of the pathophysiology of esophageal problems. This had led to his expertise and to a worldwide reputation in this particular area of gastroenterology. His knowledge and enthusiasm have stimulated other gastroenterologists and scientists to pursue similar objectives, and this has produced a greater awareness of the complexity of symptom patterns and the pathophysiology of esophageal diseases. The development of new techniques of diagnosis, new monitoring equipment, and new medical and surgical treatments have all combined to give the esophageal specialist a greater understanding of the fundamentals of esophageal function and hence greater power in the control of esophageal diseases.

In the preceding chapter Dr. DeMeester discusses the problems that have arisen in the search for normal physiologic mechanisms as differentiated from symptomatic pathologic conditions.

DeMeester's fame originated from his work on the development of 24-hour esophageal pH monitoring, although it is clear from his present research and from the preceding chapter of this book that he has developed many other techniques and investigations to study diseases of the esophagus. This has given him a wider knowledge of basic scientific principles in order to gain a fuller understanding of esophageal pathology. His chapter highlights a number of points that are important to the study of the principles of esophageal function and the relationship between symptoms and findings during investigation and the subsequent choice of treatment. These factors can be discussed best in their order of presentation.

BENIGN ESOPHAGEAL DISEASE PROFILES

One of the problems in understanding the pathophysiology of the esophagus is the difficulty in identifying the primary cause of the condition. The author emphasizes that since gastroesophageal reflux (GER) accounts for more than 75% of all conditions of the esophagus, this is the area that should receive the most attention. However, in the course of investigating patients for GER, the esophageal specialist is likely to find many other diseases not primarily related to GER. For example, during investigation of symptoms of dysphagia the gastroenterologist is likely to order upper gastrointestinal endoscopy to exclude malignancy, but of course this investigation also enables the endoscopist to identify esophagitis, peptic strictures, and lower esophageal sphincter abnormalities.

Similarly, given its availability, esophageal manometry may be requested. Although this investigation will not "diagnose" in the accepted sense of the word, it is still extremely useful in building a profile of esophageal pathology. For instance, a reduced lower esophageal sphincter pressure may be indicative of reflux, but one would need to confirm this either by endoscopic findings or by 24-hour pH monitoring (preferably both!). However, when dysphagia is the primary symptom, esophageal manometry will identify hypertensive, nonrelaxing sphincters, aperistaltic esophagi, and other related motor abnormalities.

Gamma scintigraphy is a technique becoming more widely available in the investigation of GER. Like manometry, gamma scintigraphy not only will detect refluxed gastric contents (albeit labeled with an isotope) but also is very useful in the measurement of esophageal transit, thus facilitating a diagnosis of poor esophageal clearance in the course of an investigation of GER. In a similar way, barium swallow radiology will produce a very presentable picture (sometimes with cine or video) of clearance problems as well as diagnosing GER.

Twenty-four hour pH monitoring will primarily identify GER. However, in the absence of a positive test, the record of multiple symptoms indicated by event markers and a daily diary is useful in identifying symptom patterns in relation to normal daily behavior patterns.

Thus, a series of investigations primarily devised to diagnose the presence of GER have other useful secondary diagnostic power in the investigation of nonreflux esophageal disease.

It remains for the investigator to decide, given the availability, how many and which particular tests are required in order to achieve an accurate diagnosis with the minimum discomfort and inconvenience to the patient and with the maximum possible efficiency.

INTERPRETATION OF REFLUX

Dr. DeMeester is probably best known in esophageal circles for the "DeMeester scoring system" in the evaluation of pathologic GER,

although, as I am sure he would agree, the technique might be more accurately entitled the "DeMeester-Johnson scoring system." The work by Johnson and DeMeester pioneered our ideas about 24-hour pH monitoring of the distal esophagus.[1] Since that time, with the advent of an increased awareness of the importance of GER disease, together with the introduction of sophisticated measuring equipment with computerized analysis, there has been considerable discussion about the objective evaluation of GER and its relationship to the normal.

A number of controversial areas still exist. Although, as the author pointed out, there was considerable agreement at the Zurich meeting about the definitions of reflux episodes, there are still some areas in which there is not a consensus. For example, many gastroenterologists feel that the rigid criteria of pH 4 for detection of a reflux episode is not always appropriate. We know from our own experiences that some patients complain of symptoms when the pH falls below 5, and some workers in Europe have demonstrated better normal/abnormal discriminant scores using 5 instead of 4. Perhaps we should consider the use of both 5 and 4 in the evaluation of symptomatic GER. With the availability of computerized analysis, this now only entails the press of a button to achieve a different discriminatory analysis.

Another area of controversy is whether scoring systems per se are always as useful as the interpretation of the raw data from 24-hour recordings. Some workers regard percent exposure time upright and supine as the most sensitive marker of GER and better than scoring systems in the evaluation of symptomatic reflux. In our unit we have developed a "frequency duration index" (FDI) to evaluate GER, and although this is a useful discriminant in most cases, there are some areas in which the raw data are considered more useful. For example, in patients who have predominantly long-duration but low-frequency night reflux, the FDI tends to underestimate the severity of reflux, and duration per hour is therefore a more useful measurement.

My final comment regarding analysis and discriminant scoring systems is the problem of definitions of normality. Many centers, including DeMeester's and mine, have devised limits of normality from young, healthy, asymptomatic volunteer subjects, who are classically chosen from the student population because these persons are those most likely to come forward when approached. This type of volunteer raises two considerations. The first is the problem of age match. Most volunteers will be in their early twenties, whereas patient populations are usually in middle age. There has been some evidence suggesting that middle-aged asymptomatic volunteers reflux to a degree similar to that of their younger counterparts, but this evidence is far from conclusive.

The second problem arises from the definition of "asymptomatic" or "normal." It has been shown that at least 40% of the general population has some reflux symptoms from time to time. This suggests that there may be a proportion of our so-called normal subjects who reflux silently and who may even have some esophagitis. This would result in raising the upper limits of normal and therefore might exclude some symptomatic patients who truly have abnormal reflux.

AMBULATORY MONITORING VERSUS HOSPITAL MONITORING

Professor DeMeester correctly points out that there is now a veritable plethora of portable monitoring equipment for the measurement of GER in ambulatory subjects. He also comments that there is no evidence to suggest that there were differences in reflux according to whether studies were performed in hospital or at home. In 1981 we performed one of the first ambulatory versus hospital pH monitoring studies on a group of 20 patients with proven reflux. The results of this study showed quite clearly that patients who were fully ambulatory at home refluxed more severely than they did when studied in the hospital environment. This conclusion has been supported by work performed by others, and it would thus seem important in some patients that tests be performed in as near a physiologic setting as possible.

There has been some doubt in the past as to the reproducibility of 24-hour pH monitoring when performed in both normal individuals and symptomatic patients. In our own experience, reproducibility, or the ability to obtain a positive test on patients, some of whom have severe esophagitis, is dependent on the cyclical nature of the disease and on whether they are having a "good" or "bad" week. Indeed, I have in the past had a totally negative test result in some patients, to be followed shortly by a highly positive result on another occasion.

A final factor to consider in the choice of home or hospital tests is the motivation factor of patients, some of whom may not prefer home monitoring because of embarrassment or self-consciousness. This may be important in considering patients for investigation by home monitoring and may be the final influencing factor in choosing the method of pH measurement.

LOWER ESOPHAGEAL SPHINCTER COMPETENCE

Professor DeMeester has been involved in extensive research in order to characterize the lower esophageal sphincter high-pressure zone. This work was primarily performed not as a means of defining the predisposition to GER but as an investigation to determine the most suitable forms of treatment given that patients had already demonstrated a positive reflux.

DeMeester advocates that in order to identify those patients most suited to surgery, esophageal manometry is mandatory as well as esophageal pH monitoring. This is required in order to document pressure profiles across the lower esophageal sphincter and will, therefore, determine whether surgical correction is likely to be successful. DeMeester has performed extensive in vitro tests on models of the lower esophageal sphincter and has produced a formula based on pressures and sphincter lengths such that the competence of the lower esophagus can be assessed. This formula relies not only on sphincter pressure but also on intraabdominal length and total length. DeMeester suggests that only patients with an incompetent lower esophageal sphincter should be offered surgical correction, the premise being that if the sphincter is normal a mechanical repair would be of little benefit.

I believe this approach to treatment of reflux, using objective scientifically based measurements, will increase the success rate of antireflux surgery. One sees many patients re-referred after antireflux operations because they have continuing symptoms of reflux. These patients have had surgery performed mainly because of long-standing esophageal reflux symptoms that have been resistant to medical therapy but without any objective evidence of reflux or sphincter incompetence. This has inevitably led in some cases to a poor result and the subsequent frustration of the patient, a situation that would not have arisen had the DeMeester approach been adopted.

OTHER CAUSES OF GER DISEASE

Two other pathophysiologic causes of GER disease are cited by the author—poor esophageal clearance and gastric function abnormalities. Poor esophageal clearance caused by a motility defect is either a primary condition, as in achalasia or diffuse esophageal spasm, or secondary to GER.

As the author states, the former condition is rare, even after dilatation of the esophagus for dysphagia. In a study performed recently in our unit, patients underwent 24-hour pH monitoring before and after pneumatic dilatation for achalasia. There was no significant GER in any patients either before or after dilatation. There was, however, an increase in acid exposure times indicated by periods of nontypical reflux falling to less than pH 4 after the procedure, particularly in patients without any esophageal food residue before dilatation. This study demonstrates the close association between all functions of the distal esophagus.

In the case of a motility disorder thought to be secondary to GER, attention to the primary problem of reflux should in theory be followed by an improvement in motility and hence clearance. Because clearance and motility and GER are so closely interactive, it is difficult to conceive where the problem arises. More studies of the history of the disease may enlighten us further.

The third cause of GER discussed by DeMeester is gastric funtion abnormalities. Thus the GER in these patients is a secondary problem. Treatment of the primary condition should lead to a resolution of the GER. The difficulty in these circumstances is the diagnosis of the gastric abnormality. It is only in the last 10 years that we have begun to understand the physiology of the motility of the gastrointestinal tract. New techniques have been developed to monitor gastric emptying, motility, and secretion. This has enabled clinicians to evaluate more fully conditions in which gastric dysfunction is suspected.

It would seem difficult to establish rigid guidelines as to the procedure one should adopt in these cases, since each case may be unique. However, one approach might be as follows. Given a patient with a positive 24-hour pH test and symptoms suggestive of gastric involvement, the first investigation might be barium follow-through to identify the region where a delay might be present, and to visualize any potentially obstructing upper gut lesions. This could be followed by a scintigraphic dual-phase gastric emptying study together with a small-bowel hydrogen breath test to evaluate upper gastrointestinal transit. Then a gastroduodenal motility study could be done to identify motor abnormalities, and possibly special tests such as a pentagastrin acid secretion test or an HIDA scan to highlight specific abnormalities like hyperacidity or duodenogastric reflux.

Clearly this is an area of investigation that needs further development. As new noninvasive techniques are evaluated, our knowledge of these special cases will become wider and improve the treatment of patients with these special problems.

SYMPTOM PATTERNS

I read the section on symptom development with great interest. Clearly the relationship between demonstrable abnormalities and symptoms is complex, varying not only between individuals but also chronologically in the same patients as the disease pattern develops. The various findings relating to pain type and sensation as well as sensitivity demonstrate the difficulties involved in diagnosis of esophageal disorders when symptoms only are used as a guideline.

It is clear that there is no consensus regarding the cause of symptoms and their relationship to specific abnormalities in the esophagus. The term "heartburn" is itself confusing. Some patients with severe esophagitis never admit to having heartburn as one of their symptoms, but complain of chest pains identical to those in cardiac conditions. The confusion between cardiac and esophageal pain is well known and has been for many years, but we still see patients in our esophageal clinics who have been treated for a cardiac disorder that on investigation is found to be esophageal.

The relationship between symptoms and abnormalities should be regarded with caution, and only objective evidence of GER and its complications should be used in the determination of specific therapy.

COMPOSITION OF REFLUXED MATERIAL

The measurement of pH in the distal esophagus detects hydrogen ions that are present at the level of the glass bulb of the electrode. In normal subjects the pH in the distal esophagus lies between 6 and 7; the slightly acid value is caused by an acidic saliva. Variations in the pH in the esophagus result from the passage of ingested food or the reflux of gastric contents into the esophagus. If refluxed gastric contents contain only parietal cell hydrochloric acid secretions, the pH electrode will accurately measure the hydrogen ion activity. More realistically, the gastric juice contains not only hydrochloric acid but also mucus, bicarbonate, pepsin, and residual materials from ingested food, thus producing an acidic "cocktail" whose pH may be higher than pure acid but nevertheless equally damaging to the esophageal mucosa. This is further complicated by the possibility of alkaline reflux from the duodenobiliary glands, this producing an even more complex refluxate.

The investigator should therefore take special

care in interpretation and quantification of "acid" reflux episodes when complications such as alkalinization of the gastric juice might be expected. For example, after the ingestion of a meal the gastric contents are buffered to a higher pH value by the components of the meal. This leads to a mixture with a pH of 3 to 5 even though gastric acid output is at a maximum. There is no doubt that postprandial reflux causes symptoms. Thus a problem in interpretation arises. Should the threshold of acid exposure (above pH 4) be raised when reflux episodes are measured in the postprandial period? This might give a better correlation between symptoms and reflux in this important period of monitoring, but obviously causes difficulties in analysis. Some researchers suggest discarding the 2-hour postprandial reflux as being irrelevant and commonplace. Others suggest that this period may be the most important period of measurement, especially in upright reflux.

The argument can be continued if one considers duodenobiliary acid refluxate. Professor DeMeester discusses at length the potential damaging effects of alkaline-acid mixtures, and although much work is quoted there is still little convincing evidence as to the nature of the role of nonacid reflux in the etiology of esophagitis.

Although measuring systems are now available to detect gastric and esophageal pH simultaneously, thus giving some indication of duodenogastric and gastroesophageal reflux, these systems still rely on a glass or antimony hydrogen ion–sensitive electrode to detect the refluxate. Perhaps a new approach should be considered. It is now possible to obtain ion-selective glass electrodes for the laboratory pH meter. It should therefore be possible to develop an ion-selective electrode that is sensitive to a representative component of alkaline refluxate. One possibility is a primary bile acid electrode that is selective for biliary reflux only. Another approach might be to sample refluxed material by aspiration through a fine tube attached to the pH electrode. This aspirate could be analyzed for bile acids, enzymes, and other possible damaging alkaline substances.

It is clear from DeMeester's chapter that much work is still to be done in this area, and I look forward to the development of further technology to facilitate the solution of this problem in the study of benign esophageal disease.

SUMMARY

The preceding chapter is a comprehensive evaluation of the spectrum of conditions likely to be met by physicians investigating patients with esophageal problems. The approach to diagnosis and management described by Professor DeMeester is based on sound scientific investigations relating to the pathophysiology of the disease. This ensures that the correct and most appropriate treatment is offered to the patient in order to control the disease progression. We are indebted to Professor DeMeester for his contribution to the field of esophageal disorders and look forward to continued research from his center.

REFERENCE

1. Johnson, L.F., and DeMeester, T.R.: Twenty-four-hour pH monitoring of the distal esophagus, Am. J. Gastroenterol. **62**:325-332, 1974.

CHAPTER 9

Principles of surgical treatment of gastroesophageal reflux

Mark K. Ferguson and David B. Skinner

Gastroesophageal reflux was recognized as a surgically remediable entity as early as the 1950s.[1] During the ensuing years, many procedures and subsequent modifications evolved for the treatment of reflux. Of the operations commonly employed currently, all have an acceptable rate of success and a low degree of morbidity. All these procedures share the same basic physiologic principles that underlie the successful operative treatment of gastroesophageal reflux.

DIAGNOSIS

Accurate diagnosis of gastroesophageal reflux (GER) prior to operation is essential, since 25% of patients with typical symptoms of reflux will have normal results of esophagoscopy and 24-hr pH monitoring.[2] Over 10% of patients presenting to our institution with a poor outcome from antireflux surgery were operated upon with an incorrect diagnosis. The classic symptom of reflux, substernal burning pain occurring postprandially or when supine, can be mimicked by a variety of other disorders, both gastrointestinal and cardiac. These include peptic ulcer disease, chronic cholecystitis, esophageal spasm, and coronary artery disease. These disorders should be considered at all times when the diagnosis of reflux is entertained, and appropriate evaluations should be performed when indicated. In a small percentage of patients, more than one disease process is active. This occurs with coronary artery disease and gastroesophageal reflux,[3] with reflux and peptic ulcer disease, and with reflux and gastritis. Thus, the documentation of reflux pathology does not obviate the need for clinical evaluation of potential problems in other organ systems suggested by a patient's symptom complex. In patients with symptoms of gastroesophageal reflux, the diagnosis is confirmed by objective findings of reflux, either endoscopic evidence for esophagitis (grade 2 or worse) or pathologic reflux on extended esophageal pH monitoring. In patients with atypical symptoms and no esophagitis, extended esophageal pH monitoring is essential to document the presence of reflux.

Esophageal pH monitoring also determines the pattern of acid reflux, and is helpful when considering surgical therapy. Upright refluxers, those whose reflux is usually secondary to aerophagia and belching, infrequently develop esophagitis and do well with medical management. When operated upon they have a high incidence of gas bloating symptoms postoperatively and rarely notice symptomatic improvement. Pure supine refluxers have a high incidence of esophagitis, but normally respond well to medical management and infrequently require operation. Patients with combined upright and supine reflux have the highest incidence of esophagitis and are unlikely to achieve satisfactory long-term results from conservative therapy.[4] Thus, it is important to document the existence of reflux and to determine the pattern of reflux prior to recommending definitive therapy. Knowledge of the pattern of reflux helps determine the duration of conservative therapy allowed before surgical treatment is recommended and helps predict the likelihood of success of an antireflux operation.

INDICATIONS

The initial treatment of GER remains conservative medical management, including strict diet control, head elevation during sleep, antacids, and suppression of gastric acid production. This treatment regimen should be closely monitored by a primary care physician to ensure adequate patient compliance and to confirm success of the treatment. In some patients, trials of metoclopramide or bethanecol are indicated to improve esophageal clearance, enhance gastric emptying, and increase distal esophageal sphincter pressure.[5,6,7] Indications for surgical treatment of gastroesophageal reflux include persistent symptoms following an extended trial of medical management, persistent esophagitis despite improvement in symptoms during medical therapy, and the inability to maintain a satisfactory medical regimen.

Other relative indications for antireflux surgery include stricture, aspiration pneumonitis, and Barrett's esophagus. Stricture occurs in a small percentage of patients with GER, as a result of chronic severe esophagitis. Although symptoms of reflux may improve after development of a stricture, because of its tendency to block acid reflux, local inflammation and scarring normally continue. Dilatation to relieve dysphagia usually results in worsening of acid reflux and esophagitis. Although the use of dilatation and antacid therapy alone yields good results in some,[8] we believe that the development of a stricture signifies a more severe form of reflux, for which medical therapy often ultimately fails, and is a strong relative indication for operation.

Pulmonary symptoms resulting from acid reflux occur less often than esophagitis or stricture. Nearly 50% of patients with proven GER have a history suggestive of aspiration, including nocturnal cough, morning hoarseness, recurrent pneumonia, or asthma. When present, respiratory symptoms should be correlated with objective evidence of reflux, and extended esophageal pH monitoring is ideally suited for diagnosis in these patients. The selection of patients for antireflux operations to alleviate aspiration depends upon the demonstration of pulmonary symptoms that closely follow episodes of acid reflux. Although 20% of refluxers have aspiration or episodes signifying potential aspiration, 5% of patients with reflux and respiratory symptoms have reflux episodes induced by a primary respiratory disorder.[9] This high incidence of GER is seen in patients with true asthma in the absence of pulmonary aspiration and is thought to be due to neural reflex mechanisms. Antireflux repair in these patients improves symptoms of asthma and can permit withdrawal of steroid therapy in some cases.[10]

The management of the patient with Barrett's epithelium and GER remains controversial. Reflux symptoms often regress after the development of Barrett's type of metaplasia, and this may lull the physician and the patient into a false sense of accomplishment during medical therapy. Nevertheless, the premalignant nature of Barrett's epithelium cannot be ignored. Case reports suggest that regression of columnar metaplasia can occur after antireflux repair,[11] and our own studies support this finding.[12] We believe that the demonstration of pathologic reflux in patients with Barrett's esophagus is an indication for antireflux surgery regardless of symptoms.

Gastroesophageal reflux in infants and children presents special problems in both medical and surgical management. In this age group reflux is very common, and normally responds well to dietary management, head elevation, and the use of pharmacologic agents to increase gastrointestinal motility. The complications of reflux in children are far more serious than those in adults, including intractable vomiting, failure to thrive, and severe respiratory symptoms.[13] Documentation of a near-miss episode of sudden death in the presence of reflux, which cannot be proven to be secondary to another cause, is an indication for antireflux surgery without a trial of conservative management.[14] Although esophagitis is no more common in this age group than in adults, the rapid progression to stricture that occurs in children makes this a more urgent indication for operation in the younger population.[15] The presence of esophageal stricture caused by reflux in children is a contraindication to a trial of conservative therapy because of the low rate of success of this modality.

PRINCIPLES OF SURGERY

The importance of adaptability in the operative approach to the patient with GER cannot be overemphasized. A major decision is whether to approach the hiatus transabdominally or transthoracically. The transabdominal approach allows a smaller incision, eliminates the need for an intercostal drainage catheter, and is less painful, but has a 10% incidence of reoperation for ventral hernia and a higher risk of wound infection. In some instances the transabdominal approach is dictated by the presence of other intraabdominal disease requiring intervention, particularly peptic ulcer disease or gallbladder disease. In a small number of patients, poor pulmonary function makes the risk of a transthoracic approach prohibitive.

In many cases a transthoracic approach is necessary, particularly in an obese patient and in a patient with a very large hiatal hernia. In patients with peptic esophageal strictures, there is frequently shortening of the esophagus, and a more complete mobilization of the esophagus is possible with the transthoracic approach, an important step in maintaining an intraabdominal wrap without tension. Patients with recurrent reflux following antireflux surgery present special problems during reoperation. In the vast majority of these patients a transthoracic approach to reoperation is indicated to ensure good postoperative results and minimize complications.[16]

The factors that play a role in maintaining the normal competence of the cardia and the mechanisms by which gastroesophageal acid reflux occurs are outlined elsewhere in this book. Successful operations to prevent reflux incorporate principles that restore normal function of the cardia. All the currently successful operations for control of reflux incorporate the maintenance of an intraabdominal segment of esophagus as a feature necessary for good results. Anatomic studies show that the length of the intraabdominal segment of esophagus is directly related to the presence or absence of reflux.[17,18] This concept is also supported by clinical studies performed in our laboratory.[19]

Another mechanism that is believed to play a role in the control of reflux is the calibration of the esophageal orifice at the junction of the esophagus with the stomach. An abrupt change in diameter between esophagus and stomach brings into play the forces governed by the law of Laplace. Creation of such a narrow orifice usually involves a fundoplication of stomach around the esophagus, which also creates an inkwell or flap valve mechanism. Although such a valve does not play a role in the normal control of reflux, it is incorporated into each of the successful reflux operations. Such valves promote an increase in resting distal esophageal sphincter pressure. Experimentally, altering the angle at the gastroesophageal junction has a similar effect, as occurs with a variety of mechanical devices.[20] The fact that antireflux operations can prevent reflux even when a wrap is located intrathoracically supports the concept that an adequate wrap is an independent determinant of competence of the cardia.[21]

Selection of specific operative procedures depends to some extent on each surgeon's training and experience. Nevertheless, each individual should have more than one antireflux repair at his or her command to ensure the appropriate treatment of selected clinical problems. Although the Nissen fundoplication is the most frequently performed antireflux operation, it produces a higher incidence of gas bloating in the early postoperative period and introduces the greatest sphincter pressure increase, which may cause dysphagia. In patients who have a significant degree of aerophagia or in whom the peristaltic function of the body of the esophagus is abnormal, a fundoplication of less than 360 degrees should be done. We find the Hill operation particularly useful in patients who have had prior gastric surgery, particularly antrectomy, and in whom a total fundoplication would unnecessarily limit the size of the gastric reservoir. In patients requiring esophageal myotomy or in whom intrinsic esophageal body function is abnormal, a Belsey repair, or partial fundoplication, is indicated.

SUMMARY

This chapter serves as a brief outline of the basic principles involved in antireflux surgery. We wish to emphasize the importance of accurate diagnosis and the necessity for a program of conservative medical management of these problems to prevent precipitous and unwarranted surgical procedures. When operation is indicated, consideration of both the underlying pathophysiology of gastroesophageal reflux and the accompanying surgical problems is necessary. Each surgeon then should maintain adequate flexibility in the approach to antireflux surgery to provide each patient with the maximum benefit of the surgical procedure.

REFERENCES

1. Allison, P.R.: Reflux esophagitis, sliding hiatal hernia, and the anatomy of repair, Surg. Gynecol. Obstet. **92:**419, 1951.
2. DeMeester, T.R., Wang, C.-I., Wernly, J.A., Pellegrini, C.A., Little, A.G., Klementschitsch, P., Bermudez, G., Johnson, L.F., and Skinner, D.B.: Technique, indications and clinical use of 24 hour esophageal pH monitoring, J. Thorac. Cardiovasc. Surg. **79:**656-667, 1980.
3. DeMeester, T.R., O'Sullivan, G.C., Bermudez, G., Midell, A.I., Cimochowski, G.E., and O'Drobinak, J.: Esophageal function in patients with angina-type chest pain and normal coronary angiogram, Ann. Surg. **196:**488-498, 1982.
4. DeMeester, T.R., Johnson, L.F., Joseph, G.J., Toscano, M.S., Hall, A.W., and Skinner, D.B.: Patterns of gastroesophageal reflux in health and disease, Ann. Surg. **184:**459-469, 1976.
5. Russell, C.O., and Hill, L.D.: Gastroesophageal reflux, Curr. Probl. Surg. **20**(4):205-278.
6. Johnson, L.F.: New concepts and methods in the study and treatment of gastroesophageal reflux disease, Med. Clin. North Am. **65:**1195-1222, 1981.
7. Cooper, J.D., and Jeejeebhoy, K.N.: Gastroesophageal reflux: medical and surgical management, Ann. Thorac. Surg. **31:**577-593, 1981.
8. Wesdorp, I.C., Bartelsman, J.F., den Hartog Jager, F.C.A., Huibregtse, K., and Tytgat, G.N.: Results of

conservative treatment of benigh esophageal strictures: a follow-up study in 100 patients, Gastroenterology **82**:487-493, 1982.

9. Pellegrini, C.A., DeMeester, T.R., Johnson, L.F., and Skinner, D.B.: Gastroesophageal reflux and pulmonary aspiration: incidence, functional abnormality, and results of surgical therapy, Surgery **86**:110-118, 1979.

10. Lorrain, A., Carrasco, J., Galleguillos, J., and Pope, C.E., II: Reflux treatment improves lung function in patients with intrinsic asthma, Gastroenterology **80**:1204, 1981.

11. Brand, D.L., Ylvisaker, J.T., Gelfand, M., and Pope, C.E., II: Regression of columnar esophageal (Barrett's) epithelium after antireflux surgery, N. Engl. J. Med. **302**:844-848, 1980.

12. Skinner, D.B., Walther, B.C., Riddel, R.H., Schmidt, H., Iascone, C., and DeMeester, T.R.: Barrett's esophagus: comparison of benign and malignant cases, Ann. Surg. **198**:554-565, 1983.

13. Johnson, D.G., Jolley, S.G., Herbst, J.J., and Cordell, L.J.: Surgical selection of infants with gastroesophageal reflux, J. Pediatr. Surg. **16**:587-594, 1981.

14. Johnson, D.G., and Jolley, S.G.: Gastroesophageal reflux in infants and children: recognition and treatment, Surg. Clin. North Am. **61**:1101-1115, 1981.

15. Belsey, R.H.R.: Gastroesophageal reflux, Am. J. Surg. **139**:775-781.

16. Little, A.G.L., Ferguson, M.K., and Skinner, D.B.: Reoperation for failed antireflux surgery, J. Thorac. Cardiovasc. Surg. (In press.)

17. Bombeck, C.T., Dillard, D.H., and Nyhus, L.M.: Muscular anatomy of the gastroesophageal junction and role of phrenoesophageal ligament: autopsy study of sphincter mechanism, Ann. Surg. **164**:643, 1966.

18. Henderson, R.D.: Gastroesophageal junction in hiatus hernia, Can. J. Surg. **15**:63, 1972.

19. O'Sullivan, G.C., DeMeester, T.R., Joelsson, B.E., Smith, R.B., Blough, R.R., Johnson, L.F., and Skinner, D.B.: Interaction of lower esophageal sphincter pressure and length of sphincter in the abdomen as determinants of gastroesophageal competence, Am. J. Surg. **143**:40-47, 1982.

20. Benjamin, S.B., Knuff, T.K., Fink, M., Woods, E., and Castell, D.O.: The Angelchik antireflux prosthesis: effects on the lower esophageal sphincter of primates, Ann. Surg. **197**:63-67, 1983.

21. Maher, J.W., Hocking, M.P., and Woodward, E.R.: Supradiaphragmatic fundoplication: long-term follow-up and analysis of complications, Am. J. Surg. **147**:181-186, 1984.

Principles of surgical treatment of gastroesophageal reflux

DISCUSSION

John Bancewicz

This review of the principles of the surgical treatment of gastroesophageal reflux is, as one would expect from the authors, succinct, appropriate, and practical. However, it would be wrong to imply that there is no controversy in this maturing branch of surgery. My intention is not, therefore, to criticize those whose previous writings have helped my own understanding of reflux disease, but rather to highlight areas of debate and point to those aspects of the subject that still require clarification.

In my own part of the world reflux esophagitis is now the commonest finding at upper gastrointestinal endoscopy. The incidence is greater than that of duodenal ulcer and gastric ulcer combined, and there is no reason to suppose that this experience is unique. Of course, most of the time no operation is required, but because it is so common many surgeons have to grapple with the problems that these patients may pose. Unfortunately, a large number of medical gastroenterologists do not share the rosy view expressed by the authors in their opening paragraph that the operations currently employed have an acceptable rate of success and a low degree of morbidity.

Why should there be this difference between published surgical data and popular perception? Ferguson and Skinner deal nicely with the principles of diagnosis, patient selection, and technique of operation, but omit one extremely important issue, namely variations in individual surgical performance.

It is impossible to argue with the authors' basic premise that accurate diagnosis is essential. My own experience is that physicians do not think of the esophagus often enough as a cause of atypical symptoms, but the reverse seems to be the case in the United States. Whatever the popular local failing, the message is the same: this apparently simple condition can cause great diagnostic confusion. One of the problems is that minor esophageal symptoms are so common in the general population that dual pathology is therefore to be expected frequently. There are two essential stages in making an assessment of an individual patient. First, is the esophagus abnormal? Second, is that abnormality responsible for the symptoms? Investigation must be directed to both of these issues.

Twenty-four-hour pH recording is a particularly valuable tool, since it deals with both of these elements of diagnosis. It allows one to distinguish with reasonable accuracy between the normal and the abnormal and also to record symptoms in relation to documented reflux episodes. I have been less impressed with the clinical value of making the distinction between supine and upright reflux. To my knowledge there has been no independent confirmation of DeMeester's thesis that upright reflux is due to aerophagia and belching. My own experience with 24-hour pH recording now extends to over 800 patients; some 200 of whom have subsequently had an operation to control reflux. Very few have had reflux that occurs only in the supine position, and the majority have had either upright reflux or combined reflux. Combined refluxers certainly seem more likely to have severe esophagitis or stricture, but I cannot confirm that those with upright reflux do badly with surgery. Indeed, many of our most dramatic successes after Nissen fundoplication have been in patients with upright reflux, and there has been no difference in the incidence, type, or severity of side effects. This may reflect differing methods of clinical case selection.

Patients with gastrointestinal disorders other than reflux who happen to have a little heartburn will almost always reflux only in the upright position. If 24-hour pH recording is done on a relatively unselected group of patients, it is inevitable that there will be some positive tests in those whose reflux is not a serious clinical problem. Obviously such patients are not candidates for an operation, but this is quite different from saying that everybody with upright reflux will do badly with an operation.

With such considerations in mind I think it is much more rational to assume that combined reflux simply represents more advanced disease. Within the upright group are many who have severe symptoms and who will in time develop progressive disease. There is every reason to try to identify and treat these patients at an early stage.

In general I agree with the indications for surgery outlined by Ferguson and Skinner, but I would take issue with them on the question of Barrett's esophagus. They have acknowledged that this is a controversial topic, and I think it is likely to remain so for some time. Many authors have made the fundamental mistake of confusing incidence with prevalence. It is quite true that a large number of patients with Barrett's esophagus have a cancer when they first see a surgeon (prevalence). However, what matters for the future of the others is their risk of subsequently developing a cancer (incidence). Few large series address this issue, but what little information there is suggests that the incidence of cancer is much lower than the prevalence.[1, 2] In addition to this difficulty in quantifying the risk of cancer, there is the difficulty of determining whether the natural history can be influenced by surgery to control reflux. Skinner et al.[3] have produced some provocative evidence that it may be, but more information is required. Finally, any suggestion that prophylactic surgery reduces risk must take into account the deleterious effects of surgery, including postoperative mortality. My own feeling is that the issue is far from settled and that a great deal of further study is required.

The final topic is the nature and technique of surgery. I thoroughly agree with the authors' advocacy of adaptability. Some patients, particularly those who have had previous gastrointestinal surgery and those with panmural esophagitis, pose formidable problems for the surgeon. It is essential that those who perform this sort of surgery feel equally happy working on either side of the diaphragm. I am less happy about the suggestion that every surgeon should have a number of antireflux repairs at his command. Although reflux is, as I have indicated, a very common condition, most surgeons will not have a vast experience. This is reflected in part by the relatively small numbers in many published series. If this experience is further diluted by a piecemeal approach, the results of surgery are hardly likely to improve. Conversation with many surgeons and gastroenterologists indicates to my own satisfaction that the biggest problem with reflux surgery at the moment is its variability from one surgeon to another. It is therefore desirable that surgeons be thoroughly familiar with their own results and use this information to try to produce a consistently satisfactory surgical result.

My own practice has been to use the floppy Nissen operation, which can easily be done via the chest or thorax and combined with a Collis gastroplasty if necessary. Abnormal peristaltic function of the body of the esohagus has not been associated with poor results. I suspect that much of the information that says it is simply reflects inadequate surgical technique. Dysphagia may be produced by a wrap that is too tight or too long or by one that is poorly constructed and does not control reflux.

In the hands of experienced surgeons, operations for gastroesophageal reflux are now highly effective. Ferguson and Skinner have nicely encapsulated the state of the art, but fortunately the subject has not ossified. There is still debate and room for further research, and every prospect that matters will continue to improve.

REFERENCES

1. Cameron, A.J., Ott, B.J., and Payne, W.S.: The incidence of adenocarcinoma in columnar-lined (Barrett's) esophagus, N. Engl. J. Med. **313:**857-859, 1985.
2. Spechler, S.J., Robbins, A.H., Rubins, H.B., Vincent, M.E., Heeren, T., Doos, W.G., Colton, T., and Schimmel, E.M.: Adenocarcinoma and Barrett's esophagus: an overrated risk, Gastroenterology **87:**927-933, 1984.
3. Skinner, D.B., Walther, B.C., Riddell, R.H., Schmidt, H., Iascone, C., and DeMeester, T.R.: Barrett's esophagus: comparison of benign and malignant cases, Ann. Surg. **198:**554-565, 1983.

CHAPTER 10 Personal reflections on standard antireflux procedures

Ronald H. Belsey

Current antireflux procedures can be classified into three main groups: one historic, three abdominal procedures, and two thoracic.

1. Allison repair
2. Total fundoplication (Nissen)
3. Posterior gastropexy (Hill)
4. Angelchik antireflux prosthesis
5. Mark IV antireflux procedure
6. Collis gastroplasty

There are probably as many modifications of these procedures as there are surgeons practicing antireflux surgery. No attempt will be made to describe all these modifications in detail. The principles underlying the three groups will be reviewed.

Controversy persists regarding the relative merits of the abdominal and thoracic routes. Certain indications have been generally accepted. The advantages of the abdominal route are as follows:

1. Familiarity. The majority of surgeons active in this field are primarily abdominal surgeons with no thoracic training
2. Easy access for management of coexisting upper abdominal pathology
3. Less risk of persisting postoperative pain
4. May be indicated in patients with serious chronic aspiration pneumonitis with impairment of pulmonary function

The following are disadvantages of the abdominal route:

1. Does not permit adequate mobilization of the esophagus
2. Inadequate exposure in the obese patient
3. Contraindicated in patients with chronic esophagitis with impending stenosis or in patients with recurrent reflux following previous surgery.

Advantages of the thoracic route are as follows:

1. Permits the adequate mobilization necessary for a physiologic repair

2. In patients with chronic esophagitis and acquired shortening, the choice between a Collis gastroplasty and resection and reconstruction is immediately available at thoracotomy
3. Permits the mobilization of the cardia in patients with recurrent reflux following previous surgery
4. Excellent exposure in the obese
5. Good exposure of the upper abdomen through the extended thoracotomy incision for the management of coexisting upper abdominal pathology

The following are disadvantages of the thoracic route:

1. Postthoracotomy pain
2. Incidence of lung hernia
3. Postoperative respiratory complications

The choice of approach will be governed by the basic principles of antireflux surgery favored by the individual surgeon.

There is no "best" operation. The procedure indicated in any individual patient is that which in the hands of the surgeon fulfills all or the majority of the criteria demanded of any technique to be acceptable:

1. Provides complete and permanent relief of all symptoms and complications of reflux
2. Provides the ability to belch voluntarily, to relieve gas distention of the stomach
3. Provides the ability to vomit when necessary
4. Shows objective evidence of the control of reflux
5. Allows the patient to return to a normal life-style with no further medical, postural, or dietetic therapy
6. Permits synchronous correction of other upper abdominal pathologic conditions
7. Is applicable to the control of reflux fol-

lowing esophageal myotomy for functional disorders

8. Is applicable to the correction of recurrent reflux and recurrent hiatal herniation
9. Is suitable for the correction of seriously complicated cases of reflux
10. Has applications in infants and children
11. Can be communicated to the resident or trainee surgeon of average ability

THE ALLISON REPAIR

The Allison repair[1] was based upon the principle that an anatomic reduction of the hernia, with narrowing of the hiatus, and exaggeration of the esophagogastric angle of His would automatically control the reflux by the hypothetical pinchcock action of the right crus. The operation is no longer performed in its original form as described by Allison, since the admitted recurrence rate approaches 50%, but many modifications of the technique are still favored by European surgeons.

ABDOMINAL PROCEDURES
The abdominal total fundoplication (Nissen)

As originally intended by Nissen,[2] the principle was a gastroesophageal fundoplication to enlist the hypothetical sphincteric action of the circular muscle fibers of the gastric fundus to replace an inadequate lower esophageal sphincter, and furthermore to funnel intragastric pressure to the sphincter. Owing to the inadequate mobilization of the esophagus possible by the abdominal route, the fundoplication eventually becomes a gastrogastric wrap in some patients.

The technique is too well known to require repetition. The popularity of the procedure stems from the technical ease with which some form of fundoplication can be achieved and its ready acceptance by the average trainee surgeon with no experience of thoracotomy technique. Early success in the control of reflux in 95% or 100% of cases has frequently been claimed by exponents of this technique, who have used pH studies and manometry to confirm the control. However, if prevention of reflux were the sole aim of surgery, then a simple ligature around the cardia could guarantee success. As mentioned before, essential criteria are permanent control of the reflux and restoration of the patient's ability to eat and drink a full normal meal without discomfort, to belch voluntarily to relieve gas distention in the stomach, and to vomit when necessary. Regretta-

bly, dysphagia and the gas bloating syndrome are common early complications. Much has been said about the size of bougie to be inserted to "stent" the esophagus during the fundoplication. Some surgeons favor a snug wrap, others a loose wrap. The increasing number of modifications now appearing suggests that some of the prior claims for success may have been premature. It is still accepted by the majority of surgeons that one does not "change a winning team."

A fundamental design fault in the procedure is tension on the repair resulting from inadequate mobilization of the esophagus and the precarious hold the wrap obtains on the lower sphincter region of the esophagus, thus promoting a return of the sphincter to the low-pressure, intrathoracic position. There are still no long-term surveys of the late results supported by objective evidence. On the debit side there are now appearing reports of catastrophic and life-threatening complications resulting from obstruction, strangulation, perforation, fistulae, recurrent herniation, and hemorrhage, to name but a few.[3-5]

The major problem besetting antireflux surgery today is recurrent reflux after one or many previous attempts. Management of recurrent reflux is a technically difficult exercise, and the difficulty increases with each intervention. The commonest previous procedure recorded is an abdominal total fundoplication, but this may merely reflect the greater frequency with which this procedure is currently performed. At further operation, preferably by the thoracic route, little evidence of the original fundoplication can be found, suggesting that a complete dissolution is responsible for the recurrent reflux. Evidence of any encroachment into the mediastinum is rarely encountered, suggesting that no attempt to mobilize the esophagus was ever made.

The Nissen fundoplication will undoubtedly continue to be the most popular technique until such time as a realistic and objective assessment of the long-term results has been reported, and an alternative of comparable technical ease and with more assurance of long-term satisfaction has been devised.

Posterior gastropexy (Hill)

The second standard antireflux procedure performed by the abdominal route is the Hill posterior gastropexy.[6] Theoretically this procedure is based upon sounder physiologic principles. The lower sphincter segment is restored to the high-pressure subdiaphragmatic region at least partially and is retained in that position by anchorage to the tough arcuate ligament and preaortic fascia. Hill has advanced the interesting theory that the longitudinal stretching imposed on the esophagus by the low fixation of the cardia may increase the propulsive efficiency of the esophageal pump and so aid the acid-clearing mechanism, an essential element in the prevention of peptic esophagitis. So far, so good. Placement of the anchoring sutures to the arcuate ligament involves some degree of rotation of the organ. Twisting any tubular structure creates a variable degree of obstruction, and in this context the risk of postoperative dysphagia. Hill resolves this problem by insisting on the routine use of intraoperative manometry, and the adjustment of the repair until a pressure of 30 to 50 mm Hg in the high-pressure zone has been achieved. If the necessary apparatus is unavailable, the Hill gastropexy should presumably not be attempted. The exposure necessary to permit the more thorough dissection of the arcuate ligament without damage to the important adjacent vascular structures is more difficult to achieve, especially in an obese patient, than that necessary for the Nissen procedure or its modifications.

The long-term results of the Hill procedure are difficult to assess. Hill has published excellent results, but there is little independent objective confirmation from other centers. Rather more difficult to accept is Hill's claim for a higher success rate in patients with chronic esophagitis and peptic strictures, in whom acquired shortening is regularly encountered and in whom extensive mobilization by the thoracic route may still fail to restore the sphincter to the high-pressure, intraabdominal region, the very essence of a physiologic repair.

The Angelchik antireflux prosthesis

The Angelchik procedure[7] must be reviewed in this context in view of the frequency with which the operation is currently performed. The mechanism by which an inert prosthesis can bolster the incompetence of a highly complex physiologic sphincter mechanism such as the gastroesophageal junction has not been explained. Undoubtedly, the ease and simplicity of the procedure excite acceptance as the long-sought alternative to the Nissen fundoplication. Final assessment of the value of the procedure, the indications, and the late complications that can be anticipated must be deferred until long-term objective follow-up surveys are available. Reports on migration of the prosthesis to the thorax or the pelvis and ulceration into the lumen of the bowel are already appearing, but the incidence of these complications as reported is presently low compared with the 10,000 or more prostheses that have been inserted. However, it has long been recognized

that any ligature of foreign material applied to a hollow viscus, be it major blood vessel or bowel, will demonstrate a propensity to migrate into the lumen of that structure. No antireflux procedure is completely immune to late complications and failure. In the event of failure, further information on the technical difficulties involved in removing the device and correcting the situation will play an essential role in the appraisal of the indications. Passage per rectum may prove the easier answer to the problem for the patient. Any patient about to be subjected to the procedure should be fully warned of the possible complications.

TRANSTHORACIC PROCEDURES

The transthoracic antireflux procedures involve the problems inherent in any thoracotomy, as well as the possibility of persisting postoperative pain, and demand training in the management of postthoracotomy complications. The advantages of the thoracic approach are fourfold. First, the extensive mobilization of the esophagus necessary for a physiologic repair and restoration of 4 to 5 cm of the lower sphincter zone to the high-pressure region is possible even in the presence of some degree of acquired shortening of the organ. Second, excellent exposure of the upper abdomen, often superior to that available by laparotomy, can be obtained by the extended left thoracotomy approach with peripheral detachment of the diaphragm. Third, a variety of reconstructive procedures are immediately available in the event of a physiologic repair proving technically impossible because of acquired shortening or previous surgical adventures. Fourth, with attention to certain technical details, persisting postthoracotomy pain is avoidable. These details, in summary, are as follows: (1) a high thoracotomy, no lower than the sixth interspace; (2) division of the corresponding neurovascular bundle if any rib is divided, before insertion of the rib spreaders; (3) only sufficient rib distraction to permit the procedure and avoidance of the aggressive use of rib spreaders; and (4) avoidance of close rib approximation during closure of the thoracotomy incision. The pericostal sutures should merely restore the ribs to their original anatomic relationship.

The standard transthoracic antireflux procedures are as follows:

1. Total fundoplication with extensive esophageal mobilization and restoration of the wrap to the infradiaphragmatic position
2. The Mark IV Procedure

3. The Collis gastroplasty and various modifications.

The "transthoracic Nissen," a misuse of eponymous designation, differs from the Mark IV procedure only in the 360-degree fundoplication, as opposed to a partial wrap of 240 degrees, and in the mode of anchoring the wrap to the lower esophagus. Woodward[8] has recommended retaining the fundoplication within the thorax, but this modification would appear to have no theoretical advantages and may promote the dire complications of the type II hernia situation. Woodward has stressed the importance of enlarging the hiatus if the wrap is to be retained within the thorax.

The Mark IV procedure

The Mark IV procedure has been described in detail elsewhere,[9,10] and only the basic principles and salient technical details will be reviewed. The basic principle is the restoration of 4 to 5 cm of the lower sphincter zone to the high-pressure region. The important step in the technique is the mobilization of the esophagus up to the point where the vagus nerves join the organ from the lung roots, close to the aortic arch. This is only possible through the thoracotomy approach. The second step is complete mobilization of the cardia by division of the thick band of tissue forming the upper limit of the gastrohepatic omentum and containing "Belsey's artery." The third step is the creation of a 240-degree fundoplication around the lower 4 to 5 cm of the sphincter zone of the esophagus after removal of the fat pad from the anterior aspect of the cardia. The fourth step is the approximation of the two halves of the right crus to form a posterior buttress to exert counterpressure on the lower sphincter zone when it is restored to the abdomen. The fifth step is the restoration of the fundoplication to the abdomen along with 4 to 5 cm of the sphincter zone and its permanent maintenance in that situation by the second row of fundoplication sutures, which have been passed through the diaphragm at the point where the muscle ring of the hiatus joins the central tendon. The sixth and final step is the easy passage of a finger through the hiatus behind the esophagus to exclude excessive narrowing of the hiatus. It is better to leave the hiatus rather too loose than too tight, and this may involve cutting out one or more of the buttressing sutures in the right crura.

Possible errors in technique in the hands of the surgeon or resident inexperienced in the procedure are inadequate mobilization of the esophagus, faulty placement of the fundoplicating mattress sutures, too aggressive tying of these sutures, and, finally, excessive and unnecessary narrowing of the hiatus. No dramatic or life-threatening late complications have been reported following the Mark IV operation. The long-term results have been documented. Orringer and Skinner[11] reviewed the results of the standard Mark IV procedure in 892 consecutive cases, of which 682 had been followed up for 5 years or longer. In this series the incidence of unsatisfactory results was 5.9% in patients operated upon by experienced faculty members and 14.5% in patients operated upon by residents and interns in a busy training program.

The main disadvantage to the Mark IV procedure is the greater demand for technical precision in its correct performance and the necessity for an apprenticeship in a center where the technique is in routine use.

The Collis gastroplasty

The Collis gastroplasty[12] and its modifications constitute a further commonly performed standard procedure available on certain specific indications. The procedure was originally designed by Collis to permit a repair in cases in which acquired shortening resulting from chronic esophagitis rendered it technically difficult or impossible to perform a physiologic repair. The operation is basically a stomach-lengthening procedure and in fact creates an iatrogenic Barrett's esophagus possibly prone to the late complications associated with that condition. The practical indication is dilatable peptic stenosis, in which case the procedure is performed as an alternative to resection and reconstruction. Unfortunately, a malignant stricture cannot be excluded by a negative biopsy examination, a risk that has been increased by the often inadequate biopsy specimens obtainable through the flexible scope. The introduction of the mechanical stapler, a "shortcut" tool that exercises a compelling fascination for some surgeons, has led to the use of the gastroplasty combined with a partial or total fundoplication as a routine antireflux procedure in cases in which a more physiologic correction is possible. The procedure is not without risk. Orringer and Sloan[13] reported on 77 cases with two operative deaths, gastrocutaneous fistulae in two, ischemic necrosis of the esophagus in two, perforation in two, late major bleeding in three, and recurrent reflux in 30% as shown by pH testing.

There have been references to a "Collis-Belsey" procedure, a further misuse of eponymus nomenclature. This operation bears no relationship to the Mark IV antireflux procedure, and in fact I have not found it necessary to resort to this technique. Pearson has reported satisfactory results in the management of dilatable peptic strictures but has also reported five cases of adenocarcinoma in the iatrogenic Barrett's esophagus created by the gastroplasty.[14]

SUMMARY

Nissen transabdominal total fundoplication will undoubtedly continue to be the most popular antireflux procedure on account of the ease of performance and the lack of demand for any subtleties in operative technique rather than on account of the long-term results as recorded so far, and in spite of the catastrophic late complications that have been reported. The wider adoption of the Hill posterior gastropexy, in theory a more physiologic procedure, will be deterred by the necessity for intraoperative manometry and the technical difficulty of obtaining adequate exposure of the arcuate ligament. Unlike the Nissen procedure, the Hill operation may prove satisfactory in the presence of dismotility of the esophageal pump, a situation in which a Nissen total fundoplication is contraindicated by the high incidence of persisting dysphagia.

The Mark IV antireflux procedure has proved its ability to satisfy the 11 criteria demanded of an acceptable technique. It may never supersede the transabdominal procedures on account of the greater technical precision demanded in its performance. It may, however, prove to be the procedure of choice in the management of recurrent reflux following previous surgical adventures, a situation in which the thoracic approach is obligatory to permit adequate mobilization in the face of the traumatic adhesions, the legacy of previous surgery.

The Collis gastroplasty and its modifications are a reasonable alternative to resection and reconstruction in cases of easily dilatable peptic strictures in which malignancy has been excluded beyond all reasonable doubt.

REFERENCES

1. Allison, P.: Reflux esophagitis, sliding hiatal hernia and anatomy of repair, Surg. Gynecol. Obstet. **92:**419-431, 1951.
2. Nissen, R.: Gastropexy and fundoplication in surgical treatment of hiatal hernia, Am. J. Dig. Dis. **6:**954-961, 1961.
3. Hill, L.D., Ilves, R., Stevenson, J.K., and Pearson, J.M.: Reoperation for disruption and recurrence after Nissen fundoplication, Arch. Surg. **114:**542-548, 1979.
4. Leonardi, H., Crozier, R., and Ellis, F.: Reoperation for failed Nissen fundoplication, J. Thorac. Cardiovasc. Surg. **81:**50-56, 1981.
5. Mansour, K., Burton, H., Miller, J., and Hatcher, C.R., Jr.: Complications of the intrathoracic Nissen wrap, Ann. Thorac. Surg. **32:**173-178, 1981.
6. Hill, L.: An effective operation for hiatal hernia: an 8 year appraisal, Ann. Surg. **166:**681-692, 1967.
7. Angelchik, J.P., and Cohen, R.C.: A new surgical procedure for the treatment of gastroesophageal reflux and hiatal hernia, Surg. Gynecol. Obstet. **148:**246-248, 1979.
8. Woodward, E.R.: Surgical treatment of gastroesophageal reflux and its complications, World J. Surg. **1:**453-460, 1977.
9. Belsey, R.H.R.: Hiatal herniorrphaphy. In Malt, R., editor: Surgical techniques illustrated, Philadelphia, 1985, W.B. Saunders Co.
10. Skinner, D., and Belsey, R.: Surgical management of esophageal reflux and hiatus hernia: long term results with 1030 patients, J. Thorac. Cardiovasc. Surg. **53:**33-54, 1967.
11. Orringer, M., Skinner, D., and Belsey, R.: Long term results of the Mark IV operation for hiatal hernia and analyses of recurrences and their treatment, J. Thorac. Cardiovasc. Surg. **63:**25-33, 1972.
12. Collis, J.: Gastroplasty, Thorax **16:**197-206, 1961.
13. Orringer, M., and Sloane, H.: Complications of the Collis gastroplasty, J. Thorac. Cardiovasc. Surg. **71:**295-303, 1976.
14. Pearson, F., Langer, B., and Henderson, R.D.: Gastroplasty and Belsey hiatus hernia repair: an operation for the management of peptic stricture with acquired short esophagus, J. Thorac. Cardiovasc. Surg. **61:**50-63, 1971.

Personal reflections on standard antireflux procedures

DISCUSSION

F. Henry Ellis, Jr.

Like all of Mr. Belsey's contributions, this chapter on standard antireflux procedures is interesting and informative. It is always refreshing to read the words of a master of the art. Mr. Belsey has never been shy about his beliefs, and in this chapter he states them very clearly. Based on years of clinical experience, his preference for the Mark IV procedure is only thinly disguised.

My role as a discusser, however, is not primarily to compliment the author but to bring up points for discussion, so I will proceed to function as a "devil's advocate" and advance a few contrary opinions that I hope will be received in the constructive manner in which they are intended. As Mr. Belsey will be the first to admit, our disagreements regarding esophageal surgery are numerous, and I had only to read his first sentence to realize that our differences of opinion persist. He lists six procedures that he classifies as antireflux techniques. However, neither the Allison repair nor the Collis gastroplasty is an antireflux operation, for as he points out later in the chapter, each was designed specifically to restore normal anatomy, not normal physiology. This accounts for the failure of the Allison repair to correct the physiologic abnormality of a hypotensive lower esophageal sphincter (LES). Similarly, the Collis gastroplasty, which does nothing more than lengthen the esophagus by tubing the lesser curvature of the stomach, does not restore LES pressure to normal.[1]

As a matter of historic interest, it is worth recalling that neither the Hill nor the Mark IV procedure was devised for the purpose of restoring normal physiology. In fact, in Hill's initial publication,[2] he stresses that he is restoring normal anatomy by placing stitches in the sturdiest tissue available. Only later did the concept of "calibration of the cardia"[3] and intraoperative manometry[4] reveal that this "anatomic repair" was in essence a form of fundoplication. Likewise, the early papers describing the development of the Mark IV procedure emphasized its role in

providing an intraabdominal segment of esophagus.[5] In actual fact, this procedure is successful because it restores normal LES pressure by virtue of its fundoplication features, although, to be sure, the wrap is an incomplete one. Only the Nissen fundoplication was designed to restore normal function rather than normal anatomy. Just how the Angelchik prosthesis fits into all of this is difficult to say. It does not restore normal physiology in any way, yet it apparently is successful in some cases in preventing reflux, although its reported complications have deterred many of us from using it.

These preliminary comments represent only minor and relatively unimportant differences of opinion between the two of us, and there are more important points of difference in our approaches to the management of medically recalcitrant gastroesophageal reflux disease that I would like now to discuss. In my opinion, Mr. Belsey overstates the disadvantages of the Nissen procedure whether done transabdominally or through the chest. He states, "There are still no long-term surveys of the late results [of the Nissen procedure] supported by objective evidence." I will refer to two carefully followed series that negate this statement.

DeMeester and associates[6] have reported the results of the Nissen fundoplication performed on 100 consecutive patients. The patients underwent operation between 1972 and 1984 and were followed up from 1 to 13 years, with an average period of close to 4 years. The improvement rate calculated by the actuarial method based on success in controlling reflux symptoms was 91%. Objective documentation of the results of the procedure was provided by esophageal manometry and pH reflux testing. Side effects, such as "gas bloat" syndrome and dysphagia, were minimal with the technique of a loose wrap over a large-bore indwelling stent and a relatively short length of esophagus (1 cm in recent cases).

Crozier and I[7] described almost identical results recently, reporting follow-up studies of 82 Nissen fundoplications for periods of 1 to 13 years, with an average of almost 6 years. Reflux control was effective and permanent in 90.2% of cases, and approximately four fifths of the patients stated that they were able to belch. Recurrent reflux was the commonest cause of poor results and has all but been eliminated in the past 10 years by the use of a large-bore indwelling stent (42F), much as advocated by DeMeester and associates.[6] These two long-term surveys of the late results of the Nissen procedure are supported by objective evidence of its effectiveness.

Mr. Belsey goes on to provide a laundry list of catastrophes that can accompany the Nissen fundoplication. These have been reported primarily by Hill and associates.[8] Fortunately, these catastrophes must be few and far between, for other reports on reoperations after the failed Nissen do not support this catalogue of horrors. In a recent review by Leonardi and me,[9] we described 54 reoperations on patients who had undergone the Nissen fundoplication previously, all but a few of whom underwent their original operations elsewhere. The commonest reason for reoperation was postoperative dysphagia, present in 35 patients. In 15 of these patients, the dysphagia was related to an underlying motility disorder previously undiagnosed, which was accounted for in most patients by achalasia and in about one third by diffuse spasm and scleroderma. Seven patients had a "slipped" Nissen. Quotation marks are used because, in my opinion, most of these patients had the initial wrap placed around the stomach rather than the esophagus. Three patients with strictures had persistent dysphagia, and I do not believe that a wrap of any sort around a hard panmural fibrous stricture can effectively control reflux symptoms. In 10 of 35 patients no obvious cause of the dysphagia could be identified, but by dismantling the original wrap and redoing it according to the technique that I have described,[10] which resembles that reported by DeMeester et al.,[11] the symptoms were relieved. Presumably, in these 10 patients the wrap had been made too tight. Recurrent reflux, paraesophageal hernia, and the gas bloat syndrome accounted for the remaining reoperative procedures. Interestingly enough, only two of the 54 patients required reoperation for the gas bloat syndrome. Other authors[12] have reported similar indications for reoperation, suggesting further that the disastrous consequences of the Nissen procedure have been overemphasized.

Mr. Belsey believes that the procedure involves a fundamental fault in design that causes intrathoracic migration of the wrap as a result of inadequate mobilization of the esophagus by the abdominal route. Anyone who has carried out a transhiatal esophagectomy for carcinoma is aware that the intrathoracic esophagus can be mobilized, much of it under direct vision, as high as the tracheal bifurcation through the abdominal route. Therefore, this criticism is, in my opinion, ill founded. I do agree, however, that if the wrap migrates into the chest, there may be serious consequences. This complication usually occurs when the esophagus has become shortened by scarring. For these patients, I prefer a transthoracic approach. If the wrap cannot be made around the distal esophagus and returned to the abdomen, then the esophagus should be lengthened with a Collis gastroplasty and the wrap made around the neoesophagus and returned to the abdomen, thus avoiding postoperative development of a paraesophageal hernia with its potential hazards.

As further support for my bias in favor of the Nissen procedure, I must enlist the support of the literature. Both experimentally[12] and clinically,[13] reports repeatedly document the superiority of this operation over other antireflux procedures in restoring the competence mechanism and relieving patients' symptoms.

In conclusion, I wish in no way to denigrate the contributions of Mr. Belsey and agree with him that the Mark IV antireflux procedure has, indeed, proved its place as an entirely satisfactory antireflux maneuver. In my opinion, it is particularly applicable to patients in whom for one reason or another normal peristalsis is absent or defective. In such patients, a partial wrap, such as that advocated by Mr. Belsey, is far preferable to the complete, 360-degree wrap provided by the Nissen fundoplication.

REFERENCES

1. Ellis, F.H., Jr., Leonardi, H.K., Dabuzhsky, L., et al.: Surgery for short esophagus with stricture: an experimental and clinical manometric study, Ann. Surg. **188:** 341-350, 1978.
2. Hill, L.D.: An effective operation for hiatal hernia: an eight year appraisal, Ann. Surg. **166:**681-692, 1967.
3. Hill, L.D.: Progress in the surgical management of hiatal hernia, World J. Surg. **1:**425-436, 1977.
4. Hill, L.D.: Intraoperative measurement of lower esophageal sphincter pressure, J. Thorac. Cardiovasc. Surg. **75:**378-382, 1978.
5. Skinner, D.B., and Belsey, R.H.: Surgical management of esophageal reflux and hiatus hernia: long-term results with 1,030 patients, J. Thorac. Cardiovasc. Surg. **53:**33-54, 1967.
6. DeMeester, T.R., Bonavina, L., and Albertucci, M.: Nissen fundoplication for gastroesophageal reflux disease: evaluation of primary repair in 100 consecutive patients, Ann. Surg. **204:**9-20, 1986.

7. Ellis, F.H., Jr., and Crozier, R.E.: Reflux control by fundoplication: a clinical and manometric assessment of the Nissen operation, Ann. Thorac. Surg. **38:**387-392, 1984.

8. Hill, L.D., Ilves, R., Stevenson, J.K., et al.: Reoperation for disruption and recurrence after Nissen fundoplication, Arch. Surg. **114:**542-548, 1979.

9. Leonardi, H.K., and Ellis, F.H., Jr.: Reoperative surgery for gastroesophageal reflux. In Jamieson, G.G., editor: Surgery of the esophagus, Edinburgh, Churchill Livingstone. (In press.)

10. Ellis, F.H., Jr., and Gibb, S.P.: Fundoplication for hypotensive lower esophageal sphincter, Hosp. Pract. **9:**80-85, 1974.

11. DeMeester, T.R., Johnson, L.F., and Kent, A.H.: Evaluation of current operations for the prevention of gastroesophageal reflux, Ann. Surg. **180:**511-525, 1974.

12. Maher, J.W., Hocking, M.P., and Woodward, E.R.: Reoperations for esophagitis following failed antireflux procedures, Ann. Surg. **210:**723-727, 1985.

13. Leonardi, H.K., Lee, M.E., et al.: An experimental study of the effectiveness of various antireflux operations, Ann. Thorac. Surg. **24:**215-222, 1977.

CHAPTER **11** Use of a prosthetic device to
control gastroesophageal
reflux

Jean Pierre Angelchik and Paul David Angelchik

We are now in the era of the bionic man. The past 25 years have witnessed an exponential growth in the use of implantable bioprostheses in virtually every field of surgical endeavor. Emerging technologies include artificial organs, implantable drug delivery systems, vascular grafts, cardiac valves and pacemakers, and artificial joints, to give a few examples.

While other surgical disciplines are actively exploring these new horizons, gastrointestinal surgeons have been notably slow in the development and acceptance of implantable devices. Perhaps their reluctance derives from a historic fear of infection secondary to the presence of foreign bodies in the peritoneal cavity. At this time the only prosthesis in general clinical use in the gastrointestinal field is the antireflux device described in this article. Herein a comprehensive review of the antireflux prosthesis (ARP) will be presented.

Numerous operations have been previously described for the correction of gastroesophageal reflux; however, no single procedure is entirely successful. The most widely accepted surgical procedures for the treatment of hiatal hernia and reflux, including the Nissen fundoplication, Belsey Mark IV, and Hill posterior gastropexy techniques, enjoy variable measures of efficacy. These procedures decrease peptic esophagitis primarily by enhancing resting lower esophageal sphincter pressure (LESP) through a "valvuloplasty" effect and by maintaining the gastroesophageal junction (GEJ) within the positive pressure environment of the abdominal cavity.[1,2]

Nevertheless, associated operative morbidity and recurrence of reflux symptomatology following these approaches required the development of an easily performed, standardized procedure yielding effective, reproducible, and permanent relief of reflux symptoms in association with a diminished operative morbidity.

Because of the numerous approaches utilizing autologous tissue to enhance LESP, it was decided that the next logical step in treatment would be the use of an implantable bioprosthesis. The first attempt at use of synthetic materials in the treatment of gastroesophageal reflux employed Teflon mesh as a buttress of the hiatal margins. This technique never gained wide acceptance.[3]

Four factors were considered important in the design of an ARP. First, it was felt that the reestablishment of distal esophageal wall apposition by a posterior reinforcement or padding was central to correction of pathologic reflux, since many patients with gastroesophageal reflux had patulous lower esophageal sphincters. Second, opening of the distal esophageal sphincter by gastric dilatation and progressive skirting of the sphincter[4,5] could be limited by a circumferential ring. Third, a padded ring design might also induce a ball-valve closure mechanism when antral contraction projected the apical gastric mucosal rugae against the GEJ. Finally, autogenous LESP would be enhanced by replacement of the lower esophagus into the positive pressure environment of the abdominal cavity, as observed with earlier approaches.

DESIGN

The ARP is a collar-shaped device fabricated from surgical grade polysiloxanes (silicones) (Figs. 11-1 and 11-2). A silicone rubber shell 0.4 mm in thickness and of equal diameter throughout its length envelops an internal silicone gel composed of various-length polymer chains. The ARP is elliptical with outer dimensions of 6 × 7 cm. The internal diameters are 2.5 and 3.1 cm when the tie-straps are approximated. The device weighs 45 g. A Dacron tie-strap 0.5 cm in width is bonded circumferentially to the exterior sur-

147

face, and extends 15 cm beyond each end of the body. Embedded with the tie strap in the outer shell is a radiopaque tantalum-filled marker strip for roentgenographic localization. A previous model employing Dacron tie-straps vulcanized just to the ends of the body was discontinued in early 1982 after reports of strap dehiscence and ARP displacement (see "Complications").

Initial design studies in 1971 and 1972 were performed utilizing cadaver preparations. The stomachs of fresh autopsy specimens were filled with fluid and contracted externally to effect reflux into the distal esophagus. Attempts to prevent reflux were made by placing a thumb and forefinger about the lower esophagus and varying the aperture between them. The largest inner dimension yielding abolition of reflux was 2.5 × 3.1 cm, and this was used in designing the device. The original device had greater central thickness, tapering toward the ends. An equal-thickness model was first produced in 1976.

The ARP became available for general use in 1979 following approval by the Food and Drug Administration. This was granted after studies by eight collateral groups in different areas of the United States, involving 108 patients undergoing ARP implantation, were presented. The longest follow-up period at the time was 6 years. We reported the first clinical series utilizing the ARP in 1979.[6]

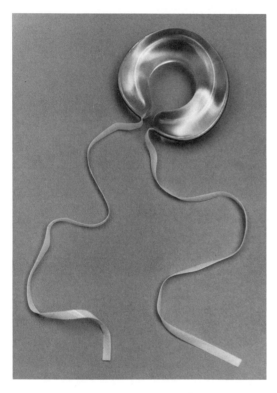

Fig. 11-1. Prosthetic device.

INDICATIONS AND CONTRAINDICATIONS TO ARP PLACEMENT

The majority of patients suffering from gastroesophageal reflux symptoms are well managed with medical measures and do not require corrective surgery. Administration of antacids, histamine receptor blockers, and other pharmacologic agents (metaclopramide, cholinergic agonists), combined with dietary modification, weight loss, and elevation of the head of the bed at night, constitute the core of the medical regimen.[7,8] ARP placement is indicated in patients whose disease is refractory to a reasonable trial period of such therapy. The appropriate length of medical management is determined by

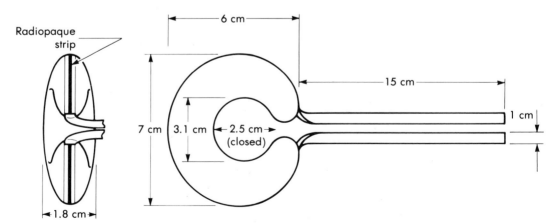

Fig. 11-2. Measurements of the prosthesis.

the nature and severity of the patient's presentation. Those individuals with frequent "pseudoanginal" substernal pain, bleeding, obstructive dysphagia as a result of stricture formation, or chronic regurgitation with pulmonary aspiration might be expected to come to surgery sooner than patients suffering from intermittent bouts of moderate pyrosis. Patients with a significant surgical or anesthetic risk might well be better served by the shorter, less traumatic insertion of an ARP as opposed to conventional valvuloplasty.[9] In patients in whom a concomitant procedure is planned, or other factors such as obesity or a history of previous failed antireflux surgery are present, ARP implantation may greatly facilitate the safety and ease of operation. Use of the prosthesis is contraindicated in the setting of infection, small pediatric cases, and concurrent opening of the gastrointestinal tract or esophagus, with the exception of a pyloroplasty.[10]

TECHNIQUE OF ARP IMPLANTATION

One of the true advantages of the ARP is the ease of implantation. Minimal dissection is required; in fact, the less dissection performed, the better.[10a] In the hands of a competent surgeon experienced with the device, an uncomplicated insertion may generally be accomplished in less than 45 minutes.[11]

The abdomen is entered through a vertical midline incision from the xiphoid process to the umbilicus. In some patients the incision is extended to the left of the umbilicus. Following abdominal exploration, the left lobe of the liver is retracted cephalad without transecting the triangular ligament. Overholt and Balfour retractors are used for exposure. The stomach and esophagus are placed under traction, and if a hiatal hernia is present, it is reduced. The peritoneum is incised at the GEJ anteriorly. A 36F Maloney bougie is introduced into the stomach by the anesthesiologist to provide easier identification of the esophagus by feel. The surgeon bluntly dissects with his finger circumferentially around the esophagus from left to right, and using the finger as a guide, the ARP is inserted about the GEJ. The fibers of the vagus nerve are undisturbed, and no attempt is made to include or exclude them during the circumferential dissection of the esophagus. The ARP is tied in place with four ties of the straps and a hemoclip is placed adjacent to the knot. Properly inserted, the device fits loosely about the GEJ, allowing the passage of one or two fingers between the esophagus and the prosthesis (Figs. 11-3 to 11-5). In

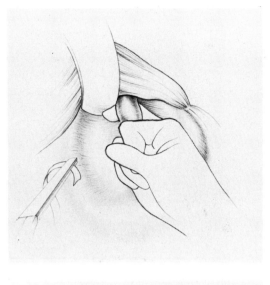

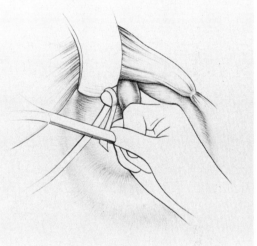

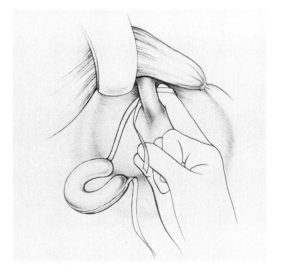

Fig. 11-3. Passing the strap behind the esophagus.

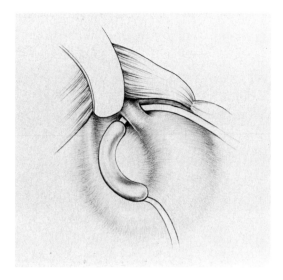

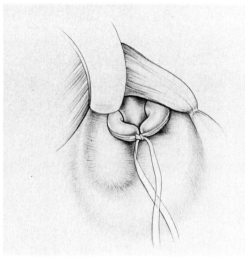

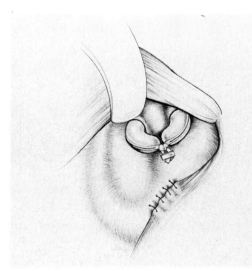

Fig. 11-4. Device passed and tied around the esophagus, and gastropexy.

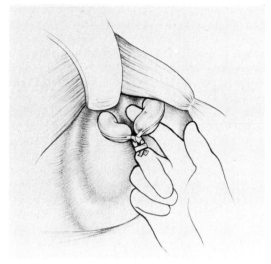

Fig. 11-5. Drawings showing space between the esophagus and the device. Finger fits loosely.

patients with esophageal strictures, dilatation is carried out prior to ARP placement, with manual and visual control of the area. Bougies of progressive size are passed through the mouth by the anesthesiologist.[12]

Crural approximation is not necessary, and it may cause persistent dysphagia in some patients. In the last 2 years we have been performing an anterior gastropexy on individuals with a large hiatus. The lesser curvature of the stomach is sutured to the anterior abdominal wall, under traction, with three or four nonabsorbable sutures before closure of the abdomen. An especially important consideration is close inspection of the ARP for structural integrity prior to placement, in order to avoid migration. Similarly, careful inspection of the GEJ should be done prior to insertion, to exclude inadvertent enterotomy and inappropriate ARP insertion.

Postoperatively a liquid diet is generally begun on the second day and advanced to a soft mechanical diet over the next twenty-four hours, which is maintained for the next 3 to 4 weeks. Patients are followed up with frequent office visits and by chest roentgenograms at 6 weeks, 6 months, and annually thereafter.

RESULTS OF TREATMENT

From May, 1973, to June, 1985, we have treated 228 patients (110 male, 118 female) for reflux esophagitis by ARP implantation. The mean follow-up period is 63 months, with 129 patients now beyond 5 years. Twelve patients

TABLE 11-1. Symptomatic results of surgery

Visick I	184 patients (80.60%)
Visick II	39 patients (17.20%)
Visick III	3 patients (1.32%)
Visick IV	2 patients (0.88%)

TABLE 11-2. Intervals of follow-up

Interval	No. of patients
Over 12 yr	2
11 yr	2
10 yr	10
9 yr	10
8 yr	20
7 yr	34
6 yr	24
Over 5 yr	27
4 yr	31
3 yr	28
2 yr	30
Over 1 yr	9
Under 1 yr	1

TABLE 11-3. Concomitant procedures

Procedure	No. of patients
Cholecystectomy	26
Vagotomy and pyloroplasty	13
Pyloroplasty	4
Vagotomy	4
Gastrojejunostomy	1
Hemigastrectomy	2
Esophageal dilatation	51
Anterior gastropexy	22

TABLE 11-4. Unrelated mortality

Cause	Time after operation
Myocardial infarction	2-4 mo, 4 yr
Metastatic cancer	2-8 mo, 6 yr
MVA	1½ years
CVA	2-2 mo, 8 yr

TABLE 11-5. Postoperative studies

Studies	No. of patients
Radiography	223
Esophagoscopy/Biopsy	71
Esophagoscopy over 5 years	30
Esophagitis by Bx	1 (replaced ARP)
pH and motility studies	14

have been lost to follow-up. The average length of preoperative symptoms was 6½ years (range, 3 months to 30 years). The mean duration of medical therapy preoperatively was 5½ years (range, 2 months to 30 years). Fifty-six patients presented with esophageal strictures; 41 patients had recurrence of symptoms and hiatal hernia following prior failed antireflux procedures. Several of these patients had multiple previous antireflux operations.

Preoperative studies included upper gastrointestinal barium study in all 228 patients; esophagoscopy/biopsy in 156, and pH and motility studies in 30.

Ninety-eight percent of the patients in our series report good results after surgery. These data are tabulated on the Visick scale in Table 11-1.

The intervals of follow-up are listed in Table 11-2, and concomitant procedures performed are listed in Table 11-3.

Surgical morbidity includes one gastric perforation on the first postoperative day requiring subsequent removal of the ARP, one incidental splenectomy, and one wound dehiscence with evisceration on the fourth postoperative day.

Surgical mortality is limited to one case, a cardiac arrest during removal of a displaced ARP 4 years after insertion. Unrelated mortality occurred in 8 patients (Table 11-4).

Displacement of the prosthesis occurred in 10

patients (4%), and the device was replaced in seven. In 28 patients (12%), the prosthesis moved above the hiatus; this event was not associated with the return of reflux.

Postoperative results have been confirmed with radiography, esophagoscopy, and pH and motility studies, as shown in Table 11-5. The excellent results in our group of patients have been corroborated in numerous other publications of smaller series.[9,13,14,15] Several recent randomized prospective trials comparing the ARP to the Nissen procedure have found similar rates of success.[11,16,17,18] Gear et al. reported 96% satisfactory or excellent results in 26 patients receiving the ARP (follow-up, 3 months to 2 years), with no failures to control reflux. An 81% success rate was obtained in an equal number of subjects after floppy Nissen fundoplication. Of the Nissen patients, six (23%) had failure to control reflux after operation.[11] Gourley and collaborators at the University of Wisconsin randomized 30 developmentally disabled patients between ARP and Nissen groups. Equally good results at 6 months were obtained in both sets, as judged by multiple parameters.[17] Similar outcomes have been reported in randomized trials by Siewert and Weiser[18] and by Dawson et al.,[16] with 20 and 40 patients, respectively; 90% to 100% good results have been standard.

In 18 studies involving 529 patients, not including our series, good or excellent results were obtained in 485 patients (91.7%).* Forty-four patients classified as treatment failures (Visick III or IV) were divided into two groups: (1) 30 patients undergoing device removal and (2) 14 patients in whom the ARP failed to control reflux or resulted in persistent dysphagia or gas bloatings. Of the 30 explants, 11 were old-model prostheses that became displaced,[19,28,29,31] 3 ARP's eroded into the gastrointestinal tract,[11,23] and the remainder were removed for severe postoperative dysphagia or mediastinal migration with recurrent symptoms. Two of the eroded devices were inserted in proximity to suture lines[23] (Table 11-6). If the 11 early-model ARPs and two inappropriately inserted ARPs are eliminated, 31 (6%) cases remain in which the prosthesis failed to provide good results. Potential reasons for prosthesis failure are addressed in the complications section that follows.

Of note is the fact that more than one half of all treatment failures occurred at three centers.[21,28,30]

COMPLICATIONS

Complications of ARP implantation generally may be divided into two groups: those associated

---

*References 11, 13, 14, 15, and 19-31.

TABLE 11-6. Reported primary indications for removal of 30 ARPs in 529 implant cases

No. of cases	Indication
11*	Displacement of ARP after tie-strap disruption
14[†,‡]	Dysphagia
3[§]	Erosion into gastrointestinal tract
2[‖]	Persistent or recurrent symptoms

* Noncircumferential strap design.
[†,‖] Three devices herniated into mediastinum, with straps intact.
[‡] Crural approximation in seven patients.
[§] Two devices placed in proximity to anastomosis.

with celiotomy and intraoperative maneuvers and those resulting as a direct consequence of device insertion. Included in the former category would be incidental splenectomy or enterotomy, superficial and deep wound infection, ventral herniations, pneumonia, thromboembolism, and so on. In the second category are case descriptions of prosthetic migration within the peritoneal cavity or into the mediastinum, as well as erosion into the gastrointestinal tract. An additional reported complication is dysphagia of either a transient or a persistent nature.[29,30]

Scattered reports of prosthetic detachment have been somewhat sensationalized in the surgical literature, often to the exclusion of larger series with favorable results and documented follow-up data.[32,33,33a] Perhaps the novel presentation of the rarely displaced ARP is more compelling than the more common failed Nissen or Belsey repair, conservatively said to occur in 7% to 23% of cases.[11,31,34] Significantly, not a single mortality has been reported in direct association with ARP insertion after approximately 25,000 implantations worldwide. Mortality rates for alternative procedures are on the order of 1%, with a much greater rate for reoperation of failed primary repairs.[35]

In the first three years of ARP commercial availability (November, 1979, to January, 1982) approximately 7700 implants were sold. Two hundred forty-four complaints have been registered with the manufacturer concerning removed devices of this era (3.2%),[36] including published cases of dislocation and migration. A majority of case reports in the world literature describing prosthetic disruption and movement are attributable to strap failure of an early design. The particular model implicated utilized peripherally vulcanized tie-straps rather than the initially used circumferential strap. Circumferential strap placement was resumed at the end of 1981 with discontinuation of the earlier design. From January, 1982, to May, 1985, 16,757 new-model ARPs were sold, with only 6 (.0003%) reported complaints involving removal.[36] In patients who had documented erosion of the prosthesis into the bowel lumen, there was a high incidence of inadvertent esophageal and gastric lacerations, concomitant procedures in which the bowel was opened, or operative trauma to the gastroesophageal junction during its mobilization, particularly in patients who had had a previous operation.[23,33,37,38] In these instances, prosthetic erosion is far more likely to occur. Prosthesis insertion in the setting of simultaneous gastrointestinal anastomosis or enterotomy is contraindicated.

Non-ARP procedures

Analysis of operative morbidity in 17 series of 2,821 patients undergoing nonprosthetic antireflux surgery reveals a range of 5% to 46%, with a mean morbidity of 12%. In eight series employing the Nissen fundoplication (770 patients), the mean morbidity was 14% (range, 7% to 23%). The mean incidence of incidental splenectomy in nine studies of the Nissen procedure (868 patients) was 7% (range, 0% to 25.8%). Pulmonary complications in 12 studies (2,446 patients) averaged 4% (range, 0% to 20.7%). Reported postoperative infections averaged 3.0% in 14 studies (2,890 patients). Postoperative dysphagia requiring dilatation occurred in 8% of 1,894 patients in 14 studies. Mortality in 18 non-ARP studies (2879 patients) averaged 1%, with a range of 0% to 4.6%. Other postoperative problems commonly encountered include gas bloating and inability of eructation or regurgitation. These complications are more prevalent after Nissen fundoplication than after other valvuloplasty procedures.[38a] Treatment failure was seen in 12% of 2,728 patients in 16 studies. In 12 studies of the Nissen operation (1235 patients), 14% of patients were classified as treatment failures. Results and references are summarized in Table 11-7.

ARP studies

In ten series (538 patients), overall operative morbidity with ARP placement was 9%. Pulmonary complications were encountered in 3% of 544 patients in 10 series. Postoperative infections of any type were noted in 5% of 634 patients in 12 series. Splenectomy was required in only 0.3% of 646 cases in 13 series. Dysphagia necessitated dilatation after surgery in 5% of 375 patients in 7 series. In 19 studies, including our own, treatment failure as judged by clinical criteria was present in 6% of 757 cases. These data and references are summarized in Table 11-8.

Postoperative dysphagia is a common complaint after prosthesis placement, being reported in approximately one third of patients. The vast majority of these patients go on to have complete resolution of dysphagia within 1 to 3 months, and generally within 6 weeks. In patients with persistent dysphagia, several mechanisms may be operative. In those individuals with long-standing preoperative symptoms of a severe nature, esophageal stricture formation may be contributory and necessitate dilatation postoperatively. In two patients, acute "angulation" of the ARP has been reported to cause dysphagia, which resolved after ARP removal.[21,39] In a much greater number of patients, high-grade or persistent dysphagia may be the result of tight hiatal closure by crural approximation. It is probable that the additive effects of the ARP and crural apposition affect esophageal motility adversely. In patients with a wide hiatus and risk of recurrent herniation, an

TABLE 11-7. Complications in nonprosthetic antireflux procedure studies: results in 3937 cases

Complication	References	Reported percent	Total no.	Percent
Operative morbidity[*]	2, 40-42, 11, 43, 44-52, 34	5-45.9	334/2821	11.8
Nissen only[†]	23, 27-28, 42, 44	7-23.0	105/770	13.6
Incidental splenectomy (Nissen only)	41, 11, 43, 46, 50, 52, 53, 2, 40, 41, 11, 43, 54, 49, 50, 53	0-25.8	64/868	7.4
Pulmonary	40, 41, 11, 43-48, 34, 53, 35	0-2.7	92/2446	3.7
Infection	2, 42, 11, 43, 44, 49, 50, 34, 53, 35	0-10.4	95/2890	3.3
Dysphagia requiring dilatation	2, 42, 43, 45-50, 53	0-16.1	156/1894	8.2
Mortality	55, 2, 40-45, 56, 46-50	0-4.6	34/2911	1.2
Nissen only	57, 38, 34, 53, 52, 55, 41, 43, 46, 49, 50, 52, 53	0-3.7	9/840	1.1
Treatment failure	40, 41, 11, 43-46, 48, 49, 51, 34, 52, 53	0-36.0	326/2728	12.0
Nissen only	55, 40, 41, 11, 43, 46, 58, 49, 53, 52, 59	0-36.0	172/1235	13.9

[*]Includes all reported surgical morbidity and early complications. Antireflux procedures performed include Nissen fundoplication and various modifications (Collis, Rosetti, anchored), Belsey Mark IV, Collis-Belsey, Hill, Allison, and crural repair.

[†]Includes Nissen, Nissen-Rosetti, Anchored Nissen, and concomitant procedures such as supraselective vagotomy, cholecystectomy, and hernia repair. Does not include Collis-Nissen.

TABLE 11-8. Complications in ARP studies: results in 807 cases[*]

Complication	References	Reported percent	Total no.	Percent
Operative morbidity[†]	12, 21, 11, 22, 14, 27, 31, 9, 30, 23	0-29.2	46/538	8.6
Incidental splenectomy	12, 19, 20, 11, 22, 14, 27, 31, 9, 23, 24, 15, 60, 30	0-4.2	2/646	0.3
Pulmonary	19, 16, 21, 11, 22, 27, 30, 31, 9, 23	0-14.0	15/544	2.8
Infection	12, 19, 11, 22, 15, 18, 27, 31, 9, 21, 23, 60, 30	0-26.8	29/634	4.6
Dysphagia requiring dilatation	12, 19, 11, 22, 27, 31, 9	0-10.0	17/375	4.5
Mortality[‡]	13, 12, 19, 20, 21, 11, 22, 23, 24, 14, 25, 26, 15, 27-30, 31, 9, 60	0-2.4	2/807	0.3
Treatment failure	13, 12, 19, 20, 21, 11, 22, 23, 24, 14, 25, 26, 15, 27-30, 31, 9	0-19.5	48/757	6.3

[*]Includes ARP implantation with concomitant procedures such as cholecystectomy, supraselective vagotomy, crural repair, etc.
[†]Includes all reported surgical morbidity and early complications.
[‡]Mortalities unrelated to ARP implantation. One case was an intraoperative cardiac arrest not associated with the prosthesis. One case was a postoperative pneumonia in an elderly patient.

anterior gastropexy may be performed if deemed necessary. Crural closure is not advised (see section on technique).

Should an ARP become displaced or not function effectively, the obvious remedy is to remove or replace it, as we have done in 10 of our patients. If the device is within the gastric lumen, the optimal approach is via a gastrotomy without breaching the integrity of the external capsule surrounding the ARP. If the capsule is incised, an enteral fistula is created that will be difficult to close and may require a gastroesophageal resection for adequate repair. Opening the stomach through a minimal incision and directly removing the device is a safe, effective, and short procedure. If the device is located within the small bowel, then an enterotomy will suffice. Successful endoscopic removal of an intragastric ARP has been reported.[38,61]

We have come full circle with established authorities in esophageal surgery and believe the principal danger associated with use of the ARP stems from the ease of implantation. In this respect we are in complete agreement with Bombeck,[62] who has stated:

. . . when all directions which accompany the prosthesis are observed, it can be put in place during an operation lasting no more than an hour. The device is simply slipped around the esophagus and tied loosely in place. It is obvious that the simplicity of the procedure is not justification for its indiscriminate use.

The comparison data assembled above are not suitable for the rigorous statistical analysis reserved for carefully controlled randomized prospective trials. Rather they reflect the spectrum of experience of a wide variety of surgeons with the commonly performed antireflux procedures. Nevertheless, we believe the lower complication rate and superior efficacy seen with the ARP procedure to be representative of worldwide results to date. Further corroborative study is currently going on at a number of centers.

POSTULATED MECHANISMS OF ACTION OF THE ARP

The reported efficacy of the ARP in clinical trials has prompted attempts by several investigators to determine its mechanism(s) of action in animal models. Interest has been focused primarily on the well-documented rise of LESP following ARP implantation.

Theoretically, any action of the device at the LES must be a purely mechanical phenomenon; neurohormonal factors have no postulated effect. Alterations in motility of the lower esophageal sphincter have been reported after ARP placement, probably reflecting the beneficial resolution of esophagitis-associated disordered motor activity, and/or limitation of peristaltic amplitude at the level of the implant with large boluses. Disordered or spastic motility patterns may be noted in patients with postoperative dysphagia or persistent reflux. Benjamin et al.,[63] employing a supine primate model, were able to demonstrate a statistically significant rise in baseline LESP with ARP placement at the GEJ in normal rhesus monkeys (n = 4) and in baboons with experimentally induced acute esophagitus (n = 4). Pressure changes in the normals were from 12.7 ± 3.1 mm Hg to 62.5 ± 20.7 mm Hg. (p < 0.05). Animals with induced esophagitus had preoperative LESP of 5.7 ± 1.3 mm Hg, which rose to 17.8 ± 1.5 mm Hg after application of an ARP (p < 0.05). This effect could be simulated alternatively to a variable extent with posterior positioning of wooden dowel rods or Maloney dilators of different sizes at the GEJ. A significant increase in intraabdominal esophageal length was also noted, but only with ARP at the GEJ (1.4 cm ± 0.08 cm to 3.2 cm ± 0.5 cm; p < 0.05). The authors interpret these data as indicative of a posterior padding of the GEJ at the level of the LES, causing a change in the length-tension relationship of the esophageal musculature. They go on to suggest that a similar mechanism may be operative after a Hill or Nissen repair.

Cohen et al.[64] randomly assigned myotomized adult rhesus monkeys with confirmed esophageal reflux to four treatment groups: (1) sham operation; (2) Nissen fundoplication; (3) ARP; or (4) modified ARP (a strap-like structure with the same internal circumference as the ARP). Postoperative studies at 1, 3, and 6 months demonstrated objective evidence of efficacy in all antireflux treatment groups. LESP was elevated concomitantly. Intraabdominal length of the esophagus and gastroesophageal angle remained unchanged. The modified prosthesis was associated with intraluminal erosion, fibrous stricture formation, and slippage over the stomach.

A collaborative effort undertaken by researchers at the Universities of Göttingen and Illinois demonstrated equal effectiveness in preventing gastroesophageal reflux in LES-myomectomized dogs between the ARP and Nissen-Rosetti procedures.[5] Of note, the LESP of the fundoplication group animals responded to hormonal stimulation with pentagastrin and atropine in physiologic fashion, whereas a tonic elevation of LESP unresponsive to humoral influences from 3.6 ± 1.6 mm Hg to 11.7 ± 5.8 mm Hg was documented, as expected, in the ARP group. Corollary in vitro experiments utilizing canine gastroesophageal preparations with circular ligatures of different sizes placed 3 cm distal to the GEJ showed an increase in stimulated lower esophageal sphincter opening pressure (LESOP) above control during continuous gastric infusion and increasing intragastric pressure.

LESOP varied in an inverse linear fashion with ligature circumference. These investigators invoke the law of Laplace ($P = 2T/R$) and earlier work by Petterson and Bombeck[4] to suggest that the ARP functions by interrupting the transmission of gastric wall tension to the LES during gastric distention.

In the most extensive clinicoradiologic study to date, Wyllie and Edwards assessed the results of ARP implantation in 15 poor-risk patients in whom medical therapy failed.[9] Twelve patients had esophageal strictures. The average follow-up period was 12 months (range, 6 to 24 months). Through the use of special radiographic techniques, stricture bore and length, ARP position, "hiatal flow," and gastroesophageal reflux were evaluated.

Clinically, 14 of 15 patients reported subjective improvements of heartburn and cessation of regurgitation. Eleven of twelve patients reported decreased dysphagia. The prosthesis worked equally well in the chest (n = 8) or in the abdomen (n = 7). The only postoperative complication was a wound dehiscence. One ARP was removed for persistent dysphagia, which did not resolve after removal. Consistent evidence of slight reflux could be obtained in only one patient. Stricture bore in 12 patients increased from 7.93 ± 0.74 mm to 11.3 ± 1.19 mm, with length decreasing from 7.08 ± 1.46 mm to 2.92 ± 1.08 mm (p < 0.01).

Of most interest, the authors were able to demonstrate that the prosthesis was at least 12 mm below the LES in 14 of 15 patients, thus making the reported increase in LESP seen after implantation difficult to explain on the basis of a direct effect at the LES. A posterior padding effect was not seen. The sole consistent roentgenographic finding was a drastic reduction in barium flow across the hiatus with the patient in a slight Trendelenburg position.

The work cited raises several questions. All investigators were able to demonstrate the effectiveness of the ARP in preventing reflux under experimental and clinical conditions. The variety of mechanisms suggested for prosthesis action implies that multiple factors may be responsible. The applicability of the law of Laplace to the issue is not entirely clear, since this physical law was conceived with regard to the properties of passive vessels, which are clearly not represented by the stomach or the esophagus. Gastric distention is not invariably present in patients with peptic esophagitis, and other factors influence gastric wall tension and compliance beyond gastric volume. Moreover, it is unlikely that wall tension is uniform throughout the stomach during the phases of peristalsis. The highly original work by Wyllie and Edwards should serve to provoke further study into the mechanisms of ARP action.

HOST-PROSTHESIS INTERACTION

With all foreign implantable materials a potential exists for interaction at the host-implant interface. The most worrisome aspect of such an interaction is the increased risk of tissue damage and/or infection leading to sepsis. Implant properties affecting host-tissue response include chemical composition, contour (sharp versus smooth), site of implantation, mechanical factors such as friction, and particle size as a function of surface area.[65] Host responses range from fibrous encapsulation with implant acceptance to abscess formation and chronic inflammatory changes.[66] In certain instances host responses may cause corrosion or polymer scission of implant materials.[65]

The ARP is made of medical grade (no additives) silicones, except for a Dacron tie-strap and a Tantalum marker. The dimethylpolysiloxanes are inert, nonimmunogenic, biocompatible inorganic polymers.[59] Although the host reaction to other silicone implants, such as breast prostheses, has been clearly described, Sapala et al,[57] have recently conducted the first study examining the ARP-host interaction with respect to morphologic changes of the device and the histopathology of local tissue response after implantation. In 19 of 142 patients with ARPs requiring laparotomy for disease unrelated to reflux, 10 (53%) formed periprosthetic capsules. Grossly, all capsules were complete and composed of fibrous tissue of uniform thickness. No capsule demonstrated constrictive fibrosis with esophageal lumen compromise. Capsular formation was not related to length of implantation. All 19 patients had a pronounced foreign-body reaction to the silk suture material used to secure the Dacron tie-straps.

Histologically, capsular biopsy specimens (n = 10) revealed a predominantly mature connective tissue consisting of fibrocytes with laminar collagen deposition. Focal sites of proliferating fibroblasts and rare areas of perivascular inflammation consisting of lymphocytes, histiocytes, and plasma cells were noted. Foreign-body giant cells were uniformly absent. Cytoplasmic inclusions in biopsy specimen histocytes were negative for lipid stains, and presumably represent ingested silicone droplets "bled" from the fluid phase of the internal gel. In contrast, in four

prostheses removed from patients undergoing gastrointestinal anastomotic procedures, a characteristic intense granulomatous process was associated with the silk suture material. In one case the reaction extended beneath Glisson's capsule into hepatic parenchyma.

Morphologic changes were seen in removed implants examined grossly and by scanning electron microscopy (SEM). SEM of unimplanted elastomer shells demonstrated a smooth surface topography with occasional scattered elevations and rare convex silicone droplet configurations. In the four devices removed (implantation time, 12 to 37 months), there were no major surface defects. However, surface elevations consistent with gel droplet extrusion were observed with greater frequency over implantation time. Further corroboration of silicone fluid phase microleakage is provided by elevated levels of silicone in capsular tissue in a patient whose ARP was removed at 27 months. Silicone content was 58 μg/g of tissue (normal = 20 to 40 μg/g). Slight discoloration and opacification were seen in the gel of two removed ARPs, which the authors speculate may be secondary to lipid accumulation through the microporous shell. Pseudocrystalline inclusions observed in one device are of unknown origin. Penetrometer measurements of the explanted ARPs revealed no significant changes in gel viscosity as compared with controls.

The excellent data assembled by Sapala's group indicate that the structural integrity of the ARP is preserved over time after implantation. Microscopic gel polymer extrusion probably occurs very gradually, and the elevated levels of the capsular silicone at 27 months were less than twice the upper limit of normal. There were no adverse effects correlated with the elevated level, such as capsular constriction or distant fibrosis within the peritoneum. Although the authors suggest that capsular formation is in part due to silicone bleeding, the additional effects of surgical insertion with tissue dissection, prosthetic mobility with generation of slight friction, dessicatory effects of the silicone shell on adjacent soft tissue, and host factors are likely to be contributory to the internal wound healing surrounding the ARP.[57,66] It is interesting to note that, anecdotally, following removal of ARPs, certain patients with capsules have not experienced recurrence of symptoms, nor has there been objective evidence of gastroesophageal reflux. This phenomenon is probably related to the "phantom" antireflux action of the capsule itself, which forms a mold with a configuration close to that of the ARP. Importantly, infection related to prosthesis insertion has not emerged as a significant problem.

CONCLUSIONS

The ARP was created to fill the need for an effective, safe, and simple solution to refractory gastroesophageal reflux. In our experience over the last 12 years, and as is becoming evident in the world literature presented here, the prosthesis has fulfilled these goals. Notable advantages over earlier antireflux procedures include (1) improved efficacy, (2) rapidity and ease of implantation, (3) decreased associated morbidity and mortality, and (4) shorter postoperative hospitalization.

Reoperation after ARP implantation for recurrent symptoms is far less involved than after other accepted procedures. Should the device fail to provide a good result, it is simply removed, with replacement or, alternatively, repair by other techniques. We believe the simplicity of the ARP to be commensurate with the benign pathologic entity for which it was devised, and although not a panacea, it represents the logical surgical approach to reflux after medical treatment.

Nevertheless, the ARP has not met with the widespread acceptance anticipated upon its introduction. Early controversy focused on the lack of preliminary animal experimentation preceding clinical use, short available follow-up, and hypothetical concerns about the ARP as a foreign body. More recently, case reports of prosthesis displacement and intraluminal erosion have been noted in print, accompanied by caustic, if somewhat inaccurate, editorials.[32,33a]

In addressing these issues, we rely upon the body of data presented in this article. The principal reason why early animal studies were not conducted was the difficulty of enlisting support within the academic sector for such a project. Studies by other investigators, performed after commercial approval, have not yet elucidated a clear explanation for the ARP mechanism(s) of action, perhaps reflecting our still growing understanding of the pathophysiology of reflux esophagitis. Before FDA approval of the device, clinical trials were conducted by eight collateral study groups in 108 patients. Strap design problems have been successfully resolved for several years and greatly overemphasized. Host-prosthesis interaction has not eventuated in catastrophic, or even moderate, complications. What remains to be corrected is the mistake of inserting the ARP when specifically contraindicated or not required by the condition of the individual patient.

We now have follow-up periods averaging greater than 5 years in our series, longer than most comparably sized series reported by authors employing other techniques. In fact, there is a true paucity of long-term multicenter studies of the Belsey, Hill, and Nissen procedures, despite the anecdotal reports emerging from each technique's major advocates. We await with great interest the long-term results of the randomized trials being conducted at several centers between the ARP and Nissen techniques. We believe the ARP procedure will prove the more durable repair.

It is our hope that the ARP will encourage other investigators to actively take innovative approaches to the many unresolved problems confronting general surgeons and their patients. By taking advantage of powerful new technologies and the expanding frontiers of medical knowledge, general surgeons may envision a significant augmentation of their therapeutic repertoire. From electronically regulated endocrine systems to gastrointestinal pacemakers and weight loss devices, what can be conceptualized is coming increasingly within our grasp. Vision and creativity, rather than dogmatic reliance on established concepts, will lead the way toward better diagnosis and treatment of the surgical patient. Through carefully applied study, the digestive system will be effectively integrated into the bionic man.

REFERENCES

1. Bombeck, C.T., Aoki, T., and Nyhus, L.M.: Anatomic etiology and operative treatment of peptic esophagitis: an experimental study, Ann. Surg. **165**:752-764, 1967.
2. DeMeester, T.R., Johnson, L.F., and Kent, A.H.: Evaluation of current operations for the prevention of gastroesophageal reflux, Ann. Surg. **180**:511-525, 1974.
3. Merendino, K.A., and Dillard, D.H.: Permanent fixation by Teflon mesh of the size of the esophageal diaphragmatic aperture in hiatus hernioplasty: a concept in repair, Am. J. Surg. **110**:416-420, 1965.
4. Petterson, G.B., Bombeck, C.T., and Nyhus, L.M.: The dynamics of lower esophageal sphincter function, Curr. Surg. **37**:143-145, 1980.
5. Samelson, S.L., Weiser, H.F., et al.: A new concept in the surgical treatment of gastroesophageal reflux, Ann. Surg. **197**:254-259, 1983.
6. Angelchik, J.P., and Cohen, R.: A new surgical procedure for the treatment of gastroesophageal reflux and hiatal Hernia, Surg. Gynecol. Obstet. **148**:246-248, 1979.
7. Russell, C.O.H., and Hill, L.D.: Gastroesophageal reflux, Curr. Prob. Surg. **20**:209-277, 1983.
8. Henderson, R.D.: Medical management of hiatal hernia: general measures—drug therapy and bougienage. In The esophagus, Baltimore, 1980, The Williams & Wilkins Co.
9. Wyllie, J.H., and Edwards, D.A.W.: A quantitative assessment of results with the Angelchik prosthesis, Ann. R. Coll. Surg. **67**:216-221, 1985.

10. Mentor Corporation: Angelchik antireflux prosthesis product information sheet, Goleta, Calif.

10a. Sapala, M.A., Sapala, J.A., et al.: A technique for anatomic placement of the Angelchik anti-reflux prosthesis, Surg. Gynecol. Obstet. **158:**178-180, 1984.

11. Gear, M.W.L., Gillison, E.W., and Dowling, B.L.: Randomized prospective trial of the Angelchik antireflux prosthesis, Br. J. Surg. **71:**681-683, 1984.

12. Angelchik, J.P., and Cohen, R.: A silicone prosthesis for gastroesophageal reflux: long term results, Contemp. Surg. **26**(1):29-34, 1985.

13. Anfossi, A., Arnulfo, G., et al.: Evaluation of the functional changes of the lower esophageal sphincter (LES) after application of Angelchik's prosthesis, Chir. Ital. **35**(3):332-341, 1983.

14. Montori, A., Pietropaolo, V., et al.: Current surgical treatment of gastroesophageal reflux: the Angelchik prosthesis, Arch. Att. Soc. Ital. Chir., pp. 181-186, 1984.

15. Sapala, M.A., and Hurtado, M.H.: Correction of reflux esophagitis with the Angelchik silicon prosthesis: a preliminary report in 26 patients (abstract), Am. J. Gastroenterol. **78:**695, 1983.

16. Dawson, K., Ryan, R., et al.: Prospective randomized trial of Angelchik prosthesis versus Nissen fundoplication (abstract), Gut. **26**(5):A555, 1985.

17. Gourley, G.R., et al.: Randomized prospective double-blind study of gastroesophageal surgery: Nissen fundoplication vs. Angelchik prosthesis (abstract), Gastroenterology **86**(5):1095, 1984.

18. Siewert, J.R., and Weiser, H.F.: A randomized prospective trial of the Angelchik antireflux prosthesis versus Nissen fundoplication. (In preparation.)

19. Beland, L., et al.: Preliminary report on the use of the Angelchik prosthesis in the treatment of esophageal reflux. Presentation at Symposium on ARP, American College of Surgeons Clinical Congress, San Francisco, 1981.

20. Deitel, M., Basi, S.S., and Ilves, R.: The Angelchik antireflux prosthesis, Can. J. Surg. **282:**176-179, 1985.

21. Durran, D., Armstrong, C.P., and Taylor, T.V.: The Angelchik antireflux prosthesis: some reservations, Br. J. Surg. **72:**525-527, 1985.

22. Kozarek, R.A., Phelps, J.E., et al.: An antireflux prosthesis in the treatment of gastroesophageal reflux, Ann. Intern. Med. **93:**310-315, 1983.

23. Malik, M.A., Tahir, M.A., and Sawyna, V.: Treatment of symptomatic reflux esophagitis with the Angelchik prosthesis and its complications. Scientific exhibit, 1982 American College of Surgeons Clinical Congress, Chicago, October 25-29, 1982.

24. McGinty, C.P., Kasten, M.C., et al.: Experience with the Angelchik antireflux prosthesis. Presentation, Missouri Chapter of the American College of Surgeons, Kansas City, 1982.

25. Olivero, S., and Juliani, G.: Surgical treatment of the hiatal hernia and gastroesophageal reflux in adult patients, using the Angelchik antireflux prosthesis (translation), Minerva Chir. **36:**1382-1390, 1981.

26. Ruffo, A., Ferraris, R., and Nahum, M.: Some remarks about the use of the Angelchik ring, Minerva Med. **73:**171-174, 1982.

27. Starling, J.R.: Experience with the antireflux prosthesis: effects on oesophageal function. ARP Symposium, Royal Postgraduate Medical School, London, 1983.

28. Temple, J.G., Taylor, T.V., and Alexander-Williams, J.: A simple operative prosthetic treatment for gastroesophageal reflux, J. R. Coll. Surg. Edin. **29:**16-17, 1984.

29. Varon, D.N., and Silverman, L.M.: The Angelchik prosthesis in the treatment of refractory gastroesophageal (GE) reflux (abstract), Am. J. Gastroenterol. **78:**699, 1983.

30. Wale, R. J. Royston, C.M.S., Bennett, J.R., and Buckton, G.K.: Prospective study of the Angelchik antireflux prosthesis, Br. J. Surg. **72:**520-524, 1985.

31. Willekens, F.G.J., et al.: Treatment of symptomatic gastroesophageal reflux using the Angelchik antireflux prosthesis: a preliminary report. (In preparation.)

32. Condon, R.E.: More misadventures with the esophageal collar (editorial), Surgery, **93**(3):477-478, 1983.

33. Lackey, C., and Potts, J.: Penetration into the stomach; a complication of the antireflux prosthesis, J.A.M.A. **248**(3):350, 1982.

33a. Mansour, K.A., and McKeown, P.P.: Disastrous complications of the Angelchik prosthesis, Am. Surg. **49**(11):616-618, 1983.

34. Skinner, D.B., et al.: Surgical management of esophageal reflux and hiatus hernia, J. Thorac. Cardiovasc. Surg. **53:**33-54, 1967.

35. Zucker, K., Peskin, G.W., and Saik, R.P.: Recurrent hiatal hernia repair, Arch. Surg. **117:**413-414, 1982.

36. Data on file with Mentor Corporation, Goleta, Calif.

37. Lees, C.D., Steiger, E., and Cosgrove, D.M.: Esophageal perforation: a complication of the Angelchik prosthesis, Cleve. Clin. Q. **50:**449-451, 1983.

38. Schultz, K.A., Pickleman, J., et al.: Endoscopic removal of an intragastric Angelchik antireflux prosthesis, Surgery **972:**234-246, 1985.

38a. Henderson, R.D., et al.: Dysphagia complicating hiatal hernia repair, J. Thorac. Cardiovasc. Surg. **88:**922-928, 1984.

39. Battaglini, J.W., Schorlemmer, G.R., and Frantz, P.T.: Intractable dysphagia following placement of Angelchik prosthesis for reflux esophagitis, Ann. Thorac. Surg. **35**(5):551-552, 1983.

40. Ferraris, V.A., and Sube, J.: Retrospective study of the surgical management of reflux esophagitis, Surg. Gynecol. and Obstet. **152:**17-21, 1981.

41. Garcia-Rinaldi, R., and Lanza, F.: Hiatal hernia with severe reflux esophagitis: treatment by superselective vagotomy and Nissen fundoplication, South. Med. J. **77:**418-422, 1984.

42. Gardner, R.J., Bonnabeau, R.C., and Warden, H.E.: Surgical repair of gastroesophageal reflux with sliding hiatal hernia, Am. J. Surg. **13:**554-556, 1977.

43. Gregorie, H.B., Cathcart, R.S., and Gregorie, R.J.: Surgical treatment of intractable esophagitis, Ann. Surg. **199:**580-587, 1984.

44. Henderson, R.D., and Marryatt, G.: Total fundoplication gastroplasty: long term follow-up in 500 patients, J. Thorac. Cardiovasc. Surg. **85:**81-87, 1983.

45. Hermreck, A.S., and Coates, N.R.: Results of the Hill antireflux operation, Am. J. Surg. **140**(6):764-767, 1980.

46. Matikainen, M.: Nissen-Rosetti fundoplication for the treatment of gastroesophageal reflux, Acta. Chir. Scand. **148:**173-177, 1982.

47. Nicholson, D.A., and Nohl-Oser, H.C.: A comparison between two methods of fundoplication by evaluation of the long-term results, J. Thorac. Cardiovasc. Surg. **72**(6):938-943, 1976.

48. Orringer, M.B., and Orringer, J.S.: The combined Collis-Nissen operation: early assessment of reflux control, Ann. Thorac. Surg. **33**(6):534-539, 1982.

49. Polk, H.C.: Fundoplication for reflux esophagitis: misadventures with the operation of choice, Ann. Surg. **183:**645-652, 1976.

50. Rogers, D.M., Herrington, J.L., and Morton, C.: Incidental splenectomy associated with Nissen fundoplication, Ann. Surg. **191:**153-156, 1980.

51. Sillin, L.F., et al.: Effective surgical therapy of esophagitis, Arch. Surg. **114:**536-540, 1979.

52. Stahlgren, L.H., Pagana, T.J., and Costantino, G.N.: Fundoplication for major reflux in patients with gallstones, Surg. Gynecol. and Obstet. **150:**875-877, 1980.

53. Washer, G.F., Gear, M.W.L., et al.: Randomized prospective trial of Roux-en-Y duodenal diversion versus fundoplication for severe reflux oesophagitis, Br. J. Surg. **71:**181-184, 1984.

54. Menguy, R.: A modified fundoplication which preserves the ability to belch, Surgery **84**(3):301-307, 1978.

55. Burnett, H.F., Read, R.C., et al.: Management of complications of fundoplication and Barrett's esophagus, Surgery **82:**521-530, 1977.

56. Maher, J.W., Hollenbeck, J.T., and Woodward, E.R.: Recurrent esophagitis following gastropexy (Hills), Ann. Surg. **187:**227-230, 1978.

57. Sapala, M.A., et al.: Evaluation of the Angelchik antireflux prosthesis in vivo: early clinical and microscopic findings. (In preparation.)

58. Negre, J.B.: Post-fundoplication symptoms: do they restrict the success of the Nissen fundoplication? Ann Surg. **198**(6):698-700, 1983.

59. Woodward, E.R., Thomas, H.F., and McAlhany, J.C.: Comparison of crural repair and Nissen fundoplication in the treatment of esophageal hiatus hernia with peptic esophagitis, Ann. Surg. **73:**782-792, 1971.

60. Sessions, H.R., Haynie, C.C., and Kingsley, J.R.: Reflux esophagitis: clinical experience with the Angelchik antireflux prosthesis. (In preparation.)

61. Brandt-Graede, V., Huibregtse, K., and Tytgat, G.N.: Endoscopic removal of an antireflux prosthesis, Acta Endoscopica **13**(1):47-50, 1983.

62. Bombeck, C.T.: The choice of operations for gastroesophageal reflux. In Watson, A., and Celestin, L.R., editors: Disorders of the oesophagus: advances and controversies, London, 1984, Pitman Books, Ltd. p. 126.

63. Benjamin, S.B., Knuff, T.K., et al.: The Angelchik antireflux prosthesis: effects on the lower esophageal sphincter of primates. Ann. Surg. **197:**63-67, 1983.

64. Cohen, D.J., Benjamin, S.B., et al.: Evaluation of the Angelchik antireflux prosthesis using a model for esophageal reflux in rhesus monkeys. Presentation at Southwestern Surgical Congress, Hawaii, April, 1984.

65. Dougherty, S.H., and Simmons, R.L.: Infections in bionic man: the pathology of infections in prosthetic devices, part I, Curr. Prob. Surg. **19**(5):220-264, 1982.

66. Habal, M.B.: The biologic basis for the clinical application of silicones, Arch. Surg. **119:**843-848, 1984.

Use of a prosthetic device to control gastroesophageal reflux

DISCUSSION

John G. Temple

That many operations have been described for correcting gastroesophageal reflux is perhaps a testimony to the fact that no simple and universally successful operation has yet been devised. The addition of the Angelchik antireflux prosthesis to the surgical armamentarium is, therefore, of interest.

The ideal operation for gastroesophageal reflux should be easily performed, effective, and reproducible, should produce permanent relief of symptoms, and should be associated with a decreased operative morbidity and mortality. Unfortunately, in stating these aims the authors have rather dismissed the results of other antireflux procedures as not falling easily within these criteria. A careful search of the literature shows that in fact the standard antireflux procedures such as the Nissen and Belsey operations do produce reliable and safe results in competent hands. They have, however, never been the procedures for the occasional operator and never will be, if good and lasting results are to be achieved. The same limitations should also be applied to any new procedure for gastroesophageal reflux. The selection of patients for such operations and the efficacy of the operative methods will always be equally important.

Angelchik's approach to the problem has been refreshingly direct and simple. This device has been widely available since 1979, and many centers throughout the world are now reporting their results. However, the device has always been manufactured in only one size, even though the anatomic variations at the gastroesophageal junction are diverse. It is perhaps, therefore, surprising that a single-sized device can be or should be expected to produce uniformly good results in all patients.

The technique is easily performed and is, or should be, entirely reproducible. Certainly in Angelchik's hands it has been exceedingly effective, and a 98% symptomatic improvement, with

Visick grades I or II in his 228 patients, is quite remarkable. A major criticism of this series, however, is that objective assessment of the patient by means other than radiology was infrequently carried out. In fact, only 30 patients had pH and motility studies preoperatively, and an even smaller number (14, [6%]) had postoperative studies, and none of these results are actually included in the discussion. The literature does not record such good clinical results in other hands. Even ardent protagonists of the procedure only report an overall good symptomatic improvement somewhere in the region of 80% of cases, and all their series reports are of short-term follow-up. Other published work does, however, show good objective evidence that the ARP does prevent reflux when correctly positioned at the cardia.[1]

Although in many cases this prosthetic device does produce satisfactory and potentially long-lasting results, there have been complications that have been much publicized, and perhaps overemphasized. Without doubt, it is a very safe technical operation with a very low operative mortality. Because of the minimal mobilization, it is quite likely that the overall mortality will be less than for other antireflux procedures, and the evidence to date supports this.

Unexplained modifications to the original technique are described. Anterior gastropexy is advanced as a solution to the problem of the wide hiatus, but the authors have only used it in the last 2 years. Since there have been so few failures with the technique in their hands in previous years, why do they need to suggest anterior gastropexy at all? Equally, concomitant procedures with the exception of pyloroplasty, but which involve opening the gastrointestinal tract, are condemned by the authors, and yet of 46 such procedures carried out, only 17 in fact were pyloroplasty procedures. Therefore, concomitant procedures were performed that did involve other parts of the gastrointestinal tract, particularly the stomach and biliary tract, in 29 cases and yet these were not associated apparently with any significant postoperative problems. Despite these modifications to the surgical procedure, only five patients were graded Visick III or IV.

Failure of the device does cause concern. The problem of prosthetic disruption caused by tearing of the vulcanized straps leading to dislocation and migration was not an inherent fault in the device, but one of manufacture. This has now been overcome, and probably all the failures related to this have been detected and corrected. However, it would be interesting to know how many prostheses of this design were implanted or removed because of failure worldwide. In my own series of 27 patients, this problem was encountered twice.

Problems and complications of the prosthesis not directly related to technical failure of the device itself are a cause for greater anxiety. Displacement of the device occurred in 10 patients, and the device actually had to be replaced in 7, and yet, as stated, poor symptomatic results were obtained only in 2% of the 228 patients. However, the device migrated into the chest in 28 patients, or 12%. Surely this represents displacement. Apparently none of these patients had any return of symptoms or dysphagia. This has not been the experience of several other authors. Host-prosthesis interaction has not led to any clear or well proven complications other than the variable fibrosis that occurs around any silicone prosthesis upon implantation. Often this may be beneficial in fixing the prosthesis in place, although in two of my own cases this fibrous capsule produced severe dysphagia necessitating removal of the device.

Few comparisons between the ARP and Nissen fundoplications have been reported, and these are all early studies with very short follow-up periods. In 18 other studies in which ARPs are reported, the mean number of patients in any of the series can only be 30, and these are, therefore, very small series with very short follow-up periods.

The postulated mechanism of action is as yet ill defined. Undoubtedly when correctly positioned at the gastroesophageal junction below the diaphragm, the device constitutes a bulky posterior buttress, angulating the cardia forward and obliquely. This in itself increases the manometrically determined barrier to reflux at this site. If, however, the device rotates so that the collars and strap-knot lie posteriorly, this effect can be lost,

leading to a return of reflux or even dysphagia, if the esophagus becomes trapped between the two collars themselves.[2] Wyllie and Edwards' paper[3] is of particular interest in that the device was situated below the lower esophageal sphincter in nearly all their patients and yet a good symptomatic response was obtained. In conjunction with my radiological colleague Dr. John Lee in Birmingham, I have found that in a group of patients in whom the device produced a good symptomatic and objective response as evidenced by esophagoscopy, manometry, and pH measurements, a variable knuckle of fundus had herniated through the prosthetic ring. Thus we believe that when the fundus distends with air postprandially, this knuckle likewise distends and, being contained within the semi-rigid ring, actively compresses the lower esophagus, thus preventing reflux.

This paper is largely a compilation of uncontrolled reports of the use of the Angelchik prosthesis. The assembled information cannot, therefore, accurately be compared with reported series of other antireflux procedures. What is needed is prospective trials of the ARP compared with other antireflux procedures, or even consecutive series from the same center where operations are being performed under the same conditions by the same group of surgeons. This would be more helpful than the totally random and sporadic reporting at present taking place.

It may be that the ARP is a useful addition to the surgical armamentarium for the treatment of gastroesophageal reflux. However, although thousands of the devices have now been implanted, properly controlled objective scientific evaluation is still lacking, and the ARP should certainly not undergo widespread use at the present time, until the results of well controlled and conducted comparative trials have been presented.

REFERENCES

1. Weaver, R.M., and Temple, J.G.: The Angelchik prosthesis for gastroesophageal reflux: symptomatic and objective assessment, Ann. R. Coll. Surg. Engl. **67:**299-302, 1985.
2. Morris, D.L., Jones, J., Evans, D.F., Foster, G., Smart, H., Gregson, R., Amar, S., Doran, J., and Hardcastle, J.D.: Reflux versus dysphagia: an objective evaluation of the Angelchik prosthesis, Br. J. Surg. **72:**1027-1020, 1985.
3. Wyllie, J.H., and Edwards, D.A.W.: A quantitative assessment of results with the Angelchik Prosthesis, Ann. R. Coll. Surg. Engl. **67:**216-221, 1985.

Gastric secretion suppression and duodenal diversion: the Roux-en-Y principle in the management of complex reflux problems

W. Spencer Payne, Geoffrey B. Thompson, Victor F. Trastek, Jeffrey M. Piehler, and Peter C. Pairolero

The role of acid-peptic gastric secretions in the genesis of the symptoms and complications of gastroesophageal reflux has received major attention in the medical and surgical literature during the past 40 years. The role of biliary-pancreatic secretions has been less well appreciated.[1-5] There is now sufficient information to state that biliary-pancreatic secretions, irrespective of pH, can be equally as noxious to esophageal mucosa as acid-peptic secretions.[6-19] Confusion regarding the relative roles of upper digestive secretions has stemmed in part from the misconception that if duodenal contents are refluxed into the esophagus, intraluminal pH detectors should register alkalinity. Thus, the elusive "alkaline reflux esophagitis" is often sought, but rarely encountered.

That duodenogastric reflux normally occurs[20] and that bile refluxes along with acid into the esophagus under the usual circumstance of gastroesophageal incompetence have been repeatedly demonstrated by the use of bile indicators such as sulfobromophthalein[21] and indocyanine green[22] and more recently by scintiscanning using imidodiacetic acid (HIDA).[23] The detection of acid in the esophagus is merely a convenient indicator of gastroesophageal reflux; acid is not necessarily the sole agent responsible for the symptoms and complications of gastroesophageal reflux. Similarly, positive results of acid perfusion tests only indicate the presence of erosive esophagitis, and do not necessarily reveal its cause. For example, patients with esophagitis do not avoid citrus fruits because such fruits are the cause of the esophagitis but because they are irritating to a previously injured mucosa. Similarly, a positive result on an acid perfusion test is seen in patients with lye burns, medication burns, or stasis esophagitis as readily as in patients suffering from reflux esophagitis. The test is specific for esophagitis but not for its cause.

We, as well as others, have documented continued subjective symptoms and objective signs of severe reflux esophagitis in patients in whom gastric acids have been effectively eliminated by medication, surgery, or disease.[*]

In clinical and surgical practice, it is usually not important to determine which of the upper digestive secretions are responsible for esophageal injury, because almost all patients selected for surgical management will be subjected to an antireflux procedure. This type of procedure provides a nonselective interruption of all potentially injurious secretions, thus preventing them from having retrograde contact with esophageal mucosa. However, patients selected for surgical management have failed to respond either subjectively or objectively to medical treatment, and many of them have been rendered achlorhydric by H_2-blocking agents.

---

[*]References 4, 5, 10, 13, 14, 21, 22 and 24-26.

EVOLUTION OF THE OPERATION AND CLINICAL APPLICATIONS

At the Mayo Clinic, more than 25 years ago, we attempted to control reflux esophagitis and its complications in selected patients by surgically suppressing gastric acid secretion alone,[24,25,27] without notable success. Thus, it became apparent that factors other than acid-peptic secretions were responsible for the failure of these procedures on long-term follow-up. Largely through that experience and the experimental studies of Mann and Williamson[28] and the later studies of Musgrove et al.[15] with biliary diversion by the Roux-en-Y procedure, we came upon the concept of combined duodenal diversion and gastric-acid suppression (see Fig. 12-1). Our early successes were encouraged by the 1961 report of Holt and Large.[16] During the succeeding decade, one of us (W.S.P.)[17] successfully managed 15 patients by a combination vagotomy, antrectomy, and Roux-en-Y procedure, some of whom required conversion of previous Billroth I or II procedures (see Fig. 12-2).

Subsequently, the long-limb Roux-en-Y principle[18] was extended to patients undergoing total gastrectomy[29,30] (Fig. 12-3) and esophagogastrectomy[26] (Fig. 12-4), and more recently it has been employed after total esophagogastrectomy with colon interposition[31] (Fig. 12-5). The validity of the long-limb Roux-en-Y principle has been repeatedly confirmed by others[32-36] (Table 12-1). Of the patients previously reported on, 92% had had one to seven previous operations for either reflux control or reduction of gastric acid secretion. The 22 patients reported by Washer et al.[34] are not included in this percentage because their series involved primary operations in a prospective randomized trial comparing the Roux-en-Y procedure with Nissen fundoplication. With that exception, most of the procedures were truly salvage operations, often performed under circumstances for which there were few therapeutic alternatives. Despite the relatively desperate status of the remaining 66 patients, 88% experienced "excellent" or "good" results, with only one death.

Although dilatable esophageal stenoses were the most frequent cause for surgical intervention, these almost always responded to bougienage during the first postoperative year. Marginal ulcers with bleeding were seen in three patients

Fig. 12-1. A, Truncal vagotomy, gastric antrectomy, and, when esophageal stenoses are not dilatable, conservative stricture resection. **B,** Reconstruction using the 18-inch-long Roux-en-Y gastric drainage procedure to divert biliary and pancreatic secretions away from the stomach. (From Payne, W.S.: Prevention and treatment of biliary-pancreatic reflux esophagitis: the role of long-limb Roux-Y, Surg. Clin. North Am. **63:**851, 1983.)

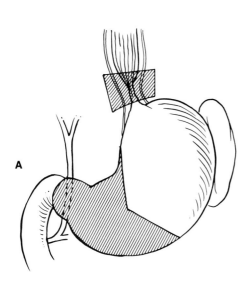

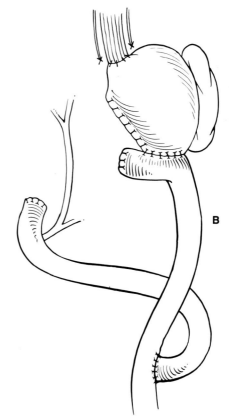

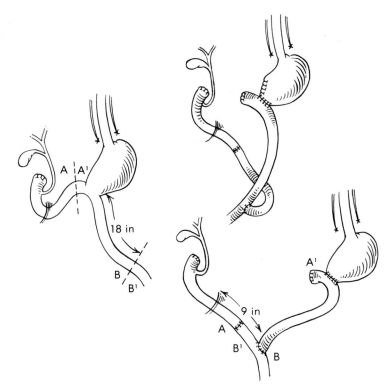

Fig. 12-2. In patients in whom a Billroth II anastomosis has been performed along with truncal vagotomy, and in whom an antireflux procedure cannot be performed, the long-limb Roux-en-Y gastric drainage anastomosis can be constructed by using one of the two methods illustrated on the right. (From Payne, W.S.: Prevention and treatment of biliary-pancreatic reflux esophagitis: the role of long-limb Roux-Y, Surg. Clin. North Am. **63:**851, 1983).

Fig. 12-3. A, Two commonly employed techniques of esophagoenteric reconstruction after total gastrectomy. *Top left,* End-to-side esophagojejunostomy. *Bottom left,* Distal side-to-side enteroenterostomy. Approximately 20% of patients undergoing reconstruction by these means experience intractable biliary reflux and esophagitis and its complications despite achlorhydria. **B,** Revision, by conversion to 18-inch-long Roux-en-Y, is a reliable means of correcting "bile" reflux esophagitis. (From Payne, W.S.: Prevention and treatment of biliary-pancreatic reflux esophagitis: the role of long-limb Roux-Y, Surg. Clin. North Am. **63:**851, 1983.)

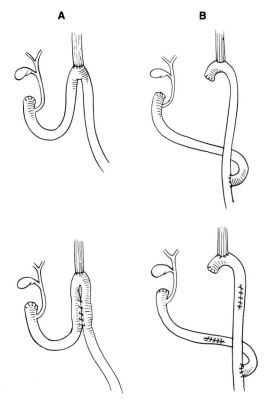

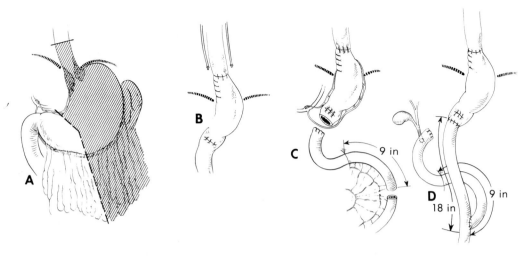

Fig. 12-4. Sequence of procedures: **A** and **B**, Patient's primary operation for cancer of cardia, which was followed by intractable gastroesophageal reflux and severe objective esophagitis despite achlorhydria. **C** and **D**, Subsequent procedure, years later, to correct biliary pancreatic esophagitis. **A**, Esophagogastrectomy for malignant disease at gastric cardia. Shading shows tissues resected, including proximal blood supply to stomach, along with distal portion of esophagus, vagi, spleen, greater omentum, gastrohepatic omentum, and proximal part of stomach with its parietal cell mass. **B**, Reconstruction complete with end-to-end esophagogastrostomy and closure of lesser curvature. Pyloroplasty was performed to minimize postvagotomy gastric retention. When the patient had reflux esophagitis, the following procedure was performed. **C**, Transection of duodenum distal to pyloroplasty with closure of distal duodenal stump. Note preservation of right gastric and right gastroepiploic vessels as the only remaining blood supply for the gastric remnant. The jejunum was transection 9 inches (23 cm) distal to the ligament of Treitz in preparation for Roux-en-Y anastomosis. **D,** Completed procedure. Distal cut end of jejunum has been brought through small defect in transverse mesocolon (not shown) and anastomosed end-to-end to duodenum distal to pyloroplasty. The Roux-en-Y is completed with end-to-side jejunojejunostomy 18 inches (45 cm) distal to the pylorojejunal anastomosis. The proximal jejunal segment distal to the ligament of Treitz is about half the length of the long-limb gastric drainage segment and passes behind and to the left of it to prevent distortion of radian of small-bowel mesentery and obstructive angulation of bowel at the site of end-to-side jejunojejunostomy. Biliary and other duodenal secretions are diverted into more distal upper small bowel. The 18-inch (45-cm) isoperistaltic segment of jejunum is an effective peristaltic barrier against reflux of bile and pancreatic secretions into the stomach and esophagus. (From Smith, J., and Payne, W.S.: Surgical technique for management of reflux esophagitis after esophagogastrectomy for malignancy: further application of Roux-en-Y principle, Mayo Clin. Proc. **50:**588, 1975. By permission of Mayo Foundation.)

and were relieved by complete vagotomy. The early morbidity of small-bowel obstruction was seen in the earlier series by Payne[17] and has been completely avoided since a 9-inch (23-cm) afferent limb (see Fig. 12-4) was used to prevent obstructive angulation at end-to-side jejunojejunostomy. An 18-inch-long (45-cm) Roux-en-Y gastric drainage limb is generally favored by all authors for effective diversion of duodenal contents from the stomach.

Dumping and diarrhea, although uncommon, appear to be unavoidable complications of vagotomy and any gastric drainage procedure. In the series by Payne[17,39] 6 of the 28 patients experienced postoperative respiratory aspiration despite resolution of esophagiis, stenosis, and heartburn. Most patients so afflicted were experiencing this complication before the Roux-en-Y procedure was done. This complication detracted from the otherwise favorable results in these patients.

To the present time, we have employed these basic Roux-en-Y principles in the treatment or prevention of esophagitis in more than 100 patients in the previously listed categories as well as in circumstances to be described.

We believe that the surgical suppression of gastric secretion and Roux-en-Y diversion of pancreatic-biliary secretions should not be performed when an effective antireflux procedure

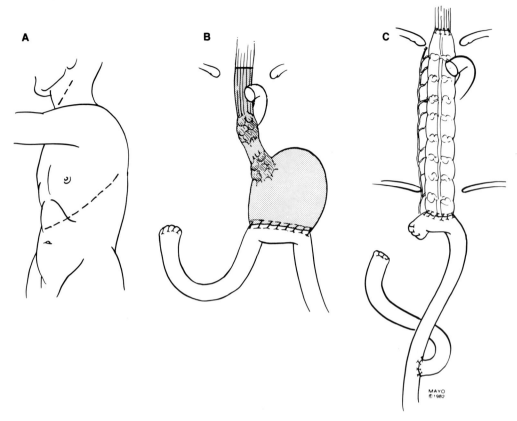

Fig. 12-5. In patients requiring total esophagectomy and total gastrectomy, as is required in the case shown in **B**, in which there are distal esophageal malignant disease and previous Billroth II procedures, it is preferable to anastomose the interposed colon to a long-limb Roux-en-Y, **C**, to prevent postoperative oral regurgitation and aspiration of biliary-pancreatic secretions. Such resection and reconstruction can be achieved, as shown in **A**, through a left thoracoabdominal incision and a left cervical incision. Even long segments of isoperistaltic colon provide an unreliable barrier to retrograde flow of biliary-pancreatic secretions, unless they are diverted as shown. (From Payne, W.S.: Prevention and treatment of biliary-pancreatic reflux esophagitis: the role of long-limb Roux-Y, Surg. Clin. North Am. **63**:851,1983. By permission of W.B. Saunders Co.)

can be done.[18,30-35,39,40] Usually, even patients with failed antireflux procedures can be managed more effectively and more safely by a well-planned and executed fundoplication, even if the reoperation is the second or third attempt.[39,40] As effective as the combined vagotomy–antrectomy–Roux-en-Y procedure may be, the procedure is not devoid of dumping and diarrhea, as implied by others.[34,41] Furthermore, when gastroesophageal competence is not restored, esophageal reflux continues, and though bland in terms of esophageal injury, respiratory aspiration can and does occur in a small percentage of patients and detracts from an otherwise satisfactory result.[39]

However, there are specific though uncommon circumstances when antireflux procedures cannot be carried out at reoperation. Some of these will

be in patients who have undergone previous, unsuccessful antireflux procedures. These include patients in whom, on reexploration, no fundus can be developed or defined with careful dissection; patients in whom, on reexploration, neither the distal segment of the esophagus nor the proximal portion of the stomach is approachable because of dense inflammatory reaction to previous surgery, radiation therapy, or resolved sepsis; patients who have undergone such radical previous distal gastric resections with either Billroth I or II anastomosis in whom no fundus is available for plication; and the rare patient with a truly shortened esophagus so fixed to the thoracic vertebrae or aorta that an esophageal lengthening procedure cannot be performed.[42]

A more obvious indication for conversion to

TABLE 12-1. Summary of reported cases of vagotomy–antrectomy–Roux-en-Y for reflux esophagitis

Year	Author	No. of cases	Mortality	Morbidity		Average follow-up (yr)	Results[*]
				Early	Late		
1966	Cenni et al.[35]	3	0	0	0	3.2	E 3
1970	Weaver et al.[32]	7	0	0	Diarrhea, 1 Dumping, 1	15.3	E 5 G 2
1970	Payne[17]	15†	0	Marginal ulcer, 1 Small-bowel obstruction, 2 Myocardial infarction, 1 Dysphagia, 2	Respiratory aspiration, 4 Dumping, 1 Diarrhea, 1 Nausea, 1	3	E 6 G 5 P 4
1973	Himal and MacLean[37]	3	0	0	0	1.4	E 3
1973	Coppinger et al.[38]	11	0	Marginal ulcer, 1 Wound infection, 1 Delayed gastric emptying, 1	No weight gain, 1	1.3	E 10 G 1
1975	Royston et al.[33]	8	1	Dysphagia, 4	Diarrhea and stricture, 1	1.6	E 2 G 4 F 1
1976	Herrington and Mody[36]	6	0	0	Abdominal fullness, 1	1.1	E 5 G 1
1984	Washer et al.[34]	22	0	Stroke, 1 Septicemia, 1 Marginal ulcer, 1	Incisional hernia, 1	6	E 15 G 5 F 1 Visick P 1 III or IV
1984	Payne[39]	13‡	0	0	Respiratory aspiration, 2	3.2	E 7 G 4 P 2
TOTAL		88	(1%)	(16%)	(15%)	—	E or G, 89% F or P, 11%

[*] *E*, Excellent; *G*, good; *F*, fair; *P*, poor.

†Includes 6 patients with additional resection of esophageal stricture and 2 patients with long jejunal interposition between stomach and duodenum in lieu of Roux-en-Y configuration. Excludes 15 patients without reflux esophagitis or in whom a reversed jejunal segment was employed.

‡Includes 3 patients with resection of esophageal stricture.

long-limb Roux-en-Y anastomosis is a previous total gastrectomy with nondiverting esophagojejunostomy. Conversion to Roux-en-Y anastomosis promptly resolves the esophagitis and brings dilatable stenoses under control and will resolve the oral regurgitation of bile (see Fig. 12-3). Similarly, patients with oral regurgitation of bile after total esophagogastrectomy with colon interposition will benefit from long-limb Roux-en-Y jejunal drainage of the colon interposition (see Fig. 12-5). Obviously, prevention of esophagitis by the Roux-en-Y procedure at the initial operation would have been more desirable. Many other procedures bypass or completely destroy the lower esophageal sphincter[26] and produce reflux esophagitis[43] that is amenable to the combined vagotomy–antrectomy–Roux-en-Y procedure (see Figs. 12-1 and 12-4).

Less well appreciated is the use of a long-limb Roux-en-Y anastomosis as a gastric drainage procedure after the Ivor Lewis or transhiatal esophagectomy, which on rare occasions can be complicated by reflux esophagitis or oral regurgitation of bilious fluid (see Fig. 12-4).

GASTRIC EMPTYING, GASTROESOPHAGEAL REFLUX, AND THE ROLE OF GASTRIC DRAINAGE PROCEDURES

The need for competence at the gastroesophageal junction is a compelling factor in the prevention of esophageal mucosal injury, irrespective of the specific injurious agents implicated. Even if the sphincter mechanism is normal, potent forces may hinder competence (see Fig. 12-6). In addition to the factors listed, there are dynamic vagal-vagal reflexes that increase sphincteric tone as intragastric pressures increase.

Gastric emptying has an important role in the genesis of gastroesophageal incompetence, and both overt and subtle dysfunctions of stomach and bowel can influence intragastric pressure and competence. Thus, some understanding of normal and abnormal gastric, gastroduodenal, and small-bowel function[44,45] is essential to the understanding of gastroesophageal competence. The proximal portion of the stomach (fundus) (see Fig. 12-7) receives and stores boluses of food received from the esophagus; the fundus is the site of gastric reservoir function. As boluses of food pass from the esophagus into the stomach, the proximal portion relaxes, so-called receptive relaxation.[44] This accommodation to distention of the proximal portion fortunately is associated with little change in intragastric pressure. As a consequence of this receptive relaxation and accommodation, intragastric pressure normally remains low as the stomach fills. Slow, sustained

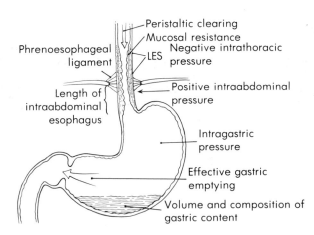

Fig. 12-6. Factors that affect gastroesophageal competence or permit gastroesophageal reflux and its complications. These include esophageal peristalsis with its clearing action, intrinsic lower esophageal sphincter tone, intra-abdominal position of part of esophagus, site of phrenoesophageal ligament insertions, intra-abdominal and intrathoracic pressures, intragastric pressure, effective gastric emptying, and concentration and composition of digestive secretions (acid-bile-pancreatic) present in the stomach and available for reflux into the esophagus. (From Payne, W.S., and Ellis, F.H., Jr: Esophagus and diaphragmatic hernias. In Schwartz, S.I., Shires, G.T., Spencer, F.C., et al., editors: Principles of surgery, ed. 4, New York, 1983, McGraw-Hill Book Co., p. 1063. By permission.)

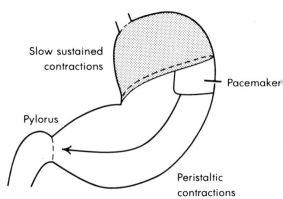

Fig. 12-7. The stomach has two motor regions, proximal fundic (*shaded area*) and distal (*clear area*). The gastric pacemaker is located in the proximal corpus along the greater curve. (From Kelly, K.A.: Gastric motility after gastric operations. In Nyhus: Surgery Annual 1974, New York, 1974, Appleton-Century-Crofts.)

fundic contractions gradually press ingested contents toward the distal portion of the stomach and the duodenum (Fig. 12-7). Peristaltic contractions of the distal two thirds of the stomach arise from the intrinsic gastric pacemaker (Fig. 12-7) and aid this slow, sustained pressure of the fundus in propelling the gastric contents aborally. The antrum acts as the gastric mixer and grinder. Its contractions thoroughly homogenize the gastric solids before allowing the liquified particulate to pass into the duodenum. As the terminal antrum contracts, the pylorus closes, permitting only the liquid homogenate to selectively pass into the duodenum. Solids, however, meet resistance at the pylorus and are retained and retropulsed into the antrum for further grinding and mixing before again being propelled toward the closed pylorus for selective passage of liquid contents into the duodenum. By repeated cycles, the stomach thus eventually completely empties of liquids and digestible solids by squeezing, retropulsion, mixing, grinding and selective passage of liquified chyme into the small intestine. Characteristic myoelectric activity parallels motor activity and changes in intragastric pressure. Motor control is largely neural, with modulation by hormonal and possibly paracrine functions, each of which may have either excitatory or inhibitory effects. The rate of gastric emptying varies directly as a function of the pressure gradient between stomach and duodenum and inversely with the resistance to flow across the pylorus.

The rate of gastric emptying in turn is carefully controlled by feedback from small intestinal receptors that sense the pH, osmolarity, and caloric density of the chyme. These trigger multimodality (neural, humoral, and so forth) responses that may be either stimulatory or inhibitory to gastric motor activity.

It has long been known that organic gastric-outlet obstruction, such as that seen with benign pyloric stenosis or gastric stasis secondary to paresis from vagotomy, can result in gastroesophageal reflux, even in the presence of a normal gastroesophageal competence mechanism. With the definitive relief of organic obstruction or with provision for adequate gastric drainage, competence can be restored in most of these patients without the need for any specific antireflux procedures. If gastric stasis is not relieved, antireflux measures may not be totally effective[46] (see Fig. 12-8).

Only in recent decades have we become aware of some of the more subtle dysfunctions of gastric, duodenal, and jejunal motility in the genesis of gastroesophageal reflux. Chief among these

are incidences of congenital and acquired dysautonomia, smooth-muscle degeneration, and other less well-defined motor abnormalities of the gut.[47-49]

It is no longer completely justifiable simply to define anatomic patency of the gut or to assume that gastric stasis is merely a dysfunction of the gastric antrum, even though these are common, more easily detected potential causes for increased intragastric pressure and esophageal reflux.

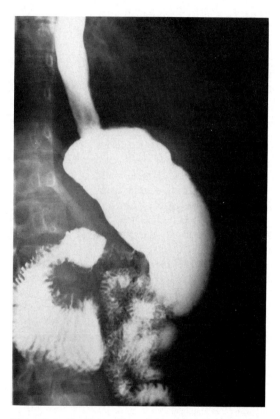

Fig. 12-8. Radiographic appearance of esophagus, stomach, duodenum, and upper small bowel of young woman with scleroderma of the esophagus with CREST syndrome, intractable heartburn, oral regurgitation, bile staining of pillow, and occasional respiratory aspiration. Manometric studies defined advanced sclerodermatous involvement of esophagus, lower esophageal sphincter, stomach, and duodenum, with feeble contractions of jejunum. Note the dilated, atonic third portion of duodenum, with normal small-bowel mucosal pattern beyond. This patient had significant gastric retention. An antireflux procedure relieved massive regurgitation and aspiration, but minor heartburn with occasional emesis remains. Antrectomy, Billroth II anastomosis, or a Roux-en-Y gastric drainage procedure might be ineffective because of the jejunal motility problem.

Most patients with gastroesophageal reflux have primary sphincter dysfunction and are appropriately managed by antireflux procedures.[18,40] It is often only when these measures fail in the presence of the persistently intact procedure that other, rare causes for reflux are sought. Because most failed antireflux procedures are corrected by reapplication of the same or similar procedure, almost all reflux is initially, and correctly, considered to be due to sphincter failure alone. Furthermore, the successful widespread application of vagotomy, antrectomy, and Roux-en-Y diversion attests to the apparent absence of small-bowel dysfunction in almost all patients so managed. Interestingly, however, the same may not be true of patients with so-called alkaline reflux gastritis (a condition rarely seen concomitantly with bile reflux esophagitis). Alkaline reflux gastritis is uncommon and has had such a varied response to Roux-en-Y diversion and such a varied gastric emptying response[50] that there may be some underlying gut motility problem not inherent in most patients with gastroesophageal reflux. Thus, before empirically applying antrectomy with a Billroth I or II *or* a long-limb Roux-en-Y gastric drainage, there should be some assurance that the bowel to which the stomach is to be anastomosed has reasonably normal motility downstream.

Although some patients with antral dysfunctions or with organic gastric-outlet obstruction and gastroesophageal reflux respond well to antrectomy, others will not, and failure usually can be traced to continued gastric stasis resulting from either narrowed anastomosis or small-bowel motor dysfunction.

Currently, we are on the threshold of a better understanding of gut motility and the complex series of resistance and capacitance elements that influence the physiologic pressure gradients that are responsible for effective and comfortable ingestion, propulsion, digestion, and elimination. In the near future, it may be possible to pace the alimentary tract electrically[51] in a manner similar to that in current practice for the heart. Clinical awareness, improved knowledge, standardization of diagnostic testing and the wider application of tests may permit even more rational management of some of the more complex motility problems that may accompany gastroesophageal reflux.

REFERENCES

1. Andersen, H.A., and Payne, W.S.: Esophageal hiatal hernia, gastroesophageal reflux, and their complications. In Payne, W.S., and Olsen, A.M., editors: The esophagus, Philadelphia, 1974, Lea & Febiger, p. 107.

2. Burgess, J.N., Payne, W.S., Andersen, H.A., et al.: Barrett esophagus: the columnar-epithelial-lined lower esophagus, Mayo Clin. Proc. **46:**728, 1971.

3. Moersch, R.N., Ellis, F.H., Jr., and McDonald, J.R.: Pathologic changes occurring in severe reflux esophagitis, Surg. Gynecol. Obstet. **108:**476, 1959.

4. Payne, W.S.: Esophageal reflux ulceration: causes and surgical management, Surg. Clin. North Am. **51:**935, 1971.

5. Windsor, C.W.O.: Gastro-oesophageal reflux after partial gastrectomy, Br. Med. J. **2:**1233, 1964.

6. Cross, F.S., and Wangensteen, O.H.: Role of bile and pancreatic juice in production of esophageal erosions and anemia, Proc. Soc. Exp. Biol. Med. **77:**862, 1951.

7. Lambert, R.: Relative importance of biliary and pancreatic secretions in the genesis of esophagitis in rats, Am. J. Dig. Dis. **7:**1026, 1962.

8. Levrat, M., Lambert, R., and Kirshbaum, G.: Esophagitis produced by reflux of duodenal contents in rats, Am. J. Dig. Dis. **7:**564, 1962.

9. Moffat, R.C., and Berkas, E.M.: Bile esophagitis, Arch. Surg. **91:**963, 1965.

10. Palmer, E.D.: Subacute erosive ("peptic") esophagitis associated with achlorhydria, N. Engl. J. Med. **262:**927, 1960.

11. Gillison, E.W., Kusakari, K., Bombeck, C.T., et al.: The importance of bile in reflux esophagitis and the success in its prevention by surgical means, Br. J. Surg. **59:**794, 1972.

12. Wickbom, G., Bushkin, F.L., and Woodward, E.R.: Alkaline reflux esophagitis, Surg. Gynecol. Obstet. **139:**267, 1974.

13. Safaie-Shirazi, S., DenBesten, L., and Zike, W.L.: Effect of bile salts on the ionic permeability of the esophageal mucosa and their role in the production of esophagitis, Gastroenterology **68:**728, 1975.

14. Salo, J.A., Kivilaakso, E.: Role of bile salts and trypsin in the pathogenesis of experimental alkaline esophagitis, Surgery **93:**525, 1983.

15. Musgrove, J.E., Grindlay, J.H., and Karlson, A.G.: Intestinal-biliary reflux after anastomosis of common duct to duodenum or jejunum: an experimental study, Trans. West. Surg. Assoc. **59:**77, 1951.

16. Holt, C.J., and Large, A.M.: Surgical management of reflux esophagitis, Ann. Surg. **153:**555, 1961.

17. Payne, W.S.: Surgical treatment of reflux esophagitis and stricture associated with permanent incompetence of the cardia, Mayo Clin. Proc. **45:**553, 1970.

18. Payne, W.S.: Reflux esophagitis with stricture: alternative methods of management. In Jackson, J.W., editor: Operative Surgery: cardiothoracic surgery, ed. 4, London, 1986, Butterworth.

19. Redo, S.F., Barnes, W.A., and de la Sierra, A.O.: Perfusion of the canine esophagus with secretions of the upper gastrointestinal tract, Ann. Surg. **149:**556, 1959.

20. Beaumont, W.: Experiments and observations on the gastric juice, and the physiology of digestion, Plattsburg, 1833, F.P. Allen.

21. Gillison, E.W., and Nyhus, L.M.: Bile reflux, gastric secretion, and heartburn (abstract), Br. J. Surg. **58:**864, 1971.

22. Duthy, B.: Personal communication.

23. Thomas, W.E.G., Jackson, P.C., Cooper, M.J., et al.: The problems associated with scintigraphic assessment of duodenogastric reflux, Scand. J. Gastroenterol. **19** (Suppl. 92):36, 1983.

24. Payne, W.S., Andersen, H.A., and Ellis, F.H., Jr.: The treatment of short esophagus with esophagitis by gastric drainage procedures with and without vagotomy, Surg. Gynecol. Obstet. **116**:523, 1963.

25. Payne, W.S., Andersen, H.A., and Ellis, F.H., Jr.: Reappraisal of esophagogastrectomy and antral excision in the treatment of short esophagus, Surgery **55**:344, 1964.

26. Smith, J., and Payne, W.S.: Surgical techique for management of reflux esophagitis after esophagogastrectomy for malignancy: further application of Roux-en-Y principle, Mayo Clin. Proc. **50**:588, 1975.

27. Ellis, F.H., Jr.: A physiologic operation for ulceration and stricture of the terminal esophagus, Proc. Staff Meet. Mayo Clin. **31**:615, 1956.

28. Mann, F.C., and Williamson, C.S.: The experimental production of peptic ulcer, Ann. Surg. **77**:409, 1923.

29. Payne, W.S.: The long-term clinical state after resection with total gasrectomy and Roux loop anastomosis. In Smith, R.E., and Smith, R.A., editors: Surgery of the esophagus (the Coventry Conference), London, 1972, Butterworth, p. 23.

30. ReMine, W.H., Payne, W.S., and van Heerden, J.A.: Manual of upper gastrointestinal surgery, New York, 1985, Springer-Verlag.

31. Payne, W.S.: Prevention and treatment of biliary-pancreatic reflux esophagitis: the role of long-limb Roux-Y, Surg. Clin. North Am. **63**:851, 1983.

32. Weaver, A.S., Large, A.M., and Walt, A.J.: Surgical management of severe reflux esophagitis: eight to seventeen year follow-up study, Am. J. Surg. **119**:15, 1970.

33. Royston, C.M.S., Dowling, B.L., and Spencer, J.: Antrectomy with Roux-en-Y anastomosis in the treatment of peptic esophagitis with stricture, Br. J. Surg. **62**:605, 1975.

34. Washer, G.F., Gear, M.W.L., Dowling, B.L., et al.: Randomized prospective trial of Roux-en-Y duodenal diversion versus fundoplication for severe reflux esophagitis, Br. J. Surg. **71**:181, 1984.

35. Cenni, L.J., Cox, W.F., and Hands, S.: Gastric surgery: the Roux-en-Y procedure for bile esophagitis, J. Kans. Med. Soc. **67**:421, 1966.

36. Herrington, J.L., Jr., and Mody, B.: Total duodenal diversion for treatment of reflux esophagitis uncontrolled by repeated antireflux procedures, Ann. Surg. **183**:636, 1976.

37. Himal, H.S., and MacLean, L.D.: Bile esophagitis, Can. J. Surg. **16**:17, 1973.

38. Coppinger, W.R., Job, H., DeLauro, J.E., et al.: Surgical treatment of reflux gastritis and esophagitis, Arch. Surg. **106**:463, 1973.

39. Payne, W.S.: Surgical management of reflux-induced esophageal stenoses: results in 101 patients, Br. J. Surg. **71**:971, 1984.

40. Piehler, J.M., Payne, W.S., Cameron, A.J., et al.: The uncut Collis-Nissen procedure for esophageal hiatal hernia and its complications, Probl. Gen. Surg. **1**:1, 1984.

41. Cade, R.J., and Kilby, J.O.: The incidence of the dumping syndrome following gastrojejunostomy with Roux-en-Y anastomosis, Postgrad. Med. J. **58**:760, 1982.

42. Ellis, F.H., Jr., and Payne, W.S. (conferee): Collis-Nissen procedure with esophageal dilation for short esophagus with stricture. In Cardiothor techniques: a pictorial review of surgical procedures, presented by Smith Kline & French Laboratories, Albany, N.Y., 1981, LTI Medica, 12 pp.

43. Ripley, H.R., Olsen, A.M., and Kirklin, J.W.: Esophagitis after esophagogastric anastomosis, Surgery **32**:1, 1952.

44. Kelly, K.A.: Motility of the stomach and gastroduodenal junction. In Johnson, L.R., editor: Physiology of the gastrointestinal tract, vol. 1, New York, 1981, Raven Press, pp. 393-410.

45. Kelly, K.A.: Gastric emptying disorders following gastric surgery. In Dubois, A., and Castell, D.O., editors: Esophageal and gastric emptying, Boca Raton, Fla., 1984, CRC Press, Inc. p. 89.

46. Stanghellini, V., and Malagelada, J.-R.: Gastric manometric abnormalities in patients with dyspeptic symptoms after fundoplication, Gut **24**:790, 1983.

47. Malagelada, J.-R., and Camilleri, M.: Unexplained vomiting: a diagnostic challenge, Ann. Intern. Med. **101**:211, 1984.

48. Malagelada, J.-R., and Stanghellini, V.: Manometric evaluation of functional upper gut symptoms, Gastroenterology **88**:1223, 1985.

49. Camilleri, M., and Malagelada, J.-R.: Abnormal intestinal motility in diabetics with the gastroparesis syndrome, Eur. J. Clin. Invest. **14**:420, 1984.

50. Pellegrini, C.A., Patti, M.G., Lewin, M., et al.: Alkaline reflux gastritis and the effect of biliary diversion on gastric emptying of solid food, Am. J. Surg. **150**:166, 1985.

51. Kelly, K.A.: Pacing the gut: possible clinical applications. In Najarian, J.S., and Delaney, J.P., editors: Advances in gastrointestinal surgery, Chicago, 1984, Year Book Medical Publishers, Inc., p. 345.

Gastric secretion suppression and duodenal diversion: the Roux-en-Y principle in the management of complex reflux problems

DISCUSSION

John Spencer

Dr. Spencer Payne and his colleagues give a detailed and balanced account of the value of combined acid suppression and duodenal diversion in the treatment, and indeed prevention, of reflux esophagitis. This operation was first described by Wells and Johnston in Liverpool in 1955.[1] Disappointed at the high recurrence rate that followed the operations then used to reduce hiatal hernias, they adopted a new approach. They wrote:

> We accept the incompetent cardia but seek to prevent regurgitation by securing rapid emptying of the stomach. We also produce achlorhydria and divert the bile and pancreatic stream so that such regurgitation as may persist does no harm. These desiderata are achieved by vagotomy, partial gastrectomy, and re-anastomosis by the Roux-en-Y method.

They used an abdominal approach, and mention that obtaining a complete vagotomy may be difficult in some patients; a two-thirds gastric resection was used. Excellent results were described in twelve patients.

Subsequent work, to which Dr. Spencer Payne has contributed so much, has confirmed these early results. In early series, resection of the esophageal stricture was often added to the procedure. That this is now known to be unnecessary is in itself strong evidence of the efficacy of duodenal diversion. Modern techniques for esophageal dilatation have helped to avoid resection and reduce mortality.

Originally an extensive gastric resection was utilized, but today the principle is to perform an antrectomy only, with vagotomy. The success of the combined resection and Roux-diversion is undoubted, and my colleagues and I have confirmed this in a series of 57 patients.[2] This series included 22 patients who were randomized to have the procedure as part of a controlled clinical trial and 6 patients with irreducible hernias in whom a more extensive procedure was deemed unwise. In 13 patients previous operations on the hiatus had failed; in this situation in particular Roux-diversion should be considered, in view of the high morbidity and mortality associated with repeated attempts at hiatal herniorrhaphy. The small group of patients who develop reflux problems and stricture after operations for achalasia are also very problematical. We have obtained good results from diversion in such cases. Overall we have obtained excellent or good results in 86% of patients, unsatisfactory results in 5%, and poor results in 9%. Four of the five failures were due to stomal ulceration, emphasizing the need for vagotomy, which was initially done only in patients with relatively high acid secretion. It is of particular interest that even in patients who developed stomal ulcer, stricture and esophagitis resolved completely.

Small series elsewhere in Europe have given support to this approach.[3] Not all authors, however, have had uniform success with this procedure, the problem being the occasional unpredictable failure.[4]

Why does this combined operation succeed? It seems clear that the diversion of duodenal juices is the most important factor. We cannot at present say how important the reduction of acid-peptic secretion is, except to say that this alone gives poor results.

It has occasionally been noted after diversion without vagotomy that esophagitis persisted but that the inflammation resolved after truncal vagotomy.[4] Thus in some patients, at least, acid-peptic factors predominate. At the present time we cannot elucidate in an individual which factors are most important. We need both to reduce acid secretion and to divert duodenal secretions to get good results.

It is of interest that very early on, Tanner improved the results of a Billroth II gastrectomy for reflux by the use of a jejunojejunal (afferent to efferent loop) anastomosis to divert bile.[5] Does rapid gastric emptying really help, as Wells and Johnston suggested? It probably plays a part, since, although reflux of secretions may still be troublesome after the combined procedure, it is surprising how uncommon this is.

Why does the operation fail? Inadequate vagotomy may give rise to stomal ulcer. Today this may be treated by acid suppression without resort to transthoracic vagotomy. Other postgastrectomy sequelae have been surprisingly uncommon in our own experience. Cade and Kilby have produced evidence that dumping is less common after a "Roux" than after partial gastrectomy.[6] Further evidence is needed on this curious observation, which is difficult to explain but consistent with the good clinical results. The small-stomach syndrome may occur, but has not been a problem in our patients.

Although in a randomized controlled trial of patients with severe esophagitis the Roux procedure gave overall results as good as those of a fundoplication,[7] we would agree with the assertion that it is not to be considered as a primary operation in cases in which an antireflux procedure can be performed.

The logical management of the reflux of secretions is to prevent reflux. In clinical practice, however, the symptoms associated with reflux vary considerably. In some patients, the mechanical presence of reflux dominates the picture; these patients notice liquid reflux: they awake choking at night and may suffer respiratory problems in consequence. They have predominantly a "volume reflux" problem. Such patients clearly need control of reflux as the primary aim. A combined

Roux procedure would reduce secretion and help most such patients, but its results would be very unpredictable. It is not the logical treatment.

In many patients, however, particularly among the elderly, the principal symptom is heartburn. Often this has been intermittent and mild for years, and suddenly becomes worse; dysphagia may rapidly supervene. It would appear that in such patients the nature of the refluxed material may have changed, probably by the addition of duodenogastric reflux. In patients with such a history we have found that Roux-diversion gives good results, almost universally. Even in such patients, however, if an antireflux procedure can be performed readily, it should be the first line of treatment. Otherwise, diversion can be performed in such cases with every confidence of a good result.

REFERENCES

1. Wells, C., and Johnson, J.H.: Hiatus hernia: surgical relief of reflux oesophagitis, Lancet **268**:937, 1955.
2. Washer, G.F., Gear, M.W.L., Dowling, B.L., et al.: Duodenal diversion with vagotomy and antrectomy for severe or recurrent reflux and stricture: an alternative to operation at the hiatus, Ann. R. Coll. Surg. Engl. (In press.)
3. deMiguel, J.: Tratamiento de ciertas estrecheces pepticas del esofago mediante vagotomia, gastrectomia parcial y anastomosis gastroyeyunal en "Y" de Roux, Rev. Esp. Enf. Ap. Dig. **67**:511, 1985.
4. Matikainen, M.: Antrectomy, Roux-en-Y reconstruction and vagotomy for recurrent reflux oesophagitis, Acta Chir. Scand. **150**:643, 1984.
5. Tanner, N.C., and Westerholm, P.: Partial gastrectomy in the treatment of esophageal stricture after hiatal hernia, Am. J. Surg. **115**:449, 1968.
6. Cade, R.J., and Kilby, J.O.: The incidence of the dumping syndrome following gastrojejunostomy with Roux-en-Y anastomosis, Postgrad. Med. J. **58**:760, 1982.
7. Washer, G.F., Gear, M.W.L., Dowling, B.N.L., et al.: Randomised prospective trial of Roux-en-Y duodenal diversion versus fundoplication for severe reflux oesophagitis, Br. J. Surg. **71**:181, 1984.

Robin Barker Smith

Gastroesophageal reflux (GER), with its classical symptoms of heartburn and regurgitation, usually directs the eye of the clinician to the investigation of the lower esophageal sphincter, in an attempt to measure the inadequacy of the barrier to reflux provided by the lower esophageal high-pressure zone and its position in relation to the diaphragm. The majority of patients with reflux have simple mechanical explanations for their problems. This chapter is intended to explore the association of reflux with other disorders that might cause or exacerbate this mechanical problem and contribute to GER either directly or indirectly. The treatment of such associated disorders is an essential part of the treatment of the reflux, although such treatment frequently involves the addition of antireflux procedures.

CHOLELITHIASIS AND CHOLECYSTECTOMY

The simultaneous occurrence of gallbladder disease and GER is well known and accounts for the clinical dilemma as to the origin of symptoms in patients with both anomalies. Several authors have documented the occurrence of "esophageal symptoms," namely heartburn and regurgitation.[1,2,3] Some have suggested that these symptoms are often relieved by cholecystectomy.[2,3] The rationale for such an approach has been that an inflamed gallbladder impinges on the first part of the duodenum and the pylorus, causing pyloric dysfunction and bile regurgitation into the stomach and the esophagus.[4] Medical students for generations have been told of Saint's triad, the association of gallstones, hiatal hernia, and diverticular disease. There appear to be few objective data to support such an association. Work in Chicago involving a retrospective survey of patients admitted for evaluation of their reflux showed that patients with gallstones or who had

had a previous cholecystectomy had no more severe symptoms of reflux or endoscopic esophagitis, or no higher 24-hour pH reflux scores, than those with normal gallbladders.[5] Neither cholecystectomy nor gallstones affected the lower esophageal high-pressure zone, and any change in intestinal hormone secretion produced by cholecystectomy had no demonstrable effect on the high-pressure zone. Pressure changes noted by Giles et al.[6] may have been pharmacologic rather than physiologic in origin. Abnormal alkaline reflux was more common in refluxing patients with gallstones than after cholecystectomy or in refluxing controls.[5] It has been suggested by Rains that gallstones may in some way alter the function of the pylorus, allowing duodenogastric reflux of alkaline material and subsequent gastroesophageal reflux.[4] Such regurgitation has been shown radiologically by Johnson in patients with gallbladder disease.[7] The Chicago study produced no evidence to support the concept of increased incidence of either alkaline or acid GER and concluded, on the basis of a prospective study, that in the presence of gallstones a combined operation of cholecystectomy and an antireflux procedure was necessary to relieve the symptoms of reflux in the presence of gallstones. The study emphasized the need for objective evaluation with 24-hour pH studies of the symptoms of reflux in the presence of combined disease.

SCLERODERMA

Scleroderma is a collagen vascular disorder most frequently found in females between 30 and 40 years of age. This condition may occur in isolation or as part of the CREST syndrome. The high mortality, 50% dying within five years,[8] has influenced the management of some of the complications of the disease, particularly those affecting the esophagus. The clinicopathologic features of scleroderma of the esophagus have been well described by Hurwitz et al.[9] Cohen, in a study of scleroderma esophagitis, suggests an ischemic cause for the changes seen in esophageal muscles and nerves.[8] Muscle atrophy probably occurs late in the disease process. The effects of the disease on the esophagus are to reduce motility in the body of the esophagus and to reduce the pressure in the high-pressure zone. Thus two problems occur, namely gastroesophageal reflux and poor clearance of the refluxed material. These combine to produce severe degrees of esophagitis, with subsequent stricture formation.

Netcher and Richardson, using barium studies, state that distal esophageal strictures and hiatal hernias occur in 25% of patients with scleroderma and that a further 18% have reflux.[10] It is likely that with the use of more objective tests of reflux, such as 24-hour pH monitoring, a much higher incidence of reflux would be demonstrated. In my own experience of such tests in 14 patients from the Royal National Hospital for Rheumatic Diseases in Bath, all patients referred with symptoms of reflux or dysphagia exhibited abnormal reflux on 24-hour pH monitoring. Manometric measurements show a complete loss of high-pressure zone pressure in one third or more of patients and a loss of peristalsis in the distal two thirds of the body of the esophagus.[10] Virtually all patients show impaired acid clearance. Esophageal manometry and 24-hour pH testing should be considered essential investigations in such patients.

The initial treatment of patients with scleroderma who reflux has traditionally been medical. This is due partly to the reluctance of the physician or rheumatologist to consider surgical treatment in patients with a limited life expectancy and partly to the efficacy of H_2 receptor blockading drugs. Petrokubi and Jeffries reported improved symptoms and superior healing of esophagitis with cimetidine when compared to conventional antacids.[11] Our experience with ranitidine would confirm that finding, although stricture formation and the length of time between dilatations have not been significantly reduced.

McLaughlin and his colleagues were among the first to describe surgical treatment for esophageal stricture in scleroderma and combined resection of the stricture and reanastomosis of the stomach to the esophagus.[12] Vagotomy and pyloroplasty were part of the procedure, but subsequent problems with alkaline reflux led to the abandonment of the latter. Various authors have described the use of the Thal fundic patch, either alone or with the addition of a 360-degree Nissen wrap.[13-15] Standard antireflux operations such as the Belsey or the Nissen, often modified to include lengthening of the constricted esophagus by a Collis gastroplasty, have been advocated by several groups in the United States.[16-18] Henderson and Pearson[17] advocated the Collis-Belsey procedure for scleroderma, but subsequent work by Orringer and Sloan[19,20] suggested that better results could be obtained using a Collis-Nissen 360-degree wrap. Unfortunately, most series of these procedures do not separate patients with scleroderma from other patients with stricture, but it would seem likely that the current fashion for a "slack" Nissen would allow the poorly clearing esophagus of the scleroderma refluxer to empty, while still preventing reflux. There are no available studies as yet on the use of the Angelchik device in such patients, but my own experience with three such patients with a 6-month follow-up period would indicate a favorable course. Clearly, surgical treatment should be considered at an early stage in these poor-risk patients if severe stricturing is to be avoided.

SYMPTOMS AFTER GASTRIC SURGERY

The evaluation of patients who complain of recurrent pain, nausea, vomiting, or the classical heartburn and regurgitation after either gastric resection or vagotomy and drainage is usually difficult. All forms of gastric surgery for peptic ulceration, with the exception of highly selective vagotomy, render the stomach incontinent and liable to allow retrograde flow of alkaline duodenal or small bowel secretions. The chief difficulty is to decide whether the symptoms are due to such duodenogastric reflux, to gastroesophageal reflux, or to a combination of the two. Endoscopy is of considerable value in this regard, enabling the clinician to exclude recurrent or stomal ulceration as the cause of symptoms. Bile is frequently found in the stomach of normal people, and its presence after gastric surgery may not be of diagnostic significance. The use of isotopes can be of help in establishing such reflux, but confusion in the region of the hiatus because of the overlap of the liver renders the diagnosis of biliary gastroesophageal reflux difficult. Twenty-four pH tests are undoubtedly the best tool to evaluate GER and may be combined with pH studies of the stomach or stomach remnant. O'Sullivan and his colleagues described the use of 24-hour pH monitoring of the esophagus in patients after truncal vagotomy and gastric resection or drainage.[21] They found a mixed pattern of reflux, with the majority of patients having abnormal acid reflux but one third having acid-alkaline reflux, which is particularly damaging to the esophagus. Few patients had pure alkaline reflux. Supine reflux occurred more commonly in these patients, a fact attributed by the authors to the rapid upright emptying of the stomach aided by gravity, previously reported by McKelvey.[22] Supine reflux, occurring mainly at night, when swallowing is less frequent, leads to more severe esophagitis.

The defect in the competence of the cardia that allows gastroesophageal reflux is the same in patients who have reflux after gastric surgery as it is in those who have not had previous surgery. Several authors[23,24] have failed to demonstrate any change in high-pressure zone pressure after vagotomy or gastric resection, and O'Sullivan et al.[21] concluded that GER was present before the gastric surgery, but was undiagnosed. Medical treatment of such reflux is generally of limited success. The difficulty lies mainly in the elimination of the alkaline component of reflux, although bile salt binding agents such as cholestyramine may be of benefit. Conventional medical therapy is aimed at the acid component of reflux and may indeed mask mixed or alkaline reflux by reducing the symptoms of heartburn, generally accepted as being caused by acid reflux.

Surgical therapy must therefore be considered early in such patients. Standard antireflux procedures, such as the Nissen, Hill, or Belsey, will all be of benefit. When mixed or alkaline reflux can be documented, biliary diversion using a long-limb Roux-en-Y procedure should be added. Before the latter, O'Sullivan et al.[21] recommend the presence of a triad of symptoms or signs: (1) epigastric pain and nausea aggravated by meals, (2) gastritis on endoscopic examination, and (3) objective evidence of severe intestinogastric reflux as determined by 24-hour pH monitoring of the stomach and/or by direct bile acid reflux measurement.[25]

OBESITY

When one thinks of the wide range of diseases that are exacerbated or indeed caused by obesity,[26] it is perhaps not unreasonable to accord obesity the title of a disease. In my own practice, weight reduction is one of the most essential first-line treatments for gastroesophageal reflux, a view supported more scientifically by O'Brien[27] and by Chernow.[28]

Beauchamp presented a review of the Montreal experience in 13 obese patients with GER.[29] He concluded that medical treatment should be employed for at least 1 year, with a genuine attempt at weight reduction, but he found that surgery produced no greater rates of failure or complications in that group than in patients of normal or near-normal weight. There is a need for more prospective data to support the general feeling among clinicians that obesity leads to increased GER.

RESPIRATORY DISEASES

Since the advent of objective investigations such as 24-hour pH monitoring and isotope scintigraphy, the relationship of chronic respiratory diseases, both in children and adults, to gastroesophageal reflux has been well established. Spitzer and his colleagues documented a clear association between GER and awake apnea in children, using pH monitoring combined with a cardiopneumogram and nasal thermistor.[30] Their results contrasted with those of two previous studies.[31,32] Spitzer et al. explained their different findings on the basis of more sophisticated nasal thermistor measurements. Martin and his colleagues correlated GER with nocturnal wheezing in children with asthma, and Orenstein and his colleagues showed a similar relationship between GER and stridor in infants.[33,34] The subject has been extensively reviewed by Nelson.[35] Overall, 71% to 100% of children with reflux-related respiratory disorders were improved by medical or surgical control of their reflux.[36-38]

The association between chronic pulmonary fibrosis and reflux in adults has been more difficult to prove, with authors reporting different findings.[39,40]

Bronchial asthma in adults seems more commonly associated with GER. Early studies by Urschel[41] and Overholt[42] showed a reduction in respiratory symptoms after surgical correction of reflux. Few studies have used 24-hour pH monitoring in adults—with the exception of Perpina and his colleagues, who found no association with reflux.[43] Mays showed an incidence of GER on barium meal of 46% in patients with severe asthma.[39] Kjellen showed greatly reduced symptoms of asthma and reduced need for asthma medication when patients with esophageal symptoms defined by motility studies and clinical evaluation had their reflux treated medically.[44]

The mechanism by which asthma attacks are triggered by reflux may not be as straightforward as was thought. Aspiration of gastric contents was assumed by many[39,42,45] to be the cause of the attack. Mansfield and Stein demonstrated deterioration in pulmonary function when Bernstein acid-perfusion tests were carried out.[46] Further evidence from the same authors[47] and from Kjellen[48] supported the concept of bronchoconstriction in response to acid perfusion of the esophagus. Orringer suggested that a number of respiratory symptoms experienced secondary to reflux may be due to a reflux spasm in the esophagus giving rise to a feeling of a lump in the throat, cough, and hoarseness.[49] There is a clear need for more careful evaluation of respiratory disease and its association with reflux, particularly in adults, using the more sophisticated methods currently available.

CORONARY ARTERY DISEASE

The dearth of literature documenting an association between angina and gastroesophageal reflux is surprising given that esophageal pain caused by reflux may be atypical in many patients.[50,51] Mellow and his colleagues investigated this association in 27 patients who had been fully investigated for angina.[52] Their symptoms of GER were graded using the questionnaire of DeMeester, Johnson, et al.[53] The patients underwent a modified Bernstein acid-perfusion test. The authors concluded that acid-induced esophageal pain may serve as a source of confusion with angina, resulting in incorrect classification of angina. GER may well even induce true angina. They concluded that GER in such patients should be treated aggressively with H_2 receptor antagonists.

CONCLUSION

It can be seen from the foregoing that gastroesophageal reflux is often associated with other disorders and that the diagnosis of GER should be considered perhaps more frequently than before. With the advent of sophisticated objective tests for the evaluation of reflux and widely available endoscopic expertise, the precise relationship of GER to other diseases can now be fully appreciated.

REFERENCES

1. Price, W.H.: Gallbladder dyspepsia, Br. Med. J. **2**:138-141, 1963.

2. Rhind, J.A., and Watson, L.: Gallstone dyspepsia, Br. Med. J. **1**:32, 1968.

3. Barker, J.R., and Alexander-Williams, J.: The effect of cholecystectomy on esophageal symptoms, Br. J. Surg. **61**:346-348, 1974.

4. Rains, A.J.H.: Gallstones, causes and treatment, London, 1964, Heinemann, p. 101.

5. Smith, R.B., DeMeester, T.R., O'Sullivan, G.C., Johnson, L.R., and Skinner, D.B.: Studies on the relationship of cholelithiasis and cholecystectomy to gastroesophageal reflux in man. (In preparation.)

6. Giles, G.R., Mason, M.C., Humphrey, C.S., and Clark, C.G.: Action of gastrin on the lower esophageal sphincter in Man, Gut **10**:730-734, 1969.

7. Johnson, A.G.: Pyloric function and gallstone dyspepsia, Br. J. Surg. **59**:449-454, 1972.

8. Cohen, S.: The gastro-intestinal manifestations of scleroderma: pathogenesis and management (clinical conference), Gastroenterology **79**:155-166, 1980.

9. Hurwitz, A.L., Duranceau, A., and Haddad, J.K.: Disorders of esophageal motility, Philadelphia, 1979, W.B. Saunders Co.

10. Netscher, D.T., and Richardson, J.D.: Complications requiring operative intervention in scleroderma, Surg. Gynecol. Obstet. **158**:507-512, 1984.

11. Petrokubi, R.J., and Jeffries, G.H.: Cimetidine versus antacid in scleroderma with reflux esophagitis, Gastroenterology **77**:691-695, 1979.

12. McLaughlin, J.S., Roig, R., and Woodruff, M.F.: Surgical treatment of strictures of the esophagus in patients with scleroderma, J. Thorac. Cardiovasc. Surg. **61**:641-646, 1971.

13. Murray, G.F.: Operation for motor dysfunction of the esophagus, Ann. Thorac. Surg. **29**:184-191, 1980.

14. Maher, J.W., Hocking, M.P., and Woodward, E.R.: Long term follow up of the combined fundic patch fundoplication for the treatment of longitudinal peptic strictures of the esophagus, Ann. Surg. **194**:64-69, 1981.

15. O'Leary, J.P., Hollenbeck, J.I., and Woodward, E.R.: Surgical treatment of esophageal stricture in patients with scleroderma, Ann. Surg. **41**:131-135, 1975.

16. Pearson, F.G., Langer, B., and Henderson, R.D.: Gastroplasty and Belsey hiatus hernia repair, J. Thorac. Cardiovasc. Surg. **61**:50-63, 1971.

17. Henderson, R.D., and Pearson, F.G.: Surgical management of esophageal scleroderma, J. Thorac. Cardiovasc. Surg. **66**:686-692, 1973.

18. Orringer, M.B., Dabich, L., Zarafonetis, C.J.D., and Sloan, H.: Reflux in esophageal scleroderma, Ann. Thorac. Surg. **22**:120-129, 1976.

19. Orringer, M.B., and Sloan, H.: Complications and failings of the combined Collis-Belsey operation, J. Thorac. Cardiovasc. Surg. **74**:726-735, 1977.

20. Orringer, M.B., and Sloan, H.: Combined Collis-Nissen reconstruction of the esophagogastric junction, Ann. Thorac. Surg. **25**:16-21, 1978.

21. O'Sullivan, G.C., DeMeester, T.R., Smith, R.B., Ryan, J.W., Johnson, L.F., and Skinner, D.B.: Twenty-four-hour pH monitoring of esophageal function: its use in evaluation in symptomatic patients after truncal vagotomy and gastric resection or drainage, Arch. Surg. **116**:581-590, 1981.

22. McKelvey, S.T.: Gastric incontinence and post-vagotomy diarrhoea, Br. J. Surg. **57**:741-747, 1970.

23. Mann, C.V., and Hardcastle, J.D.: The effect of

vagotomy on the human gastroesophageal sphincter, Gut **9:**688-695, 1968.

24. Mazur, J.M., Skinner, D.B., Jones, E., et al.: Effect of transabdominal vagotomy on the human gastroesophageal high pressure zone, Surgery **73:**818-822, 1973.

25. Ritchie, W.P.: Alkaline reflux gastritis: an objective assessment of its diagnosis and treatment, Ann. Surg. **192:**288-298, 1980.

26. Mann, G.V.: The influence of obesity on health, N. Engl. J. Med. **291:**178-184, 1974.

27. O'Brien, T.F.: Lower esophageal sphincter pressure (LESP) and esophageal function in obese humans, J. Clin. Gastroenterol. **2:**145-148, 1980.

28. Chernow, B., and Castell, D.O.: Diet and heartburn, JAMA **241:**2307-2308, 1979.

29. Beauchamp, G.: Gastroesophageal reflux and obesity, Surg. Clin. North Am. **63**(4)**:**869-876, 1983.

30. Spitzer, A.R., Boyle, J.T., Tuchman, D.N., and Fox, W.W.: Awake apnea associated with gastroesophageal reflux: a specific clinical syndrome, J. Pediatr. **104**(2)**:**200-205, 1984.

31. Walsh, J.K., Farrell, M.K., Keenan, W.J., et al.: Gastroesophageal reflux in infants: relation to apnea, J. Pediatr. **99:**197-201, 1981.

32. Ariagno, R.L., Guillenminault, C., Baldwin, R., et al.: Movement and gastroesophageal reflux in awake term infants with "near miss" SIDS, unrelated to apnea, J. Pediatr. **100:**894-897, 1982.

33. Martin, M.E., Grunstein, M.M., and Larsen, G.L.: The relationship of gastroesophageal reflux to nocturnal wheezing in children with asthma, Ann. Allergy **49:**318-322, 1982.

34. Ovenstein, S.R., Ovenstein, D.M., and Whitington, P.F.: Gastroesophageal reflux causing stridor, Chest **84**(3)**:**301-302, 1983.

35. Nelson, H.S.: Gastroesophageal reflux and pulmonary disease, J. Allergy Clin. Immunol. **73**(5)**:**547-555, 1984.

36. Jolley, S.G., Herbst, J.J., Johnson, D.G., Matlak, M.E., and Book, L.S.: Esophageal monitoring during sleep identifies children with respiratory symptoms from gastroesophageal reflux, Gastroenterology **80:**1501-1506, 1981.

37. Berquist, W.E., Rachelefsky, G.S., Kadden, M., Siegel, S.C., Katz, R.M., Fonkalstud, E.W., and Ament, M.E.: Gastroesophageal reflux-associated recurrent pneumonia and chronic asthma in children, Pediatrics **68:**29-35, 1981.

38. Christie, D.L., O'Grady, L.R., and Mack, D.V.: Incompetent lower esophageal sphincter and gastroesophageal

reflux in recurrent acute pulmonary disease of infancy and childhood, J. Pediatr. **93:**23-27, 1978.

39. Mays, E.E.: Intrinsic asthma in adults, JAMA **236:**2626-2628, 1976.

40. Vraney, G.A., and Pokorny, C.: Pulmonary function in patients with gastroesophageal reflux, Chest **76:**678-680, 1979.

41. Urschel, H.C., Jr., and Paulson, D.L.: Gastroesophageal reflux and hiatal hernia, J. Thorac. Cardiovasc. Surg. **53:**21-32, 1967.

42. Overholt, R.H., and Voorhees, R.J.: Esophageal reflux as a trigger in asthma, Dis. Chest **49:**464-466, 1966.

43. Perpina, M., Ponce, J., Marco, V., Benlloch, E., Miralbes, M., and Berenguer, J.: The prevalence of asymptomatic gastroesophageal reflux in bronchial asthma and in non-asthmatic individuals, Eur. J. Respir. Dis. **64:**582-587, 1983.

44. Kjellen, G., Tibbling, L., Wranne, B.: Effect of conservative treatment of esophageal dysfunction on bronchial asthma, Eur. J. Respir. Dis. **62:**190-197, 1981.

45. Babb, R.R., Notarangelo, J., and Smith, V.M.: Wheezing: a clue to gastroesophageal reflux, Am. J. Gastroenterol. **53:**230-233, 1970.

46. Mansfield, L.E., and Stein, M.R.: Gastroesophageal reflux and asthma: a possible reflux mechanism, Ann. Allergy **41:**224-226, 1978.

47. Spaulding, H.S., Jr., Mansfield, L.E., Stein, M.R., Sellner, J.C., and Aremillion, D.E.: Further investigation of the association between gastroesophageal reflux and bronchoconstriction, J. Allergy Clin. Immunol. **69:**516-521, 1982.

48. Kjellen, G., Tibbling, L., and Wranne, B.: Bronchial obstruction after esophageal acid perfusion in asthmatics, Clin. Physiol. **1:**285-292, 1981.

49. Orringer, M.B.: Respiratory symptoms and esophageal reflux, Chest **76:**618-619, 1979.

50. Roberts, R., Henderson, R.D., and Wigle, D.: Esophageal disease as a cause of severe retrosternal chest pain, Chest **67:**523-526, 1975.

51. Henderson, R.D., Wigle, E.D., Sample, K., and Maryatt, G.: Atypical chest pain of cardiac and esophageal origin, Chest **73:**24-27, 1978.

52. Mellow, M.H., Simpson, A.G., Watt, L., Schoolmeester, L., and Haye, O.L.: Esophageal acid perfusion in coronary artery disease, Gastroenterology **85:**306-312, 1983.

53. DeMeester, T.R., Johnson, L.F., and Kent, A.H.: Evaluation of current operations for the prevention of gastroesophageal reflux, Ann. Surg. **180:**511-525, 1974.

Reflux associated with other disorders or lesions

DISCUSSION

Hiram C. Polk, Jr., and Gerald M. Larson

The material by Dr. Smith regarding associated illnesses is an important component of modern understanding of reflux esophagitis and its surgical treatment. The author thoroughly describes six conditions that can either contribute to gastroesophageal reflux or cause reflux-like symptoms. Correctly, he gives primary attention to the issue of associated biliary tract disease and provides a scholarly and articulate examination of physiologic effects of such associated disease. As a matter of fact, this is even more important in terms of clinical practicality when both biliary lithiasis and sliding hiatal hernia coexist. Although there is a defined set of symptoms associated with biliary tract disease and another set that describes reflux esophagitis, as pointed out by the author, the symptomatology frequently overlaps.

We have always preferred to let the endoscopic evaluation and the 24-hour pH study of the patient guide our treatment of gastroesophageal reflux. If there is no esophagitis present, then we can confidently attack the biliary tract as the primary disease. If esophagitis is present, then we uniformly recommend a combined approach with conduct of an antireflux operation and simultaneous cholecystectomy through an abdominal incision. In our opinion, there is virtually no justification for neglecting documented biliary tract disease with its known likelihood, however modest, of progression to more serious disease. It is, however, crucial that the clinician realizes that there is a real overlap of symptoms in these illnesses, and he or she needs to carefully consider the options before deciding which, if either, of the illnesses warrants primary surgical attention.

The issue of scleroderma has been similarly addressed in a constructive fashion, and it is difficult to disagree with any of the comments or recommendations of the author, with the exception of his tentative endorsement of the Angelchik device. Current publications suggest that recognition of the unacceptability of this device is growing and that we certainly should not apply it in scleroderma involvement of the esophagus.[1,3] We do, however, concur with his thoughts that one should earlier, rather than later, address the potential reflux-related complications such as ulcerative esophagitis, esophageal stricture, aspiration pneumonia, and odynophagia in the scleroderma patient.[4,5] Although the long-term survival is limited, patients with this systemic illness are particularly vulnerable to these serious complications.[6] Properly applied, antireflux operations have given good results in more than 80% of patients.[7]

The impact of gastric surgery upon reflux esophagitis is complex and has been the source of a number of studies. It is easy to hypothesize why the anatomic dissection related to vagotomy might actually promote gastroesophageal reflux. On the other hand, this is an infrequent clinical event, and manometric and reflux studies demonstrate that lower esophageal sphincter function is not altered by vagotomy.[8] We cannot accept the concept of Roux-en-Y conversion when there remains so much honest skepticism about both the prevalence and the significance of bile reflux gastritis and when there is so little evidence that this is a significant threat to the patient with occult reflux.[9] Certainly, the patient with possible alkaline bile gastritis or esophagitis deserves thorough evaluation with 24-hour pH studies, analysis of gastric juice for bile, measurement of gastric emptying, motility studies, and endoscopy before this poorly understood diagnosis can be considered.

The issue of obesity, particularly increasing obesity, is a very challenging one to the surgeon who deals with reflux esophagitis and will, in most people's opinion, provide for a slightly higher failure rate over time, in part because of increased intraabdominal pressure, but also in part, no doubt, because of some anatomic difficulties involved in the operation itself.

The association with pulmonary illness is a crucial one and one that is widely misunderstood. We think most gastroenterologists, and certainly all surgeons, interested in reflux disease appreciate the variant of gastroesophageal reflux that produces aspiration and thereby acute respiratory distress and/or chronic pulmonary infection.[10] The real issue is the failure of pulmonary medical specialists to be alert to this identifiable complication of an underlying disease; it is currently all too seldom considered. It is perhaps wise and proper that surgeons interested in reflux disease continue to carry this message to the pulmonary physicians just as we have done for the gastroenterologists over the last decade.

Coronary artery disease is in and of itself an important issue in gastroesophageal reflux. As with the case of biliary tract disease, there are precise examples of one symptom complex resembling another.[11,12] In some patients with chest pain, there is a distinct overlapping of symptoms, and the possibility for a serious error and patient harm is considerable. If, after a careful history, the issue remains in doubt, the surgical consultant should carefully consider preoperative coronary stress testing and angiography, depending upon the individual circumstances. We have on two occasions carried out an antireflux procedure successfully in patients whom we believed had primary reflux esophagitis and later proved to have angina pectoris as well. We have now also operated upon seven patients who had been treated for angina by balloon angioplasty or coronary artery bypass when, in retrospect, what they surely had was reflux esophagitis.

The consultant surgeon involved in the care of these complex patients needs to consider all these issues and his or her educational and diagnostic interrelationships with other physicians. For the patient with esophageal symptoms and associated diseases, a complete evaluation by pH testing, endoscopy, motility, manometry, and gastric emptying is indicated in most cases, as discussed by Mr. Smith.

REFERENCES

1. Benjamin, S.B., Kerr, R., Cohen, D., Motaparthy, V., and Castell, D.O.: Complications of the Angelchik antireflux prosthesis, Ann. Intern. Med. **100:**570-575, 1984.

2. Mansour, K.A., and McKeown, P.P.: Disastrous complication of the Angelchik prosthesis, Am. Surg. **49:**616-618, 1983.

3. Smith, R.S., Chang, F.C., Hayes, K.A., and deBakker, J.: Complications of the Angelchik antireflux prosthesis, Am. J. Surg. **150:**735-738, 1985.

4. Wale, R.J., Royston, C.M.S., Bennett, J.R., and Buckton, G.K.: Prospective study of the Angelchik antireflux prosthesis, Br. J. Surg. **72:**520-524, 1985.

5. Durrans, D., Armstrong, C.P., and Taylor, T.V.: The Angelchik antireflux prosthesis—some reservations, Br. J. Surg. **72:**525-527, 1985.

6. Netcher, D.T., and Richardson, J.D.: Complications requiring operative intervention in scleroderma, Surg. Gynecol. Obstet. **158:**507-512, 1984.

7. Orringer, M.B., Orringer, J.S., Dabich, L., and Zarafonetis, C.J.D.: Combined Collis gastroplasty-fundoplication operations for scleroderma reflux esophagitis, Surgery **90:**624-630, 1981.

8. Csendes, A., Oster, M., Moller, J.T., Flynn, J., Funch-Jensen, P., Overgaard, H., and Amdrup, E.: Gastroesophageal reflux is duodenal ulcer patients before and after vagotomy, Ann. Surg. **188:**804-808, 1978.

9. Vogel, S.B., Vair, B., and Woodward, E.R.: Alterations in gastrointestinal emptying of 99m-technetium labeled solids following sequential antrectomy, truncal vagotomy and Roux-Y gastroenterostomy, Ann. Surg. **198:**506-515, 1983.

10. Bancewicz, J., Bernstein, A., Cooper, D.N., and Pierry, A.: Medical and surgical treatment of gastroesophageal reflux in patients with asthma, World J. Surg. **6:**646, 1982.

11. Benjamin, S.B., and Castell, D.O.: Chest pain of esophageal origin: where do we go from here? Arch. Intern. Med. **143:**772-776, 1983.

12. DeMeester, T.R., O'Sullivan, G.C., Bermudez, G., Midell, A.I., Cimochowski, G.E., and O'Drobinak, J.O.: Esophageal function in patients with angina-type chest pain and normal coronary angiograms, Ann. Surg. **196:**488-498, 1982.

CHAPTER 14

Management of failed
antireflux procedures

Mark B. Orringer

BACKGROUND AND CURRENT CLINICAL EXPERIENCE

The earliest descriptions of the surgical treatment of hiatal hernia emphasized anatomic correction of the hernia rather than the need to control gastroesophageal reflux. Harrington's classic monograph from the Mayo Clinic on diaphragmatic hernia "lumped" together both traumatic hernias through the leaf of the diaphragm and those through the diaphragmatic hiatus. Restoration of the stomach into the abdominal cavity and closure of the hiatus were felt to be the important elements of repair.[1] Similarly, although clearly establishing the concepts of gastroesophageal reflux and reflux esophagitis and their role in causing symptoms in patients with hiatal hernia, Allison also stressed the need for anatomic, rather than physiologic, reconstruction of the cardia.[2] Other surgeons soon followed suit.[3,4] The result was a variety of "hiatal hernia" operations intended to control reflux by anatomic correction of the defect at the cardia. These procedures, based upon an erroneous assumption, did not recognize the importance of a valve mechanism at the cardia in preventing gastroesophageal reflux. Thus, at its inception, surgery designed to control reflux was not based upon valid theory, and the foundation for recurrent reflux and failed antireflux operations was established as the first anatomic hiatal hernia repair for gastroesophageal reflux was performed.

The development of fundoplication procedures by Nissen[5,6] and Belsey[7,8] introduced the concept of physiologic operations to control reflux. The Hill transabdominal posterior gastropexy is currently the third of the most commonly performed physiologic operations for reflux control.[9,10] Although it is now recognized that anatomic correction of the hernia is not absolutely essential for reflux control, and that in fact restoration of lower esophageal sphincter competence can be achieved even in the presence of a hiatal hernia, establishing an intraabdominal segment of distal esophagus wrapped in some fashion by the stomach is the common denominator in most effective antireflux operations.

A successful antireflux operation eliminates symptoms caused by gastroesophageal reflux (heartburn and regurgitation) and results in resolution of reflux esophagitis, if present, without producing undue adverse effects (dysphagia and "gas bloats" secondary to inability to eructate). Most often a "failed" antireflux operation is manifested by persistence or recurrence of reflux symptoms, but intractable dysphagia resulting from too tight a fundoplication, distortion of the gastroesophageal junction, or excessive narrowing of the diaphragmatic hiatus is equally indicative of an unsuccessful repair. For many years, lack of *objective* evaluation of the efficacy of an operation in controlling gastroesophageal reflux has prevented any meaningful statement as to the *actual* failure rate of any specific antireflux repair. Long-term results have not consistently been reported, and the success of an operation has been measured in terms of "patient satisfaction," the postoperative barium swallow examination, or occasionally endoscopic follow-up. However, the absence of endoscopic reflux and/or esophagitis postoperatively may not establish that reflux has been controlled. Furthermore, the notoriously poor correlation between the barium esophagogram and the presence of gastroesophageal reflux is well known. Allison, for example, reporting a 20-year experience with his operation, indicated that 82% of his patients were completely relieved of reflux symptoms and 5% were improved.[11] Yet 49% had radiographic findings of either a recurrent hernia or gastroesophageal reflux. Urschel and Paulson reported a 10% incidence of recurrent hernia and a 25% incidence of reflux on barium studies following 182 Allison repairs, in contrast to a 2% incidence of anatomic recurrence and a 7% incidence of reflux after 208 Belsey operations.[12]

A number of reports have presented preoperative and postoperative manometric records of distal esophageal sphincter pressures.[13-20] Unfortunately, all investigators have found a wide variety of pressures in the distal high-pressure zone (HPZ) both before and after operation, and some patients with symptomatic reflux control do not show elevations of their distal HPZ pressures after operation. Therefore, although it is generally recognized that distal HPZ pressure should increase after an antireflux operation, its failure to do so may not necessarily indicate a failed operation. In other words, no specific distal HPZ pressure per se is absolutely indicative of sphincter competence or incompetence.

It is difficult, then, to define the magnitude of the problem of the "failed antireflux operation" because neither the numerator nor the denominator of the equation is the same in various reported series. Results vary not only with the experience of the surgeon performing a particular operation, but also according to the degree of esophagitis present at the time of operation. Hoffman and Sumner, reporting 1- to 10-year follow-up of 232 Allison repairs, indicated that 76% of their patients were completely relieved of reflux symptoms and 18% were partially relieved; in their 204 patients without strictures preoperatively, the failure rate was only 2.5%.[21] Hill has modified his originally described operative technique, and since 1973 has introduced the routine use of intraoperative manometry for his procedure.[22] With his current approach, he reports an excellent clinical result (no reflux symptoms) in 62% of his patients, a good result (minimal symptoms that do not require medication) in 27%, and a fair result (improved symptoms or symptoms derived from surgery that require medication) in 11%.[23] Postoperative pH reflux testing in these patients has shown good reflux control in 98%. In 79 patients with strictures who were operated on since 1969, with a mean follow-up period of 59 months, excellent or good results have been obtained in 67% and poor results in 12%.

A review of the long-term results of the Belsey Mark IV operation by Orringer, Skinner, and Belsey constituted one of the most comprehensive and complete analyses of the efficacy of any antireflux operation available at that time.[24] In this study, 892 patients were followed for 3 to 15 years after operation with regular interviews, barium swallow, and esophagoscopy when indicated, and complete follow-up was available in 761, or 85% of the patients. Clinical status was graded as follows: A, completely asymptomatic; B, no reflux symptoms, but mild nonspecific complaints; C, symptoms suggesting reflux, but no objective evidence of recurrence on barium swallow or esophagoscopy; and D, documented recurrent hiatal hernia or reflux. The recurrence rate for patients followed more than 3 years was 12%; for those followed more than 5 years, 12%; for those followed more than 7 years, 12%; and for those followed from 10 to 15 years, 15%. The overall recurrence rate for all 883 operative survivors was 11%. Had the intraesophageal pH electrode been available to evaluate these patients, however, the conclusions regarding the efficacy of this procedure might well have been altered. For if the patients whose status was "C" (symptomatic with complaints suggesting reflux, but without objective evidence of recurrence on barium swallow or esophagoscopy) had been proven to have abnormal reflux with the intraesophageal pH electrode, the reported recurrence rates would have been altered to 19% for those followed more than 3 years, 5 years, and 7 years, and 24% for those followed more than 10 years.

Rossetti and Hell reported the results of 1,400 Nissen fundoplications performed over 20 years at the University of Basel, where the procedure was devised.[25] This is the largest series of Nissen fundoplications that has been described. Among 590 patients with long-term follow-up, 516 (87%) were symptom free, and 62 (10.5%) had "postfundoplication syndrome." A reoperation had been required in only five patients. McAlhaney and associates, comparing the results of 127 Allison repairs with 103 fundoplications, reported recurrent symptoms and radiographic hernias in 18% and 39%, respectively, of the former and in 7.5% and 6%, respectively, of the latter.[26] An update of this fundoplication series in 1977[27] reported recurrent symptoms in 9% of 139 patients, and gas-bloat syndrome in 13%. In the United States, Polk's series of Nissen fundoplications is the largest, and with an average follow-up period of 3.8 years among 400 patients, the failure rate was 4.5%.[28] Others have reported equally good results with the Nissen fundoplication.[17,29-33] Postlethwait's report of 202 patients undergoing various hiatal hernia repairs, about half of whom had been followed for more than 10 years, indicates a clear superiority of the Nissen repair in controlling reflux symptoms.[34] Among his patients treated with a Nissen, Belsey, Hill, or Allison repair, heartburn was totally eliminated in 100%, 77%, 80%, and 75%, respectively, and regurgitation in 100%, 63%, 69%, and 69%, respectively. Conversely, recurrent regurgitation or heartburn occurred with about equal frequency (in approximately 10% to 20%) in patients undergoing an Allison, Hill, or Belsey repair. Dysphagia was marked or severe in 25% of the Nissen patients, 10% of the Belsey patients, 6% of the Hill patients, and 8% of the Allison repair patients.

Although the degree to which a patient is relieved of preoperative symptoms of heartburn and regurgitation is important, *subjective* improvement after operation may not necessarily correlate with actual reflux control. Insistence upon objective long-term documentation of the results of an antireflux operation, by means of esophageal manometry and intraesophageal pH monitoring both preoperatively and postoperatively, must become the mark of the modern esophageal surgeon if the relative merit of one operation over another is to be determined with accuracy.[35,36] Current long-term reports, many based primarily upon subjective questioning of the patients, indicate that reflux is controlled in approximately 85% to 90% of patients undergoing the standard antireflux operations (Hill, Belsey, Nissen) and that approximately 10% to 25% of patients undergoing these procedures develop new adverse symptoms, not necessarily related to reflux.[24,32,37-39] The management of the patient with a failed antireflux operation is the subject of the remainder of this chapter.

PREVENTION

As is often the case, prevention is one of the most important facets of therapy, and in certain patients with reflux, persistence or recurrence of the problem after one of the standard operations (Belsey, Nissen, or Hill repair) is *predictable* and at least potentially avoidable. When an antireflux operation succeeds in establishing a distal esophageal high-pressure zone of sufficient amplitude and length to control gastroesophageal reflux, the result from the patient's standpoint should be immediate. Within several days of operation, despite postoperative incisional discomfort and use of analgesics, the patient typically reports that heartburn and effortless regurgitation have been eliminated and that he can assume the supine position without reflux. Review of the clinical courses of patients with failed antireflux operations indicates that there is a population of patients who have reflux symptoms before being discharged from the hospital, presumably because adequate reflux control was not achieved from the outset. The surgeon may have failed to reduce an appropriate segment of distal esophagus into the abdominal cavity. This is especially a

problem with transabdominal hiatal hernia repairs in obese patients, particularly if there is associated esophageal shortening. In the process of mobilizing the herniated stomach through the hiatus and drawing it down into the abdomen, the upper stomach and fundus may be elongated by the surgeon and thus give the false impression of being the distal esophagus. A fundoplication is then performed around the proximal stomach rather than the distal esophagus, resulting in the postoperative radiographic appearance of the "slipped Nissen" (Fig. 14-1). In such a case, the wrap has *not* slipped; it was never performed around the distal esophagus in the first place. Thus, in markedly obese patients, the gastroesophageal junction is more readily identified through a *transthoracic* approach, which therefore minimizes the chance of recurrence resulting from inability to clearly see the distal esophagus through the abdomen.

Another cause of early postoperative recurrence of a hiatal hernia is disruption of the posterior crural repair, which approximates the medial and lateral crura of the diaphragmatic hiatus behind the reconstructed cardia. Such disruption may occur if inadequate bites of crural tissue are taken during the operation, or if the patient is permitted to "buck" violently and involuntarily against the endotracheal tube at the conclusion of the operation (see Fig. 14-2). The force generated by a voluntary cough in a patient who has a recent abdominal or thoracic incision and is "splinting" the operative site is clearly not so great as that of an involuntary cough of a semiconscious patient whose tracheobronchial tree is being irritated by an endotracheal tube. Thus, patients should either have their endotracheal tubes removed promptly after a hiatal hernia repair or should be sedated adequately so that they tolerate the tube without "bucking."

Vagal nerve injury may occur during an antireflux operation, particularly one that is being performed for recurrent reflux. Periesophageal or hiatal adhesions may prevent accurate identification of the vagi, which can be injured inadvertently. Resultant pylorospasm or gastric-outlet obstruction in the patient with a newly constructed competent lower esophageal sphincter mechanism is a disastrous complication. The over-distended stomach, which cannot empty and is only further stretched by swallowed air, stresses the sutures placed in performance of an antireflux operation and may disrupt the repair, resulting in recurrent reflux (see Fig. 14-3). If vagal nerve injury is recognized during a hiatal hernia repair, it is usually safer to perform a gastric drainage procedure (pyloromyotomy or pyloroplasty) than

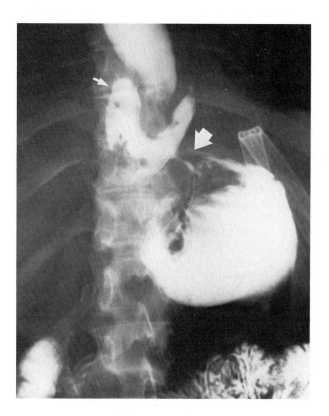

Fig. 14-1. Failure to reduce the gastroesophageal junction below the diaphragm during transabdominal fundoplication. This obese patient was referred 1 week after attempted transabdominal fundoplication with "obstruction of the stomach." Her esophageal shortening had prevented adequate reduction of her hiatal hernia into the abdomen, and unintentionally, the gastric wrap (*large arrow*) had been performed around the high stomach rather than the distal esophagus, leaving the herniated stomach (*small arrow*) above the diaphragm.

Fig. 14-2. An esophagogram taken 1 week after a combined Collis gastroplasty–Nissen fundoplication. A portion of the fundoplication (*arrow*) has slipped into the chest through the diaphragmatic hiatus because of disruption of the posterior crural sutures. Although this patient was asymptomatic, reoperation and reduction of the herniated fundus below the diaphragm were carried out to prevent the potential complications of this "paraesophageal" hernia, which occurred when the patient was permitted to "buck" forcefully against his endotracheal tube prior to extubation in the operating room. Retrospectively, he had evidence of the recurrent hernia on a chest roentgenogram taken the night of operation. Although asymptomatic, this patient was reoperated upon, his intrathoracic stomach was reduced back into the abdomen, and his crural sutures were replaced. (Reproduced with permission of the J.B. Lippincott Company from *Complications in Surgery and Trauma*, edited by Lazar J. Greenfield, M.D., Philadelphia, 1984. Figure 23-15. Page 275.)

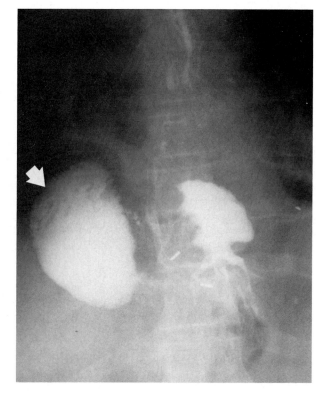

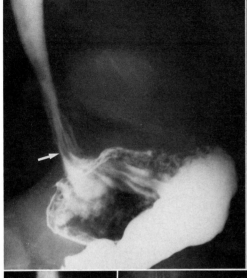

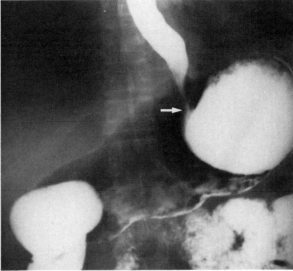

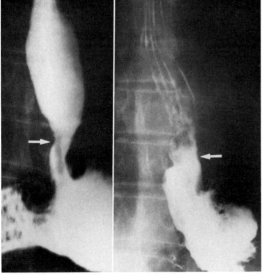

Fig. 14-3. Disruption of hiatal hernia repair secondary to postoperative gastric dilatation. (Arrows indicate the gastroesophageal junction.) **A,** A preoperative esophagogram shows a small, recurrent sliding hiatal hernia 2 years after a Belsey Mark IV repair. **B,** A postoperative esophagogram taken 1 week after a Belsey Mark IV repair shows not only good reduction of the gastroesophageal junction below the diaphragm, but also gastric dilatation resulting from poor emptying. Periesophageal fibrosis had prevented identification of the vagus nerves at reoperation. **C,** A recurrent hiatal hernia 1 year after this patient's second hiatal hernia operation, with the gastroesophageal junction again above the diaphragm. Vagal nerve injury at the time of repair of the recurrent hiatal hernia produced delayed gastric emptying, which should have been treated with pyloromyotomy or pyloroplasty. (Reproduced with permission of the J.B. Lippincott Company from *Complications in Surgery and Trauma*, edited by Lazar J. Greenfield, M.D., Philadelphia, 1984. Page 274.)

to risk the possibility of subsequent gastric-outlet obstruction and recurrent gastroesophageal reflux. Similarly, if a patient demonstrates gastric-outlet obstruction during the first week after operation, prompt reoperation and a gastric drainage procedure may not only minimize the length of hospitalization, but also the chance of disruption of the repair.

IDENTIFYING THE PATIENT PRONE TO RECURRENT REFLUX: "RECURRENCE RISK FACTORS"

Most patients with failed antireflux operations present with recurrent reflux symptoms within months to a few years of the repair, after an initial symptom-free interval. The exact reason why long-term reflux control is not achieved in these patients is unknown, but postoperative esophagograms and results of esophageal manometry and pH reflux testing usually indicate a distinct change in the configuration of the gastroesophageal junction as compared with that of the immediate postoperative period. It is recognized that most successful antireflux operations result in a 2- to 4-cm-long distal esophageal high-pressure zone with an amplitude of 10 to 20 mm Hg. This is achieved by reducing a 3- to 5-cm segment of distal esophagus beneath the diaphragmatic hiatus, where it is under the influence of positive intraabdominal pressure, further augmented by some type of fundoplication. When reflux recurs, the length of intraabdominal distal esophagus is typically found to be shorter than it was immediately after operation, and HPZ amplitude is similarly less. The barium esophagogram no longer shows the "correct" postoperative appearance of the reconstructed gastroesophageal junction,[40,41] and there is either anatomic recurrence of the hiatal hernia or shortening of the intraabdominal distal esophageal segment. The repair has not "held."

The long-term results of the Belsey Mark IV operation reported in 1972 indicated that the incidence of recurrence among patients with strictures or severe esophagitis undergoing the Belsey repair was 45%, compared with an 11% incidence in those without esophagitis or stricture.[24] This seemed a clear demonstration of the fact that esophageal shortening and inflammation from reflux esophagitis jeopardize the success of this repair. Based on these data, Belsey in fact recommended distal esophagectomy and reconstruction with colon rather than a standard repair in the presence of significant esophagitis and shortening. Similarly, Donnelly and associates reported a 75% incidence of recurrent reflux when the Belsey repair was performed in a

patient with a reflux stricture.[42] Mural inflammation, esophagitis, and esophageal shortening, which are characteristic of peptic esophageal strictures, prevent the *tension-free* reduction of 3 to 5 cm of distal esophagus below the diaphragm and require that fundoplication sutures be placed between stomach and inflamed distal esophagus. It is not surprising, therefore, that standard antireflux operations in these patients do not "hold," and recurrence in the presence of stricture is more common. And since the Belsey and Nissen fundoplications, as well as the Hill posterior gastropexy, all require an intraabdominal location of the gastroesophageal junction and sutures in the distal esophageal or periesophageal tissues, the long-term success of any of these standard antireflux procedures *must* be jeopardized if mural inflammation and esophageal shortening are present (see Fig. 14-4).

Nevertheless, treatment of reflux strictures with a combination of dilatation and a standard antireflux procedure, either a Hill posterior gastropexy[43-44,45] or a Nissen fundoplication,[27,46] is commonly performed. Even if the esophagus is not shortened, when there is mucosal or submucosal stricture from reflux and the inevitably accompanying mural inflammation, it would

A **B** **C**

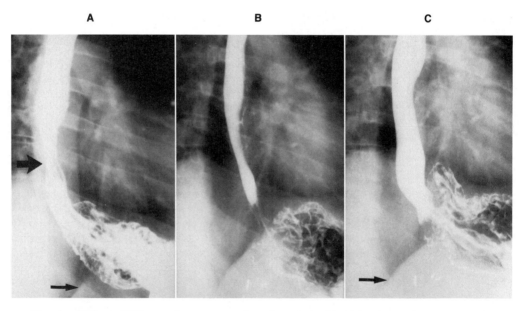

Fig. 14-4. Failure of Hill posterior gastropexy for reflux esophagitis with stricture. **A,** A large sliding hiatal hernia above the diaphragm (*small arrow*). This patient was obese and had distal esophagitis, a stricture (*large arrow*), and relative esophageal shortening, all "recurrence risk factors." **B,** One week after a Hill repair, there was little evidence of an intraabdominal distal esophageal segment. **C,** One year later, the repair, which had been performed under tension, had pulled loose, and the stomach is again seen above the level of the diaphragm (*arrow*). (Reproduced with permission of the J.B. Lippincott Company from *Complications in Surgery and Trauma*, edited by Lazar J. Greenfield, M.D., Philadelphia, 1984. Page 262.)

seem that healing of the esophageal sutures of the standard operations in these patients is jeopardized. As an alternative, others have favored a Nissen fundoplication with the stomach remaining above the diaphragm in the thorax.[47-51] Although conceptually simple, this approach results in a man-made paraesophageal hiatal hernia with its attendant mechanical complications— strangulation, perforation, ulceration, and bleeding—and each of these disastrous occurrences has been reported after an intrathoracic fundoplication.[39,52-54] The Thal cardioplasty operation[55] not only relies on the healing of the diseased, opened esophagus to which the gastric fundus is sutured, but also requires the addition of an intrathoracic fundoplication to control reflux,[56,57] both major disadvantages of this approach to the short esophagus. Although there is no question that effective reflux control can be achieved whether the hiatal hernia repair is intraabdominal or intrathoracic, the advantages of an intraabdominal location of the reconstructed gastroesophageal junction, avoiding the numerous potential complications of an intrathoracic fundoplication, are clear.

In 1971, Pearson and associates reported the efficacy of the combination of the esophagus-lengthening Collis gastroplasty and the Belsey repair in controlling reflux in patients with strictures.[58] The rationale for this approach followed logically the conclusions of the long-term Belsey study: recurrence can be minimized in a patient with a peptic stricture undergoing an antireflux operation if additional distal esophageal length is gained and if suturing to the diseased esophagus is avoided. The Collis gastroplasty tube provides a healthy "neoesophagus" of resilient stomach rather than inflamed or scarred distal esophagus around which to perform the fundoplication, and tension on the repair is eliminated since no effort is made to reduce the squamocolumnar junction below the diaphragm. Pearson and associates, using the combined Collis-Belsey operation, have subsequently reported excellent results in controlling reflux in patients with strictures.[59] Others, because of the finding of unsatisfactory reflux control with the Collis-Belsey operation,[36,60] have combined the Collis gastroplasty procedure with a 360-degree Nissen-type fundoplication[61-63] and have reported gratifying results in patients with difficult reflux problems.

My current preference is to perform the combined esophagus-lengthening Collis gastroplasty–Nissen fundoplication procedure (Fig. 14-5) not only in patients with strictures from reflux, but also in those demonstrating what we have come to identify as "recurrence risk factors."[64] In

general, the factors responsible for disruption of a hiatal hernia repair can be divided into (1) those that jeopardize the healing of sutures placed into either the esophageal or the periesophageal tissues and (2) those that result in increased tension on the repair. The presence of *reflux esophagitis* with intramural esophageal inflammation or *periesophagitis*, secondary either to reflux esophagitis or to prior operations at the gastroesophageal junction, jeopardizes the reliable placement of esophageal sutures into healthy muscle or submucosal layers. *Esophageal shortening* may be absolute, as in the case of a reflux stricture with secondary fibrous contracture of the esophagus, or relative, as occurs with many long-standing hiatal hernias. In either instance, the surgeon performing one of the standard hiatal hernia repairs may find that a moderate degree of tension is required to reduce the gastroesophageal junction the prerequisite 3 to 5 cm *below* the hiatus into the abdomen. This is much more apparent when the hiatal hernia repair is performed transthoracically, for the amount of tension on the lower esophagus that results after the reduction of the stomach into the abdomen can be better appreciated. When the surgeon recognizes that such tension on the distal esophagus will result from a standard hiatal hernia repair, he or she must be prepared to alter the operation if the risk of recurrent reflux from disruption of the repair is to be minimized. It has been recommended that to reduce undue tension on the repair in these cases, the esophagus be mobilized to the level of the aortic arch.[8] I believe that if there is enough shortening to require such extensive mobilization, the esophagus-lengthening Collis gastroplasty in combination with a Nissen fundoplication is probably a better option for ensuring a tension-free repair. Patients who are markedly *obese* or who suffer from *chronic obstructive pulmonary disease* and repeated coughing have elevated intraabdominal pressure, which is responsible for their well-recognized increased incidence of abdominal wall hernias (incisional and inguinal). It is logical to reason that the same intraabdominal forces that stress the anterior abdominal wall in these patients exert a similar effect at the diaphragmatic hiatus, where recurrent herniation may occur. Thus any technical maneuver that can minimize tension on the reconstructed gastroesophageal junction in these patients would seem desirable, in the same manner in which a "relaxing" incision is used in an inguinal hernia repair. Again, the esophagus-lengthening Collis gastroplasty combined with a fundoplication would seem appropriate in the markedly obese patient or the patient with chronic obstructive pulmonary

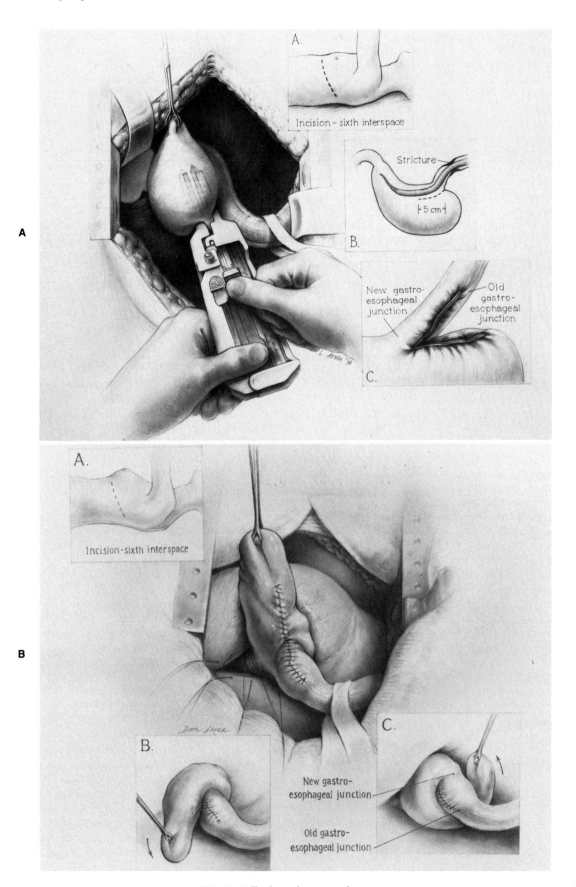

A.

Incision ~ sixth interspace

Stricture

5 cm

New gastro-esophageal junction

Old gastro-esophageal junction

C.

B.

A.

Incision-sixth interspace

B.

C.

New gastro-esophageal junction

Old gastro-esophageal junction

Fig. 14-5. For legend see opposite page.

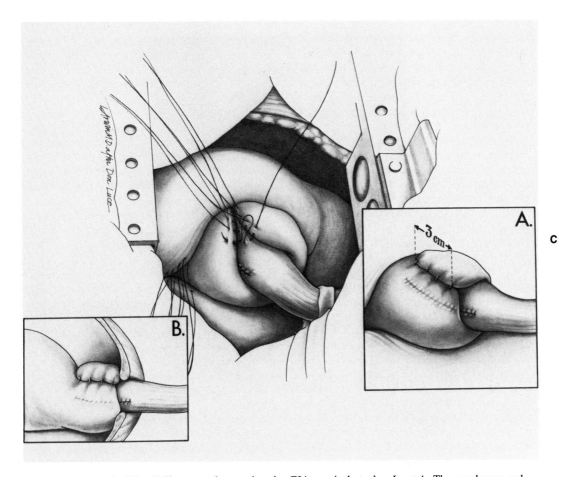

Fig. 14-5. A, The Collis gastroplasty using the GIA surgical stapler. *Inset A,* The esophagus and fundus of the stomach are mobilized through a lateral thoracotomy in the sixth or seventh left intercostal space. *Inset B,* A No. 54 or 56 French Hurst-Maloney dilator is passed through the esophageal stricture and displaced against the lesser curvature of the stomach as the stapler is applied. The knife assembly is advanced (*main drawing*), and the stapler is removed. *Inset C,* The result is a 5-cm-long gastric tube extension of the functional esophagus. An additional 2 to 3 cm can be gained by a second, partial application of the stapler, if necessary. **B,** The elongated, narrowed gastric fundus available for the fundoplication after completion of the Collis procedure. *Insets B and C,* The gastric fundus is wrapped around the gastroplasty tube. Note that the posterior crural sutures are left untied at this time. **C,** Placement of the seromuscular sutures from the gastric fundus to the gastroplasty tube to the gastric fundus in construction of the fundoplication. Approximately four sutures, 1 cm apart, are placed, resulting in a 3- to 4-cm fundic wrap (*inset A and main drawing*). The fundoplication, reduced into the abdomen, rests below the diaphragm without tension on the distal esophagus after the posterior crural sutures are tied (*inset B*). (**A** from Orringer, M.B., and Sloan, H.: J. Thorac. Cardiovasc. Surg. **68:**2989, 1974; **B** from Orringer, M.B., and Sloan, H.: Ann. Thorac. Surg. **25:**16, 1978.)

disease, to minimize the chance of failure of the hernia repair.

TREATMENT OF RECURRENT GASTROESOPHAGEAL REFLUX

As at the time of the first operation, the most common indications for reoperation for gastroesophageal reflux are (1) intractability of symptoms and (2) persistent ulcerative esophagitis despite maximal medical therapy. In addition, postoperative dysphagia may occur after any of the standard antireflux operations, and although this is generally a transient early postoperative phenomenon, it may persist, become more severe, and eventually require reoperation.

The operative approach to the patient with recurrent reflux is influenced in part by (1) the type of initial repair, (2) the existing anatomy at the gastroesophageal junction as determined by barium esophagogram, and (3) the degree of esophagitis seen at esophagoscopy. Esophageal manometry and acid reflux testing with the intraesophageal pH electrode are important in the evaluation of the patient with recurrent symptoms after a prior antireflux operation, not only to document abnormal reflux and to objectively quantitate the amplitude and length of the distal high-pressure zone, but also to exclude any unrecognized *esophageal motor disturbance* such as spasm, achalasia, or scleroderma. Whenever possible, the operative report describing the initial procedure should be obtained. This may provide important clues to the feasibility of reoperation. For example, knowledge that a fundoplication was performed with fine absorbable suture, combined with a barium esophagogram showing a large hiatal hernia with no evidence of a fundoplication, is a fairly good indication that the wrap has disrupted completely and that reoperation may not be difficult. Similarly, if the hiatus was either not closed or inappropriately closed with fine suture at the last operation, and the fundoplication has migrated into the chest, correction may involve mobilization and reduction of the wrap into the abdomen and proper reapproximation of the crura with heavy (no. 1 or 2) nonabsorbable sutures. It is also helpful to know if extensive upper abdominal adhesions from prior operations were encountered initially or if a gastrostomy was performed, either of which increases the degree of difficulty of a reoperation. Knowledge of the initial operation also facilitates the "takedown" that is needed for a subsequent repair. After a Hill posterior gastropexy, for example, there may be firm adhesions between the gastroesophageal junction and the region of the median arcuate ligament. Care must be exercised to avoid injury to the celiac axis vessels in this area as these adhesions are divided. With a Belsey operation, the two rows of three sutures each must be taken down carefully, since a division of adhesions between the gastric fundus and the diaphragm resulting from the sutures may result in holes in the stomach and a fundus that is unsuitable for another fundic wrap. Although the Nissen repair typically involves no stitches between the diaphragm and the stomach, meticulous division of any intact fundoplication sutures must be carried out to prevent entry into either the esophagus or the stomach.

The barium esophagogram provides important information in the patient with recurrent reflux. Each of the standard repairs (the Belsey, the Nissen, and the Hill) has characteristic roentgenographic patterns of recurrence,[24,40,41] which

have direct implications for subsequent operations. In general, in patients with the most extensive disruptions of their repairs and recurrent hiatal hernias, with little remaining roentgenographic evidence of the initial operation, reoperation is easier because not as much dissection is required to "take down" the repair. In contrast, patients with recurrent reflux but repairs that appear to be intact require dismantling of a "normal" hiatus and "unwrapping" of the cardia, and devascularization of the gastric fundus occurring in this process may ultimately contraindicate another fundoplication.

Regardless of the type of the initial antireflux operation, complete mobilization of the gastroesophageal junction in the patient with recurrent gastroesophageal reflux is as important as it was the first time and is facilitated by adherence to certain basic principles. An *intraesophageal dilator* (40 French or larger) across the gastroesophageal junction facilitates identification of the distal esophagus and proximal stomach. When mobilizing the stomach away from the liver or the diaphragm, in order to minimize the chance of devascularizing it, the surgeon should conscientiously *avoid dissecting into the wall of the stomach*—if necessary, allowing some of the liver capsule or diaphragmatic muscle fibers to remain adherent to the stomach. It is usually, but by no means always, possible to redo a hiatal hernia operation at least once. With a third or fourth antireflux procedure, however, the potential need for partial esophageal or gastric resection is much greater, and the surgeon must be prepared to undertake a larger operation. If after mobilization of the gastric fundus and distal esophagus, there is extensive disruption or devascularization of either of these organs, resection and distal esophageal substitution with either colon or jejunum is far safer than attempted local repair and repeat fundoplication. This is usually best achieved through a left thoracoabdominal incision and is the reason that operations for recurrent reflux are generally best performed through a *left thoracotomy*, which can be extended into the upper abdomen if necessary. In these patients, a preoperative barium enema is obtained to assess the suitability of the colon as an esophageal substitute, and the colon is prepared preoperatively in the evident that it is needed as an esophageal replacement. An isoperistaltic short segment of left colon based upon the ascending branch of the left colic artery is an excellent distal esophageal replacement in patients with recurrent reflux esophagitis.[65] The alkaline colonic mucus resists gastric acid, and good symptomatic reflux control is usually obtained. Similarly, a jejunal interposition, although more limited in length and dependent upon a more precarious blood supply than the colon, functions well in this situation.[50,66] It is often a difficult decision to begin a distal esophagectomy and either colonic or jejunal interposition after having struggled for several hours to mobilize an esophagus and upper stomach that are surrounded by adhesions and acute inflammatory reaction only to find that a "redo" hiatal hernia repair is not possible. It may seem a more expedient solution to resect the irreparably damaged esophagus or stomach and then perform a low intrathoracic esophagogastric anastomosis to reestablish continuity of the alimentary tract. Rationalization of this approach on the basis of a shorter operative time and "greater patient safety" is unfortunately not prudent. Not only is the patient subjected to the hazards of a postoperative intrathoracic esophagogastric anastomotic disruption, but he is left with certain gastroesophageal reflux and esophagitis, which inevitably follow resection of the lower esophageal sphincter mechanism and esophagogastrostomy. Reflux esophagitis occurs in *at least* 40% of patients undergoing an intrathoracic esophagogastrostomy, and for this reason this operation should virtually *never* be performed for the treatment of gastroesophageal reflux or its complications lest the patient finish with the same disease process for which he was operated upon.

Since in the majority of patients with gastroesophageal reflux requiring reoperations it is possible to mobilize the stomach and esophagus away from adjacent structures so that a standard antireflux procedure (Belsey, Nissen, or Hill) is possible, the unanswered question is "Which operation is *best* in the treatment of *recurrent* reflux?" There are a few published reports that address the topic of the surgical management of recurrent reflux. As a rule, surgeons who prefer the Belsey, Nissen, or Hill repair for the initial treatment of gastroesphageal reflux and its complications, when confronted with a patient with recurrent reflux, simply advocate redoing "their" operation. Thus, Orringer, Kinner, and Belsey, reporting 892 patients undergoing the Belsey Mark IV operation and followed 3 to 15 years, found 98 patients with documented hiatal hernia or gastroesophageal reflux (11% recurrence rate).[24] Eleven of these were asymptomatic, 10 required no treatment, 32 were treated by standard medical management, and 45 required a second surgical procedure. Among the 45 patients with recurrences treated surgically, 33 had a second Mark IV repair. In 14 of these, a pyloromyotomy was added because periesophageal fibrosis

caused difficulty identifying and preserving the vagus nerves. An esophageal resection (with esophagogastrostomy in 4 and short segment colon interposition in 5) was required in 9 patients. Twenty-four of the 33 patients (76%) undergoing a second Mark IV repair, and 8 of 9 patients requiring esophageal resection, had either good or excellent subjective results after 1 to 5 years of follow-up.

Hill and associates discussed the management of 25 patients with failed Nissen fundoplications, all of whom had symptoms of heartburn, reflux, and/or dysphagia.[67] Twenty-four of these patients underwent a median arcuate ligament posterior gastropexy, and one required a jejunal interposition. Among 23 patients followed by questionnaire, telephone interview, or personal interview and examination for an average of 2 years, results were described as good or excellent in 20. Leonardi and associates have discussed the surgical management of 25 patients requiring reoperation for complications of the Nissen fundoplication.[68] Recurrent reflux symptoms were present in 7, dysphagia in 14, gas-bloat syndrome in 2, and paraesophageal hernia in 2. Revision of the fundoplication relieved symptoms in the 15 patients in whom it was done, with follow-up periods ranging from 3 months to 9 years (average, 2.8 years). The remaining 10 patients were treated with a variety of operations: takedown of the Nissen repair (2), conversion to a Collis-Belsey repair (2), total esophagectomy with colon interpostion (1), long esophagomyotomy (1), esophagogastrectomy (1), conversion to a Hill posterior gastropexy (1), and transabdominal reduction of a paraesophageal hiatal hernia (2).

The natural tendency of a surgeon to whom a patient with recurrent reflux is referred is to assume that the initial operation failed either because of technical reasons or because "the best" antireflux procedure was not performed the first time. The Belsey advocate then attempts to convert the patient who has had a failed Nissen or Hill repair to a Mark IV reconstruction. The Nissen advocate favors the 360-degree wrap, just as Hill is a proponent of the posterior gastropexy when other operations have failed. The logic to such reasoning is simply unsound. Experienced esophageal surgeons who follow their patients long enough will eventually see some recurrences after their antireflux operations. Whether because of initially inadequate esophageal mobilization, tension on the repair, disruption of esophageal sutures, marked obesity, chronic obstructive pulmonary disease, or as yet undetermined factors, the operation has failed to provide lasting reflux control. To repeat the attempt at reconstructing the gastroesophageal junction by using a different standard antireflux operation may simply not be recognizing the fact that a particular patient is prone to recurrence and merits an alternative approach. I, for example, have noted that many patients undergoing an antireflux operation have a history of multiple previous inguinal or abdominal incisional hernia repairs and perhaps may have an intrinsic connective tissue weakness. For this reason, I regard patients with recurrent reflux as being "at risk" for recurrence after the standard operations and believe that they are better treated with a combined Collis gastroplasty–Nissen fundoplication operation (Fig. 14-6). With careful mobilization of the cardia, as described previously, this approach is usually feasible and provides excellent reflux control in these patients.

Fundoplication operations that have "failed" because of resulting dysphagia or fistula forma-

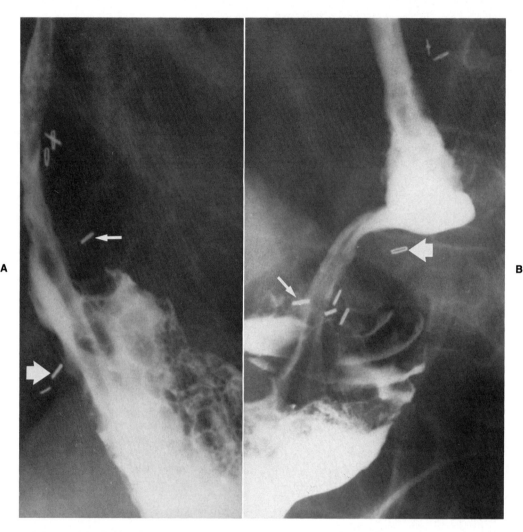

Fig. 14-6. The Collis-Nissen operation for recurrent hiatal hernia. **A**, Detail of the gastroesophageal junction in a patient with a recurrent hiatal hernia, reflux, and peptic stricture after two previous Belsey repairs. **B**, The reconstructed gastroesophageal junction following the Collis-Nissen procedure. Dense lower mediastinal fibrosis prevented application of the GIA stapler flush against the esophagus, resulting in a diverticulum-like deformity of the stomach at the proximal end of the gastroplasty tube. Nevertheless, a very satisfactory gastroplasty tube was constructed. Note the horizontal gastric folds in the fundoplication around the distal 3 to 4 cm of functional esophagus. (In both views, the large arrow is at the diaphragmatic hiatus, and the small arrow is at the gastroesophageal junction). (Reproduced with permission of Little, Brown & Company from Orringer, M.B., and Sloan, H.: Combined Collis-Nissen reconstruction of the esophagogastric junction, Ann. Thorac. Surg. **25**:16, 1978.)

tion constitute the most difficult of this group to treat surgically. Persistent fistulas at the gastroesophageal junction that fail to respond to external drainage most often require resection and visceral esophageal substitution of the esophagus. Early dysphagia after an antireflux operation may occur because of transient distal esophageal motor dysfunction, too tight a fundoplication, excessive narrowing of the diaphragmatic hiatus, or herniation of the fundoplication or gastric fundus into the chest through the hiatus or a diaphragmatic counterincision with secondary esophagogastric obstruction. Later, fibrosis in the region of the repair, perhaps the result of an occult localized perforation from a suture, may develop and cause severe dysphagia refractory to dilatation. The barium esophagogram is helpful in localizing the point of obstruction. A postoperative obstructing paraesophageal hiatal hernia requires reduction of the stomach into the abdomen and closure of the diaphragmatic defect. If the fundoplication or hernia repair is still located in its proper intraabdominal position, but the distal esophagus is obstructed, a transabdominal approach to the hiatus is indicated. The exact site of the obstruction is demonstrated by positioning a fiberoptic esophagoscope within the esophagus at the point of obstruction and transilluminating this area so that is can be localized by external examination of the hiatus and hernia repair. The problem may be as easy to manage as simply removing a single suture from the posterior crural repair. If relief of the obstruction is confirmed by endoscopic examination, a simple solution has been found. Alternatively, takedown of the fundoplication and rewrapping of the fundus with a large (46 French or larger) dilator across the gastroesophageal junction may be required. Obstructive symptoms after a fundoplication, regardless of the type of wrap, may be a reflection of marked inflammatory reaction in the region of the repair, and in these patients the surgeon should be prepared to resect the esophagus and reconstruct it if necessary. Traditionally, a distal esophagectomy and either short-segment left colon or jejunal interposition have been advocated when a "redo" hiatal hernia repair is not possible. A number of these patients with distal esophageal obstruction following a prior antireflux operation, however, present with marked weight loss and negative nitrogen balance, not unlike the patient with esophageal carcinoma. Avoidance of a thoracoabdominal operation and the potential complications of an intrathoracic esophageal anastomotic disruption is highly desirable in these patients. In recent years, when faced with the necessity of resecting the esophagus after several failed antireflux operations, particularly in a debilitated patient, I have utilized the technique of transhiatal esophagectomy without thoracotomy.[69] The entire thoracic esophagus is resected through the hiatus and a cervical incision, the stomach is mobilized through the posterior mediastinum in the original esophageal bed, and a cervical esophagogastric anastomisis is performed. Despite multiple prior operations involving the gastric cardia, it is usually possible to preserve the high greater curvature of the fundus, that portion which reaches most superiorly to the neck. Symptoms from reflux esophagitis are eliminated when the esophagus is resected, and the patient with a cervical esophagogastric anastomosis has virtually no clinically significant reflux. The stomach has proven to be an excellent visceral esophageal substitute in these patients.

CONCLUSION

The management of the patient with a failed antireflux operation remains an intellectual and technical challenge for the esophageal surgeon and clearly requires individualization of therapy. As more attention is directed toward objective long-term follow-up of the various hiatal hernia repairs, the procedure that carries the lowest recurrence rate may be identified, so that the need for reoperation will be minimized. Identification of factors predisposing certain patients to recurrence, with selection of more appropriate operations, may further obviate the problem of the failed antireflux procedure.

REFERENCES

1. Harrington, S.W.: Diaphragmatic hernia, Arch. Surg. **16:**386, 1928.
2. Allison, P.R.: Reflux esophagitis, sliding hiatal hernia, and the anatomy of repair, Surg. Gynecol. Obstet. **92:**149, 1951.
3. Lortat-Jacob, J.L., and Robert, F.: Les malpositions cardio-tuberositaires, Arch. Mal. Appar. Dig. **42:**750, 1953.
4. Sweet, R.H.: Esophageal hiatus of the diaphragm, Ann. Surg. **1:**135, 1952.
5. Nissen, R.: Eine einfache Operation zur Beeinflussung der reflux Oesophagitis, Schweiz. Med. Wochenschr. **86:**590, 1956.
6. Nissen, R.: Gastropexy and "fundoplication" in surgical treatment of hiatal hernia, J. Dig. Dis. **6:**954, 1961.
7. Baue, A.E., and Belsey, R.H.R.: The treatment of sliding hiatus hernia and reflux esophagitis by the Mark IV technique, Surgery **62:**396, 1967.
8. Skinner, D.B., and Belsey, R.H.R.: Surgical manage-

ment of esophageal reflux and hiatus hernia, J. Thorac. Cardiovasc. Surg. **53:**33, 1967.

9. Hill, L.D.: An effective operation for hiatal hernia: an eight year appraisal, Ann. Surg. **166:**681, 1967.

10. Hill, L.D., Tobia, J., and Morgan, E.H.: Newer concepts of the pathophysiology of hiatal hernia and esophagitis, Am. J. Surg. **111:**70, 1966.

11. Allison, P.R.: Hiatus hernia: a 20 year retrospective survey, Ann. Surg. **178:**273, 1973.

12. Urschel, H.C., Jr., and Paulson, D.L.: Gastroesophageal reflux and hiatal hernia, J. Thorac. Cardiovasc. Surg. **53:**21, 1967.

13. Behar, J., Biancani, P., Spiro, H.M., and Storer, E.H.: Effect of anterior fundoplication on lower esophageal sphincter competence, Gastroenterology **67:**209, 1974.

14. Brennan, T.G., Trindale, L.M., Rozycki, Z.J., and Giles, G.R.: The influence of the lower esophageal splincter pressure on the outcome of hiatus hernia repair, Br. J. Surg. **61:**201, 1974.

15. Csendes, A., and Larrain, A.: Effect of posterior gastropexy on gastroesophageal sphincter pressure and symptomatic reflux in patients with hiatal hernia, Gastroenterology **63:**19, 1972.

16. DeMeester, T.R., Johnson, L.F., and Kent, A.H.: Evaluation of current operations for the prevention of gastroesophageal reflux, Ann. Surg. **180:**511, 1974.

17. Ellis, F.H., Jr., El-Kurd, M.F.A., and Gibb, S.P.: The effect of fundoplication on the lower esophageal splincter, Surg. Gynecol. Obstet. **143:**1, 1976.

18. Higgs, R.H., Castell, D.O., and Farrell, R.L.: Evaluation of the effect of fundoplication or the incompetent lower esophageal splincter, Surg. Gynecol. Obstet. **141:**571, 1975.

19. Moran, J.M., Pihl, C.O., Norton, R.A., and Rheinlander, H.F.: The hiatal hernia–reflux complex: current approaches to correction and evaluation of results, Am. J. Surg. **121:**403, 1971.

20. Pope, C.E., II, Eastwood, L.F., and Eastwood, I.R.: Objective results of antireflux surgery (abstract), Clin. Res. **21:**208, 1973.

21. Hoffman, E., and Sumner, M.C.: A clinical and radiological review of 204 hiatal hernia operations, Thorax **28:**379, 1973.

22. Hill, L.D.: Intraoperative measurement of lower esophageal stricture pressure, J. Thorac. Cardiovasc. Surg. **75:**378, 1978.

23. Hill, L.D., and Velasco, N.: The Hill repair. In Sabiston, D.C., Jr. and Spencer, F.C., editors: Gibbon's surgery of the chest, ed. 4, Philadelphia, 1983, W.B. Saunders Co., pp. 797-804.

24. Orringer, M.B., Skinner, D.B., and Belsey, R.H.R.: Long-term resuls of the Mark IV operation for hiatal hernia and analyses of recurrences and their treatment, J. Thorac. Cardiovac. Surg. **63:**25, 1972.

25. Rossetti, M., and Hell, K.: Fundoplication for the treatment of gastroesophageal reflux and hiatal hernia, World J. Surg. **1:**439, 1977.

26. McAlhany, J.C., Thomas, H.F., and Woodward E.R.: Gastroesophageal reflux after operative procedure for sliding hiatal hernia, Am. J. Surg. **123:**657, 1972.

27. Bushkin, F.L., Neustein, C.L., Parker, T.H., and Woodward, E.R.: Nissen fundoplication for reflux peptic esophagitis, Ann. Surg. **185:**672, 1977.

28. Polk, H.C., Jr., and Zeppa, R.: Fundoplication for complicated hiatal hernia: rationale and results, Ann. Thorac. Surg. **7:**202, 1969.

29. Battle, W.S., Nyhus, L.M., and Bombeck, C.T.: Nissen fundoplication and esophagitis secondary to gastroesophageal reflux, Arch. Surg. **106:**588, 1973.

30. Dilling, E.W., Peyton, M.D., Cannon, J.P., Kanaly, P.J., and Elkins, R.C.: Comparison of Nissen fundoplication and Belsey Mark IV in the management of gastroesophageal reflux, Am. J. Surg. **134:**730, 1977.

31. Ferraris, V.A., and Sube, J.: Retrospective study of the surgical management of reflux esophagitis, Surg. Gynecol. Obstet. **152:**17, 1981.

32. Negre, J.B., Markkula, H.T., Keyrilainen, O., and Matikainen, M.: Nissen fundoplication: results at 10 year follow-up, Am. J. Surg. **146:**635, 1983.

33. Sillin, L.F., Condon, R.E., Wilson, S.D., et al.: Effective surgical therapy of esophagitis: experience with Belsey, Hill, and Nissen questions, Arch. Surg. **114:**536, 1979.

34. Postlethwait, R.W.: Surgery of esophagus, New York, 1979, Appleton-Century-Crofts, pp. 232-233.

35. Brand, D.L., Eastwood, I.R., Martin, D., Carter, W.B., and Pope, C.E.: Esophageal symptoms, manometry, and histology before and after anti-reflux surgery, Gastroenterology **76:**1393, 1979.

36. Orringer, M.B., and Sloan, H.: Complications and failings of the combined Collis-Belsey operation, J. Thorac. Cardiovasc. Surg. **74:**726, 1977.

37. Hiebert, C.A., and O'Mara, C.S.: The Belsey operation for hiatal hernia: a twenty year experience, Am. J. Surg. **13:**532, 1979.

38. Negre, J.B.: Post-fundoplication symptoms: do they restrict the success of Nissen fundoplicaton? Ann. Surg. **198:**698, 1983.

39. Polk, H.C., Jr.: Fundoplication for reflux esophagitis: misadventures with the operation of choice, Ann. Surg. **183:**645, 1967.

40. Feigin, D.S., James, A.E., Jr., Stitik, F.F., Donner, M.W., and Skinner, D.B.: The radiologic appearance of hiatal hernia repairs, Radiology **110:**71, 1974.

41. Teixidor, H.S., and Evans, J.A.: Roentgenographic appearance of the distal esophagus and the stomach after hiatal hernia repair, Am. J. Roentgenol. **119:**245, 1973.

42. Donnelly, R.J., Deverall, P.B., and Watson, D.A.: Hiatus hernia with and without stricture: experience with the Belsey Mark IV repair, Ann. Thorac. Surg. **16:**301, 1973.

43. Hill, L.D., Gelfand, M., and Bauermeister, D.: Simplified management of reflux esophagitis with stricture, Ann. Surg. **172:**638, 1970.

44. Larrain, A., Csendes, A., and Pope, C.E.: Surgical correction of reflux: an effective therapy for esophageal strictures, Gastroenterology **69:**578, 1975.

45. Maher, J.W., Hollenbeck, J.I., and Woodward E.R.: An analysis of recurrent esophagitis following posterior gastropexy, Ann. Surg. **187:**227, 1978.

46. Herrington, J.L., Wright, R.S., Edwards, W.H., and Sawyers, J.L.: Conservative surgical treatment of reflux esophagitis and esophageal stricture, Ann. Surg. **181:**552, 1975.

47. Harrison, G.K., and Compels, B.M.: Treatment of reflux strictures of the esophagus by the Nissen-Rossetti operation, Thorax **26:**77, 1971.

48. Krupp, S., and Rossetti, M.: Surgical treatment of hiatal hernias by fundoplication and gastropexy (Nissen repair), Ann. Surg. **182:**472, 1975.

49. Naef, A.P, and Savary, M.: Conservative operations for peptic esophagitis with stenosis in columnar-lined lower esophagus, Ann. Thorac. Surg. **13:**543, 1972.

50. Polk,, H.C., Jr.: Indications for, technique of, and results of fundoplication for complicated reflux esophagitis, Ann. Surg. **44:**620, 1978.

51. Safaie-Shirazi, S., Zike, W.L., Condon, R.D., and DenBesten, L.: Nissen fundoplication without crural repair: a cure for reflux esophagitis, Arch. Surg. **108:**424, 1974.

52. Balison, J.R., Macgregor, A.M.C., and Woodward, E.R.: Postoperative diaphragmatic herniation following transthoracic fundoplication, Arch. Surg. **106:**164, 1973.

53. Burnett, H.F., Read, R.C., Morris, W.D., and Campbell, G.S.: Management of complications of fundoplication and Barrett's esophagus, Surgery **82:**521, 1977.

54. Mansour, K.A., Burton, H.G., Miller, J.I., Jr., and Hatcher, C.R., Jr.: Complications of intrathoracic Nissen fundoplication, Ann. Thorac. Surg. **32:**173, 1981.

55. Thal, A.P., Hatafuku, T., and Kurtzman, R.: New operation for distal esophageal stricture, Arch. Surg. **90:**464, 1965.

56. Strug, B.S., Jordan, P.H., Jr., and Jordan, G.L., Jr.: Surgical management of benign esophageal strictures, Surg. Gynecol. Obstet. **138:**74, 1974.

57. Thomas, H.F., Clarke, J.M., Rayl, J.E., and Woodward, E.R.: Results of the combined fundic patch fundoplication operation in the treatment of reflux esophagitis with stricture, Surg. Gynecol. Obstet. **135:**241, 1972.

58. Pearson, F.G., Tanger, B., and Henderson, R.D.: Gastroplasty and Belsey hiatal hernia repair, J. Thorac. Cardiovasc. Surg. **61:**50, 1971.

59. Pearson, F.G., and Henderson, R.D.: Long-term follow-up of peptic strictures managed by dilatation, modified Collis gastroplasty, and Belsey hiatus hernia repair, Surgery **80:**396, 1976.

60. Henderson, R.D.: Reflux control following gastroplasty, Ann. Thorac. Surg. **24:**206, 1977.

61. Henderson, R.D., and Marryatt, G.V.: Total fundoplication gastroplasty (Nissen gastroplasty): five-year review, Ann. Thorac. Surg. **39:**74, 1985.

62. Orringer, M.B., and Orringer, J.S.: The combined Collis-Nissen operation: early assessment of reflux control, Ann. Thorac. Surg. **33:**534, 1981.

63. Orringer, M.B., and Sloan, H.: Combined Collis-Nissen reconstruction of the esophagogastric junction, Ann. Thorac. Surg. **25:**16, 1978.

64. Orringer, M.B., and Sloan, H.: Collis-Belsey reconstruction of the esophagogastric junction, J. Thorac. Cardiovasc. Surg. **71:**295, 1976.

65. Belsey, R.H.R.: Reconstruction of the esophagus with left colon, J. Thorac. Cardiovasc. Surg. **49:**33, 1965.

66. Polk, H.C., Jr., Jejunal interposition for reflux esophagitis and esophageal stricture unresponsive to valvuloplasty, World J. Surg. **4:**731, 1980.

67. Hill, L.D., Ilves, R., Stevenson, J.K., and Pearson, J.M.: Reoperation for disruption and recurrence after Nissen fundoplication, Arch. Surg. **114:**542, 1979.

68. Leonardi, H.K., Crozier, R.E., and Ellis, F.H., Jr.: Reoperation for complications of the Nissen fundoplication, J. Thorac. Cardiovasc. Surg. **81:**50, 1981.

69. Orringer, M.B.: Transhiatal esophagectomy for benign disease, J. Thorac. Cardiovasc. Surg. **90**(5):649, 1985.

Management of failed antireflux procedures

DISCUSSION

Hein G. Gooszen and J.L. Terpstra

In his chapter Dr. Orringer has described the present state of knowledge on the management of failed antireflux procedures and has added his current approach to this extremely difficult group of patients. Dr. Orringer starts off summarizing the accepted goal of antireflux surgery—that is, not only to reduce 4 to 5 cm of distal esophagus into the abdominal cavity but also to add some form of fundoplication. Although this concept is still valid, since its introduction by Belsey and Nissen independently, it should be emphasized that it is still entirely empirical.

As long as the pathophysiologic mechanisms leading to pathologic reflux and subsequent symptoms and/or esphagitis have not been established, antireflux surgery will not be a causal therapy. It has become clear, however, that the defect is a multifactorial one, and it may be more appropriate not to speak about sphincter incompetence but to refer to insufficiency of the cardia mechanism. Several factors, either "local" or "regional," seem to play a role in regulating the cardia mechanism; local factors are the so-called "pinchcock valve," or lower esophageal sphincter, the angle of His, and the local esophageal innervation. Regional or systemic factors are saliva production, esophageal motility, gastric motility and neural and hormone regulation. The only thing these factors have in common is that their separate roles in insufficiency of the cardia mechanism have not been established. An unknown combination of factors eventually leads to absolute or relative insufficiency of the cardia mechanism.

Absolute insufficiency means that the cardia is incapable of keeping reflux within physiologic limits in the absence of any other demonstrable defect, such as esophageal motility disorder or delayed gastric emptying. Relative insufficiency means that the cardia mechanism per se is sufficient but gastric emptying is delayed, clearance of alkaline or acid material is disturbed, or

esophageal motility is in some way interfered with.

Although with the current state of knowledge and diagnostic facilities, these different factors are difficult to unravel, they do illustrate the multifactorial cause of reflux esophagitis and are a justification for extensive investigation of patients considered for antireflux surgery.

Before we try to comment on "Management of Failed Antireflux Procedures," it seems appropriate to define what surgery is expected to accomplish, and why it is ever successful with the current lack of knowledge about the cause of reflux esophagitis. These topics cannot be adequately discussed before describing how results of surgical treatment can be scored.

In the literature a wide variety of denominators to describe the results of antireflux surgery are used. If follow-up periods are given, they are usually given as mean follow-up periods. This method leaves the reader with severe problems in getting information on actuarial data. Follow-up percentages range from 42%[1] to 85%.[2] In the studies cited by Dr. Orringer the terms "failure rate," "symptom-free interval," and "overall recurrence rate" have been used. From these data it is impossible to decide upon the merits of the different types of operation, let alone decide which type of operation should be favored.

In our analysis of 107 patients who have been operated upon, we have divided the results of surgery into four categories: clinical success or failure and objective success or failure. Clinical success means absence of symptoms, absence of esophagitis on endoscopy, and absence of demonstrable reflux on x-ray film. Clinical failure has occurred with recurrence of specific symptoms with or without esophagitis on endoscopy. Objective success implies no recurrent hernia and no esophagitis on endoscopy, whereas in contrast the presence of a hernia and/or esophagitis after surgery indicates objective failure. That such a subdivision only supplies "terms for negotiations," rather than adding to our understanding of what surgery has in fact accomplished, was shown in a recent survey which we conducted.[3]

In a small group of patients classified as clinical successes, results of 24-hour pH monitoring had greatly improved in all but were still abnormal in 25% of patients. So the reflux seemed to have been reduced to a level that was no longer pathologic for those particular patients, but were they surgical failures or had they been successfully operated upon? Do they illustrate that the more tests you carry out, the more likely you are to find an abnormal result eventually? Perhaps they illustrate that even the "gold standard" of 24-hour pH monitoring should be interpreted very critically in patients considered for surgical treatment? They do emphasize our lack of knowledge of the mechanisms causing reflux esophagitis, and hence one will have no major objections to the statement that it is unknown why and how antireflux surgery fails in 10% to 15% of carefully selected patients. Nevertheless there are factors, as described by Dr. Orringer, now very well documented to increase the chance of failure, such as the experience of the surgeon, the grade of esophageal inflammation, and the presence of esophageal shortening. Fundoplication stitches put into an edematous esophagus harbouring ulcerative esophagitis are likely to give way, and hiatal hernia repair on a shortened esophagus results in a reconstruction under tension, which is sooner or later doomed to tear out and cause recurrence. Why, then, does surgery fail in about 10% of cases in experienced hands when there is a nonedematous, nonshortened esophagus? Is this because surgery has not sufficiently raised LES pressure? If fundoplication reduces the LES diameter, one can expect the baseline pressure to rise. The importance of this accomplishment is unknown, and it is certainly not the only factor.

An increase in pressure as compared with the preoperative value should be very cautiously interpreted, since pressures tend to show considerable fluctuations during the day.[4] It may be justifiable to state that the fundoplication performed is too loose if the pressure after surgery was not increased, based merely on the fact that the pressure of a sphincter increases with the decrease of its diameter. Has surgery failed because sphincter incompetence was not the key factor and therefore "sphincter support" by fundoplication and reposition of the cardia was not sufficient to cure the disorder? To address this question, we have compared the reflux characteristics as documented in 24-hour pH monitoring of primary cases before operation with those of another group of mostly referred patients with recurrence after previously performed antireflux surgery. It was shown that the percentage of supine time (pH < 4), the percentage of total time (pH < 4), and the mean duration of reflux episodes were all significantly higher in the recurrent cases than they were in primary cases before surgery.[3] Unfortunately, in the recurrent cases preoperative data from before the primary operation, for comparison, are lacking. If the reflux characteristics shown had been similar before operation, because of concomitant delayed gastric emptying, esophageal motor function disorder, or decreased saliva production, they may well have contributed to persistence or recurrence of pathologic reflux. If, however, the reflux characteristics had deteriorated because of surgical treatment, this probably should be explained by surgical destruction of anatomic connections at the level of the cardia, by vagal nerve damage, or by unrecognized newly introduced functional defects.

The incidence and clinical importance of vagal nerve damage are not known. Only those patients with clinical symptoms of vagal nerve damage, such as diarrhea or delayed gastric emptying, are listed as such in some surveys. It is well known that these patients represent only a minority of probably 10% to 20% of the total group of patients whose vagal nerves were accidentally cut. Preoperative and postoperative pancreatic polypeptide stimulation tests can answer this question. Pancreatic polypeptide (PP) is a hormone under complete vagal control. Vagal stimulation induces a peak in plasma PP level. After vagal nerve damage this response will be completely flat. The world is waiting for prospective studies comparing preoperative data with data after failed antireflux surgery, based on 24-hour pH monitoring, gastric emptying studies, esophageal manometry, esophageal clearance tests, and PP stimulation tests, but such studies are unlikely ever to be reported.

At this discouraging stage, an effective approach to patients with recurrence after antireflux surgery has to be chosen. We have operated upon 27 patients in the last few years for this indication. Five patients had undergone the Belsey Mark IV operation, and the remaining 22 had been subjected to different sorts of reconstructions. In all but one we were able to do a Belsey Mark IV fundoplication. In quite a few patients hardly any trace of previous surgery was detectable. For the surgical treatment of recurrence we favor a thoracic approach, since with this exposure the esophagus can be palpated, mobilized up to the aortic arch, and if necessary dilated under direct vision control. The identification and dissection of the vagal nerves are easier when the thoracic approach is chosen, and the fundoplication can be performed in a "fresh operation field." Quite often it appeared to be necessary to extend the incision over the costal margin and to open the abdominal cavity in order to free the cardia from the diaphragm and/or the liver.

Although the statement of Ronald Belsey that "the treatment of recurrence is to perform a proper operation" might be true in a strict sense and although we were able to perform a Belsey Mark IV repair in most of our patients with recurrent reflux, we find ourselves confronted with a clinical failure rate of about 30%. A proper operation in our hands is therefore not the complete answer to the problem. Nevertheless, 19 out of 27 patients (70%) were successfully reoperated upon with a standard Mark IV antireflux procedure. We therefore do not agree with Dr. Orringer that a combined procedure like the Collis-Nissen repair is indicated in every patient with recurrent reflux esophagitis. We feel that this operation should be performed in two categories of patients: those in whom at reoperation the former repair was intact and the reason for failure remains unclear and those with too short an esophagus either primarily or as a result of grade IV esophagitis. Favorable results in patients with reflux stricture and esophageal shortening have been described by Pearson and Henderson.[5]

Our current strategy is that patients with recurrent esophagitis or reflux after antireflux surgery go through a full scale of investigations, including esophageal manometry, 24-hour pH monitoring, pancreatic polypeptide test, and gastric emptying studies. If we can rule out esophageal motility disorder, vagal nerve damage, and delayed gastric emptying, we feel confident to proceed to a straightforward Belsey Mark IV repair. If gastric emptying is delayed, especially if combined with vagal nerve damage, we tend to add a pyloroplasty. We do not have the answer for patients with recurrent reflux and esophageal motility disorder and can only speculate that this is the group of patients that will benefit from short-segment colonic interposition. The results of the above approach have to be awaited, and nowadays the tailoring of the approach to primary cases and recurrences is not based on objective information but is determined by the personal experience of the surgeon involved.

REFERENCES

1. Rosetti, M., and Hell, K.: Fundoplication for the treatment of gastroesophageal reflux and hiatal hernia, World J. Surg. **1**:439, 1977.
2. Orringer, M.B., Skinner, D.B., and Belsey R.H.R.: Long-term results of the Mark IV operation for hiatal hernia and analysis of recurrences and their treatment, J. Thorac. Cardiovasc. Surg. **63**:25, 1972.
3. Gooszen, H.G., Griffioen, G., and Terpstra, J.L.: Objective assessment of the outcome of surgical treatment for pathological gastro-oesophageal reflux (abstract), Gastroenterology **90**:1790, 1986.
4. Dent, J., Dodds, W.J., Friedman, R.H., et al.: Mechanisms of gastroesophageal reflux in recumbent asymptomatic patients, J. Clin. Invest. **65**:256, 1980.
5. Pearson, F.G., and Henderson, R.D. Long-term follow-up of peptic strictures managed by dilatation, modified Collis gastroplasty and Belsey hiatus hernia repair, Surgery **80**:396, 1976.

Management of failed antireflux procedures

DISCUSSION

Lucius D. Hill

One of the first reports in the United States dealing with failed antireflux procedures was compiled by our group in 1971.[1] The report included 63 patients having had 71 antireflux operations. The Allison repair was the most common procedure, comprising 56 of the previous operations. Three patients had had Nissen repairs. Over the last 15 years we have compiled two additional reports dealing with failed antireflux procedures. Our most recent report includes 303 patients who had 380 previous repairs. Whereas in our first report the Allison repair was the most common, in our most recent report[2] the Nissen procedure is by far the most common. One hundred forty-eight Nissen repairs had been done on 120 patients, whereas only 65 Allison repairs had been performed on 52 patients. There were 25 patients who had had a Belsey repair and 13 who had had a Hill repair. The remaining repairs in this latter group consisted of Angelchik prostheses in 10 and a group of patients in whom the repair could not be identified, either from the previous operative report or at the time of surgery. These were included in the indeterminate group, of which there were 75 patients.

From this experience, which appears to be the largest in the world dealing with failed antireflux procedures, we have tried to learn as much as possible in an effort to avoid failures and improve results. If we are to learn anything from our previous observations, we need to answer critical questions, such as why procedures fail, what kind of failures are common to all antireflux operations, and what kind of failures are unique to a given procedure.

It is difficult to tell from either the text or the references, in Dr. Orringer's chapter, how many failed antireflux procedures have been seen by his group. He mentions and has illustrations of anecdotal cases, but it would be nice to know what observations have been gained from first-hand experience with "redo" operations. Dr. Orringer mentions the Belsey experience of 892 operations on patients in whom 98 documented recurrences were found, but it is difficult to tell from the discussion why the procedure failed in these patients.

In all of our analyses, the most common reason for recurrent reflux was failure to construct an adequate barrier at the gastroesophageal junction. At reoperation the gastroesophageal junction was grossly patulous in these individuals. This finding, in our experience, is the most common reason for failure of antireflux operations.

In the Allison and Belsey repairs, the second most common cause of failure was inadequate fixation sutures, which allowed the stomach to again herniate back into the mediastinum.

A third type of failure common to all types of antireflux procedures occurs when the surgeon makes the gastroesophageal junction too tight so that the patient has serious dysphagia. Although this type of failure was seen in all types of antireflux operations, it appeared to be far more common with the Nissen procedure.

Another important question that should be answered is whether a given type of failure is the fault of the surgeon or whether there appear to be basic defects with an operation itself. As the Nissen repair has become more common and we are seeing more and more complications with the Nissen procedure, it would appear that there are failures that are peculiar to this operation and that occur rarely, if ever, with any other type of antireflux procedure. We reported these failures at the American College of Surgeons in October of 1985, and these have been compiled in a report that has been submitted for publication.

Gas bloating and inability to vomit after Nissen repair are well-known complications of the procedure. They may be severe but infrequently require reoperation, whereas, other complications can be life threatening. In one hundred twenty patients requiring reoperation for failed Nissen repair, 80% of the complications represented serious recurrent reflux. Sixty percent of these patients had severe dysphagia. Esophageal dysmotility was seen in 48% of patients.

The most common reason for failure of the Nissen procedure was the so-called "slipped Nissen." In these cases the sutures that were intended to hold the wrap in place pulled out of the esophageal muscularis, and either the repair slipped down around the junction of the upper and middle thirds of the stomach or, in some cases, the wrap appeared to have been constructed at this level. A slipped Nissen that occurs following a correctly done Nissen repair would appear to be a basic weakness in the operation itself. The esophagus lacks a serosal coat and is the weakest part of the gastrointestinal tract. For an operation to depend on sutures in the esophagus for its integrity indicates that there is a flaw in the procedure itself. Slipping of the wrap away from the gastroesophageal junction not only results in a failure to correct reflux but compounds the failure by producing an obstruction of the stomach. This obstruction results in poor emptying of the wrap as well as the cardia of the stomach and promotes severe gastroesophageal reflux. The slipped wrap drains poorly and is subject to gastric ulceration. Woodward's group[3] was among the first to draw attention to the occurrence of gastric ulcer after Nissen fundoplication. As a result of these ulcerations, serious and life-threatening fistulas may occur. Again, this kind of complication appears to be peculiar to the Nissen, since it has not been reported following the Belsey or the Hill repair.

The patulous Nissen was the next most common cause of failure. This complication, we believe, results from the surgeon failing to calibrate the cardia sufficiently to prevent reflux. When the procedure is done over a bougie, it is difficult to tell how tight or loose the wrap will ultimately be. It is difficult for the surgeon to tell, when the bougie is removed, whether the gastroesophageal junction will snap shut or whether it will remain patulous.

As the Nissen fundoplication has become more popular, more and more reports dealing with failed antireflux procedures have concentrated primarily on the Nissen procedure. The report of Ellis and coworkers[4] is important in that, of the 25 cases reported, 8 were from their own series. Ellis is one of the most experienced esophageal surgeons in the world, and if 8 of his own cases needed reoperation, this suggests that the surgeon who infrequently operates on the esophagus may well have more failures of the Nissen operation. Two hundred seventy-one cases of "redo" Nissen operations have been reported in large series since 1979. Many smaller series of three or four operations have also appeared. A study by Negre[5] indicates an extremely high incidence of postfun-

doplication symptoms in 226 patients followed for 5½ years. Forty-four percent of these patients had difficulty swallowing, 31% were unable to vomit, 19% were unable to belch, 12% had abdominal pain, and 10% had dyspepsia. As Negre concluded, these findings clearly restrict the success of the Nissen procedure.

The report of Little and Skinner[6] is a significant one, representing a large series of 61 patients undergoing repeat antireflux procedures. Twenty-seven of these patients had more than one Nissen repair. Eight had at least three previous attempts at repair. We agree with Little's statement that many antireflux procedures across the country are done by surgeons who rarely operate on the esophagus and who appear to lack an understanding of the basic principles of antireflux surgery. We would add, however, that the increasing number of reports pertaining to the Nissen itself may indicate that the operation is flawed for reasons that we have outlined. Many of the patients operated on by us following failed Nissens had previously had surgery by board-certified surgeons in large university centers.

Orringer states that establishing an intraabdominal segment of distal esophagus wrapped in some fashion by the stomach is the common denominator of most effective antireflux operations. Our observations are not in agreement with this thesis. The normal lower esophagus is not wrapped by the stomach, and in many of the patients who had severe recurrent reflux with esophagitis there was an obvious intraabdominal segment of the esophagus but the gastroesophageal junction was patulous. Our experience would indicate that the important factors in preventing reflux in the normal individual as well as in an antireflux operation are the lower esophageal sphincter itself and the gastroesophageal valve. There has been a great deal of evidence to support the role of the lower esophageal valve in preventing reflux. We have recently done a number of cadaver dissections and have reported out findings,[7] which suggest a role for the gastroesophageal valve in preventing reflux. We have suspected for a long time that the sphincter alone could not withstand the pressures exerted on the gastroesophageal junction by high intraabdominal pressure and that a valve mechanism was essential to reflux control. In the cadaver, we have demonstrated that there is a pressure gradient across the gastroesophageal junction and that by accentuating the valve this pressure gradient can be markedly increased. We believe it is this valve rather than the intraabdominal segment itself that prevents reflux, and, in fact, there is little direct evidence in the living human being that the intraabdominal segment of esophagus itself plays a real role in the antireflux barrier. It is for these reasons that we believe that careful assessment of the status of the barrier during surgery is the most important measurement that we can take in these patients.

Dr. Orringer stresses over and over the need for preoperative and postoperative evaluation by pH and motility studies, with which we agree. We have also made the point emphatically that there is no point in doing preoperative and postoperative pH and motility studies if, during the operation, the cardia is not calibrated at a time when the repair can be adjusted if the LES pressures are too high or low. We have found intraoperative manometry to be an invaluable part of our antireflux surgery. It enables surgeons to vary their repair according to objectively measured criteria.

Orringer states that we have modified the basic technique of our repair, which is incorrect. The basic objectives and technique of the repair have remained the same. We have continued to polish each step, and the addition of intraoperative manometrics simply brings objectivity to a repair that was yielding good results in terms of correcting reflux. As long as there are any recurrences, it is important that we strive to prevent persistent reflux. It has been a mystery to us why surgeons in this country have resisted the application of new technology to antireflux surgery.

Orringer states that subjective improvement after operation may not necessarily correlate with actual reflux control. He further states that insistence upon objective long-term documentation of the results of an antireflux operation, utilizing esophageal manometry and intraesophageal pH monitoring both preoperatively and postoperatively, must become the mark of the modern esophageal surgeon if the relative merit of one operation over another is to be determined with accuracy. We would agree with this statement emphatically and would add, "Why not proceed and add the same technology to the operative procedure itself?" We have maintained that no preoperative and postoperative tests ever corrected reflux and that the most beautiful workup and beautiful postoperative care will do little for a patient in whom the cardia is not calibrated at surgery and in whom reflux persists.

Orringer appears to indicate that if we utilized the Nissen procedure with greater frequency there would be fewer recurrences, since, as he states, the Nissen procedure has clear superiority relative to correction of reflux. He cites the report of Rossetti and Hell, which is the largest report of the Nissen procedure. Rossetti inherited Rudolph Nissen's surgical practice, and the cases reported by Rossetti and Hell represent the total Nissen-Rossetti-Hell experience up to the time of the report in 1977.[8] A critical analysis of the report by Rossetti and Hell shows that over a 20-year period the group had operated on approximately 1400 patients. In 1972, 590 patients with fundoplication were evaluated at their follow-up clinic. An x-ray examination was performed only if the patient was not satisfied with the result or if the operation had not completely relieved symptoms. There is no mention of pH and motility studies or of any objective determination of the presence or absence of reflux. An analysis such as this leaves a great deal to be desired. What happened to the other 810 patients? Very often it is the group of patients who do not return to the same surgeon who may have serious complications and total failure of the procedure. In the largest series of Nissen operations in this country, reported by Polk in 1978,[9] there is no mention of postoperative pH and motility studies or of other objective determinations in 400 patients who had the Nissen repair. Polk states that during his early experience esophagoscopy was used frequently, but it is difficult to tell from the text whether, during the later experience, esophagoscopy or any other objective determination was used in reaching the conclusion that the results were good. Orringer has stated that esophageal manometry and intraesophageal pH monitoring should be the hallmarks of reliable postoperative follow-up data. If Orringer's criteria are used, the largest series from Europe and this country lack objective data, and the statement that the Nissen procedure controls reflux rests on very weak evidence. Our experience, therefore, would not support Orringer's inference that if the Nissen procedure were used more frequently there would be fewer recurrences, and, in fact, our experience would indicate that the more frequently the Nissen procedure is used, the more we are going to see serious complications.

The serious complications that we have referred to are the fistulas that are being reported in our series. These include gastrobronchial fistulas, gastroesophageal fistulas, and gastrocutaneous fistulas, and our report includes a patient with a gastric ulcer in the slipped Nissen wrap that penetrated into the aorta, or shown in Fig. 14-7. An alert surgeon was able to evacuate a large clot from the stomach and with finger pressure on the aorta, oversewed the aorta and closed the ulcer in the stomach. This represents the only survivor of a gastroaortic fistula of whom we are aware. Another life-threatening fistula occurred in a patient who was admitted to the coronary care

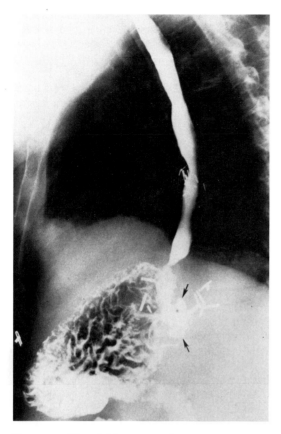

Fig. 14-7. Slipped Nissen procedure with a posterior gastric ulcer penetrating into aorta. The gastroaortic fistula was oversewn, with survival of the patient.

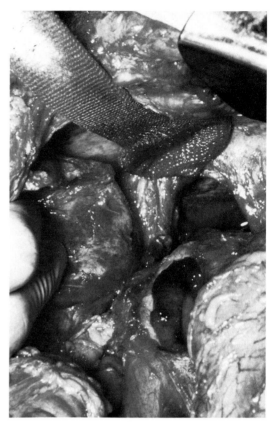

Fig. 14-8. Gastric ulcer, resulting from failed Nissen procedure, penetrating through stomach, diaphragm, and pericardium. The ulcer was closed and the gastroesophageal junction was sutured to preaortic fascia, with survival of the patient.

unit with a diagnosis of myocardial infarction. The electrocardiogram showed what was interpreted as a diaphragmatic infarction with diaphragmatic pericarditis. The surgeon, noted that the patient had had a Nissen fundoplication; a barium swallow showed barium in the pericardium, and at operation the patient was found to have a large ulcer that had penetrated through the stomach, the diaphragm, and the pericardium, and the base of the ucler was the myocardium itself (Fig. 14-8). The ulcer was taken down and closed, and the gastroesophageal junction was anchored to the preaortic fascia. This patient represents the only survivor of a gastropericardial fistula of whom we are aware. In addition to these life-threatening complications, we have seen gastrobronchial fistulas from slipped Nissens in which gastric ulcers developed and penetrated the stomach, the diaphragm, and into the lung (Fig. 14-9). These serious, life-threatening complications are further contradictions to Orringer's contention that the Nissen procedure is the superior antireflux operation.

Throughout Orringer's discussion, he insists that an intraabdominal segment of esophagus is important and that in the presence of esophageal inflammation and stricture formation one cannot get the gastroesophageal junction into its normal location without tension. In our experience with 243 patients undergoing operation for peptic esophageal stricture, we were able to get the gastroesophageal junction into its normal location without tension in all cases except those in which the esophagus had been perforated or destroyed by multiple dilatations. We therefore agree with Conrad Lam[10] that the "short esophagus" is a myth and that the term can lead to serious problems in that surgeons either recommend the Collis gastroplasty or a resection of the lower esophagus solely on the basis of the idea that the esophagus is short. This same reasoning is carried over into the repair of recurrent hernia, in which Orringer again states that if a patient has had an antireflux procedure the esophagus is undoubtedly shortened and a lengthening pro-

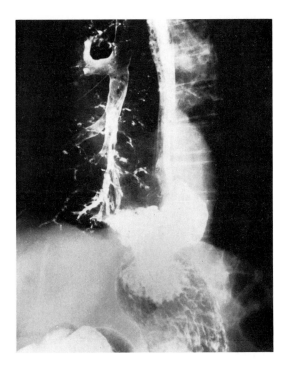

Fig. 14-9. Gastrobronchial fistula from penetrating gastric ulcer in slipped Nissen repair. Successfully corrected.

cedure or resection should be used. In our experience, many of the Nissen repairs that have slipped have left almost a virgin gastroesophageal junction with an esophagus that oftentimes appears lengthened because it is distended from partial obstruction by the slipped Nissen. We have routinely been able to get good lengths of esophagus below the diaphragm with no tension whatsoever. The results in the repair of 116 failed Nissen operations as determined by close follow-up, including motility and pH studies, showed an excellent result in 86%, fair in 11.6%, and a poor result in 5%, which is comparable to the results of the Collis-Nissen operation in primary repair. Orringer reported an overall objective recurrence rate, as documented with intraesophageal pH probe and standard acid reflux tests, of 13% in the combined Collis-Nissen operation in patients who had had no previous operations.[11] We therefore believe that a failed antireflux operation can be corrected by use of the Hill procedure in most cases. Twenty-seven of our patients had undergone more than one previous antireflux operation (range, 1 to 4) while 28 had undergone previous unrelated upper gastrointestinal surgery.

We have emphasized that in these difficult patients, intraoperative manometrics has been very useful, since the landmarks are obscured and it is difficult to determine whether the barrier that the surgeon has constructed is adequate or not. We believe that intraoperative manometrics will prevent many of the failures we have seen. The patulous repair, whether Nissen or otherwise, could certainly be avoided by utilizing intraoperative manometrics. A sphincter pressure of 0 at operation should alarm the surgeon that he or she has accomplished absolutely nothing in terms of correction of reflux. Unless the surgeon is willing to alter the operation according to the findings of the pressure measurements, there is no point in doing the measurements.

We agree, however, with Orringer that one should not be wedded to a single procedure. In the management of the failed antireflux operations, we used a wide variety of procedures necessitated by the disastrous findings that were present. The various fistulas were dealt with usually by transsecting the fistula with a stapling device, closing the fistula, restoring the gastroesophageal junction and calibrating the cardia, and restoring the gastroesophageal valve. Jejunal interposition was required for a patient with loss of continuity between the esophagus and the stomach, and we have used resection of the esophagus in those patients in whom the esophagus had been perforated and in whom the esophageal lumen had been obliterated. Otherwise we believe that a reconstruction of the normal anatomy can be performed.

It would be well to note that the Collis-Belsey and the Collis-Nissen operations are not small procedures. Having participated in the Collis-Belsey operation with Dr. F.G. Pearson, who popularized it, I can attest that this is a major procedure. Dr. Pearson is a reknowned master surgeon, and the patient did beautifully. I would conclude that in the hands of an outstanding surgeon like Dr. Orringer or Dr. Pearson, the Collis-Belsey operation or the Collis-Nissen operation may be very safe. In the hands of the surgeon who does few operations on the gastroesophageal junction, an operation of this magnitude could lead to serious complications involving all of the body cavities.

For completeness in a discussion of failed antireflux procedures, a word about the Angelchik prosthesis is essential. We have now removed 10 Angelchik prostheses for problems ranging from migration of the prosthesis into the chest, with obstruction of the esophagus, to erosion of the prosthesis through the stomach or through the esophagus and into the stomach, with passage of the prosthesis per rectum or obstruction of the stomach at the pylorus. Reports from around the country attest to the disastrous complications that are occurring with this prosthesis. When one recognizes that the mission of the gastrointestinal tract is to ingest and excrete foreign material that is placed in or around it, we can predict that more of these prostheses are going to be ingested and excreted. A large number of these devices have been placed, but it is too early to say whether the Angelchik prosthesis is safe. The complications we have seen with it indicate that because it is simple to place, surgeons who would not otherwise be operating on the gastroesophageal junction are placing an Angelchik prosthesis. Some of the devices we have seen were placed by nonsurgeons simply because it was felt that it was an easy procedure to do. We have seen the device placed below the left gastric artery in two instances, indicating that the surgeon had no concept of what an antireflux procedure entails.

The chapter by Orringer as well as the reports that are accumulating around the country that we have mentioned—by Little, Woodward, Ellis, and many others—indicate that reconstruction of the gastroesophageal junction to control reflux requires meticulous and careful surgery. Because surgery for hiatal hernia has been done by surgeons who have little experience in the gastroesophageal junction, surgery in this area has not enjoyed a good reputation. Many gastroenterologists are loath to send a patient to surgery because they have seen disastrous results in their patients. If we are to restore the confidence of the gastroenterologists, we must be more careful in patient selection and execution of appropriate surgery. Many of the so-called failed antireflux procedures we have seen were actually operations done inappropriately for achalasia, scleroderma, esophageal spasm, and other abnormalities of the esophagus that should have been diagnosed with even cursory preoperative evaluation. With careful preoperative evaluation and utilization of modern technology, both preoperatively and intraoperatively, the modern surgeon can indeed produce outstanding results in this area. We agree with Orringer that the modern antireflux surgeon should utilize modern technology to carefully select patients. We go a step further, however, to say that the modern surgeon should bring the new technology to the surgical procedure itself and, by so doing, improve results and restore the confidence of other physicians in our work.

REFERENCES

1. Hill, L.D.: Management of recurrent hiatal hernia, Arch. Surg. 102:296-302, 1971.
2. Low, D.E., Mercer, C.D., James, E.C., and Hill, L.D.: Post Nissen syndrome. (In preparation.)
3. Bushkin, F.L., Woodward, E.R., and O'Leary, J.P.: Occurrence of gastric ulcer after Nissen fundoplication, Amer. Surgeon 42:821-826, 1976.
4. Leonardi, H.K., Crozier, R.E., and Ellis, F.H.: Reoperation for complications of the Nissen fundoplication, J. Thorac. Cardiovasc. Surg. 81:50-56, 1981.
5. Negre, J.B.: Postfundoplication symptoms: do they restrict the success of Nissen fundoplication? Ann. Surg. 191:698-700, 1983.
6. Little, A.G., Ferguson, M.K., and Skinner, D.B.: Reoperation for failed antireflux operations, Surgery 91:511-517, 1986.
7. Thor, K.B.A., Hill, L.D., Mercer, C.D., and Kozarek, R.D.: Reappraisal of the flap valve mechanism in the gastroesophageal junction, Acta Chir. Scand. (In press.)
8. Rossetti, M., and Hell, K.: Fundoplication for the treatment of gastroesophageal reflux in hiatal hernia, World J. Surg. 1:439-444, 1977.
9. Polk, H.C.: Indications for, technique of, and results of fundoplication for complicated reflux esophagitis, Ann. Surg. 44:620-625, 1978.
10. Lam, C.R., and Gahagan, T.H.: special comment: the myth of the short esophagus. In Nyhus, L.M., and Harkins, H.N., editors: Hernia, Philadelphia, 1964, J.B. Lippincott Co., p. 450.
11. Orringer, M.B., and Orringer, J.S.: The combined Collis-Nissen operation: early assessment of reflux control, Ann. Thorac. Surg. 33:534-539, 1981.

J. Boix-Ochoa

Gastroesophageal reflux (GER) and spitting up are common problems in pediatrics and among the major complaints for which infants and children are seen by pediatricians. Contrary to adults, in whom recurrent vomiting must be considered pathologic, in early infancy this constitutes a "physiologic" event and is of little clinical consequence.[1,2] In some cases, however, the GER has its etiology in serious alterations of gastroesophageal physiology. The particular characteristics of the infant and child give place to a more varied clinical picture, including sudden death, asthma, otitis, and psychic disturbances, than is seen in the adult, and there are functional developmental problems (anorexia, failure to thrive, and so on) as well. Symptoms in the older child do not differ from those of the adult, but the etiopathogenesis and treatment of GER in early infancy and childhood are so different that they justify a separate discussion.

Our observations and conclusions on more than 2200 children affected with GER have provided us with a philosophy of the management of GER in pediatrics. Our aim in this chapter is to highlight some concepts, to present our point of view, and to review our results.

PATHOPHYSIOLOGY

Compared with adults, the biggest difference in the child is that he is a being in evolution. During development, the antireflux mechanisms mature, and 70% of children with GER improve by the age of weaning without any specific treatment[2]; they outgrow gastroesophageal reflux and do not need any kind of therapy. All these facts point to specific physiologic characteristics of this age group. Recent publications as well as other chapters of this book have well defined the cornerstones of the physiopathology of GER. Reflux occurs when opening pressure exceeds closing pressure. It is clear from this that reflux can be due to an incompetence of the closing mechanisms or to a pathologic increase of the opening pressure. Which are the special characteristics in infants and children?

Closing pressures

The closing pressures act on a zone called the lower esophageal sphincter (LES) and are the result of several factors active in this area. These factors are influenced by the age of our patients. In the very young (before maturation of the LES region) the forces promoting closure are not well developed, which leads to a lessening of adequate closing pressures and therefore facilitates the development of GER.

High-pressure zone

The pressure zone generated by the LES is one of the most effective factors of the antireflux barrier mechanism.[3] This LES pressure is higher than the intragastric pressure, and when challenged by an increase in intragastric pressure the LES responds by active contraction, exceeding the increase.[4] Most surely its effectiveness is based on the quality of the muscle mass in the high-pressure zone as well as on responsiveness to hormonal modulations.[5] The studies of Liebermann et al.[6,7] have demonstrated a thickened muscular segment located in the same area, thereby relating the muscular thickening of this zone and the manometric lower esophageal high-pressure zone, which means that these structures can be considered as the muscular counterpart of the LES. Therefore the development of this musculature is closely related to the competence of the LES.[8] This pressure zone, however, is not completely developed at birth[9,10]; a newborn can need some time to develop or put into function the musculature of this zone, as occurs in other zones of the body. During this development the infant will have a "transient gastroesophageal incompetence" together with a "physiologic" GER. Maturation of the lower esophageal sphincter exists and was demonstrated by us in 1979.[11]

Maturation of the lower esophageal sphincter

In order to determine when reflux stops being physiologic and should be considered as pathologic, we investigated the maturation of the LES by performing 4020 manometric studies in 680 infants and newborns ranging between 1 day and 6 months of age.[11,12] Statistical analysis of the results showed to our surprise that there was no correlation between esophageal pressures, gestational age, and birthweight. The postnatal age had the highest degree of significance, demonstrating that the "days of life" is the most important factor in the maturation of the LES, which in all the groups studied reached an effective maturation with demonstrated gastroesophageal competence between the fifth and seventh weeks of life (Fig. 15-1). Despite some controversy concerning these results,[13] recent data obtained from developing animals confirm these findings.[14] Hence, care must be taken in applying surgery in the first months of life to patients who have a physiologic right to vomit because they have not achieved full maturation. Surgical treatment should be rarely indicated at this age.

Intraabdominal segments

The intraabdominal segment is the key to gastroesophageal competence. It would be difficult to understand the working of the LES without the existence of an intraabdominal esophageal segment.[15] The determining factor is the length of the esophagus exposed to intraabdominal pressure. When intraabdominal pressure increases, the esophagus reacts as a soft tube and collapses.[16] In addition, the negative pressure in the thoracic esophagus results in it sucking the abdominal segment flat.[17] Furthermore, and according to Laplace's law, the pressure in a viscus is indirectly related to its radius. Assuming the ratio of the effective diameter of the esophagus to the stomach to be 1:5, the abdominal esophagus only needs to exceed in pressure one fifth of the intragastric pressure for gastroesophageal closure to occur.[18,19] The positive pressure of the abdomen acting on the intraabdominal esophagus will compensate for any further increase in the intragastric pressure. Therefore, the important determinant of function is the length exposed to the positive pressure of the abdomen. The greater the length, the more competent it becomes. DeMeester et al. showed that the minimum length was 4cm in the absence of any sphincter pressure.[15] There is no doubt about the prime importance of the length of the intraabdominal segment, and neither will there be doubt that if the intraabdominal segment of the esophagus is short or virtually nonexistent[3] in the first postnatal weeks, the important mechanical antireflux effect of having the esophagus exposed to intraabdominal pressure is lost. As the abdominal segment lengthens, an antireflux barrier is gradually established and GER disappears.

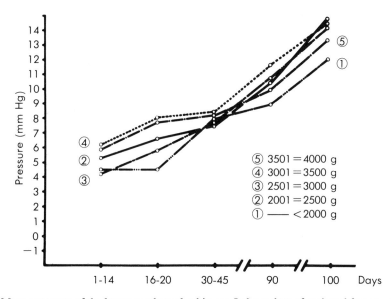

Fig. 15-1. Mean pressures of the lower esophageal sphincter. Independent of perinatal factors, all the weight groups (680 newborns) converge at 5 to 7 weeks of postnatal age to their effective maturation and gastroesophageal competence.

Gastroesophageal angle

The His angle, particularly its acuteness, plays a very important role. With an acute angle, if the patient attempts to vomit, the fluid striking the fundus decreases the angle and squeezes the esophagus closed; purely mechanical effect. If the angle is obtuse, the upper stomach is converted into a funnel, and all the fluids are directed into the esophagus. The angle principally depends on the length of the intraabdominal segment, and this is developing and lengthening during the first months of life. Only when the intraabdominal esophagus reaches adequate length will gastroesophageal competence exist. Our experimental studies[19,20] in animals show the role of the His angle in the antireflux barrier and how a minimum intraabdominal length is necessary for this to act (Figs. 15-2 and 15-3). The gastroesophageal competence is weakened in the child until this length of the intraabdominal esophagus is achieved.

Opening pressures

Very few articles have been published on the subject of opening pressures, which is of paramount importance. The surgeon has been obsessed by the reinforcement of the closing mechanisms without paying attention to the pathologic opening forces. In the infant a series of factors favor these forces.

Gastric retention

A high percentage of infants with GER have delayed gastric emptying,[21-23] placing greater stress on antireflux mechanisms.[24,25] In infants there are two facts that contribute to this delay: (1) Earlier publications have demonstrated that the fundus is of primary importance for the emptying of liquids.[26] The fundus in a sliding hernia is disturbed by displacement and cannot perform this function. (2) A normal newborn does not have a normal peristaltic wave until several weeks of age.[27] Again, a period of maturation is necessary for the normalization of gastric emptying; during this time GER is favored. This transient immaturity may involve the gastric pacemaker and the propagation of electrical activity via gastric muscle fibers.[28,29]

Lack of coordination between peristaltic waves and pyloric opening

Another factor in the early stages that raises opening pressures is lack of coordination between peristaltic waves and the pyloric opening. This situation is produced by gastritis or neurofunctional alterations leading to pyloric sphincter dysfunction and abnormal gastric responses to postprandial duodenal impulses. In small patients, ingested proteins may cause fundal or antral dysmotility with subsequent slowing of gastric emptying and an increase in the intragas-

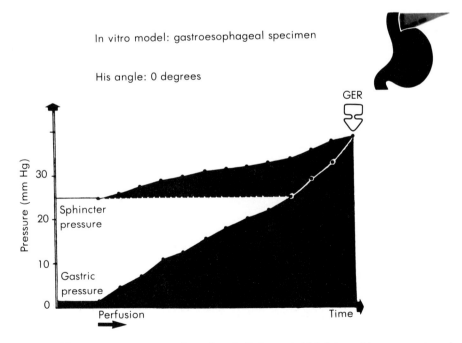

Fig. 15-2. With a very acute gastroesophageal angle (0 degrees), high intragastric pressures (opening pressures) are necessary to overcome the sphincter pressures (closing pressure) and produce gastroesophageal reflux.

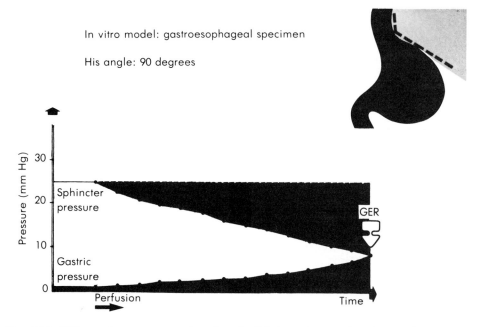

In vitro model: gastroesophageal specimen

His angle: 90 degrees

Fig. 15-3. With an obtuse gastroesophageal angle (90 degrees), very low intragastric pressures produce gastroesophageal reflux.

tric pressure.[30] The physiologic characteristics of this age clearly show that gastroesophageal reflux should be initially regarded, particularly in early infancy, as a physiologic event; only in very few cases can an operative treatment be justified.[19]

CLINICAL MANIFESTATIONS

Vomiting is the most obvious symptom of GER, but not the most important. The severity of its complications justifies the necessity of early diagnosis and treatment. We can group the clinical findings as (1) related to vomiting, (2) related to esophagitis, and (3) related to aspiration. The age of the patient and the possibility of being able to describe what he feels make the symptomatology different from one group to another.

Infants
Vomiting

Vomiting in the infant is the principal symptom. Few conclusions can be drawn from the nature of the vomitus, chronology, position in which vomiting is effected, or the type of expulsion. The important thing is that the patient vomits; how he does it is of little importance. Recurrent vomiting causes "failure to thrive." It is often the only symptom that the parents care about, since they are unaware of other complications. Severe abnormalities associated with de-

layed development in patients below the tenth percentile for weight and growth are often described.[31-33] Early recognition and specific therapy normalize the weight curve with favorable consequences for normal growth and neurologic development. Otitis is usually frequent in infants, as a consequence of the introduction of food particles into the eustachian tube when the vomit explodes into the pharynx. Dystrophy, infections (otitis), slight anemia, and anorexia worsen the clinical picture and make the parents desperate. In some cases, the surgeon has to deal with a severe social problem caused by the family's turning away from caring for a child with "feeding problems," who is chronically ill and staining the parent's clothes, furniture, and carpets with vomitus. This situation obliges the surgeon to evaluate the patient for definitive treatment.

Esophagitis and stenosis

To a greater or lesser degree, esophagitis exists in all of these patients. One main difference from the adult is that the child can show an accelerated clinical course in a few weeks, producing anemia and severe stricture. This dangerous instability is probably related to the immaturity of the local defense factors, influenced by recurrent infections, as we often observe in our patients. Smaller children cannot describe the retrosternal pain, or heartburn, but we can suspect it. Restlessness, sudden crying, brusque wakening in the night, and even behavioral disorders are evident signs of pain caused by esophagitis. Peptic esophagitis leads to blood loss and iron-deficiency anemia. Blood can be investigated in stools and sometimes the mother describes vomitus with "strands of blood" or vomitus "like coffee grounds," which points to massive hemorrhage resulting from severe esophagitis most often complicated by a stricture. Stricture is the most severe complication of GER,[34] but with greater knowledge of this disease on the part of pediatricians and early diagnosis, it is now a very unusual complication in Europe and North America, but still a nightmare in other countries where pediatric surgery is not yet a reality.

In children the first symptoms of stenosis fall like a flash of lightning; often these stenoses are spectacular and are given more importance than they deserve. An organic stricture takes a long time to evolve; otherwise the subsequent dysphagia would have appeared earlier. What often happens in children is that at a certain moment an inflammation, with a severe edema and subsequent esophageal motility dysfunction, is superimposed on a benign stenosis. If this was not the case, how can we explain that with adequate treatment the symptoms regress in such a spectacular fashion? In these cases, radiology is unable to predict the extent of the organic lesion and only esophagoscopy is of value in defining esophagitis before the progression to an organic stricture.

Aspiration and respiratory complications

The relationship between GER and pulmonary aspiration,[35,36] chronic bronchopneumopathy,[37] and even the sudden infant death syndrome[38] have been emphasized of late. However, all the reports must be carefully evaluated before the findings can be enthusiastically applied to all children with asthma or recurrent pneumonia.[39] The high incidence of respiratory problems caused by GER found in the United States is not found in Europe.[19,40] To clarify this point, we surveyed 37 major pediatric surgical centers in Europe, and respiratory problems were rarely an indication for GER surgery; 70% of the surveyed European Centers operated on less than 5% of GER surgical patients for respiratory problems.[41,42] These percentages differ completely with those from publications in the United States, where between 45% and 65% of indications for surgery are based on respiratory problems. The question of "who is right" is very difficult to answer. Nothing in medicine is ultimate. Perhaps one group overestimates the frequency and the

other underestimates this complication, and the true incidence is somewhere between these extremes. In any case, it is absolutely true that an exact demonstration of coincidence does not exist and that a single, definitive, accurate, and specific diagnosis is lacking. However, a surgeon faced with a child with severe chronic recurrent pneumonia, steroid-dependent asthma, nighttime bronchitis, or apneic spells should investigate for GER even if GER symptoms are absent.

Rumination and GER: differential diagnosis

Rumination is a voluntary regurgitation followed by an apparent chewing and swallowing, similar to the physiologic act of fractioned digestion of ruminating animals. However, there is a clear difference; the baby does not chew the regurgitated food but keeps it in his mouth, making new movements with his tongue for further regurgitation. Whereas the animal does this with a certain calm and satisfaction, the baby does it with great tension, and he looks absent and concentrated, indifferent to anything else. Rumination can lead the baby to a state of malnutrition and marasmus, which makes him prone to infections, leading to death in many cases if the condition is not diagnosed in time.

Until now only a psychologic factor has been considered the cause of this rare affectation. After studying 30 cases we arrived at the conclusion that this factor is often not the only one. It is important to determine whether either of two other factors is present, a cerebral dysfunction and a digestive factor such as "locus minore resistentia."

Psychologic factor. First, a psychologic factor is always present in a greater or lesser form. Psychoanalytic factors can be assumed in a baby who at 3 months cannot establish the first exterior contact because of lack of attention from his mother. The child then loses all interest in the outside world (objects), and he retreats inside himself and stays in the oral phase of his first months of life, when the only thing that gave him pleasure was food; with regurgitation he lengthens this pleasure past mealtimes. He becomes an autist, and other autoerotic manifestations are easily found, such as thumb sucking, hair eating, and playing with clothes and the sexual organs. The mother can also be disturbed and show signs of infantilism, narcissism, and aggressiveness.

Cerebral dysfunction. In nearly all our observations we have found an electroencephalographic alteration in the form of transitory, irritative single or multifocal points, often clinically translated as convulsive crisis. The importance of this neurologic factor has been demonstrated when some of our children have been cured through treatment of the cerebral focus.

The digestive factor. For a baby to ruminate he must have conditions that favour vomiting and regurgitation. In 22 cases we have found 5 with gastroesophageal reflux, one with gastric plicature, and another with mericism in the first months of life. We should not confuse the concept of mericism with rumination. The former appears around 2 to 3 months in an infant in a good general state. Milk trickles from the sides of the mouth with no effort from the child, and he is overfed. The differences are as follows:

Mericism	Rumination
From 3 months	Between 6 and 8 months
Good general state	Rapid malnutrition
Normal psychologic state	Neuropathic state
Passive emesis	Provoked regurgitation
No pseudomastication	False mastication and regurgitation

• • •

The cerebral dysfunction should be treated by the child neurologist with tranquilizers. Psychotherapy should be applied, and the child should be cared for by someone who shows him affection, plays with him, and gives him confidence in the outside world. The digestive anomaly, if it exists, should be treated, together with reparation of the poor general state.

Children

In children who can explain their symptoms there is not a great difference compared to the clinical picture described in adults. Abdominal pain, finger clubbing, and a protein-losing enteropathy have been described in these patients. The Sandifer syndrome is a torticollis-like anomalous posture that could be interpreted as an attempt to improve esophageal clearance. Other symptoms, such as dystonia, dysphagia, developmental retardation, irritability, seizures, and psychiatric syndromes, have been described as GER mimicking neuropsychiatric syndromes.[43]

DIAGNOSIS
Radiology

Radiology is the first line of study, and in the majority of cases it is the cornerstone for diagnosis. Roentgenography can show the existence of anatomic malpositions and serious mucosal le-

sions, but it is not conclusive in the diagnosis of GER because it shows the dynamics of the esophagus during only a short period of time[44] and because of the high incidence of false-negative results.[45,46] Nevertheless, roentgenography is an obligatory examination because of the valuable information that it supplies.

Esophagoscopy

Esophagoscopy can document lesions and their degree. It is an excellent method for evaluating mucosal lesions and the severity of a stricture. In children, however, it gives a high frequency of false-negative results.[47,48]

Esophageal biopsy

The use of esophageal biopsy in pediatric surgery has not been generalized, since it does not clarify which is the predominant factor (serious reflux or weak defense), it gives no prognosis about the complications, and it does not indicate the therapy to be followed.[49] It can give false-negative results, since the appearance of the lesions can be delayed, leading to errors as to the importance of the lesion. However, since it is a harmless procedure, it can be added to the arsenal of diagnosis.

Manometry

Manometry is useless as a diagnostic method (see Tables 15-1 and 15-2). The standard deviations are wide,[50,51] and it does not permit any conclusions, in the majority of cases, nor does it provide a reference concerning the results of medical or operative treatment.[52] However, the study of the morphology of the tracings and its alterations can be useful. In 28% of our surgical patients the tracings were morphologically altered. Manometry does have advantages, such as in locating the LES in order to place the pH elecrode in the exact position for the monitoring of reflux, to study the preoperative and postoperative lengths of the intraabdominal segment, and to study the motility disturbances related with impaired clearance.

Twenty-four hour pH monitoring of the esophagus

In 1979, five years after Johnson and De-Meester developed and standardized 24-hour pH monitoring into a useful clinical test,[53] we published the normal pattern for the pediatric age group.[54] Today, our experience with more than 250 patients is very satisfactory. When this test is used in newborns and infants, a new parameter must be added to those published for the adult,

TABLE 15-1. Statistical analysis of manometric results

Group	Results (mm Hg)
Control (n = 35)	11.8 ± 3.6
GER presurgical (n = 44)	11.22 ± 4.14
GER presurgical (n = 44)	10.72 ± 3.1
Postsurgical (n = 42)	10.90 ± 4.82
Beginning postural therapy (presurgical (n = 44)	11.22 ± 4.14
End postural therapy (n = 35)	12.66 ± 3.21
Control (n = 20)	11.8 ± 3.6
End postural therapy (n = 35)	12.66 ± 3.21

TABLE 15-2. Manometry in GER*

Group	Results (mm Hg)
Control (n = 20)	11.8 ± 3.6
Postsurgical (n = 24)	10.90 ± 4.28
Beginning postural therapy, presurgical (n = 44)	11.22 ± 4.14
End postural therapy (n = 35)	12.66 ± 3.21

*Manometry did not prove useful in the diagnosis of GER or in evaluating results of treatment.

TABLE 15-3. Normal values for 24-hour pH monitoring of the esophagus*

24-hr component	Children	Adults
Percent time pH 4		
Total period	1.86 ± 1.60	1.5 ± 1.4
Upright position	0.8 ± 1.3	2.3 ± 2
Supine position	1.59 ± 2.9	0.3 ± 0.5
Prone position	3.28 ± 3.5	
No. of reflux episodes	10.6 ± 8.2	20.6 ± 14.8
No. of reflux episodes of 5 min or longer	1.73 ± 2.05	0–6 ± 1–3
Longest reflux episodes	8.07 ± 7.19	3.9 ± 2.7

From Boix-Ochoa, J., Lafuente, J.M., and Gil Vernet, J.M.: J. Pediatr. Surg. **15:**74, 1980.
*Mean ± SD.

the prone position (see Table 15-3). Once again, in our investigations, the comparison between children and adults shows important differences: (1) While the adult tends to reflux in an erect position, the child does so in a supine or prone position. (2) In the child the prone position gives fewer but longer refluxes, of more than 5 minutes, showing that in this position the esophageal clearance is anatomically impaired. The usefulness and accuracy of this test for diagnosis, control, and investigation of the failure of postural treatment have been confirmed in our studies with 235 patients.[55] Esophageal pH monitoring also shows the effectiveness of the esophageal clearance in the pediatric field. The fact that the number of refluxes of more than five minutes is directly related to esophagitis ($p < 0.001$) is very interesting, showing once more that esophagitis depends more on the duration of the reflux than on the number of attacks. The greater the exposure, the greater the damage (see Fig. 15-4). Experience with these patients allows us to conclude that of all the parameters studied, the

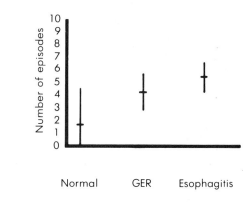

	Normal	GER	Esophagitis
N	20	44	12
Mean	1.73	4.25	5.34
±SEM	2.65	1.38	1.08

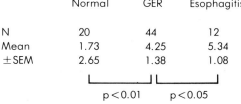

Fig. 15-4. Twenty-four-hour pH intraesophageal monitoring shows that the number of reflux episodes of more than 5 minutes (and pH<4) is significantly related (*p*<0.05) to esophagitis.

percentage of reflux time in comparison to the total period and the number of refluxes give us the diagnosis, and the number of refluxes of more than 5 minutes gives the severity. Altered esophageal clearance that does not improve with medical treatment is a serious sign and can be the deciding element for surgery. However, we do not use esophageal pH monitoring in all patients with GER. We reserve it for those cases in which there are problems of diagnosis or doubts as to the election or follow-up of therapy.

Maximal acid output

In 1975 we investigated the influence of the quantity of the reflux in the medical follow-up. We studied the influence of the amount of gastric secretion and its influence on the clinical evolution of GER.[56-58] We analyzed the relationship between maximal acid output (MAO) and the medical outcome in 125 children with GER who were undergoing medical treatment. Today our experience covers more than 600 cases. The conclusions of the study are clear and statistically significant (see Table 15-4). In infants with a high MAO—that is, with a secretion of hydrochloric acid greater than 5 mEq/L/hr/10 kg of weight after stimulation with pentagastrin—medical treatment failed significantly, whereas in those with values lower than 5 mEq the medical treatment was satisfactory (see Table 15-5). To draw conclusions from this study is a delicate matter; we do say that a high MAO (hypersecretion, hyperacidity) points to failure of medical

treatment, but in our experience, if the medical treatment fails, usually it happens with a high MAO. Actually, we perform this test only in patients in whom postural treatment has failed. The result is a complement that helps us make a decision about surgery. An unsatisfactory medical outcome with a high MAO results in performing surgery. With a normal MAO we insist on further medical treatment. Another application is that when the clinical symptoms have disappeared and the radiologic findings persist with a high MAO, we continue with the medical treatment.

Gastroesophageal scintiscan

A gastroesophageal scintiscan is a good test because of the data it offers, its scarce radiation, and the fact that it can be done in the outpatient department. It provides information regarding not only the presence of GER[59] but also alterations in gastric emptying and esophageal clearance.[60,61] It can also document the relationship between GER and respiratory symptoms.

Since one year ago we in our department have been using a gammagraphical study of the dynamics of deglutition and its alterations. The technique is based on deglutition of technetium 99m sulphur colloid. By means of the parametric composition of the images obtained it allows us to study the time of esophageal transit, the percentage of esophageal retention with alterations of esophageal clearance, and the velocity of progression of the bolus. The excellent results obtained (see Figs. 15-5 to 15-7) in more than 40 children

TABLE 15-4. Basal and maximal acid output*

| Group | No. of cases | Acid output (mEq/hr/10 kg) | |
		Basal	Maximal
Cardiohiatal anomalies			
Good response	64	0.53 ± 0.57	3.62 ± 1.65
Poor response	41	1.07 ± 0.77	6.06 ± 2.28
Control	20	0.72 ± 0.84	3.83 ± 1.31

*Mean ± SD.

TABLE 15-5. MAO differences

Group	mEq/hr/10 kg	p
Cardiohiatal anomalies (good response)	3.62 ± 1.65	NS*
Control	3.83 ± 1.31	
Cardiohiatal anomalies (poor response)	6.06 ± 2.28	<0.001
Control	3.83 ± 1.31	
Cardiohiatal anomalies (good response)	3.62 ± 1.65	<0.001
Cardiohiatal anomalies (poor response)	6.05 ± 2.28	

From Casasa, J.M., and Boix-Ochoa, J.: Surgery **82:**573, 1977.
*NS, not significant.

make us use this technique systematically for all the problems in which we suspect alterations of motility. The technique's lack of morbidity, its minimal radiation, its rapidity, and its accuracy have convinced us of its usefulness.

THERAPY

Medical or surgical? This is the problem. The percentages of patients treated medically and surgically vary enormously from one publication to another, confusing more than a few. Perhaps the choice of therapy has depended on whether the patient has been seen at the onset of symptoms by a pediatric surgeon, or whether he has been referred by a pediatrician after therapy has been tried. However, the truth remains that the therapeutic decisions vary according to the surgeon's philosophy.

In pediatrics, our philosophy is based on a series of fundamental facts, which Carré emphasized and which we have presented in this chapter[1, 2,19]:

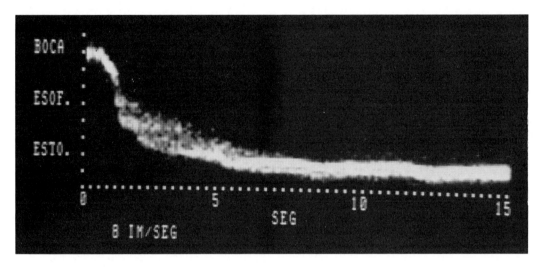

Fig. 15-5. Swallowing image: normal. Esophageal transit of 3 to 4 seconds without posterior retention of tracing. *BOCA*, Mouth; *ESOF.*, esophagus; *ESTO.*, stomach; *SEG*, seconds. Posterior retention-delayed retention in the tracing.

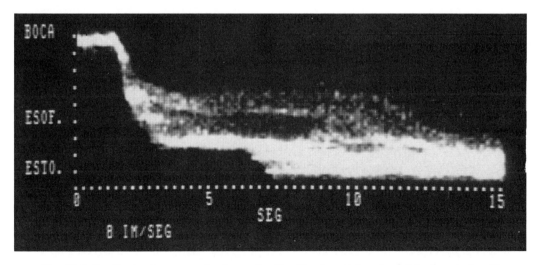

Fig. 15-6. Swallowing image: moderate esophagitis. Esophageal transit of 5 to 6 seconds with division of the bolus midway and retention of the tracing in the lower half of a 10-second duration.

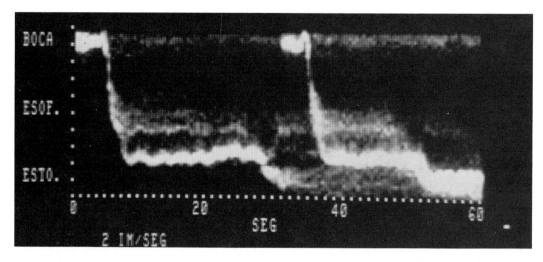

Fig. 15-7. Swallowing image: severe esophagitis. In the two deglutitions studied, a transit time of 25 seconds is observed, with division of the bolus midway in the esophagus and various zones of retention of the tracing of more than 30 seconds' duration.

1. Reflux does not mean incompetence. It is important to know the difference between what is acceptable as physiologic and what might be called pathologic. In the first months of life all conditions for reflux are normally present. A surgical decision in this period must be based on a very firm argument.
2. A displaced healthy sphincter may become incompetent; therefore incompetence does not mean sphincter pathology. In children a displaced healthy sphincter is often observed.
3. A physiologic closing pressure can be overcome by a pathologic opening pressure. Maturation of the gastric emptying and gastric wall peristalsis in the first months of life can require a certain period of time.
4. By stopping esophagitis and breaking the vicious circle we can give the LES a chance for maturation and normalization.
5. The main thing is to gain time so that a weak or displaced but healthy sphincter can recover its function.

Our therapy tends to be conservative during the first 12 months of life (only 4.2% of interventions in 1525 children less than 1 year old); from this age onward our therapy is more aggressive (surgery in 20%) (see Fig. 15-8).

Nonoperative treatment

Nonoperative treatment is based on three pillars: postural, feeding, and drugs.

Postural treatment

Since Carré's and Roviralta's publications on the natural history of GER in children,[1,62,63] postural treatment has consisted of placing the patient at an angle of 45 to 60 degrees.[64-66] In our European survey of 37 major children's hospitals, this position was successfully used in 97% of the centers. Recent publications have stressed the advantage of a prone position at 45 degrees, but our experience, our results, and our own investigations do not convince us that we should change our attitude. The high percentage of success (95%) is influenced by certain regulations: (1) Continuous treatment for 24 hours a day for a minimum of 3 to 6 months is of paramount importance. (2) Disappearance of symptoms does not mean that the reflux has disappeared. Treatment has to be continued as established.

Feeding

Frequent small feedings should be given to maintain the stomach in a half-empty state. Only in severe cases have we used a continuous nasogastric drip. We do not thicken feedings, although other authors recommend it.

Drugs

In the presence of esophagitis, it is reasonable to administer antacids. Drugs must be used if the improvement is slow or the patient is older. In severe cases we use cimetidine to break the vicious circle; however, when treatment is discontinued, care must be taken because of the rebound

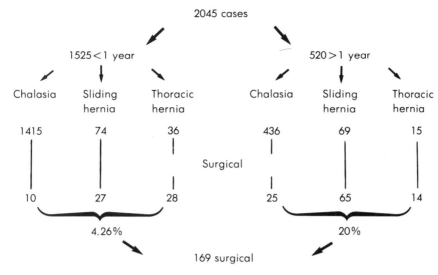

Fig. 15-8. Between 1966 and 1983, 2045 patients with GER were seen at our hospital. After 1 year of age, 20% received surgical therapy; under 1 year our therapy tends to be conservative.

effect. Mild sedatives in irritable patients are used, and in patients who do not respond to postural treatment, domperidone or bethanecol is a big help, pontentiating or normalizing gastric emptying.

• • •

We believe that nonoperative treatment should be tried in most patients of less than 16 months of age, but there are absolute indications for operation at any age, based on the impossibility or failure of medical treatment or on some severe respiratory complications. Our policy for infants of less than 16 months is to perform an operation if medical treatment controlled by 24-hour pH monitoring fails and the MAO is too high.

Operative treatment

The pediatric surgeon has at his or her disposal a variety of surgical techniques that offer good results, low mortality (1% to 3%) and few complications. Today, the most widely used procedure is that originally described by Nissen and adapted for children. The Belsey Mark IV procedure, the Hill posterior gastropexy, and the Collis gastroplasty are similar and satisfy the basic requirements for any antireflux operation. By contrast, the Boerema gastropexy in children has been rejected because of the high rate of failures it presents. The disadvantages of these techniques in children are the inability to vomit or to burp and the "gas bloat" syndrome, which can be avoided with the Thal-Ashcraft procedure, which minimizes the risk of complications.[42]

Our philosophy is very clear: we are aware that all of these techniques give excellent results, create ingenious valves, are easily performed, and have very low mortality. However, we think that the Nissen technique, although excellent, is not appropriate for children, since the conditions of the adult differ greatly from those of the infant. Therefore, in surgical treatment our philosophy is that in the child we are treating a patient with a LES that is altered because of displacement but that can be competent since it is not seriously damaged. Therefore, an operation that restores its anatomic minimums, the growth and evolution, will restore its physiology.[67] This situation is contrary to that in the adult, who can only expect a more or less perfect repair of an altered and lesioned LES.

Pediatric surgery is based on the principle that children are not "small adults" and on the potential possibilities for recuperation of a developing being. Therefore, the question is very clear: shall we try to restore and improve the function of an organ, or shall we try to replace it?

Our technique is to reinforce the anatomic relationship based on the described physiology.

1. Restore the length of the intraabdominal esophagus (Fig. 15-9, *A*).
2. Tighten the hiatus and anchor the esophagus there (Fig. 15-9, *B*).
3. Restore the angle of His by a suture from the fundus at the level of the first short gastric to the rim of the right hiatus (Fig. 15-9, *C*). After we place the important angle of His suture, we then place a few reinforcing sutures from the fundus to the

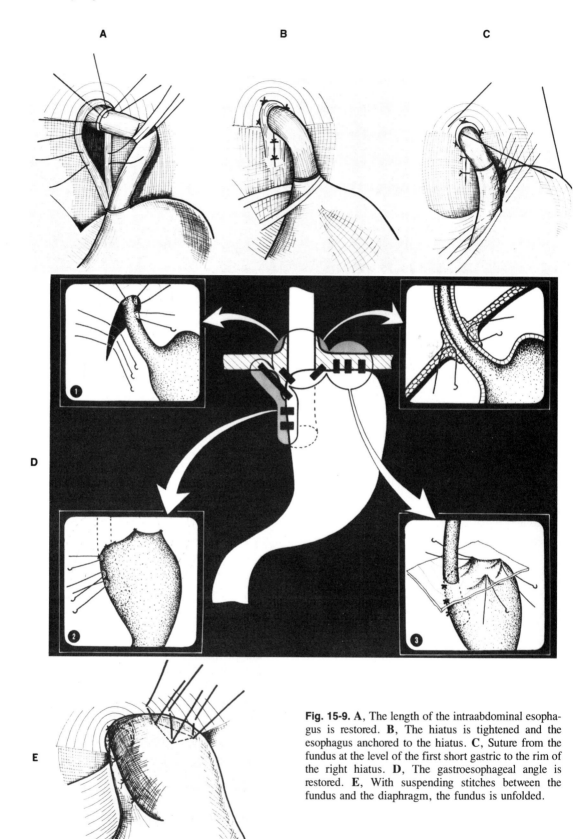

Fig. 15-9. A, The length of the intraabdominal esophagus is restored. **B**, The hiatus is tightened and the esophagus anchored to the hiatus. **C**, Suture from the fundus at the level of the first short gastric to the rim of the right hiatus. **D**, The gastroesophageal angle is restored. **E**, With suspending stitches between the fundus and the diaphragm, the fundus is unfolded.

TABLE 15-6. Results of operative treatment
(follow-up: 2 to 16 years, 165 of 169 patients*)

	Number of patients	Percent
Initial good result	163	98
Failure first procedure[†]	2	1.2
Radiologic recurrence (symptom free)	10	6

*Includes 4 lost to follow-up.
[†]Paraesophageal hernia and too short intraabdominal esophagus.

anterior wall of the esophagus (Fig. 15-9, *D*).

4. Now we have accomplished the following things: (a) narrowed the hiatus, (b) lengthened the intraabdominal esophagus, (c) restored the angle of His. The final step is in opening up or unfolding the fundus much as we would open up an umbrella. We do this with suspending stitches between the fundus and the diaphragm (Fig. 15-9, *E*).

In summary, what have we achieved with this operation? An intraabdominal segment of the esophagus has been developed, which restores normal closing pressures; the sharpening of the His angle ensures the mechanical action of compressing the esophagus and closing it; and unfolding the fundus of the stomach causes buffering of intragastric pressure and mechanical closing of the esophagus. The excellent results achieved with follow-up periods of up to 16 years have convinced us that this physiologic approach to the management of GER is a sound one (see Table 15-6).

REFERENCES

1. Carré, I.J.: Natural history of partial thoracic stomach ("hiatus hernia") in children, Arch. Dis. Child. **34:**344, 1959.
2. Carré, I.J.: Clinical significance of gastroesophageal reflux, Arch. Dis. Child. **59:**911, 1984.
3. Fyke, F.E., Code, C.F., and Schlegel, J.F.: The gastroesophageal sphincter in healthy human beings, Gastroenterologia (Basel) **86:**135, 1956.
4. Winans, C.S., and Harris, L.D.: Quantitation of lower esophageal sphincter competence, Gastroenterology **52:**773, 1967.
5. Rattan, S., and Goyal, R.K.: Neural control of the lower esophageal sphincter, J. Clin. Invest. **54:**899, 1974.
6. Liebermann, D.: Anatomie des gastroesophagealen Verschluss organs. In Blum, A.L., and Siewert, J.R., editors: Reflux therapie, Berlin, 1981, Springer.
7. Liebermann, D., Allgower, M., Schmid, P., et al.: Muscular equivalent of the lower esophageal sphincter, Gastroenterology **76:**31, 1979.
8. Liebermann-Meffert, D.: Muscular equivalent of the lower esophageal sphincter: pathological gastroesophageal reflux. In van Heukelem, H.A., editor: Proceedings of the Workshop on Diagnosis and Treatment of GER, Leiden, November 1982, pp. 9-16.
9. Creamer, B., and Pierce, J.W.: Observations on the gastroesophageal junction during swallowing and drinking, Lancet **2:**1309, 1957.
10. Gryboski, J.D.: The swallowing mechanism of the neonate: esophageal and gastric motility, Pediatrics **35:**445, 1965.
11. Boix-Ochoa, J., and Canals, J.: Maturation of the lower esophageal sphincter, J. Pediatr. Surg. **11:**749, 1979.
12. Boix-Ochoa, J.: Diagnosis and management of gastroesophageal reflux in children, Surg. Ann. **13:**123, 1981.
13. Koenig, W., Kehrer, B., and Bettex, M.: Le sphincter inferieur de l'oesophage chez le nouveau-né, Etude manometrique, Chir. Pediatr. (Paris) **23:**357, 1982.
14. Cohen, S.: Developmental characteristics of lower esophageal sphincter function: a possible mechanism for infantile chalasia, Gastroenterology **67:**252, 1978.
15. DeMeester, T.R., Wernly, J.A., Bryant, C.H., et al.: Clinical and in vitro analysis of gastroesophageal competence: a study of principles of antireflux surgery, Am. J. Surg. **137:**39, 1979.
16. Edwards, D.A.W., Thompson, H., Shaw, D.G., et al.: Symposium of gastroesophageal reflux and its complications, Gut **14:**233, 1973.
17. Johnson, H.D.: The antireflux mechanism in the cardia and hiatus, Springfield, Ill., 1968 Charles C Thomas, Publisher, pp. 57-59.
18. Winans, C.S., and Harris, L.D.: Quantitation of lower esophageal sphincter competence, Gastroenterology **52:**773, 1967.
19. Boix-Ochoa, J.: Physiological management of GER in children, J. Pediatr. Surg. **21:**1032, 1986.
20. Bardaji, C., and Boix-Ochoa, J.: Importancia del angulo de Hiss en la competencia del esofago terminal, 1986. (In preparation.)
21. Hillemeier, A.C., Lange, R., McCallum, R. et al.: Delayed gastric emptying in infants with gastroesophageal reflux, J. Pediatr. **98:**190, 1981.
22. Hillemeier, A.C., Gribosky, J.D., Lange, R., et al.: Gastric emptying in gastroesophageal reflux in infancy, J. Pediatr. **98:**190, 1981.
23. Andres, J., Hamsley, L.S., and Mathias, J.R.: Measurement of gastric emptying in infants with technetium-99m-labelled solid phase meal, Pediatr. Res. **14:**495, 1980.
24. Cavell, B.: Gastric emptying in infants, Lancet **2:**409, 1969.
25. Cavell, B.: Gastric emptying in infants, Acta Pediatr. Scand. **60:**370, 1971.
26. Dozois, R.R., Kelly, K.A., and Code, C.F.: Effects of distal antrectomy on gastric emptying of liquids and solids, Gastroenterology **61:**675, 1971.
27. Tornwall, L., Lind, J., Peltonen, and Wegebis.: The gastrointestinal tract of the newborn, Ann. Pediatr. Finn. **4:**219, 1958.
28. Hunt, J.N., and Knox, M.T.: Regulation of gastric emptying. In Code, C.F., editor: Handbook of physiol-

ogy, Washington, 1968, American Physiological Society, section 6, vol. 4, Ch. 94.

29. Kelly, A.K.: Motility of the stomach and gastroduodenal junction. In Johnson, L.R., editor: Physiology of gastrointestinal tract, New York, 1981, Raven Press, Ch. 12.

30. Code, C.F.: The mystique of the gastroduodenal junction, Rendic. R. Gastroenterol. **2:**20, 1970.

31. Euler, A.R., and Ament, M.E.: Gastroesophageal reflux in children: clinical manifestations, diagnosis, pathophysiology and therapy, Pediatr. Ann. **5:**678, 1976.

32. Voss, A., and Boerema, I.: Surgical treatment of gastroesophageal reflux in infants and children: long term results in 28 cases, J. Ped. Surg. **6:**101, 1971.

33. Randolph, J.G., Lilly, J.R., and Anderson, K.D.: Surgical treatment of gastroesophageal reflux in infants, Ann. Surg. **180:**479, 1974.

34. Boix-Ochoa, J., and Rehbein, F.: Esophageal stenosis due to reflux esophagitis, Arch. Dis. Child. **40:**197, 1965.

35. Danus, O., Casar, C., Larrain, A., et al.: Esophageal reflux: an unrecognized cause of recurrent obstructive bronchitis in children, J. Pediatr. **89:**220, 1976.

36. Darling, D.B., McCauley, R.G.K., et al.: Gastroesophageal reflux in infants and children: correlation of radiological severity and pulmonary pathology, Radiology **127:**735, 1978.

37. Herbst, J.J.: Gastroesophageal reflux and pulmonary disease, Pediatrics **68:**132, 1981.

38. Leape, L.: Gastroesophageal reflux as a cause of the sudden infant death. Ross Conference on Gastroesophageal Reflux, Sydney S. Gellis, March 1978.

39. Walsh, J.K., Farrell, M.K., Keenan, W.J., et al.: Gastroesophageal reflux in infants: relation to apnea, J. Pediatr. **99:**197, 1981.

40. Leape, L., Holder, T., Franklin, J., et al.: Respiratory arrests in infants secondary to gastroesophageal reflux, Pediatrics **60:**924, 1977.

41. Jolley, S.G., Herbst, J.J., Johnson, D.G., et al.: Surgery in children with gastroesophageal reflux and respiratory symptoms, J. Pediatr. **96:**194, 1980.

42. Ashcraft, K.W., Holder, T.M., and Amoury, R.A.: Treatment of gastroesophageal reflux in children by Thal fundoplication, J. Thorac. Cardiovasc. Surg. **82:**706, 1981.

43. Bray, P.F., et al.: Childhood GER: neurologic and psychiatric syndromes mimicked, JAMA **237:**1342, 1977.

44. Benz, L.J., Hootkin, L.A., Margulies, S., et al.: A comparison of clinical measurements of gastroesophageal reflux, Gastroenterology **62:**1, 1972.

45. Edwards, D.A.W., Thompson, H., Shaw, D.G., et al.: Symposium of gastroesophageal reflux and its complications, Gut **14:**233, 1973.

46. Johnson, D.G., Herbst, J.J., Oliveros, M.A., et al.: Evaluation of gastroesophageal reflux surgery in children, Pediatrics **59:**62, 1977.

47. DeMeester, T.R., and Johnson, L.F.: The evaluation of objective measurement of gastroesophageal reflux and their contribution to patient management, Surg. Clin. North Am. **56:**39, 1976.

48. Katz, D., and Hoffmann, F.: The esophagogastric junction, Excerpta Medica Symposium, November 1969.

49. Leape, L.L., Bhan, I., and Ramenofsky, M.L.: Esophageal biopsy in the diagnosis of reflux esophagitis, J. Pediatr. Surg. **16:**379, 1981.

50. Herbst, J.J., and Johnson, D.G.: Gastroesophageal manometry in children with gastroesophageal reflux, Clin. Res. **8:**108, 1974.

51. Euler, A.R., and Ament, M.E.: Value of esophageal manometric studies in the gastroesophageal reflux of infancy, Pediatrics **59:**1, Jan. 1977.

52. Boix-Ochoa, J.: Gastroesophageal reflux in pediatrics: experience in 2000 cases. In DeMeester, T.R., and Skinner, D.B., editors: Esophageal disorders: pathophysiology and therapy, New York, 1985, Raven Press, pp. 459-468.

53. Johnson, L.F., and DeMeester, T.R.: Twenty-four hour pH monitoring of the distal esophagus: quantitative measure of gastroesophageal reflux, Am. J. Gastroenterol. **63:**325, 1974.

54. Boix-Ochoa, J., Lafuente, J.M., and Gil Vernet, J.M.: 24-hour esophageal pH monitoring in gastroesophageal reflux, J. Pediatr. Surg. **15:**74, 1980.

55. Boix-Ochoa, J.: Pediatric aspects of 24-hour pH monitoring. In DeMeester, T.R., and Skinner, D.B., editors: Esophageal disorders: pathophysiology and therapy, New York, 1985, Raven Press, pp. 617-620.

56. Jepson, J.B., et al.: Acid and pepsin response to gastrin, pentagastrin, tetragastrin and histamine, Lancet **20:**159, 1962.

57. Lari, J., Lister, J., and Duthie, J.G.: Response to gastrin pentapeptide in children, J. Pediatr. Surg. **3:**6, 1968.

58. Casasa, J.M., and Boix-Ochoa, J.: Surgical or conservative treatment in hiatal hernia in children: a new decisive parameter, Surgery **82:**573, 1977.

59. Fisher, R.S., Malmud, L.S., Roberts, G.S., et al.: Gastroesophageal scintiscanning to detect a quantitate G.E. reflux, Gastroenterology **70:**301, 1976.

60. Heymann, S., Kirkpatrick, J.A., Witnes, H.S., et al.: An improved radionuclide method for the diagnosis of gastroesophageal reflux and aspiration in children (milk scan), Radiology **131:**479, 1979.

61. Rudd, T.G., and Christie, D.L.: Demonstration of gastroesophageal reflux in children by radionuclide gastroesophagography, Radiology **131:**483, 1979.

62. Roviralta, E.: El lactante vomitador, Barcelona, 1950, Jané Ed.

63. Roviralta, E., Martinez Mora, J., and Casasa, J.M.: Malformaciones esofago-diafragmaticas, Rev. Esp. Ped. **16:**835, 1960.

64. Meyers, W.F., and Herbst, J.J.: Effectiveness of positioning therapy for gastroesophageal reflux, Pediatrics **69:**768, 1982.

65. Orenstein, S.R., Whitington, P.F., and Orenstein, D.M.: The infant seat as treatment for gastroesophageal reflux, N. Engl. J. Med. **309:**760, 1983.

66. Carré, I.J.: Postural treatment of children with partial thoracic stomach ("hiatus hernia"), Arch. Dis. Child. **35:**569, 1960.

67. Boix-Ochoa, J., Casasa, J.M., and Gil Vernet, J.M.: Une chirugie phisiologique pour les anomalies du secteur cardiohiatal, Chir. Pediatr. **24:**117, 1983.

Children and reflux

DISCUSSION

Raymond A. Amoury

In "Children and Reflux" Dr. Boix-Ochoa has clearly outlined several aspects of gastroesophageal reflux as seen in pediatric patients, especially in those under 1 year of age.[1,2]

PATHOPHYSIOLOGY

The pathophysiology of GER can be examined in the light of normal esophageal anatomy and function. Several anatomic factors have been cited as playing a role in preventing GER.[3] These are (1) the phrenoesophageal ligament; (2) the mucosal choke, consisting of folds of gastric mucosa that are presumed to close the gastroesophageal junction; (3) the muscular contractions of the diaphragmatic crus; (4) the acute angle of entry of the esophagus into the stomach (angle of His); (5) the intraabdominal position of the esophagus (or lack of it in young infants); and (6) the lower esophageal sphincter mechanism.

The first three factors are of uncertain importance in preventing GER.[3] Boix-Ochoa has focused on the role of the LES and the length of the intraabdominal esophagus in serving as barriers to GER. The pioneering concept of maturation of the lower esophagus in very young infants was derived from the careful and extensive studies carried out by Dr. Boix-Ochoa and his coworkers at The Children's Hospital Vall d'Hebron, Barcelona, Spain. These studies greatly added to our knowledge of GER, both its evolution in very young infants and the natural history of GER to regress with increasing postnatal age, without any therapy.

Most authors do not recognize an anatomic LES, since distinct sphincteric fibers are not grossly or histologically identifiable in the lower esophagus. Physiologically, however, a high-pressure zone is normally present and can be identified manometrically in the lower esophagus above and below the diaphragm. An exception to the lack of recognition of an anatomic LES is the work of Liebermann-Meffert, et al.[4] who have identified a thickened, asymmetrical, muscular segment located in the same area as the manometrically determined high-pressure zone of the distal esophagus. Boix-Ochoa considers this structure as the possible muscular counterpart of the LES, and closely relates its development to the competence of the LES. This is presumably the most definitive anatomic correlate of the LES, and it can also be related to Boix-Ochoa's concept[2] of maturation of the lower esophageal sphincter, which is not completely developed at birth.

The majority of authors consider the LES to be the most important barrier to GER in normal individuals.

Closing pressures
High-pressure zone, sphincter pressures, and length

On the basis of Boix-Ochoa's manometric studies, the length of the intraabdominal esophagus increases with days of postnatal age as compared with the length of the intrathoracic esophagus.[1] This lengthening of the intraabdominal segment, along with maturation of the musculature of the lower esophageal sphincter region, allows for the achievement of higher closing pressures of the esophagus. This serves as a barrier against the "opening pressures" generated by those forces also outlined by Boix-Ochoa. These forces are chiefly intragastric. They relate largely to gastric peristalsis, fundal and antral motility, and pyloric contractility.

Recent experimental and clinical work by Bonavina et al.[5] has attempted to integrate the length of the distal esophageal sphincter, sphincter pressures, and competence of the cardia. For example, these authors showed that resistance to flow through the cardia is related to the integrated effect of distal esophageal sphincter pressure and length. Gastric dilatation has an adverse effect on the degree of competence achieved by a given distal esophageal sphincter length. The dilated stomach may incorporate some of the sphincter into the cardial mechanism and thereby shorten it. The authors concluded that patients with an overall distal esophageal sphincter length of 2 cm or less (measured at rest in the fasting state) are subject to reflux caused by gastric dilatation and increased intragastric pressure, independent of intraabdominal pressure. This type of precise study is important in our evolving understanding of GER.

Role of innervation, neurotransmitters, hormones, and related agents in GER

Other factors that appear important include innervation and the effects of neurotransmitters and multiple hormones in modulating the functions of the LES region. Boix-Ochoa has noted the intragastric forces, and it is appropriate here to add a comment on the above factors, which have been reviewed as they apply to the LES.[3]

Innervation. The innervation of the sphincter appears to be important. The intimate relationship of the vagus nerves to the esophagus and the gastroesophageal junction as well as to the sympathetic nerve supply has been examined. The effect of the vagus nerves on the sphincter zone is controversial. Some investigators believe that stimulation of these nerves can cause either contraction or relaxation of the LES, depending upon the rate and intensity of the stimulus, and the state of tone of the sphincter at the time of impulse propagation. In regard to the sympathetic nervous system, most workers feel that this part of the autonomic innervation plays little or no part in regulating the tone of the esophagogastric sphincter region.

It is pertinent here to note the well-recognized clinical relationship between the central nervous system and the LES, as is suggested in infants and children with severe brain damage and gastroesophageal reflux. In these children GER may be mediated from higher centers through the innervation of the esophagus. Experiments producing chronic brain injury in cats by elevating intracranial pressure with balloon catheters have demonstrated reduced LES pressures when intracranial pressure was elevated.[6] Another interesting observation is the appearance of GER in neurologically impaired children following gastrostomy.[7] The mechanisms explaining these findings are unclear. Clinically, the evolution of GER is a real possibility, and serious consideration should be given to complementing a gastrostomy with an antireflux procedure in these patients, whether or not GER is demonstrated preoperatively.

In summary, a physiologic sphincter is present at the gastroesophageal junction. It is the main barrier to reflux of gastric contents. The angle of His and the oblique gastric sling fibers do not appear important in the prevention of gastroesophageal reflux, although Boix-Ochoa adds greater emphasis to the angle of His and includes its reconstitution in his operative correction for GER.

Neurotransmitters, hormones, related agents, and other factors increasing LES pressures. Acetylcholine, urecholine, metoclopramide, gastrin, and certain peptones—all have the property of increasing LES pressures, as do inceased intragastric pressure and alkalinization of the stomach.

NEUROTRANSMITTERS. The responses of the sphincter zone to the neurotransmitter acetylcholine and the effect of adrenergic drugs have not been uniform. In some experimental animals acetylcholine causes contraction of both the circular and longitudinal muscles of the sphincter, while epinephrine relaxes the circular muscle. The role of parasympathomimetic drugs on the pathogenesis of lower esophageal sphincter incompetence has been studied by Lipshutz et al.[8] Two groups of adults were examined—the first with symptomatic gastroesophageal reflux, and the second with no symptoms, whose members served as controls. In both the symptomatic and control groups the lower esophageal sphincter response to direct muscle stimulation by the parasympathomimetic drug bethanechol chloride was identified. There was a significant increase in LES pressures above basal levels, and the effect of the cholinesterase inhibitor edrophonium chloride was identical in the two groups.

GASTRIN. Gastrin has been the most extensively studied hormone with a regulatory effect on LES pressure. The serum gastrin level is increased following the instillation of protein or alkali into the stomach, and although an increase in LES pressure can be seen in control and reflux patients, there is significantly less response in the reflux group to this endogenously released gastrin. In addition, the degree of serum gastrin elevation is not sufficient to account completely for the difference in LES pressures in the two groups.[9] In the study of Lipshutz et al.[8] the response to endogenous gastrin release was also diminished in those patients having reflux. This was in contrast to the dose-response curves of LES pressure resulting from administration of exogenous intravenous pentagastrin, which showed similar responses in patients with symptomatic reflux and in control subjects.

The role of gastrin as a major determinant of basal LES pressure has been further studied in opossums by the experimental reduction of 90%

of circulating gastrin by antibody binding. This did not result in modification of basal LES pressures, although it did antagonize or abolish the stimulating effect of gastrin on lower esophageal sphincter pressure.[10]

In short, it is unlikely that defects in the synthesis or release of gastrin, or in the sensitivity of the sphincter to it, can account entirely for LES incompetence.[11]

Opening pressures

Boix-Ochoa has highlighted the "other side" of GER, namely the forces and factors leading to the "opening" of the antireflux barrier. These include gastric retention, acidification, and lack of coordination between peristaltic waves and the opening of the pyloric sphincter. To these factors should be added the hormones that facilitate "opening" by relaxing the LES. Secretin, prostaglandin, cholecystokinin, glucagon, vasopressin, and gastric inhibitory peptide all cause a decrease in LES pressure and, presumably, favor reflux.

CLINICAL MANIFESTATIONS

Boix-Ochoa describes the clinical manifestations of GER in infants and older children. He discusses vomiting, otitis media, esophagitis and stenosis, and mericism and rumination. The incidences of otitis media and esophagitis are not well defined in our patients. We have seldom seen roentgenographic evidence of esophagitis and carry out esophagoscopy and mucosal biopsy only in selected patients. Stenosis of the esophagus as a result of a peptic stricture is decidedly uncommon in our experience.

Aspiration and respiratory complications

Respiratory complications constitute a major indication for operative management of our patients with GER. It is appropriate to present our experience with this group in some detail, since it varies considerably from Boix-Ochoa's, and from that of other European centers.

The association between gastroesophageal reflux and pulmonary disease is well established, with some of the mechanisms clearly recognized, while others are less certain, or speculative. The subject has been reviewed in detail by Boyle and co-workers.[12] The authors focused on bronchospasm as a consequence of GER, with various modes of activation of the airways without roentgenographic or clinical evidence of pneumonitis. They also indicated that the high frequency of coexistence of the two conditions (20% to 65%)

suggests that bronchospasm itself may be important in the pathogenesis of GER. The authors note that potential mechanisms whereby acidic gastric contents can trigger bronchospasm include (1) overt macroaspiration of gastric contents associated with chemical pneumonitis; (2) microaspiration of gastric fluid, causing stimulation of upper airway (tracheal) receptors with marked increase in total lung resistance; and (3) stimulation of esophageal mucosal receptors by intraesophageal acidification alone. In experiments carried out by Boyle et al.[12] the latter mechanism produced a much smaller airway response than did intratracheal acidification. Such studies underscore the high incidence and clinical importance of respiratory complications of GER in North America.

Ashcraft et al.[13] have reviewed and presented the data derived from 146 patients seen at The Children's Mercy Hospital, Kansas City, Missouri. These patients represent almost one third of those in our hospital who have undergone fundoplication for all indications. This number did not include patients who had acute respiratory complications of GER—primarily aborted sudden infant death syndrome (SIDS) or severe apnea.

FUNDOPLICATION FOR CHRONIC RESPIRATORY DISEASE IN CHILDREN

Ashcraft et al.[13] reported the manifestations of chronic respiratory disease seen secondary to GER and divided them into two patterns:

1. A crouplike syndrome without fever or other evidence of infection. This often occurs acutely following an afternoon nap. In the same category are patients with chronic night coughing or choking episodes, which may or may not be associated with overt reflux. In addition, some children present with a clinical picture of asthma with wheezing but without other findings of chronic bronchial asthma, such as a well-defined allergic history.

2. Continuous or recurrent pneumonitis. Many of these patients have multiple lobes involved, and many have had multiple hospitalizations for pneumonia.

Treatment is the same in each group. After an appropriate workup aimed at documenting GER as the probable cause of the lung disease, nonoperative management is attempted by the use of thickened feedings and positional therapy. In patients under 6 months of age this is usually successful. In older patients there is considerable difficulty in keeping them in a near-upright position, and prolonged medical therapy is not pursued. Fundoplication is indicated in cases of failure of nonoperative management.

At The Children's Mercy Hospital, our preference for an antireflux procedure is the anterior fundoplication described by Thal[14] and modified for use in children by Ashcraft.[15]

Results

One hundred and forty-five patients underwent Thal-Ashcraft fundoplications for chronic respiratory symptoms attributed to GER. Results were evaluated as follows:

1. Excellent. An excellent result was attributed to patients whose reflux was stopped, as shown either by barium study or clinically. This group had complete symptomatic relief from respiratory complications.
2. Good. A good result was attributed to patients who had mild, persistent gastro-esophageal reflux, but were asymptomatic.
3. Fair. A fair result was assigned to patients who had improvements in other manifestations of reflux but whose croup, cough, or choking continued.
4. Poor. A poor result was recorded in patients whose conditions were completely unimproved by fundoplication.

The latter two categories can be considered as "errors in selection." The categories and results are summarized in Table 15-7.

Crouplike syndrome: croup, cough, choking, and asthma

Fifty-six patients had croup, cough, choking, or asthma as their respiratory symptoms. Fifty-one had no further GER either clinically or by postoperative barium study. Three patients were demonstrated to have developed a hiatus hernia within 4 months of operation. They underwent secondary operation with restoration of competence in all. Two had low-grade GER postoperatively.

Four of the 56 patients were not improved and are considered "errors in selection." They all had GER, but it was not the cause of their respiratory problems. In all of these patients, reflux did not seem related to the clinical symptoms, but this was discernable only "after the fact" of an adequate fundoplication. They represent 7% of the patients, and GER had been diagnosed by a markedly abnormal barium study alone. All four of these patients had severe concomitant lesions.

Ninety-three percent of these patients were successfully treated by fundoplication, with good or excellent relief of their respiratory disorders. The 53 surviving patients were followed for a total of 1736 patient months, for an average of 33 months (range, 1 to 96 months).

Continuous or recurrent pneumonitis

In Ashcraft's review[13] 89 patients underwent 90 fundoplications because of continuous or recurent episodes of pneumonitis.

Continuous pneumonitis. Twenty-five of the patients had virtually continuous pneumonitis. The median age in this group was 3 months at the time of fundoplication, with ages ranging from 2 weeks to 9 months. Six of these patients had severe congenital heart disease; two had esophageal atresia and tracheoesophageal fistula. Five patients had severe mental-motor retardation, with four succumbing from complications of their retardation at 2 weeks, 6 months, 8 months, and 11 months, respectively, following operation.

Five patients required parenteral nutrition and nasogastric suction to allow for clearing of their pneumonitis prior to fundoplication. Sixteen pa-

TABLE 15-7. Results of Thal-Ashcroft fundoplications for chronic respiratory symptoms attributed to GER

	No. of patients	Errors in selection	Fundoplication failure	Average follow-up
Crouplike syndrome				
Croup, cough, choking, asthma	56	4 (7%)	3 (3%)	33 mo
Pneumonitis	89			
Continuous	(25)	4 (16%)	1 (4%)	24 mo
Recurrent episodes	(64)	4 (6%)	2 (6.3%)	30 mo
TOTALS	145	12 (8%)	6 (4%)	

From Ashcraft, K.W., et al.: Fundoplication as treatment for chronic respiratory disease in children. Presented at the International Congress of Paediatric Surgery, Perth, Australia, March 7, 1984.

tients were felt to have an excellent result from fundoplication.

Four of the 25 patients were listed as "errors in selection." All four had severe congenital heart disease and did not improve after fundoplication.

In summary, the group with continuous pneumonitis responded well. The selection error rate was 16% (4 of 25), but of the remaining 21 patients only one hospital admission was recorded for pneumonitis following operation. These 25 patients were followed for 612 patient months, or an average of 24 months per patient (range, 5 to 72 months).

Recurrent pneumonitis. Sixty-four of the 89 patients had episodes of recurrent pneumonitis. Their ages ranged from 2½ months to 169 months, with a median age of 24 months at time of operation. In 39 of these patients specific numbers of episodes of pneumonitis were identifiable, 223 episodes were identified, or an average of nearly six episodes per patient. The 64 patients in this group were followed for 1922 patient months, or an average of 30 months. Two patients required a second fundoplication to control the GER.

One episode of pneumonitis occurred in each of 10 patients postoperatively. Three of these had "multiple" episodes prior to operation, while seven patients, who had collectively accounted for 24 preoperative illnesses, had only one postoperative illness each. These patients were followed for an average of 45 months each.

Fundoplications were done in four patients who were subsequently deemed to have been "errors in selection" for operation. One had a ventricular septal defect and severe pulmonary hypertension. The second was a severely retarded boy who did not reflux but aspirated saliva and oral intake. The third patient had 15 episodes of pneumonitis in 13 preoperative years and 3 episodes in 5 postoperative years. The fourth patient had two Thal-Ashcraft fundoplications for recurrent GER, and although she had no further GER she continued to have recurrent pneumonitis. She was converted to a Nissen fundoplication, which made no change whatsoever in her clinical course.

In summary, of the fundoplications done in 89 patients for continuous or recurrent pneumonitis, eight were considered to be "errors in selection" (9%). In three patients the Thal-Ashcraft fundoplication came apart and was redone. There were 10 deaths (11%), four as a result of complex congenital heart disease and 6 as a result of severe mental-motor retardation. All cases are summarized in Table 15-7.

The foregoing emphasizes that fear of failure of fundoplication because of associated disorders should not exclude patients with GER from the opportunity for effective operative treatment. In this view, it may be necessary to accept a certain level of "errors in selection," provided the risk of operation is low. We have adopted this attitude and, for example, have accepted a significant number of patients referred from our section of neurology who have problems such as apnea and in whom GER is demonstrated, but in whom the association is not absolutely demonstrated.

THE THAL-ASHCRAFT ANTERIOR FUNDOPLICATION

It is appropriate here to describe and illustrate our procedure of choice.

Over the past 12 years we have performed the Thal-Ashcraft fundoplication in over 800 patients for all manifestations of gastroesophageal reflux. There have been no deaths related to the fundoplication directly, and the incidences of postoperative wound infection, intestinal obstruction, and recurrent gastroesophageal reflux have been reported[15] and are comparable to those after other operative procedures used in the management of GER in children. The operation is somewhat simpler than Boix-Ochoa's procedure. It has the advantage of allowing the patient to vomit and avoid the "gas bloat" syndrome, since it is a partial wrap. The steps of the procedure are noted here, and specific features are further outlined in Figs. 15-10 and 15-11.

A transverse upper abdominal incision is preferred (Fig. 15-10, *inset*). The esophagus is mobilized, and an additional length of intraabdominal esophagus is gained in standard fashion as for any fundoplication. These preliminary steps are not shown but are mentioned here to aid in understanding the fundoplication technique shown as later steps in the illustrations (Fig. 15-11).

The liver is first dissected sharply from the underside of the left hemidiaphragm to expose the esophagus at the hiatus. An indwelling nasogastric tube aids in palpating the esophagus. The liver is retracted to the right by folding the left lobe under a Deaver retractor, protecting it with a pad. The peritoneum over the hiatus is then incised transversely to expose the esophagus with its anterior vagal branch. The esophagus is bluntly freed laterally and posteriorly at the level of the gastroesophageal junction, so that a tape may be passed around for traction purposes. Downward traction is exerted via the tape. The lateral attachments of the hiatus to the esophagus

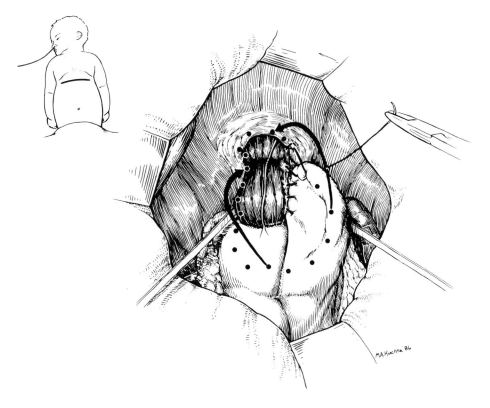

Fig. 15-10. *Inset*, Transverse upper abdominal incision is shown in a 1-year-old child. This incision is used whenever possible, extending from the costal margins between the nipple lines. This allows for exposure of the abdominal contents above the transverse colon, thereby minimizing exposure and handling of the small intestine.

The left lobe of the liver has been retracted, and the peritoneum over the esophageal hiatus has been incised. The esophagus has been encircled with an umbilical tape to facilitate its mobilization. The esophagus, as shown here in a 1-year-old infant, is slightly exaggerated in size, for purposes of illustration. In younger infants it is significantly smaller. As shown, increased length of the intraabdominal esophagus has been achieved during its mobilization. As noted in the text, the esophagus has been anchored posteriorly below the diaphragm by a crural suture. (See Fig. 15-11, *longitudinal cross section.*) Following this, the fundoplication is carried out. Each end of the tape has been grasped in a separate hemostat. This allows for continued traction with the two limbs of the tape wide apart and allows for exposure of the stomach in between. A 2-0 prolene suture on a cardiovascular needle is used for the fundoplication.

We have used two different running suture techniques for the fundoplication. The first method is to begin the suture at the lesser curvature of gastroesophageal junction, leaving the tail of the running suture to be tied to the completed fundoplication stitch. The initial stitch is run over and over across the gastroesophageal junction without actually plicating stomach to esophagus. Once the greater curvature gastroesophageal junction is reached, the suture line is directed up the patient's left lateral esophageal border, incorporating stomach and esophagus. Suture placement for the anterior fundoplication is shown by the heavy black dots in the wall of the gastric fundus, hiatal rim, and esophageal wall. The stomach is picked up a centimeter below the gastroesophageal junction and approximated to the left lateral aspect of the esophagus a centimeter above. This running suture is then continued, going down on the stomach a centimeter further and then back up to the lateral wall of the esophagus so that, in effect, a patch of stomach 3 to 4 cm distal to the gastroesophageal junction is turned up against the lower end of the exposed esophagus and sutured to it. The "folding over" effect of the suture line and the direction of deployment of the fundus over the anterior surface of the esophagus are indicated by the arrows. The incorporation of the stomach, hiatal ring, and esophagus in the uppermost "bite" of the running suture is shown before it is continued across from the greater curvature to the lesser curvature side of the esophagus. This fixes the anterior aspect of the intraabdominal esophagus below the diaphragm. (See also Fig. 15-11, *vertical cross section.*) The anterior vagus nerve is clearly seen, while the posterior vagus nerve (not shown) has been identified, and included in the umbilical tape that encircles the esophagus.

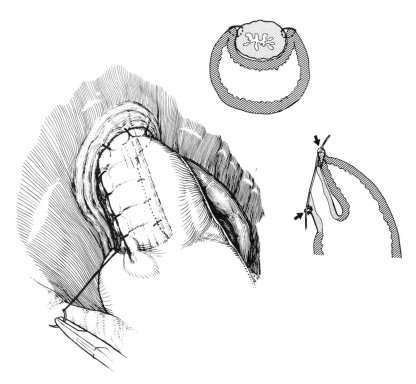

Fig. 15-11. The anterior fundic patch should be at least as wide as half the circumference of the esophagus. The hiatus has been reached and transversed, and the suture line has been carried from the patient's left, across the anterior aspect of the hiatal ring, and to the right side of the esophagus, with the anterior vagus nerve being carefully avoided. The suture is then "run down" to attach stomach to the right side of esophagus. When the running suture reaches the gastroesophageal junction, as shown here, it is tied to the tail of the original suture—or to itself, when the alternative technique of omitting the gastroesophageal junction suture is used. Shown is the nearly completed fundoplication from a somewhat lateral and oblique view to indicate the position of the suture line as it approximates stomach to the right lateral esophageal wall.

The last stitch has been placed before being tied down, thereby completing the fundoplication. The distal esophagus can be seen projecting into the upper stomach, which is partially enclosed by the fundoplication. The illustration attempts to show the fundoplication distended, thereby narrowing or closing the distal esophagus by its valve-like mechanism. The insert shows a horizontal cross-section through the fundoplication and indicates the anterior position of the fundic patch over the esophagus. It encloses somewhat more than half of the circumference of the esophagus. The vertical cross-section again shows the anterior deployment of the fundic patch over the esophagus. The lower arrow shows the position of the figure-of-eight crural-esophageal suture anchoring the mobilized intraabdominal esophagus posteriorly and "snugging up" the hiatus. The upper arrow shows one stich (or "bite") of the running suture as it crosses the upper part of the fundoplication. As indicated, the suture incorporates stomach wall, hiatal ring, and esophagus.

The alternative method of placing the running suture is to begin at the greater curvature of the gastroesophageal junction (omitting the gastroesophageal junction suture) but plicating stomach to esophagus as before. The suture line is ended at the lesser curvature side of the gastroesophageal junction. This technique has the advantage that the suture line is an inverted U and not a closed rectangle, which could potentially limit the growth of the area under the fundoplication. There have not been any obvious differences in the results in using either technique.

are freed by grasping the crura and pushing upward. The lateral and anterior aspects of the esophagus are thus exposed a distance of 2 to 4 cm, depending upon the size of the patient.

A dissector is then introduced behind the esophagus once again, making sure that the posterior vagus nerve is included in the tape. If it is not, the tape is replaced. The loose tissue at the back of the esophagus is pushed upward, exposing the posterior wall of the mobilized esophagus. A small retractor is used to lift the esophagus forward and to the patient's left so that the two limbs of the crura are exposed. A single figure-of-8 suture of 2-0 silk is used to approximate the crura posteriorly, leaving enough room in the hiatus for esophagus and nasogastric tube. The suture is tied but not cut. It is passed into the back wall of the esophagus, carefully avoiding the posterior vagus nerve.

After tying, this suture fixes the intraabdominal segment of esophagus posteriorly. (Fig. 15-11, *vertical cross section*). We feel this is important in preventing the occurrence of hiatal hernia postoperatively. In our earlier experience this suture was not placed if the hiatus was normal, and several patients thereafter developed a hiatal hernia with loosening and/or slippage of the fundoplication and recurrence of GER. The specific features of the Thal-Ashcraft fundoplication are illustrated.

Following surgery, a nasogastric tube is left in place for continuous suction during the night after the operation. The following morning it is removed and the patient is started on a liquid diet. The following day the patient is advanced to a diet for age and, if it is tolerated, he is usually dismissed the next day. Follow-up thereafter consists of an outpatient visit 1 week following dismissal; another usually 6 weeks after operation; and another 4 months postoperatively, when a barium study is obtained to determine if the fundoplication is intact. The patient is then seen at approximately 2-year intervals.

REFERENCES

1. Boix-Ochoa, J., and Canals, J.: Maturation of the lower esophageal sphincter, J. Pediatr. Surg. **11**:749, 1979.
2. Boix-Ochoa, J.: Gastroesophageal reflux. In Welch, K.J., et al., editors: Pediatric Surgery, ed. 4, Chicago, 1986, Year Book Medical Publishers, Inc., pp. 712-720.
3. Amoury, R.A.: Structure and function of the esophagus in infancy and early childhood. In Ashcraft, K.W., and Holder, T.M., editors: Pediatric Esophageal Surgery, New York, 1986, Grune & Stratton, pp. 1-28.
4. Liebermann-Meffert, D., Allgower, M., Schmid, P., et al.: Muscular equivalent of the lower esophageal sphincter, Gastroenterology **76**:31, 1979.
5. Bonavina, L., Evander, A., DeMeester, T.R., et al.: Length of the distal esophageal sphincter and competency of the cardia, Am. J. Surg. **151**:25, 1986.
6. Vane, D.W., Shiffler, M., Grosfeld, J.L., et al.: Reduced lower esophageal sphincter (LES) pressure after acute and chronic brain injury, J. Pediatr. Surg. **17**:960, 1982.
7. Mollitt, D.L., Golladay, E.S., and Seibert, J.J.: Symptomatic gastroesophageal reflux following gastrostomy in neurologically impaired patients, Pediatrics **75**:1124, 1985.
8. Lipshutz, W.H., Gaskin, R.D., Lukosh, W.M., et al.: Pathogenesis of lower-esophageal-sphincter incompetence, N. Engl. J. Med. **289**:182, 1973.
9. Farrell, R.L., Castell, D.O., and McGuigan, J.E.: Measurements and comparisons of lower esophageal sphincter pressures and serum gastrin levels in patients with gastroesophageal reflux, Gastroenterology **67**:415, 1974.
10. Goyal, R.K., and McGuigan, J.E.: Is gastrin a major determinant of basal lower esophageal sphincter pressure? J. Clin. Invest. **57**:291, 1976.
11. Sturdevant, R.A.L.: Is gastrin the major regulator of lower esophageal sphincter pressure? Gastroenterology **67**:551, 1974.
12. Boyle, J.T., Tuchman, D.N., Altschuler, S.M., et al.: Mechanisms for the association of gastroesophageal reflux and bronchospasm, Am. Rev. Respir. Dis. **131**(Suppl.):516-520, 1985.
13. Ashcraft, K.W., Holder, T.M., Amoury, R.A., et al.: Fundoplication as treatment for chronic respiratory disease in children. Presented at the International Congress of Paediatric Surgery, Perth, Australia, March 7, 1984.
14. Thal, A.P.: A modified approach to surgical problems of the esophagogastric junction, Ann. Surg. **168**:542, 1968.
15. Ashcraft, K.W., Holder, T.M., and Amoury, R.A.: Treatment of gastroesophageal reflux in children by Thal fundoplication, J. Thorac. Cardiovasc. Surg. **82**:706, 1981.

CHAPTER 16 Barrett's esophagus

Cedric G. Bremner

Norman Barrett, C.B.E., was a consultant thoracic surgeon at St. Thomas's and the Brompton Hospital, London. He was known to be a sound clinician, as well as a brilliant teacher, historian, editor, examiner, and artist, and he made many contributions to thoracic surgery in general. He died in 1979.

Barrett first described what he thought to be a congenitally short esophagus, with intrathoracic stomach, in 1950,[1] and Allison and Johnstone, in 1953,[2] correctly pointed out that the organ lined by gastric mucous membrane was indeed esophagus and not stomach. They still assumed that the columnar lining was the result of a congenital failure of the embryonic cuboidal cells to reach maturity. Allison and Johnstone suggested that the gastric "ulcer" in the esophagus be referred to as Barrett's ulcer; hence the eponym "Barrett's esophagus and ulcer." Remarkably, in 1961, Haywood stated his belief that the columnar lining of the esophagus was the result of long-continued gastroesophageal reflux, and opposed the congenital theory.[3] Since that time, arguments have been made for both the congenital theory and the acquired theory of origin of the columnar lining.

DEFINITION

A circumferential segment of the lower esophagus that is lined by columnar epithelium in continuity with the gastric lining constitutes Barrett's esophagus. There is argument about what length of segment is necessary before qualifying for the diagnosis. Because the normal esophagus may have 1 to 2 cm of columnar lining,[3] we have stipulated that a 3-cm segment of columnar lining is necessary to qualify for a diagnosis of Barrett's esophagus,[4] and have excluded shorter segments from our series. Iascone et al. also required the minimum of a 3-cm length, and also excluded equivocal cases with only small tongues of columnar epithelium.[5] This rigid definition does exclude early cases, but still helps eliminate overdiagnosis. The tongues of pink columnar epithelium often seen at endoscopy in patients with gastroesophageal reflux obviously represent creeping substitution of squamous epithelium by columnar epithelium. We have proposed the term "creeping substitution," or stage 1, for tongues; stage 2 for a columnar segment under 2 cm but with tongues; and stage 3 for a segment more than 3 cm[4] (Fig. 16-1).

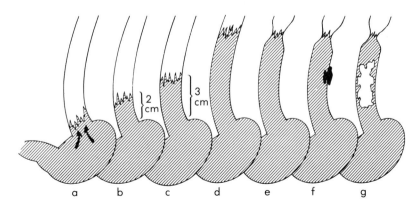

Fig. 16-1. Stages in the development of a columnar-lined esophagus. Gastroesophageal reflux results in *a,* early flame-shaped areas of columnar replacement (creeping substitution); *b,* developing Barrett's (segment under 3 cm in length); *c,* a columnar segment of 3 cm or more qualifies as a Barrett's; *d,* ascent of the columnar segment, with flattening of the squamocolumnar junction; *e,* stricture at squamocolumnar junction; *f,* penetrating "peptic" ulcer; *g,* adenocarcinoma in a columnar segment.

PATHOGENESIS

The fetal esophagus is lined by a simple columnar epithelium that gradually changes to a stratified squamous type and matures by the sixth month. Persistence of the fetal columnar epithelium would account for a congenital columnar lining, and isolated reports of columnar epithelium occurring in premature and newborn infants support this theory. Islands of heterotopic gastric mucosa have also been described in all esophageal segments, including the postcricoid area, and Weingart et al. have described such islands in the cervical esophagus of 125 patients.[6] These islands do not, however, constitute a columnar segment. Total lining by columnar epithelium in an adult esophagus is described by Hague and Merkel as evidence in favor of the persistence of a fetal type of epithelium.[7] We have also seen a total columnar lining in a patient who had reflux following an esophagogastrectomy performed 20 years previously. On the basis of a bimodal age distribution, Borrie and Goldwater have suggested that there may be a congenital type and an acquired type.[8] It has also been noted that the squamocolumnar junctional zone is usually irregular or flame shaped (suggesting a reflux replacement) but may be a clear-cut straight area of change, possibly of developmental origin.

On the other hand, there is abundant evidence for an acquired nature of this epithelium. In the presence of gastroesophageal reflux in the experimental dog reflux model, an upward growth of columnar epithelium replaced a segment of the lower esophagus previously denuded of its squamous epithelium.[9] No such replacement took place in the absence of reflux in the control group of animals. These results certainly gave support to the acquired theory of origin of the columnar lining. Clinical experience also supports the acquired theory. Most patients are middle-aged (mean age in this series of 70 patients was 51.8 years), but we have treated four young patients, ages 4, 15, 27, and 28 years. Hiatal hernia is present in the majority of cases, also supporting an associated incompetent lower esophageal sphincter. Gastroesophageal reflux tests were positive in 24 of our 28 patients tested, and reflux is demonstrated in most patients in the described series. In fact, reflux was present in 19 children (age range, 8 months to 19 years), suggesting that Barrett's esophagus is an acquired lesion even in young children.[10] Esophageal manometric measurements of the lower esophageal sphincter also confirm that the lower esophageal sphincter is incompetent in the majority of patients.[11,5]

Many of our patients gave a history of reflux (heartburn) of many years' duration. Further irrefutable evidence favoring an ascent of columnar epithelium associated with gastroesophageal reflux has been documented by serial endoscopies that showed replacement of a 5-cm segment of esophagus by columnar epithelium in a 3-year period, and a 17-cm segment in 10 years.[8] A columnar segment has also been described in patients who have absent or poor lower esophageal sphincter pressures associated with "scleroderma" of the esophagus, and following esophagomyotomy for achalasia of the esophagus.[12,13] We have also seen a scleroderma patient with severe reflux and a columnar lining. Gastroesophageal reflux that follows esophagogastrectomy may result in a columnar-lined segment above the gastroesophageal anastomosis, and we have seen this in two patients 14 and 21 years following resection for a benign stricture. Naef et al.[14] and Hamilton and Yardley[15] have described similar patients who developed extensive columnar metaplasia following subtotal esophagectomy and gastroesophageal anastomosis many years previously. It is interesting to speculate as to why some patients who have gastroesophageal reflux develop a reflux stricture at the original squamocolumnar junction, whereas others have a replacement epithelium in response to the reflux insult and only develop a high stricture after the squamocolumnar junction has been relocated to a higher level. Differences in the severity of reflux, the type of reflux, and the ability of the esophagus to clear acid may play a role in each type. Iascone et al.[5] showed a slower acid clearing in patients with Barrett's esophagus than in normals and in patients with reflux esophagitis, and many patients in our series have been shown to have hypomotility of swallow responses recorded during esophageal motility studies.

CLINICAL FEATURES

In most series there is a male preponderance, and Starnes et al.[16] reported a 3:1 male preponderance. In our series there was a male preponderance of 1.26:1, and in our series and five others, there were 132 males and 76 females, or approximately 2 males to 1 female (Table 16-1).

Barrett's esophagus is a disease that presents predominantly in the fifth decade. More cases are now being diagnosed in children, probably because of the more frequent use of fiberoptic endoscopy, and the appreciation that the condition does occur in young people. Barrett's esophagus usually presents with the complications of stricture, ulceration, hemorrhage, polyp formation, and adenocarcinoma. Stricture is the most frequent of these complications. Ulceration is less

TABLE 16-1. Sex distribution and age ranges of patients with Barrett's esophagus

Author	No. of cases	Males	Females	Age range
Starnes et al.[16]	25	18	7	32-90
Paull et al.[17]	11	10	1	31-78
Borrie and Goldwater[8]	45	21	24	0-80
Radigan et al.[18]	14	10	4	35-67
Skinner et al.[19]	43	34	9	13-78
Bremner (present series)	70	39	31	4-83
TOTAL	208	132	76	0-90

common, and polyp formation is very uncommon (1 in 45 cases seen by Borrie and Goldwater).[8] Anemia was seen in one third of cases in the same series. Gross bleeding is also unusual, and we have been presented with two such cases. Most patients have a hiatal hernia, and a long history of gastroesophageal reflux. Some patients, however, present with complications related to gastroesophageal reflux and have not had associated reflux symptoms. It is well known, however, that reflux strictures may occur in the absence of reflux symptoms.

DIAGNOSIS

By keeping a high index of suspicion in regard to patients who have a long history of gastroesophageal reflux, an examiner will overlook fewer cases. The first radiologic signs of a high stricture may be very subtle, and may mark the squamocolumnar junction. High strictures and long strictures found in association with reflux are often confirmed to be Barrett's cases. Endoscopy and biopsy, however, must ultimately be carried out. Even if a squamocolumnar junction is not clearly visible well above the gastroesophageal junction, biopsy specimens should be taken. We have several patients who were thought by the endoscopist to have esophagitis, and a surprise biopsy report of columnar epithelium first drew attention to a Barrett's. Even when Barrett's is confirmed, reendoscopy may fail to show a clear zone of epithelium demarcation. The highest level of columnar epithelium seen in our series was at 16 cm from the incisor teeth. The squamocolumnar junction is, however, usually clearly defined, and may be a straight junctional zone or an irregular area with flame-shaped upward extensions of pinkish columnar epithelium. Why there should be such a difference in presentation is unclear, but Stadelman et al.[20] suggest that the straight-line type could be congenital in origin and that the irregular type could be acquired.

The presence of an ulcer in the esophagus is highly suggestive of Barrett's ulcer. Iodine introduced through the endoscope channel may be used to stain the squamous mucosa and fails to stain the columnar epithelium.[21] Motility studies are not specific but will often record a poor lower esophageal sphincter pressure and subnormal pressure responses to swallowing in the body of the esophagus. Potential difference recordings performed at the same time as motility studies may be helpful. In Barrett's the zone of change is well above the gastroesophageal junction.[22]

Isotope scanning using sodium pertechnetate, which is concentrated in gastric-type mucosa, has been used to diagnose Barrett's esophagus.[23] The presence of a hiatal hernia will confuse the diagnosis on pertechnetate scanning. We have used the technique and found it of little value.

RADIOLOGICAL FEATURES (Fig. 16-2)

Features seen in Barrett's esophagus include gastroesophageal reflux, hiatal hernia, stricture formation, ulceration, superficial nodular changes, and a reticular pattern of the mucosa.[24,27] The stricture features are variable. There may be a short stricture that is well above the gastroesophageal junction, and often in the upper third of the esophagus, or a longer stricture up to several centimeters in length. A long stricture seen above a hiatal hernia is very suggestive of the condition (see Fig. 16-3). There are very few other conditions that cause stricturing above the middle third of the esophagus. These include caustic ingestion, epidermolysis bullosa, medication in pills and powders taken without liquids (tetracyclines, emepromium bromide, and so on), webs, and the Plummer-Vinson syndrome. Early stricturing at the squamocolumnar junction may give minimal radiologic signs, which are often missed. Ulceration in the esophagus may be related to other causes, especially medication taken in pill form in elderly people.

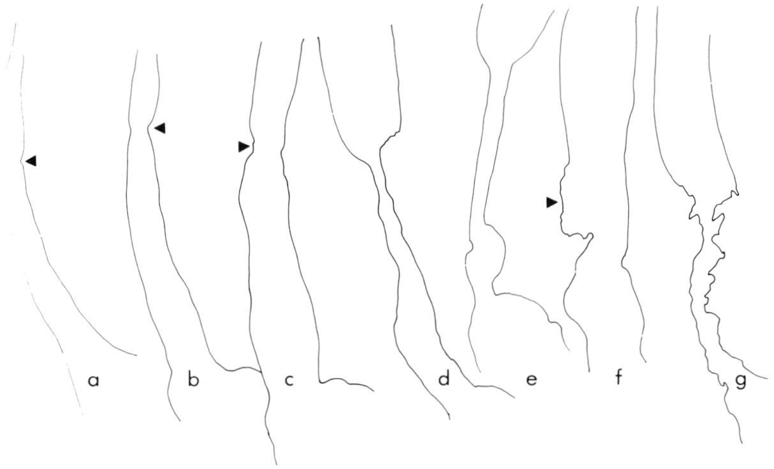

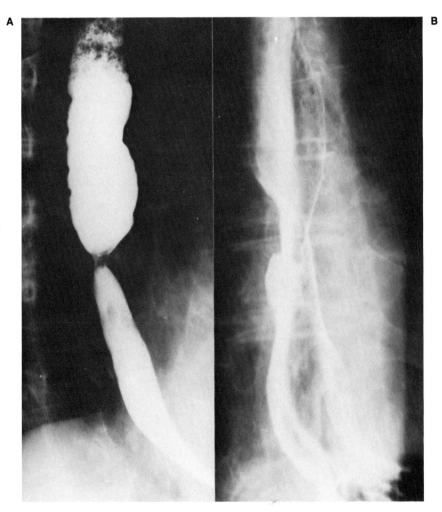

Fig. 16-2. Tracings from barium swallow studies from patients with biopsy-proven Barrett's esophagus. *a,b,c,* The sites of the squamocolumnar junction are indicated by the arrowed early strictures. *d,* A long stricture in the absence of a hiatal hernia; *e,* a long stricture above a hiatal hernia; *f,* a penetrating ulcer in the lower esophagus; *g,* the irregular outline of an extensive adenocarcinoma complicating a Barrett's epithelium.

Fig. 16-3. Examples of some radiologic features of Barrett's esophagus. **A,** Stricture at squamocolumnar junction. **B,** Ulceration in a columnar segment.

The ulceration may be solitary or multiple. Superficial mucosal nodular changes were seen in 15 of Halpert's 30 cases,[24] and a reticular pattern was seen in 26% (124 cases) of double-contrast examinations performed in Vincent's series. Vincent considered the reticular pattern to be a strong indicator of esophageal disease but not specific for Barrett's.[25]

MANOMETRIC, REFLUX, AND POTENTIAL DIFFERENCE STUDIES

In the majority of cases in our series the lower esophageal sphincter pressure (LESP) was poor (0 mm Hg in 25 cases, 1 to 5 mm Hg in 13, 6 to 10 mm Hg in 6). The pressure was normal in only four cases tested, but a normal manometric pressure also does not exclude the possibility of reflux. Reflux was shown to be present in 24 of 28 of our patients tested. Iascone et al.[5] made a careful comparison of LESP and reflux in patients with Barrett's esophagus, patients with reflux esophagitis, and persons with no esophageal pathology. Patients with Barrett's had a lower LESP, statistically more esophageal acid exposure, and a greater number of reflux episodes than patients with esophagitis and normals. Their study also suggested that the severity of acid exposure was due to a defect in the acid clearance as measured by 24-hour esophageal pH monitoring and an acid clearance test. In our series we have shown that the swallow responses in the body of the esophagus were weak in 18 cases and incoordinate or spastic in 15 cases. The squamocolumnar junction may also be defined by measuring the potential difference. The potential difference changes from a higher gastric mucosal level (approximately 36 mV) to a lower esophageal mucosal level (approximately 12 mV). In Barrett's esophagus the squamocolumnar junction is located at a higher level than usual. Although

C

D

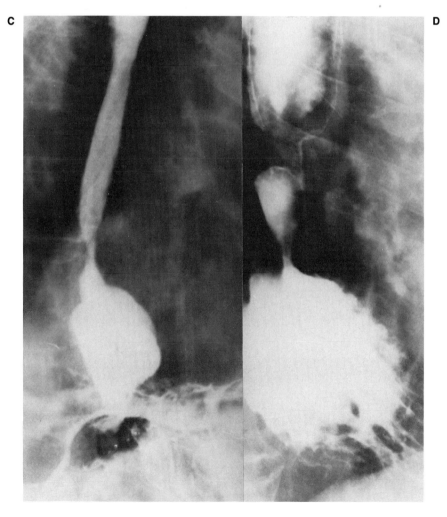

Fig. 16-3, cont'd. C, Long columnar-lined stricture proximal to a hiatal hernia. **D,** A short columnar segment with deep ulceration and associated hiatal hernia.

an abnormal potential difference has been shown to be highly specific for detecting gross esophagitis, from a practical point of view the test has limited diagnostic value in Barrett's.

ENDOSCOPY AND BIOPSY

Endoscopy and biopsy confirmation are essential for the diagnosis of Barrett's esophagus. Endoscopists should have a high index of suspicion in patients presenting with a long history (usually more than 10 years) of gastroesophageal reflux, a high stricture, or ulceration of the esophagus. The change from the whitish squamous epithelium to a pinkish columnar-type epithelium may be obvious. This junctional zone, however, may be missed when it is high in the esophagus, or the macroscopic change may be indistinct. It is therefore important to take biopsy specimens in suspected cases. We have been surprised on a few occasions to see the pathologic report of columnar epithelium when macroscopically we had not diagnosed the condition. It is necessary to document clearly the distance of the hiatus from the incisor teeth and the levels of the lower esophageal sphincter and squamocolumnar change. The level of the squamocolumnar change in a series in which the zone was clearly noted at endoscopy is presented in Table 16-2. Lackey et al.[28] have done an interesting and careful endoscopic and biopsy study in 13 patients with Barrett's stricture, and have shown that the stricture occurred below the squamocolumnar junction in 5 patients and at the junction in 6 patients. Two of their strictures were associated with malignant change. This finding suggests that the stricture took place originally at the squamocolumnar junction but that continued reflux allowed a further replacement of squamous epithelium by columnar epithelium above the stricture area.

DUODENOGASTRIC REFLUX

When a mixture of duodenal contents and acid refluxes into the esophagus, the resulting reflux esophagitis is more severe than when acid alone refluxes. It is possible that "alkaline" reflux could account for the complications that occur in Barrett's esophagus. Little attention has been focused on the pathogenesis of such complications, and the reasons why an acid-resistant epithelium should ulcerate, bleed, and constrict remains an enigma. It is my belief that duodenal contents do contribute to these complications. We have measured the bile salts in gastric aspirates

TABLE 16-2. Distance from the incisor teeth to the squamocolumnar epithelial change in 44 patients

Distance (cm)	No. of cases
15-25	8
26-30	18
31-35	16
36-37	2

from 15 patients with proven Barrett's epithelium, and 9 had an excess of bile in the fasting or post–milk-meal aspirate. Seven of these patients had strictures.[11] We also performed multiple gastric biopsies on 17 patients and showed that there was a chronic active gastritis in 9, and atrophic gastritis in 4 and mild gastritis in 3, supporting the concept that duodenogastric reflux had caused this inflammation. Duodenogastric reflux in the pathogenesis of gastric ulceration is supported clinically by du Plessis[29] and Lawson.[30]

BARRETT'S ESOPHAGUS IN CHILDREN

Dahms and Rothstein[10] reported on 13 children (ages 8 months to 19 years) seen over a 5-year period. All children presented with symptoms of gastroesophageal reflux and esophagitis, and five had a stricture. It is of interest to note that no child had a hiatal hernia, and this suggests a primary incompetence of the lower esophageal sphincter. The youngest patient in our series was 4 years old, and she presented with a stricture. One of our patients, age 28, had a history of regurgitation and reflux since birth. Seven of Borrie and Goldwater's 45 patients were under 20 years of age, and 6 were under 10 years.[8] There is thus an increasing appreciation of the condition in children, and endoscopy is considered mandatory in children with continued regurgitation and reflux symptoms.

HISTOLOGIC FEATURES

The columnar segment of Barrett's esophagus has been studied extensively by light microscopy, dissecting microscopy, scanning electron microscopy, electron microscopy, and histochemical studies. At the growing edge of a developing Barrett's in both the experimental model and humans, the columnar cell layer is only a single

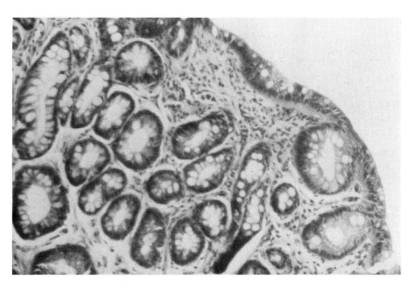

Fig. 16-4. The histologic features of the growing edge of a developing columnar segment. The cells are cuboidal in shape, and there are numerous mucus glands.

layer thick and the cells are often flattened or cuboidal (Fig. 16-4). On dissecting microscopy Thompson et al.[31] found the surface of the epithelium to be uneven and consisting of circular structures, ridges, and projections of various heights. Gland orifices were frequently large and distorted. Mangla and Lee[32] had similar findings and concluded that the shaggy, denuded, irregular configuration of this epithelium rendered it more vulnerable to ulceration, bleeding, stricture, and neoplasm. Trier[33] described a distinctive columnar secretory epithelium that was morphologically different from gastric fundic, normal junctional, and intestinal epithelium. Three cell types were distinguished, namely abundant columnar epithelial cells containing many glycoprotein granules, and a brush border with microvilli; mucus-secreting goblet cells; and enterochromaffin cells. The three epithelial zones subsequently defined by Paull et al.[17] were:

1. A proximal specialized columnar epithelium similar to small bowel, with a villiform surface, mucus glands, and goblet cells
2. A junctional epithelium without chief and parietal cells
3. A gastric fundic-like epithelium with pits, mucus glands, parietal cells, and chief cells

Residual squamous islands have also been found within the regions of the Barrett's metaplasia.[31] We have seen very few parietal cells in sections examined histologically. A notable feature on all specimens examined by us is the presence of inflammation in the submucosa.

Whether this inflammation represents an inflammatory reaction to irritant duodenal contents that reflux into the esophagus is unknown. The presence of Paneth cells suggests a form of highly differentiated intestinalization.[34] Berenson et al.[35] found that this epithelium had a uniform ultrastructural characteristic, lacked disaccharide activity, and was histochemically different from small intestine and gastric fundic epithelium. The histochemical mucin profile was also assessed in 17 patients by Peuchmar et al.[36] They found that type IIB intestinal metaplasia (with sulphomucins) was found more frequently in a columnar-lined segment than in normal epithelium. This type of metaplasia has always been considered to be a precancerous lesion, and this finding suggested that such patients had a high risk of developing cancer.

Tissue gastrin and pepsin secretion has also been demonstrated[37] but was not confirmed in the study by Dalton et al.,[38] who failed to demonstrate gastrin in specimens from 12 patients. However, immunocytochemical studies on biopsies from 20 patients did show gastrin cells, enterochromaffin cells, and somatostatin cells in approximately half of the specimens.[39] The absorptive function of the columnar epithelium was assessed as poor because of a failure to absorb a micellular lipid solution.[40] Berenson et al.[41] also compared the activity of the lysosomal enzymes β-galactosidase and β-glucuronidase in esophageal columnar, gastric fundic, and small intestinal epithelium. β-Galactosidase activity in esophageal columnar epithelium was less than that in intestinal tissue, and β-glucuronidase activity was greater than that in gastric fundic tissue. The tissue was shown, therefore, to be different from both intestinal and gastric fundic tissue, supporting a metaplastic derivation. β-Glucuronidase activity appears to be greater in tissues that are undifferentiated and undergoing growth. Neuroendocrine cells were found in the histologic studies in eight patients by Thompson et al.[31] and we have confirmed the presence of endocrine cells in electron microscopy studies on biopsy specimens from two patients.

COMPLICATIONS (Table 16-3)

Most patients present with complications, but with an increasing awareness of the condition, endoscopists are now more likely to diagnose Barrett's before complications develop. In our series stricture was the commonest complication, and was the presenting complication in approximately half of the reported series. The stricture usually occurs at the squamocolumnar junction, but as previously mentioned Lackey et al. have described the stricturing below the squamocolumnar junction in 5 of 13 cases. Lackey et al. also suggested the possibility that fibrosis and narrowing could have resulted from healing of a Barrett's ulcer in the columnar segment below the squamocolumnar junction.[28] Ulceration is less common than stricture in most series, and this may be superficial or penetrating. In the series of 40 cases reported by Starnes et al. there was ulceration in 19 cases (68%).[16] Deep ulceration is less frequently seen than superficial ulceration.

There may also be superficial liner ulceration in the squamous epithelium above the squamo-columnar junction as a result of gastroesophageal reflux. Ulcer perforation is unusual.

Bleeding from a penetrating ulcer may be severe, and in Borrie and Goldwater's case[8] urgent reconstructive surgery was necessary after a transfusion of 15 liters of blood. One third of their 45 patients had iron-deficiency anemia. Mangla et al.[37] performed an emergency Nissen fundoplication in a patient who had bleeding from a Barrett's ulcer and described severe bleeding in a further two patients who also required surgery after unsuccessful medical treatment.

ADENOCARCINOMA ARISING IN BARRETT'S COLUMNAR EPITHELIUM

The risk of developing adenocarcinoma in a Barrett's is not clearly known. The percentage of cases varies with each series; 12 of 140 patients (8.6%) in Naef's series[14] and 23 of 43 patients (46%) in Skinner's series[19] had adenocarcinoma when first seen. In a review by Sjogren[44] an overall estimate of the risk of developing adenocarcinoma was given as 10%.

These figures, however, do not reflect the true risk of developing an adenocarcinoma in the columnar segment. Many patients with uncomplicated Barrett's esophagus may not be diagnosed, either because endoscopy is not performed or because the endoscopist misses the diagnosis by failing to take routine biopsy specimens in cases of reflux esophagitis. There will also be considerable bias in the figures reported from specialized units in which only selected cases have been referred for surgery. From reported follow-up studies it would appear that the risk of developing

TABLE 16-3. Frequency of complications in Barrett's esophagus

Author	No. of Cases	Stric- ture	Ulcera- tion	Bleed- ing	Adenocar- cinoma	Esopha- gitis
Radigan et al.[18]	19	8	2		5	4
Dahms and Rothstein[10]	13	5	10	7		13
Naef and Savary[42]	62	27	4		9	
Iascone et al.[5]	22	12	3			
Starnes et al.[16]	40	19	27		15	
Robbins et al.[27]	39	32	21			29
Levine et al.[26]	29	24				14
Burgess et al.[43]	17	11	1	2		
Borrie and Goldwater[8]	45	45	1			
Bremner (present series)	70	42	9	9	10	20
TOTAL	356	183 (51%)	78 (24%)	18 (18%)	39 (20%)	80 (47%)

adenocarcinoma in diagnosed cases is small. Spechler et al.[45] followed 105 patients for a total of 350 person-years, and only two patients developed adenocarcinoma. They therefore question the value of surveillance for these patients. Only two patients in the Mayo Clinic series[46] of 104 patients with Barrett's epithelium developed adenocarcinoma—6 and 10 years after the initial diagnosis had been made (882 person-years' follow-up). We know of only one patient in our series of 60 Barrett's cases without cancer who subsequently developed adenocarcinoma while on vigorous antireflux treatment. These figures support Spechler's suggestion of a poor return from regular surveillance.[45] Most patients with adenocarcinoma in a columnar-lined esophagus are male. (Eleven of 15 in Starnes' series,[16] 18 of 20 in Skinner's series,[19] and 8 of 10 in the author's series were men.)

Is it possible to predict the development of adenocarcinoma in Barrett's epithelium? A spectrum of histologic changes ranging from a submucosal cellular infiltration to papillary hyperplasia, mild, moderate, and severe dysplasia, and finally carcinoma in situ can be found on careful examination of resected specimens. Skinner et al. found that the malignant potential of the columnar epithelium was higher in men who smoke, in patients with intestinal-type metaplasia and who continue to have severe reflux, and in patients who have dysplasia.[19] Herbst et al.[47] suggested that surface labelling with tritiated thymidine may be an indication of malignant change. We did not see surface labelling in biopsy specimens from a patient receiving medical therapy who developed adenocarcinoma within months of the biopsy being taken. The high occurrence of type IIB intestinal metaplasia in Peuchmar's study suggested a high risk of adenocarcinoma.[36]

TREATMENT

The recommended treatment of Barrett's esophagus is the prevention of gastroesophageal reflux by an antireflux operation. Our choice has been the Nissen fundoplication operation. Many patients who are elderly, frail, or have serious cardiac and pulmonary problems cannot have surgery and must be treated by vigorous antireflux measures. The use of the H_2 receptor blockers, bethanecol, and antacids has given symptomatic relief and even ulcer healing, but there are few reports with a long-term follow-up. In our series we have had difficulty in keeping deep ulcers healed in two cases, and in one patient adenocarcinoma developed after 2½ years

of medical treatment. We have noted endoscopic improvement on H_2 receptor blocker treatment but have not noted regression of the level of the squamocolumnar junction. Salzman et al.[48] reported on the progression to a stricture during cimetidine therapy. Delpre et al.[49] reported on the use of cimetidine, antacids, and metoclopramide to heal a resistant Barrett's ulcer. Medical methods are unlikely to improve the conditions of patients who have alkaline reflux, and even vigorous medical treatment using a combination of antacids, metoclopramide or domperidone, and cholestyramine to absorb bile has not given satisfactory results. Starnes et al.[16] reported on the medical management of 20 patients with Barrett's esophagus, and this included the use of cimetidine, antacids, weight reduction, and antireflux measures. Only three patients had a reasonable response. One patient had an ulcer perforation into the pleura, and another patient progressed to adenocarcinoma. Patel et al.,[50] however, reported on the resolution of severe dysplastic changes and regression of the columnar segment in one patient on medical treatment that included the use of bethanecol. Surgical correction of reflux remains the preferred treatment and should be recommended to all patients who are evaluated as being fit enough for the operation.

Choice of surgical procedure
(Table 16-4)

We have selected the Nissen fundoplication operation as the procedure of choice because a 360-degree wrap controls reflux more adequately than an incomplete wrap, such as the Hill posterior gastropexy or the Belsey Mark IV operation. The Angelchik prosthesis may be an adequate method to control the reflux, but we have not had occasion to evaluate it. Prevention of reflux gives excellent symptomatic relief, and strictures are well controlled in our experience.

In selected cases of alkaline reflux, a bile-diverting procedure should be considered. We have been very cautious in our selection of cases for such a procedure, and a combination of preoperative tests to evaluate the severity of the bile reflux has always been carried out. A history of bilious vomiting, the presence of bile in the stomach seen at endoscopy, a low acid output on pentagastrin stimulation, histologic gastritis on biopsy, and an excess of bile in the gastric aspirate (fasting and postprandial) give evidence of a bile reflux problem. Twenty-four hour pH monitoring is also a valuable tool for this investigation. As yet there are no absolute guidelines as to the severity of the "alkaline" reflux that requires bile diversion, and we have selected only

TABLE 16-4. Recommended surgical procedures to treat a columnar-lined esophagus

Condition	Procedure
1. Acid reflux	Antireflux operation (Nissen, Hill, Belsey, Angelchik)
2. Alkaline reflux (selected cases)	Vagotomy, antrectomy, Roux-en-Y (with or without antireflux procedure)
3. Associated duodenal ulcer	Parietal cell vagotomy and antireflux operation
4. Stricture	Dilate and proceed as in 1 or 2
5. Stricture (failed dilatation)	Resection
6. Penetrating ulcer	a. Vigorous conservative treatment to heal ulcers; follow with surgery as in 1 or 2
	b. Resection if ulcer fails to heal
7. Adenocarcinoma	Resection with gastric or colon replacement

the severe refluxers for surgery. Failure to treat the duodenogastric reflux may result in gastric ulceration, and this poses a further difficult problem in management.[51] We have had experience with three such cases.[52]

Associated strictures should be dilated first, and either a Celestin-type dilator or Maloney mercury bougies, or a combination of these, will prove satisfactory.[53] We have also used the Celestin dilator as the stent necessary to ensure that the wrap is not too tight. The addition of a proximal gastric vagotomy is practiced routinely by some surgeons,[16] and we have reserved this addition only if there is an associated duodenal ulcer. Esophagectomy is necessary for malignant lesions, severe dysplasia, carcinoma in situ, non-healing of Barrett's ulcers, and in some cases of failed dilatation of long strictures. We have used transhiatal esophagectomy (esophagectomy without thoracotomy) in two patients who presented with early lesions. A standard Ivor Lewis esophagectomy (two-stage) or McKeown operation (three-stage) is recommended as the usual procedure, during which the total columnar segment should be removed. Adenocarcinoma has developed in the columnar remnant following incomplete resection. A columnar-lined esophagus complicating a long-standing achalasia or scleroderma esophagus is likewise best treated by resection. Attempts to control reflux in the amotile esophagus by antireflux procedures are likely to be very disappointing.

Results of antireflux operations

Surgical control of reflux results in symptomatic improvement and control of reflux strictures. If surgery fails to control the reflux, however, the columnar lining may progress,[54] or the patient may have continued symptoms. Starnes et al.[16] had a good overall response in six of eight patients treated by a Nissen fundoplication (and proximal gastric vagotomy in six patients). One

patient continued to reflux, and a second developed an adenocarcinoma 2 years later. Ten of 13 patients who had an antireflux procedure[5] were symptom-free at follow-up (median, 34 months). Naef and Savary[42] had excellent results in 15 survivors who underwent Nissen fundoplications, and remarked on the astonishing results seen even in complicated cases when reflux is abolished.

Seventeen patients in our series had a Nissen fundoplication (together with a parietal cell vagotomy in one patient and Thal patch in two patients). Reflux was not controlled in one patient, and restricturing developed in one patient after a Thal patch that leaked. Fifteen patients were followed up, for 1 to 9 years. Symptoms were relieved in all patients. Two further patients have had bile-diverting Roux-en-Y procedures for alkaline reflux stricturing and have had a cure of the stricture.

Whether antireflux operations protect the columnar segment from malignant changes is still controversial. There is no question that a correction of reflux will prevent a recurrence of stricture formation, and ulceration has not been reported in a reflux-controlled Barrett's epithelium. There are reports, however, of adenocarcinoma that has developed after surgery. Hamilton et al.[55] reported on the development of adenocarcinoma in the remnant of a Barrett's esophagus, which occurred 8 years after a colonic interposition, and they suggest that long-term surveillance is still necessary even after antireflux surgery. The development of adenocarcinoma following antireflux surgery has been reported by others,[14,56,57] but continuous pH probing to prove the absence of reflux was not carried out as it was in Hamilton's case. It is therefore important to test the efficacy of antireflux procedures after surgery. There is also some debate as to whether the columnar segment regresses after antireflux surgery. Brand et al.[58] reported on regression of the epithelium after surgery, but this has not been a uniform finding.[59] Naef et al.[14] found no change after a follow-up of at least 5 years. Skinner et al.[19] noted squamous epithelium regeneration after surgery in zones of previous Barrett's epithelium in two patients. Following surgery there is a relocation of the squamocolumnar junction, and this level should be noted carefully soon after surgery so that follow-up detailing of the level can be made. We have not noted a regression of the columnar segment in a small group of patients followed carefully for up to 8 years.

We have also not seen a case of adenocarcinoma after antireflux surgery, during follow-up periods of up to 9 years. One of our patients receiving medical treatment, however, developed an adenocarcinoma after 2½ years of medical treatment for penetrating ulcer in a columnar segment. He died of his preexisting obstructive airways disease.

Of the 10 cases of adenocarcinoma in our series, 6 patients underwent operation. Of the 5 patients who underwent resection, 2 are alive, 27 and 5 months after surgery, respectively. The longest survivor lived 52 months. One patient died 4 weeks after surgery from a staphylococcal septicemia related to a severe postoperative pneumonia. The sixth patient was inoperable and was intubated with a Celestin tube. Four of Skinner's patients had an excellent functional result with a follow-up of 2 to 5 years after esophagectomy.

CONCLUSIONS

Barrett's esophagus is considered to be the end stage of long-continued gastroesophageal reflux, and usually presents with complications of stricture, ulceration, bleeding, polyp formation, and adenocarcinoma. Treatment is aimed at the prevention of reflux, and a 360-degree Nissen fundoplication is recommended in patients who are fit enough for surgery. Unfit patients should be treated with vigorous antireflux measures. Barrett's esophagus is a premalignant condition and approximately 10% of cases present with malignancy. However, few patients develop adenocarcinoma subsequent to diagnosis and treatment, and this discrepancy between the high incidence of adenocarcinoma seen initially and the low occurrence in diagnosed cases suggests that there are probably many undiagnosed cases, so that the true incidence of adenocarcinoma is unknown, but probably less than 10%. Surveillance programs to date have not been cost effective. The efficacy of medical and surgical treatment in the prevention of adenocarcinoma is not well established, and further careful follow-up studies are essential. There is no certain method of predicting the development of adenocarcinoma in the columnar epithelium, but histologic, histochemical, and electron microscopyic studies may be rewarding and need further evaluation.

REFERENCES

1. Barrett, N.R.: Chronic peptic ulcer of the esophagus and "esophagitis," Br. J. Surg. **38:**175-182, 1950.
2. Allison, P.R., and Johnstone, A.S.: The esophagus lined with gastric mucous membrane, Thorax **8:**87-101, 1953.
3. Hayward, J.: The lower end of the esophagus, Thorax **16:**36-41, 1961.
4. Bremner, C.G., and Hamilton, D.G.: Barrett's esophagus: controversial aspects. In DeMeester, T.R., and Skinner, D.B., editors: Esophageal disorders: pathophysiology and therapy, New York, 1985, Raven Press pp. 233-239.
5. Iascone, C., DeMeester, T.R., Little, A.G., and Skinner, D.B.: Barrett's esophagus: functional assessment, proposed pathogenesis and surgical therapy, Arch. Surg. **118:**543-549, 1983.
6. Weingart, J., Seib, H.J., Elster, K., and Ottenjann, R.: Gastric mucous heterotopias in the upper gastrointestinal tract, Leber Magen Darm **14**(4):155-60, 1984.
7. Hague, A.K., and Merkel, M.: Total columnar-lined esophagus: a case for congenital origin? Arch. Path. Lab. Med. **105**(10):546-548, 1981.
8. Borrie, J., and Goldwater, L.: Columnar cell-lined esophagus: Assessment of etiology and treatment, J. Cardiovasc. Thorac. Surg. **71:**825-834, 1976.
9. Bremner, C.G., Lynch, V.P., Ellis, F.H., Jr.: Barrett's esophagus: congenital or acquired? An experimental study of esophageal mucosal regeneration in the dog, Surgery **68**(1):209-216, 1970.
10. Dahms, B.B., and Rothstein, E.C.: Barrett's esophagus in children: a consequence of chronic gastroesophageal reflux, Gastroenterology **86**(2):318-323, 1984.
11. Bremner, C.G.: Barrett's esophagus. In Watson, A., and Celestin, L.R., editors: Disorders of the esophagus: advances and controversies, London, 1984, Pitman Books, Ltd., pp. 94-104.
12. Dill, J.E.: Barrett's epithelium in scleroderma, Gastrointest. Endosc. **29**(4):296-297, 1983.
13. Feczko, P.J., Ma, C.K., Halpert, R.D., and Batra, S.K.: Barrett's metaplasia and dysplasia in postmyotomy achalasia patients, Am. J. Gastroenterol. **78**(5):265-268, 1983.
14. Naef, A.P., Savary, M., Ozzello, L., and Pearson, F.G.: Columnar-lined lower esophagus, Surgery **70:**826-834, 1975.
15. Hamilton, S.R., and Yardley, J.H.: Regeneration of cardiac type mucosa and acquisition of Barrett's mucosa after esophago-gastrectomy, Gastroenterology **72:**669-675, 1977.
16. Starnes, V.A., Adkins, R.B., Ballinger, J.F., and Swayers, J.L.: Barrett's esophagus: a surgical entity, Arch. Surg. **119**(5):563-567, 1984.

17. Paull, A., Trier, J.S., Dalton, M.D., Camp, R.C., Loeb, P., and Goyal, R.: The histologic spectrum of Barrett's esophagus, N. Engl. J. Med. **295**:476-480, 1976.

18. Radigan, L.R., Glover, J.L., Shipley, F.E., and Shoemaker, R.E.: Barrett's esophagus, Arch. Surg. **112**:486-491, 1977.

19. Skinner, D.B., Walther, B.C., Riddell, R.H., Schmidt, H., Iascone, C., and DeMeester, T.R.: Barrett's esophagus: comparison of benign and malignant cases, Ann. Surg. **198**(4):554-566, 1983.

20. Stadelman, O., Elster, K., and Kuhn, H.A.: Columnar-lined esophagus (Barrett's syndrome): congenital or acquired? Endoscopy **13**(4):140-147, 1981.

21. Burbridge, E.J., and Radigan, J.: Characteristics of the columnar cell–lined (Barrett's) esophagus, Gastrointest. Endosc. **25**:133-136, 1979.

22. Orlando, R.C., Powell, D.W., Bryson, J.C., Kinard, H.B., Carney, C.M., Jones, J.D., and Bozymski, E.M.: Esophageal potential difference measurements in esophageal disease, Gastroenterology **83**(5):1026-1032, 1982.

23. Berquist, T.H., Nolan, N.G., Carlson, H.C., and Stephens, D.H.: Diagnosis of Barrett's esophagus by pertechnetate scintigraphy, Mayo Clin. Proc. **48**:276-279, 1973.

24. Halpert, R.D., Feczko, P.J., and Chason, D.P.: Barrett's esophagus: radiological and clinical consideration, J. Can. Assoc. Radiol. **35**(2):120-123, 1984.

25. Vincent, M.E., Robbins, A.H., Spechler, S.J. Scwartz, R., Doos, W.G., and Schimmel, E.M.: The reticular pattern as a radiographic sign of the Barrett esophagus: an assessment, Radiology **153**(2):333-335, 1984.

26. Levine, M.S., Kressel, H.Y., Caroline, D.F., Laufer, I., Herlinger, H., and Thompson, J.J.: Barrett's esophagus: reticular pattern of the mucosa, Radiology **147**:663-667, 1983.

27. Robbins, A.H., Vincent, M.E., Saini, M., et al.: Revised radiologic concepts of Barrett's esophagus, Gastroint. Radiol. **3**:377-381, 1978.

28. Lackey, C., Rankin, R.A., and Welsh, J.D.: Stricture location in Barrett's esophagus, Gastrointest. Endosc. **30**(6):331-333, 1984.

29. du Plessis, D.J.: Pathogenesis of gastric ulceration, Lancet **1**:974-978, 1965.

30. Lawson, H.H.: Gastritis and gastric ulceration, Br. J. Surg. **53**:493-496, 1966.

31. Thompson, J.J., Zinsser, K.K., and Enterline, H.T.: Barrett's metaplasia and adenocarcinoma of the esophagus and gastroesophageal junction, Human Pathol. **44**(1):42-61, 1983.

32. Mangla, J.C., and Lee, C.: Scanning electron microscopy of Barrett's esophageal mucosa, Gastrointest. Endosc. **25**(3):92-94, 1979.

33. Trier, J.S.: Morphology of the epithelium of the distal esophagus in patients with mid-esophageal peptic strictures, Gastroenterology **58**(4):444-461, 1970.

34. Schreiber, D.S., Apstein, M., and Hermos, J.A.: Paneth cells in Barrett's esophagus, Gastroenterology **74**:1302-1304, 1978.

35. Berenson, M.M., Herbst, J.J., and Freston, J.W.: Enzyme and ultrastructural characteristics of esophageal columnar epithelium, Dig. Dis. Sci. **19**(10):895-907, 1974.

36. Peuchmar, M., Potet, F., and Goldfain, D.: Mucin histochemistry of the columnar epithelium of the esophagus (Barrett's esophagus): a prospective biopsy study, J. Clin. Pathol. **37**:607-610, 1984.

37. Mangla, J.C., Schenk, E.A., Desbaillets, L., Guarasci, G., Kubasik, M.P., and Turner, M.D.: Pepsin secretion, pepsinogen, and gastrin in "Barrett's esophagus," Gastroenterology **70**(5):669-676, 1976.

38. Dalton, M.D., McGuigan, J.E., Camp, R.C., and Goyal, R.K.: Gastrin content of columnar mucosa lining the lower (Barrett's) esophagus, Am. J. Dig. Dis. **22**:970-972, 1977.

39. Buchan, A.M.J., Grant, S., and Freeman, H.: Regulatory peptide-containing cells in Barrett's esophagus (abstract), Gastroenterology **84**(5):1116, 1983.

40. Endo, M., Kobayaski, S., Kozu, T., Takemoto, T., and Nakayama, K.: A case of Barrett's epithelialisation followed up for five years, Endoscopy **6**:48-51, 1974.

41. Berenson, M.M., Herbst, J.J., and Freston, J.W.: Esophageal columnar epithelial β-galactosidase and β-glucuronidase, Gastroenterology **68**(6):1417-1420, 1975.

42. Naef, A.P., and Savary, M.: Conservative operations for peptic esophagitis with stenosis in columnar-lined lower esophagus, Ann. Thorac. Surg. **13**(6):543-551, 1972.

43. Burgess, J.N., Payne, W.S., Anderson, H.A., Weiland, L.H., and Carlson, H.C.: Barrett's esophagus, Mayo Clin. Proc. **46**:728-734, 1971.

44. Sjogren, R.W., Jr., and Johnson, L.F.: Barrett's esophagus: a review, Am. J. Med. **74**:313-321, 1983.

45. Spechler, S.J., Robbins, A.H., Rubins, H.B., Vincent, H.E., Heerer, T., Doos, W.G., Cotton, T., and Schimmel, E.M.: Adenocarcinoma in Barrett's esophagus: an overrated risk? Gastroenterology **87**(4):927-933, 1984.

46. Cameron, A.J., Ott, B.J., and Payne, W.S.: Incidence of adenocarcinoma and long term follow-up. Presented at International Meeting on Esophageal Cancer, Rome, October, 1983.

47. Herbst, J.J., Berenson, M.M., McCloskey, D.W., and Wiser, W.C.: Cell proliferation in esophageal columnar epithelium (Barrett's esophagus), Gastroenterology **75**:683-687, 1978.

48. Salzman, M., Barwick, K., and McCallum, R.W.: Progression of cimetidine-treated reflux esophagitis to a Barrett's stricture, Dig. Dis. Sci. **27**(2):181-186, 1982.

49. Delpre, G., Kadish, U., Glanz, I., and Avidor, I.: Prolonged cimetidine therapy in ulcerated Barrett's columnar-lined esophagus, Am. J. Gastroenterol. **79**(1):8-11, 1984.

50. Patel, G.K., Clift, S.A., Schaefer, R.A., Read, R.C., and Texter, C., Jr.: Resolution of severe dysplasia (ca in situ) changes with regression of columnar epithelium (CE) in Barrett's esophagus (BE) on medical treatment (abstract), Gastroenterology **82**:1147, 1982.

51. Bremner, C.G.: Gastric ulceration after a Nissen fundoplication operation for gastroesophageal reflux, Surg. Gynecol. Obstet. **148**:62-64, 1979.

52. Bremner, C.G., and Hamilton, D.: The columnar-lined (Barrett's) esophagus: surgical techniques. In Stipa, S., Belsey, R.H.R., and Moraldi, A., editors: Medical and surgical problems of the esophagus, Serono Symposium, vol. 43, New York, 1981, Academic Press, pp. 205-207.

53. Bremner, C.G.: Benign strictures of the esophagus, Curr. Probl. Surg. **19**(8):402-492, 1982.

54. Ransom, J.M., Patel, G.K., Clift, S.A., Womble, N.E., and Read, R.C.: Extended and limited types of Barrett's esophagus in the adult, Ann. Thorac. Surg. **33**(1):19-27, 1982.

55. Hamilton, S.R., Hutcheon, D.F., Ravich, W.J., Cameron, J., and Paulson, M.: Adenocarcinoma in Barrett's esophagus after elimination of gastro-esophageal reflux, Gastroenterology **86**:356-360, 1984.

56. Haggitt, R.C., Tryzelaar, J., Ellis, F.J., and Colcher, H.: Adenocarcinoma complicating columnar epithelial-lined (Barrett's) esophagus, Am. J. Clin. Pathol. **70**:1-5, 1978.

57. Smith, R.R.L., and Hamilton, S.R.: Spectrum of carcinoma arising in Barrett's esophagus: a clinicopathologic study in twenty-five patients (abstract), Lab. Invest. **46**:78A, 1982.

58. Brand, D., Ylvisaker, J.T., Gelfand, M., and Pope, C.E., III: Regression of columnar esophageal (Barrett's) epithelium after antireflux surgery, N. Engl. J. Med. **302**:844-848, 1980.

59. Mangla, J.C.: Barrett's epithelium: regression or no regression? N. Engl. J. Med. **303**:529-530, 1980.

Barrett's esophagus

DISCUSSION

F. Griffith Pearson

Dr. Bremner's chapter on Barrett's esophagus is a complete and well-referenced review of a condition that has generated much discussion and controversy during the past decade. The review is an orderly discussion of definition and historical information, pathogenesis, histologic features, clinical presentations, diagnosis, and management. Discussion of controversial areas is thoughtful, and his own opinions about controversial issues are significantly strengthened by his large and well-documented personal experience.

My report will discuss specific areas of interest or controversy, add some observations from our own personal experience, and summarize our current approach to the investigation and management of patients with this condition.

HISTORICAL CONSIDERATIONS

Bremner identifies Hayward, in 1961, as the first individual to suggest that columnar-lined esophagus was an acquired condition resulting from the effects of gastroesophageal reflux.[1] It was, in fact, Allison and Johnstone, in their classic 1953 description, "The Oesophagus Lined with Gastric Membrane," who first suggested a reflux origin. They postulated that some cases of columnar-lined esophagus may be acquired rather than congenital: "Is healing of the ulcer (in squamous epithelium) in an acid medium more likely to be by the overgrowth of the gastric rather than squamous epithelium? If this were so, it might be that some examples of gastric mucosa in the esophagus were acquired rather than congenital."[2] Indeed, in this original report, Allison and Johnstone described many of the significant characteristics of columnar-lined esophagus. They noted that these cases were usually associated with hiatal hernia, gastroesophageal reflux, and superficial ulceration of the squamous epithelium above the squamocolumnar interface as the result of reflux esophagitis, and frequently resulted in an esophageal stricture. These authors clearly distinguished the superficial ulceration of reflux esophagitis from the less common condition of chronic peptic ulcer occurring in that segment of esophagus lined with columnar, gastric-type mucosa—for which they coined the term "Barrett's ulcer." They observed that these chronic ulcers may be found at the squamocolumnar junction or in the more distal parts of the columnar-lined segment, and may result in complications of penetration with pain, intrathoracic or mediastinal perforation, massive bleeding, and esophageal obstruction. In this report, Allison and Johnstone also described one case of adenocarcinoma confined to the columnar-lined segment.

DEFINITION AND PATHOGENESIS

It is now widely accepted that the majority of cases of Barrett's esophagus are the result of a replacement by columnar epithelium of areas of superficial ulceration in the squamous mucosa immediately proximal to the squamocolumnar junction. The earliest stages of this process will be no more than minor alterations in the configuration and position of the squamocolumnar mucosal junction. It is for this reason that several authors recommend that a definition of columnar-lined esophagus be restricted to cases in which at least 3 cm of the distal esophagus is lined by a columnar epithelium. We agree with Bremner, however, that projecting tongues of columnar epithelium, which are often seen at endoscopy in patients with reflux, represent the earliest stages of the condition. Bremner and Hamilton suggested three stages: stage 1—tongues, stage 2—a columnar segment less than 2 cm in length, but with tongues; and stage 3—a segment greater than 3 cm in length. This definition offers a useful approach for standardizing observations in future reports and publications.[3]

The association of gastroesophageal reflux with columnar-lined esophagus appears incontrovertible, and the evidence is well documented in Bremner's report. It is less well appreciated that this acquired condition occurs in young children, and may complicate primary motor diseases such as scleroderma, or cases of achalasia in which reflux esophagitis develops following esophagomyotomy. We support Bremner's contention that reflux of duodenal contents may play a significant role in the pathogenesis of squamous ulceration followed by columnar replacement. Bremner's report on a study of gastric aspirates in 15 patients with Barrett's esophagus is one of the few studies that have been undertaken to support this theory.[4]

HISTOLOGY

We have not documented the detailed histology of the columnar epithelium in our own cases. Bremner's review of this subject is detailed and comprehensive, and is reinforced by a more recent report by Spechler and Goyal.[5] There is compelling evidence for an increased risk of adenocarcinoma developing in the columnar-lined segment, and it appears that malignant transformation is preceded by dysplastic epithelial changes. Spechler et al. summarized the data from three reports of retrospective analyses of experience with Barrett's esophagus,[6,7,8] and estimates that the risk for adenocarcinoma is thirty to forty times greater than in the general population. They emphasized, however, that esophageal cancer is relatively uncommon in the general population, and that a fortyfold increase in incidence still represents a much smaller increased risk of adenocarcinoma in patients with Barrett's esophagus than that suggested in earlier prevalence studies.

COMPLICATIONS
Stricture

Peptic stricture at the squamocolumnar junction is the commonest significant complication, and occurs in approximately half of reported cases, including Bremner's own series. A peptic stricture is usually the result of confluent, circumferential superficial ulceration of the distal squamous epithelium. Luminal narrowing may be due to a combination of edema, muscle spasm, and concentric scar contracture in the underlying wall of the esophagus. It may be argued that most peptic strictures will be associated with some

degree of acquired, columnar replacement, which is a natural sequence in the healing phase of ulcerative esophagitis. It is difficult, or impossible, to interpret the surface changes seen at endoscopy in cases of peptic ulceration with obstruction and stricture. Even the technique of multiple biopsy may miss an early adenocarcinoma, and it is suggested that endoscopic evaluation include cytopathologic study of circumferential brushings from the narrowed and ulcerated segment.

Barrett's ulcer

In 1950, Barrett reviewed reported cases of peptic ulcer of the esophagus and documented additional cases from his own hospital.[9] Barrett's ulcer is an uncommon lesion that behaves like any peptic ulcer in gastric mucosa and may penetrate, perforate, or bleed. We have recently reported our own experience in 11 patients.[10] An analysis of our experience indicates that the ulcer is induced by gastroesophageal reflux and will heal rapidly in most cases after adequate reflux control. Intensive medical treatment was insufficient in our cases, and ulcer healing was only achieved after antireflux surgery.

Adenocarcinoma

As previously noted, although the incidence of adenocarcinoma is significantly higher in cases of columnar-lined esophagus, it is clearly not 10% or greater, as indicated in a number of prevalence reports. The retrospective reviews by Spechler et al.[6] and Cameron et al.[7] identify a much lower risk. Spechler et al. observed one case of adenocarcinoma developing in 105 cases of columnar-lined esophagus, with 350 patient-years of follow-up. Cameron et al. reported only two cases of adenocarcinoma developing in 104 patients, with 882 patient-years of follow-up. This relatively low incidence challenges the practicality of vigorous surveillance programs employing repetitive endoscopy for follow-up. In our own series of 295 patients who have undergone antireflux surgery for ulcerative peptic esophagitis and peptic stricture, there have been five instances of the subsequent development of adenocarcinoma in the distal esophagus.[11] We might assume that at least half of our cases were associated with some degree of acquired columnar replacement. The mean follow-up time in these patients is 6 years.

SUMMARY AND CONCLUSIONS

Columnar-lined esophagus is a relatively common condition complicating gastroesophageal reflux. Both acid-pepsin and duodenal reflux may play a role in pathogenesis. The diagnosis is primarily established at endoscopy and requires biopsy for absolute confirmation. Although some patients are asymptomatic, the majority have at least some symptoms of reflux and may suffer the additional complications of peptic stricture, Barrett's ulcer, and adenocarcinoma. Although the risk of adenocarcinoma is undoubtedly significantly higher in these cases, the role of endoscopic surveillance remains controversial because the evaluation required to identify severe dysplasia or early cancer is not yet sophisticated or precise.

There is insufficient data to resolve the controversy concerning (1) regression of the columnar lining following the control of reflux by either medical or surgical treatment and (2) whether control of reflux diminishes or precludes the risk of the development of subsequent adenocarcinoma.

Treatment recommendations

1. In asymptomatic patients without endoscopic evidence of esophagitis, ulcer, or other complication, no specific treatment is recommended aside from observation. An annual follow-up visit is recommended, and endoscopy is undertaken only with the development of new symptoms.

2. To date, we have not advised additional or more radical treatment in patients with columnar-lined esophagus as opposed to any other group of patients with symptomatic reflux. Surgery is not undertaken if symptoms are adequately controlled with medical therapy, provided there are no endoscopic changes such as persistent ulcerative peptic esophagitis, which may warrant a more radical approach.

3. Bremner states, "The recommended treatment of Barrett's esophagus is the prevention of gastroesophageal reflux by an antireflux operation." He notes that surgery is only advised in patients at acceptable risk. We would restrict this recommendation to patients with symptomatic reflux that is inadequately controlled by medical treatment, and to patients with the complications of ulcerative peptic esophagitis and stricture. The presence of a Barrett ulcer that fails to heal after an adequate trial of medical treatment is a clear indication for surgery. We would not, however, recommend a resection as proposed by Bremner. Healing of the Barrett ulcer was achieved in all 10 of our cases managed by antireflux surgery.[10] Our choice of antireflux operation is a

transthoracic repair combining a modified Collis gastroplasty with a Belsey-type partial fundoplication.[11] A gastroplasty is preferred in all cases because it is assumed that some degree of acquired shortening is an almost certain accompaniment. The columnar-lined segment has been the site of previous ulceration, which implies a potential for some degree of scarring in the esophageal wall. Many of these patients have obvious acquired shortening, often in association with severe ulcerative esophagitis and stricture.

4. We advise a total thoracic esophagectomy in patients with adenocarcinoma. Adenocarcinoma in a columnar-lined esophagus frequently lies entirely within the esophagus itself, and presumably spreads like a squamous cell cancer of the distal third. A total thoracic esophagectomy should reduce the incidence of local recurrence at the anastomosis and will also remove the entire columnar-lined segment, which might otherwise be the site for a subsequent second primary.

REFERENCES

1. Hayward, J.: The lower end of the oesophagus, Thorax **16:**36-41, 1961.
2. Allison, P.R., and Johnstone, A.S.: The oesophagus lined with gastric mucous membrane, Thorax **8:**87-101, 1953.
3. Bremner, C.G., and Hamilton, D.G.: Barrett's esophagus: controversial aspects. In DeMeester, T.R., and Skinner, D.B., editors: Esophageal disorders: pathophysiology and therapy, New York, Raven Press, 1985.
4. Bremner, C.G.: Barrett's oesophagus. In Watson, A., and Celestin, L.R., editors: Disorders of the esophagus: advances and controversies, London, 1984, Pitman Books, Ltd., pp. 94-104.
5. Spechler, S.J., and Goyal, R.K.: Barrett's esophagus, N. Engl. **315:** 362-371, 1986.
6. Spechler, S.J., Robbins, A.H., Rubins, H.B., et al.: Adenocarcinoma and Barrett's esophagus: an overrated risk? Gastroenterology **87:**927-933, 1984.
7. Cameron, A.J., Ott, B.J., and Payne, W.S.: The incidence of adenocarcinoma in columnar-lined (Barrett's) esophagus, N. Engl. J. Med. **313:**857-859, 1985.
8. Sprung, D.J., Ellis, F.H., Jr., and Gibb, S.P.: Incidence of adenocarcinoma in Barrett's esophagus (abstract), Am. J. Gastroenterol. **79:**817, 1984.
9. Barrett, N.R.: Chronic peptic ulcer of the oesophagus and "oesophagitis," Br. J. Surg. **38:**175-182, 1950.
10. Pearson, F.G., Cooper, J.D., Patterson, G.A., and Prakash, D.: Peptic ulcer in acquired columnar-lined esophagus: results of surgical treatment, Ann. Thorac. Surg. **43:**241-244, 1987.
11. Pearson, F.G., Cooper, J.D., Patterson, G.A., et al.: Gastroplasty and fundoplication for complex reflux problems: long-term results, Ann. Surg. (In press.)

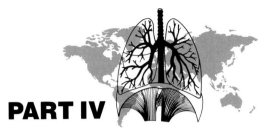

PART IV   REFLUX STRICTURES AND CHEMICAL INJURIES

CHAPTER **17** Management of reflux strictures

Anthony Watson

The first prerequisite in the effective management of reflux stricture is an accurate diagnosis confirming that the stricture is indeed reflux induced. It must be appreciated that there are many causes of benign esophageal stricture (see box, below) other than reflux esophagitis, some of which are considered in later chapters, and the application of a standard management program to all benign strictures will lead to therapeutic failures. The term "reflux stricture" can only be legitimately applied when these other causative factors have been excluded and when the presence of a benign esophageal stricture is accompanied by objectively demonstrated reflux of gastric or duodenal contents.

PATHOPHYSIOLOGY

The esophageal mucosa is extremely sensitive to damage by either acid or alkali, initially resulting in esophagitis with cellular infiltration, edema, basal cell hyperplasia, increasing depth of the vascular papillae, and a varying degree of fibrosis.[1,2] As the esophagitis progresses, erosions occur, which subsequently become con-

---

PRINCIPAL CAUSES OF BENIGN ESOPHAGEAL STRICTURE

1. Congenital
    a. Esophageal atresia
    b. Webs
    c. Tracheobronchial remnants
2. Infections
    a. Moniliasis
    b. Tuberculosis
    c. Crohn's Disease
    d. Typhoid
3. Posttraumatic
    a. Caustic burns
    b. Irradiation
    c. Nasogastric intubation
    d. Endoscopic injury
4. Postoperative
    a. Anastomosis
    b. Closure of perforation
    c. Diverticulectomy
5. Medications
    a. Tetracycline
    b. Aspirin
    c. Nonsteroidal anti-inflammatory drugs
    d. Progesterone-containing contraceptive pills
    e. Theophylline and derivatives
    f. Certain anticholinergic drugs
6. Reflux esophagitis and complications

---

fluent and extend proximally, initially as tongue-like projections but later progressing to circumferential areas of damage. If healing of such lesions takes place, it does so by replacement with columnar epithelium growing upward from the cardia, resulting in alteration in configuration of the Z line and ultimately in its proximal migration to form Barrett's esophagus.

Continued reflux in these circumstances leads to progressive tissue damage and fibrosis, commencing initially at the squamocolumnar junction, wherever that may lie, but in severe cases extending proximally over a variable length (see Fig. 17-1). In the early stages, strictures are often soft and associated principally with spasm, edema, and the laying down of immature collagen, which is usually confined to the submucosa (grade 1). Maturation of the collagen and further fibrosis result in a hard, annular stricture, the

pathologic changes still being confined to the submucosa (grade 2); more severe cases are associated with mucosal ulceration, the inflammatory and fibrotic process becoming transmural with muscular involvement and frequently periesophagitis that extends longitudinally, resulting in esophageal shortening (grade 3).

Stricture formation is almost invariably associated with severe degrees of reflux or with reflux of long duration, but depends on the balance existing between aggressiveness of the refluxate and esophageal mucosal resistance and efficiency of clearance. Patients with strictures often have the lowest values of resting lower esophageal sphincter pressure and are predominantly supine or combined refluxers.[3] They frequently have motility problems resulting in impaired clearance, these motility disturbances being exacerbated by transmural stricture formation,[4] extreme examples being the relatively early stricture formation in reflux associated with scleroderma or systemic sclerosis and following treated achalasia. Some evidence exists to suggest that alkaline reflux may be more likely to produce more severe degrees of esophagitis and stricture formation than acid-pepsin reflux.[5,6] Antroduodenal dysmotility as well as organic gastric outlet obstruction may increase reflux potential.

DIAGNOSIS

The presentation is invariably dysphagia, which frequently may be the first indication of reflux disease. In 120 cases reported from our institution (the Royal Lancaster Infirmary, Lancaster, England), 68% of cases did not have an antecedent diagnosis of gastroesophageal reflux, although a suggestive history could be elicited in 76%.[7] A careful history is essential to exclude caustic or drug ingestion, together with more obvious predisposing factors such as previous surgery, radiotherapy, endoscopy, or nasogastric intubation.

A barium swallow is useful, first in excluding other structural causes of dysphagia, such as Zenker's diverticulum, webs, or obvious neoplasm, and, second, to assess the site and length of the stricture, which complements the information obtained at esophagoscopy, especially when the stricture is impassable. Esophagoscopy allows the opportunity for mucosal visualization and histologic confirmation of the diagnosis. Our preference is to use fiberoptic endoscopy, with a combination of punch biopsies and brush cytology of smears obtained from the lumen of the stricture, which increases diagnostic accuracy to

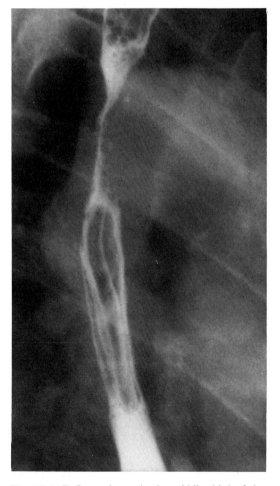

Fig. 17-1. Reflux stricture in the middle third of the esophagus at the squamocolumnar junction in a patient with columnar-lined esophagus (Barrett's esophagus).

over 90%.[8] In grade 1 and some grade 2 strictures, gentle passage of the fiberoptic pediatric endoscope will allow the lumen of the stricture and the distal esophagus and stomach beyond to be examined. In more advanced strictures, this can often be accomplished after gentle dilatation.

The demonstration of gastroesophageal reflux is essential to the diagnosis and correct management of reflux stricture. Reflux may often be suggested on barium swallow or esophagoscopy, but manometry and pH recording are necessary to quantify the reflux and categorize its type as well as to identify coexisting motility problems, all of which may have important therapeutic implications. The conduct of manometry and pH recording is facilitated by the prior dilatation of the stricture, especially if dual-probe simultaneous monitoring of gastric and esophageal pH is to be undertaken to assess the contribution of alkaline reflux.

Some of the more severe degrees of acid or alkaline reflux are seen in patients with stricture, who are often predominantly supine refluxers, patients in this category having a 25% incidence of reflux stricture.[3] Motility studies show an increased incidence of disordered motor activity, with low-amplitude contractions in the distal esophagus, these changes being progressively more marked as panmural inflammation and scarring progress.[9] A vicious circle is established if the lower esophageal sphincter (LES) is involved in the process, with progressive decrease in tone allowing more reflux. Since certain motor disorders, predominantly scleroderma, predispose patients to more severe esophagitis and stricture formation, characteristic changes of total ablation of the LES and gross diminution or loss of peristaltic activity may be found. A similar loss of peristaltic activity will be seen in achalasia complicated by gastroesophageal reflux after forcible dilatation or myotomy; in such cases organic stricture formation is common because of impaired esophageal clearing capacity, but in these circumstances LES tone may be present although relaxation remains impaired. It is clearly of vital importance, therefore, to perform careful manometric studies, especially if antireflux surgery is contemplated, to ensure that peristalsis is adequate and that LES relaxation occurs; otherwise, severe obstructive problems may be an undesirable consequence of treatment.

PHILOSOPHY OF MANAGEMENT

The development of reflux stricture is a serious condition and a consequence of severe and prolonged esophageal exposure to acid or alkaline refluxate, demanding active treatment. Such a development occurring during conservative management of gastroesophageal reflux represents failure of such treatment. In general terms, the aims of therapy are to improve swallowing and prevent further esophageal damage as effectively and safely as possible. While a surgical approach is likely to best fulfill the former criterion, the age and general condition of many patients with reflux stricture often preclude an operative approach. Of 120 patients with reflux stricture reported from our institution[7] the mean age was 69.5 years and the oldest 92. In practical terms, a balance has to be struck between the age and condition of the patient and the severity of the stricture in selecting the therapeutic modality most appropriate to the individual circumstance, acknowledging the fact that many grade 1 and some grade 2 strictures will respond to less active forms of management. In general terms, management can be categorized into nonoperative methods and operative methods.

NONOPERATIVE MANAGEMENT

Nonoperative management may be considered as an initial line of approach in grade 1 and some grade 2 strictures and in all cases in which the patient's age or general condition precludes more active intervention. The essential components of a nonoperative treatment program are (1) dilatation of the stricture, (2) control of reflux, and (3) surveillance.

Dilatation of reflux stricture

Dilatation of esophageal strictures has taken numerous forms since the first report of its use in 1922[10] (see Table 17-1). Most of the early techniques involved the unguided passage of dilators through the rigid esophagoscope, but more recently, guided techniques (Fig. 17-2) through the fiberoptic endoscope have gained popularity since their introduction in 1976,[11] largely because of the avoidance of the need for general anesthesia and the lower risk of perforation.[12] All the techniques, with the exception of the Didcott dilator,[13] have in common the application of a tangential force from above, but the recent introduction of the use of polyvinyl balloons for stricture dilatation[14] is an attempt to apply a more logical coaxial force.

Since 1975, we have treated 168 patients with benign esophageal stricture. In patients treated by dilatation, our early practice of unguided dilatation with gum-elastic bougies through the rigid

TABLE 17-1. Types of dilators used in management of benign strictures

System	Dilator used
Unguided	Gum-elastic bougies
	Chevalier-Jackson dilators
	Maloney and Hurst mercury-filled bougies
Guided	String-guided dilators
	Wire-guided dilators: Eder-Puestow, Celestin, Savary
Continuous coaxial	Didcott dilator
	Lunderquist balloon

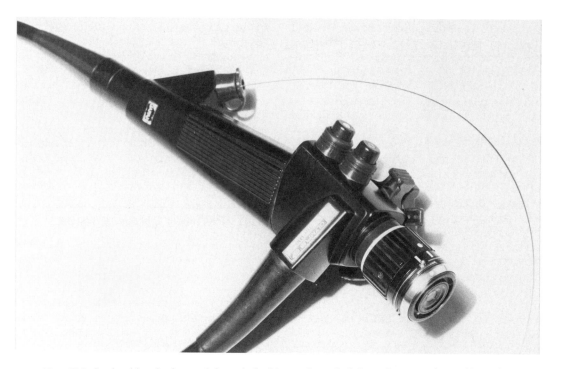

Fig. 17-2. Steel guide-wire inserted through the biopsy channel of the endoscope prior to fiberoptic endoscopic dilation.

esophagoscope was superseded in our unit in 1977 by guided dilatation using fiberoptic endoscopy, which has remained our preferred technique since then. During the first three years of our experience with fiberoptic endoscopic dilatation, we used the Eder-Puestow system (Fig. 17-3), as described by Lilly and McCaffrey,[11] but since 1980 have used Celestin bougies[15] (Fig. 17-4). These have the advantage of inducing less pharyngeal trauma, first because they are made of soft thermoplastic polyvinylchloride as opposed to metal and, second, because of progressively graded increase in diameter, such that dilatation between 12 F.G. and 56 F.G. is possible with only two insertions. Savary dilators are similarly less traumatic, although a separate dilator is used for each increment in size, making multiple passages necessary.

The principal advantages of fiberoptic endoscopic dilatation are (1) that it can be performed without general anesthesia as an outpatient procedure, sedation with diazepam and pentazocine being adequate, and (2) that the risk of perforation is low, being less than 0.05% in our unit.[16] We have performed over 500 such dilatations in 152 patients since 1976 without mortality, the only morbidity being two perforations, which were successfully treated. Such ease of performance lends itself to an "open-access" system for repeated dilatations of known patients, who in our institution telephone the endoscopy unit when their swallowing deteriorates and a further dilatation is then arranged. This, we believe, results in a more efficient use of hospital facilities and better control of the patient's ability to swallow.

Data on the efficacy of dilatation are rather

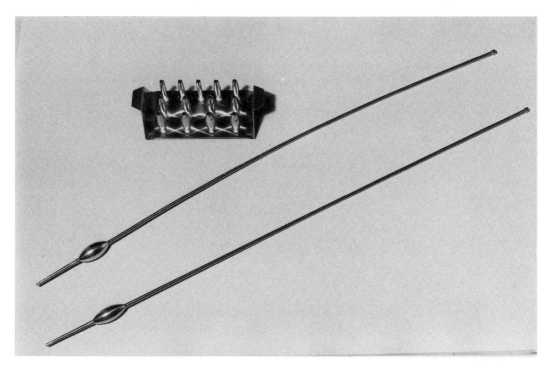

Fig. 17-3. Eder-Puestow dilating system. Progressively larger olives fit onto the hollow introducer, which is fed over the guide-wire previously passed through the stricture.

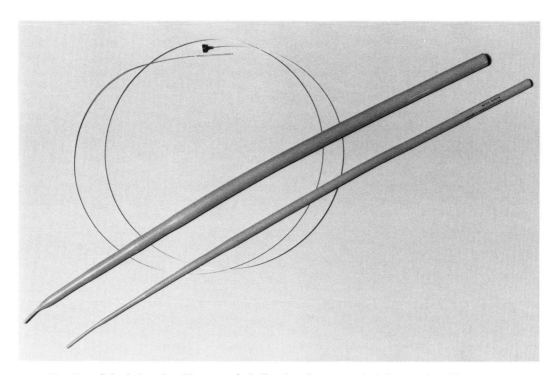

Fig. 17-4. Celestin bougies. The two soft, hollow bougies progressively increase in caliber to allow dilation up to 56 F.G. with only two passages over the guide-wire.

sparse, and mostly relate to fiberoptic endoscopic dilatation. Benedict[17] reported a success rate of 70%, Larza and Graham[18] 79%, and Wesdorp and Tytgat[19] 88%. Success in the context of these reports refers to the avoidance of surgical intervention, and the progressive increase in success rate in these series was attributed to the progressive increase in diameter to which strictures were routinely dilated. However, the avoidance of surgery does not equate with success except to the most conservative physician, and a uniform policy of dilating to a predetermined size in all circumstances may be considered inappropriate in view of the variation in types of stricture and in the stage at which they first present. Other criteria used to assess efficacy have been the effect on stricture diameter as measured by barium studies and the passage of radiopaque spheres,[20] the number of dilatations required over successive years,[21] and the mean number of dilatations over a finite follow-up period,[7,22] which allows comparison with other treatment regimens.

In the study of Ogilvie et al.[21] 40% of patients treated by dilatation and pharmacologic antireflux preparations did not need further dilatations after the initial procedure. Of those needing subsequent dilatation, the frequency of dilatation decreased with time to a mean of 0.6 dilatations per patient three years after the initial dilatation, although individual patients required up to 18 dilatations over a four-year period. In 78 patients treated in our institution by a similar regimen, 41% needed only one dilatation, the mean number of subsequent dilatations required in the remainder being 3.1 in a mean follow-up period of 3.3 years. In 42 patients in whom control of reflux was achieved surgically, 71% needed a single dilatation only, the mean number of dilatations required in the remainder over the same follow-up period being 1.6.

Of the various guided dilatation systems available, the Eder-Puestow system has been compared with the Celestin[23] and the latter with the Lunderquist balloon.[24] There was no apparent difference in efficacy between the various systems, but the Celestin system would appear to have advantages in being less traumatic than the Eder-Puestow and considerably less expensive than the polyvinylchloride balloons, which have a limited life. The most popular of the nonguided forms of dilatation is the use of Maloney tapered mercury bougies, which lend themselves to outpatient management of strictures without the need for endoscopy and are therefore useful in frail, elderly patients. Bremner[25] reported good results in selected, poor-risk patients, with approxi-

mately half requiring only a single dilatation. The principal disadvantage would appear to be the lack of surveillance if endoscopy is avoided, which in any event is of limited practical importance in the poor-risk patients in whom the technique is most appropriately used.

Control of reflux

A detailed discussion of the nonoperative treatment of gastroesophageal reflux is outside the scope of this chapter, but suffice it to say that in those patients with reflux stricture in whom surgery is inappropriate, it is illogical to perform intermittent dilatation without attempting pharmacologic reflux control. Agents employed should be appropriate to the nature of the refluxate, the pattern of esophageal exposure, and the clearing capacity of the distal esophagus.

The superiority of surgical over medical reflux control is, however, particularly reflected in the management of reflux stricture. Not only have strictures resolved with effective antireflux surgery alone, but a controlled trial conducted in our institution of medical against surgical reflux control performed in conjunction with fiberoptic endoscopic dilatation has shown a significant reduction in dilatation requirements in the surgically treated group, in whom such requirements were reduced to approximately half of those in the medically treated group (see Table 17-2).

Surveillance and the cancer risk

Many series of reflux stricture report a 2.5% to 4% incidence of the development of adenocarcinoma.[7,21,26] This is hardly surprising, since up to 76% of some series of reflux stricture comprise patients with columnar-lined (Barrett's) esophagus,[27,28] in which condition there is abundant evidence of malignant potential[29-31] (see also Chapter 16). We have seen esophageal adenocarcinoma develop in four patients undergoing intermittent dilatation and pharmacologic antireflux therapy, 1½ to 2½ years after initial diagnosis, at which time results of both punch biopsies and brush cytologic studies were negative. It seems inconceivable in these circumstances, in light of the natural history of untreated esophageal adenocarcinoma, that these could have been present from the outset.

These circumstances suggest the need for regular surveillance of patients undergoing an intermittent dilatation program, especially those with columnar-lined esophagus, although regular surveillance is clearly less of a requirement in frail elderly patients unfit for active treatment of an adenocarcinoma if this were to develop. Regular endoscopy and cytology are desirable at least

TABLE 17-2. Results of randomized controlled trial comparing the effect of medical and surgical reflux control on dilatation requirements in reflux stricture

	Medically treated group (Gaviscon 40 ml/day + cimetidine 800 mg/day) (n = 16)	Surgically treated group (n = 16)
Percent requiring single dilatation only	44	75
Mean number of dilatations over mean follow-up period of 22 months	1.8	0.3

Data from Watson, A.: (abstract) Gut **26:**553, 1985.

annually, and it is our practice to perform these at each dilatation, taking particular care in circumstances in which dilatation requirements are increasing. When adenocarcinoma supervenes, this should be treated according to normal practice, although because of the age and general condition of many patients suffering from reflux stricture, palliative management may be all that is appropriate in some instances. Two of our patients developing esophageal adenocarcinoma were suitable for resection; the other two elderly patients were treated by fiberoptic endoscopic intubation.

OPERATIVE MANAGEMENT

The last two decades have seen a swing away from resection to a more conservative approach in the majority of cases, based on dilatation of the stricture and correction of reflux. The disadvantages of resection are the operative mortality of up to 15%[32] and the fact that the potential for reflux may remain. The relative safety and efficacy of dilatation combined with antireflux surgery has allowed a more radical approach than intermittent dilatation alone to be employed in suitable patients earlier in the course of the disease; thus, resection should now rarely be necessary in benign reflux stricture. The range of surgical approaches currently used in the management of reflux stricture is as follows; each approach will be considered.

Antireflux surgery alone
Antireflux surgery plus dilatation of stricture
Gastroplasty with antireflux surgery and dilatation
Roux-en-Y duodenal diversion
Resection and interposition

Antireflux surgery alone

The beneficial effect of antireflux surgery alone in the healing of strictures was suggested by Burkhart and Sullivan in 1972,[33] with improvement of 12 of 17 patients treated. This finding was subsequently confirmed by Larrain, Csendes, and Pope,[34] who added some objectivity by measuring stricture diameter before and after Hill posterior gastropexy without dilatation. Mean stricture diameter increased from 6.3 mm preoperatively to 13.0 mm postoperatively in 24 patients, who were felt to have true fibrous stricture on the basis of endoscopic and manometric criteria.

While it is our practice to combine dilatation with antireflux surgery, we have confirmed the resolution of strictures in four patients treated by antireflux surgery alone, each of whom had true fibrous strictures impassible with an Olympus GIFQ 11-mm endoscope. (See Fig. 17-5.)

Antireflux surgery combined with dilatation

In a situation in which correction of reflux alone will heal some strictures, and in which 75% of patients having antireflux surgery and dilatation will not require subsequent dilatations, the combination of antireflux surgery and dilatation is currently the preferred form of management—providing, first, that the patient is fit to undergo surgery and, second, that the patient does not have an advanced (grade 3) stricture such that periesophagitis and shortening preclude an adequate antireflux operation.

Dilatation may be performed either immediately before surgery, by one of the techniques previously described, or intraoperatively through a gastrotomy. Most of the currently practiced antireflux operations have been performed in this context. Bremner[25] reported good results using the Nissen fundoplication in 25 patients, but Ellis et al.[35] were less enthusiastic, reporting a high incidence of residual dysphagia and the need for further dilatations, and questioned the need in stricture patients for a pro-

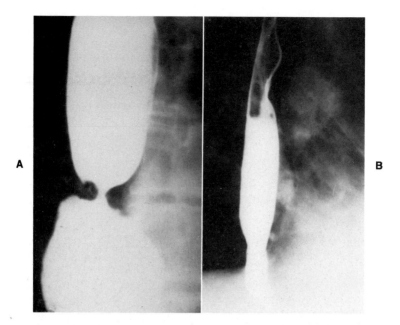

Fig. 17-5. Barium swallow of patient with fibrous reflux stricture before (**A**) and after (**B**) antireflux surgery without dilation.

cedure other than total fundoplication. Skinner[36] reported good results with the Belsey Mark IV operation, after a previous, less encouraging report. Consistently good results have been reported with the Hill gastropexy,[37,38] with Hemreck and Coates[38] reporting a success rate of 96%, although overall results of a large review of 17 pooled series including each of the above-mentioned procedures showed a mean success rate of approximately 75%.[28]

The rather lower success rate than usually achieved in uncomplicated reflux disease is due to a combination of greater difficulty in achieving complete reflux control, especially in the presence of esophageal shortening, and the accompanying motility problem producing the potential for esophageal obstruction after total fundoplication. This latter problem is most marked in patients with underlying primary motility disorders, in whom the success rate is as low as 58%.[3]

Our preferred antireflux procedure is one that depends on transhiatal mobilization and fixation of a long intraabdominal segment of esophagus (and thus the majority of the LES) to a posterior crural repair and therefore under the influence of positive intraabdominal pressure, accentuating the flutter valve at the cardia and necessitating only a 120-degree fundoplication to achieve reflux control objectively demonstrated by 24-hour pH recording. We have performed this procedure in 248 patients with gastroesophageal reflux over an 11-year period, including 68 patients with

reflux stricture, mostly transabdominally but using a thoracoabdominal approach in the presence of marked periesophagitis. There has been no mortality and minimal morbidity; in particular, there has been no gas bloating, no necessity to reoperate for mechanical complications, and no obstructive symptoms other than transient dysphagia in approximately 6%, which always resolves spontaneously prior to discharge from hospital. Subjective results have shown improvement in 97% of patients, with objective evidence of reflux control by 24-hour pH monitoring in 85%.[39] Manometric studies have shown the range of resting LES pressure to be similar to that of our asymptomatic controls,[40] as distinct from the Nissen fundoplication, which in several reports results in supraphysiologic values of resting LES pressure.[41,42] It is likely that this has a bearing on the incidence of obstructive complications, particularly when motor abnormalities coexist with reflux as in the presence of reflux stricture, and may explain the problems encountered with the Nissen fundoplication in the patients in the series of Ellis et al. In common with other workers, our incidence of good results in stricture patients was somewhat less than in uncomplicated reflux patients, but at 81%, compares very favorably with other series. (See Fig. 17-6.)

In situations in which extensive periesophagitis and esophageal shortening preclude the easy conduct of a standard antireflux procedure, a transthoracic or thoracoabdominal approach to

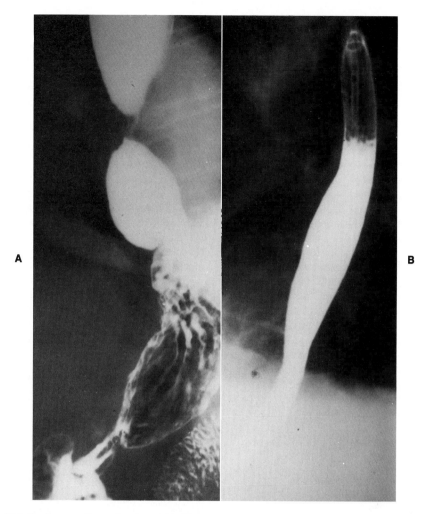

Fig. 17-6. Barium swallow of patient with fibrous reflux stricture before (**A**) and after (**B**) antireflux surgery and fiberoptic endoscopic dilatation.

those procedures normally performed transabdominally enables greater mobilization of the esophagus to be achieved. Indeed, a Nissen fundoplication situated within the chest has been shown to effectively control reflux,[43] although a disturbing incidence of gastric ulceration and even perforation has been reported in such circumstances.[44] Current opinion would now favor the combination of a gastroplasty, to gain length, and an antireflux operation when any doubt exists about the ability to conduct a safe and effective antireflux procedure in the presence of esophageal shortening.

Gastroplasty with antireflux surgery and dilatation

The most popular gastroplasty is that described by Collis,[45] which creates a 5-cm length of intraabdominal "esophagus" from a gastric tube, which aids reflux control by providing a pressure gradient between this segment exposed to positive intraabdominal pressure and the intrathoracic esophagus under the influence of negative intrathoracic pressure. This procedure also provides a structure around which a varying degree of fundoplication may be performed, most popularly a Belsey or Nissen repair, and we have combined gastroplasty with the repair described above with good effect.

Pearson[46] has reported the largest series of the Collis-Belsey procedure, 166 of his 360 procedures being performed for reflux stricture. Overall, satisfactory results were obtained in 85% of patients, with equally good results in patients with stricture, although subsequent resection was necessary in two such patients. Orringer[47] and Ellis[48] have both reported superior results in their hands with the Collis-Nissen procedure when objective measurements of reflux control have been made. In Orringer's series, 93% achieved good reflux control, but of 30 patients so treated, 50% required subsequent dilatations and two needed regular dilatations because of unsatisfactory resolution of their strictures.

Since around 95% of reflux strictures are dilatable and capable of regression with adequate reflux control,[48] the trend toward dilatation with antireflux surgery, with or without gastroplasty, has resulted in the preservation of many more esophagi that two decades ago would have been resected. This has resulted in considerable lowering of operative mortality, from around 15% to near 1%, and better control of reflux. In view of the risk of adenocarcinoma complicating reflux stricture and the fact that antireflux surgery may not result in regression of columnar-lined esophagus,[35] the carcinoma risk might be expected to persist when resection is not performed. All the cases of adenocarcinoma complicating reflux stricture reported from our institution were in medically treated patients, with no patient undergoing antireflux surgery subsequently developing carcinoma. However, Pearson[46] reported three adenocarcinomas in 166 patients treated by the Collis-Belsey procedure and dilatation, and have suggested the need for regular surveillance of these patients, and indeed Skinner[49] has advocated resection in those cases with severe dysplasia.

Resection and interposition

Greater knowledge of the behavior of reflux stricture and the application of modern dilatation techniques with well-conducted antireflux procedures have significantly reduced the need for resection in these cases. The overall incidence of resection has fallen to 5% or less, only three resections for reflux stricture having been performed in our institution in the past decade. Resection should be reserved for patients whose cases are resistant to the more conservative techniques described, who most frequently are those who have associated motor disorders or who have undergone multiple operations. Several techniques of resection and interposition have been described, using stomach, jejunum, or colon as the replacement organ.

The stomach is technically the simplest replacement organ, but when an end-to-end intrathoracic esophagogastric anastomosis is utilized, reflux is not controlled and the risk of further ulceration and stricture formation is high, reaching 27% within 6 months of resection.[50] This problem has been overcome in short segment replacement by adding a form of fundoplication[9]

and in other cases by using a reversed gastric tube,[51] although this seems to have been more widely used in children, in whom good results have been reported.[52] The use of an isoperistaltic segment of jejunum for interposition is technically more difficult, especially when long segment replacement is necessary, but good long-term results have been obtained by Polk, with an operative mortality of 4% but a significant incidence of early postoperative complications.[53]

The most popular replacement organ has been an isoperistaltic segment of colon, which is suitable for long segment replacement, as far as the neck if necessary. Its advocates claim that it is technically easier and safer to use than jejunum and more appropriate to use in childhood. The left colon based on the left colic artery is the most popular technique, its smaller bulk and its normal function being to transmit a solid bolus resulting in the likelihood of a better anatomic and functional result. However, ischemic colitis and structural and functional problems more commonly affect the left colon, and it is important to be assured of the vascularity and the absence of coexisting disease prior to its use. Belsey[54] has reported excellent results in a large series of colonic replacements, with an operative mortality of 4.2% and a low incidence of complications. The functional results of using the colon as a replacement organ have been shown to be excellent.[55]

Roux-en-Y duodenal diversion

Roux-en-Y duodenal diversion has been advocated in situations in which bile is felt to be a major component of the refluxate or in which previous multiple operations at the cardia make further dissection difficult. It is usually combined with antrectomy and vagotomy if feasible, so that both major reflux components are diminished and the risk of anastomotic ulceration is reduced, and good results have been reported in these circumstances.[56,57]

CONCLUSIONS

Reflux stricture is a serious complication of gastroesophageal reflux, demanding active treatment to reduce the risk of permanent esophageal damage. An accurate diagnosis is an essential prerequisite to effective management, and when treated early, 95% of strictures are dilatable, and resection can be avoided by combining dilatation with an effective antireflux procedure, combined with gastroplasty when necessary. This is the management of choice in patients with dilatable strictures who are fit for surgery, since surgery offers superior control of reflux and reduces the need for subsequent dilatations, with good results in over 75% of patients. However, in frail, elderly patients, in whom reflux stricture is common, good symptomatic relief can be obtained with intermittent dilatation and medical antireflux measures. Resection is necessary in the approximately 5% of patients who are resistant to more conservative methods or when multiple previous operations or superimposed motor disorders are an added problem. In these circumstances, colonic interposition is the preferred procedure, and is accompanied by good long-term and functional results. The small but definite risk of adenocarcinoma complicating reflux stricture must not be forgotten, and careful follow-up of these patients is essential.

REFERENCES

1. Palmer, E.D.: Subacute erosive ("peptic") esophagitis, Arch. Pathol. **59:**51-57, 1955.
2. Ismail-Beigi, F., Horton, P.F., and Pope, C.E.: Histological consequences of gastroesophageal reflux in man, Gastroenterology **58:**163-174, 1970.
3. DeMeester, T.R.: Management of benign esophageal strictures. In Stipa, S., Belsey, R.H.R., and Moraldi, A., editors: Medical and surgical problems of the esophagus, New York, 1981, Academic Press, p. 973.
4. Pearson, F.G.: Surgical treatment of a peptic stricture. In Stipa, S., Belsey, R.H.R., and Moraldi, A., editors: Medical and surgical problems of the esophagus, New York, 1981, Academic Press, p. 159.
5. Crumplin, M.K.H., Stol, D.W., and Collis, J.L.: The pattern of bile salt reflux and acid secretion in sliding hiatal hernia, Br. J. Surg. **61:**611-616, 1974.
6. Gillison, E.W., De Castro, V.A.M., Nyrus, L.M., et al.: The significance of bile in reflux esophagitis, Surg. Gynecol. Obstet. **134:**419-424, 1972.
7. Watson, A.: The role of antireflux surgery combined with fiberoptic endoscopic dilatation in peptic esophageal stricture, Am. J. Surg. **148:**346-349, 1984.
8. Tytgat, G.N.J.: Non-radiological investigation of the oesophagus. In Watson, A., and Celestin, L.R., editors: Disorders of the oesophagus, London, 1984, Pitman Books, Ltd., p. 24.
9. Henderson, R.D.: Management of the patient with benign esophageal stricture, Surg. Clin. North Amer. **63:**885-903, 1983.
10. Jackson, C.: Bronchoscopy and esophagoscopy, Philadelphia, 1922, W.B. Saunders Co.
11. Lilley, J.O., and McCaffery, E.D.: Esophageal stricture dilatation: a new method adapted to the fiberoptic esophagoscope, Am. J. Dig. Dis. **16:**1137-1140, 1971.
12. Katz, D.: Morbidity and mortality in standard and flexible gastrointestinal endoscopy, Gastrointest. Endosc. **15:**134-141, 1969.
13. Didcott, C.C.: Oesophageal stricture: treatment by slow continuous dilatation, Ann. R. Coll. Surg. Engl. **53:**112-126, 1973.
14. Owman, T., and Lunderquist, A.: Balloon catheter dilatation of esophageal strictures: a preliminary report, Gastrointest. Radiol. **7:**301-305, 1982.
15. Celestin, L.R., and Campbell, W.B.: A new and safe system for oesophageal dilatation, Lancet **1:**74, 1981.
16. Watson, A.: Dilatation of benign oesophageal strictures, Br. J. Surg. **72:**153-154, 1985.
17. Benedict, D.B.: Peptic stenosis of the esophagus: a study of 233 patients treated with bougienage, surgery or both, Am. J. Dig. Dis. **11:**761-770, 1966.
18. Lanza, F.L., and Graham, D.Y.: Bougienage is effective therapy for most benign esophageal strictures, JAMA **240:**844-847, 1978.
19. Wesdorp, I.C.E., and Tytgat, G.N.J.: Results of conservative treatment of benign esophageal strictures in 100 patients. In DeMeester, T.R., and Skinner, D.B., editors: Esophageal disorders: pathophysiology and therapy, New York, 1985, Raven Press, p. 221.
20. Bennett, J.R., Sutton, D.R., Price, J.R., et al.: Effects of bougie dilatation on esophageal stricture size. In DeMeester, T.R., and Skinner, D.B., editors: Esophageal disorders: pathophysiology and therapy, New York, 1985, Raven Press, p. 221.
21. Ogilvie, A.L., Ferguson, R., and Atkinson, M.: Outlook with conservative treatment of peptic oesophageal stricture, Gut **21:**23-25, 1980.
22. Watson, A.: Randomised study comparing medical and surgical reflux control in the management of peptic oesophageal stricture treated by intermittent dilatation (abstract), Gut **26:**553, 1985.
23. Hine, K.R., Hawkey, C.J., Atkinson, M., et al.: Comparison of the Eder-Puestow and Celestin techniques for dilating benign oesophageal strictures, Gut **25:**1100-1102, 1984.
24. Cox, J.C., Winter, R.K., Jones, R., et al.: Balloons against bougies for dilatation of benign oesophageal stricture: a randomised prospective trial (abstract), Gut **26:**1136, 1985.
25. Bremner, C.G.: Benign strictures of the esophagus, Curr. Probl. Surg. **19:**406-489, 1982.
26. Moghissi, K.: Conservative surgery in reflux stricture of the oesophagus associated with hiatal hernia, Br. J. Surg. **76:**221-225, 1979.
27. Hill, L.D., Gelfand, M., and Bauermeister, D.: Simplified management of reflux esophagitis with stricture, Ann. Surg. **172:**638-651, 1970.
28. Siewert, R.: Surgical therapy of peptic stenoses. In Stipa, S., Belsey, R.H.R., and Moraldi, A., editors: Medical and surgical problems of the esophagus, New York, 1981, Academic Press, p. 146.
29. Naef, A.P., Savary, M., and Ozello, L.: Columnar-lined lower esophagus: an acquired lesion with malignant predisposition, J. Thorac. Cardiovasc. Surg. **70:**826-835, 1975.
30. Moghissi, K.: Carcinoma of the cardia and thoracic oesophagus coexisting with and following sliding hiatus hernia and peptic stricture, Thorax **32:**342-345, 1977.
31. Haggitt, R.C., Tryzelaar, J., Ellis, F.H., et al.: Adenocarcinoma complicating columnar epithelium–lined (Barrett's) esophagus, Am. J. Clin. Pathol. **70:**1-5, 1978.

32. Franklin, R.H.: The advancing frontiers of oesophageal surgery, Ann. R. Coll. Surg. Engl. **59:**284-287, 1977.

33. Burkhart, K.L., and Sullivan, B.H.: Course and treatment of benign esophageal strictures, Am. J. Gastroenterol. **58:**531-536, 1972.

34. Larrain, A., Csendes, A., and Pope, C.E.: Surgical correction of reflux: an effective therapy for esophageal strictures, Gastroenterology **69:**578-583, 1975.

35. Ellis, F.H., Garabedion, M., and Gibb, S.P.: Fundoplication for gastroesophageal reflux, Arch. Surg. **107:**186-192, 1973.

36. Skinner, D.B.: Benign esophageal strictures, Adv. Surg. **10:**177-196, 1976.

37. Russell, C.O., and Hill, L.D.: Gastroesophageal reflux, Curr. Probl. Surg. **20:**209-278, 1983.

38. Hermreck, A.S., and Coates, N.R.: Results of the Hill anti-reflux operation, Am. J. Surg. **140:**764-767, 1980.

39. Watson, A.: A clinical and pathophysiological study of a simple and effective operation for the correction of gastro-oesophageal reflux (abstract), Br. J. Surg. **71:**991, 1984.

40. Watson, A.: Lower oesophageal sphincter characteristics of a simplified procedure for the correction of gastro-oesophageal reflux, Br. J. Surg. (In press.)

41. DeMeester, T.R., and Johnson, L.F.: Evaluation of the Nissen anti-reflux procedure by esophageal manometry and twenty-four hour pH monitoring, Am. J. Surg. **129:**94-100, 1975.

42. Dawson, K., Ryan, R., Donovan, M., et al.: Prospective randomised trial of Angelchik prosthesis versus Nissen fundoplication (abstract), Gut **26:**555, 1985.

43. Nissen, R., Rossetti, M., and Siewert, R.: Twenty years in the management of reflux disease using fundoplication, Chirurg. **48:**634-639, 1977.

44. Mansour, K.A., Burton, H.G., Miller, J.I., et al.: Complications of intrathoracic Nissen fundoplication, Ann. Thorac. Surg. **32:**173-178, 1981.

45. Collis, J.L.: Gastroplasty, Thorax **16:**197-206, 1961.

46. Pearson, J.G.: Collis-Belsey procedure for peptic strictures: five to fifteen year follow-up. In DeMeester, T.R., and Skinner, D.B., editors: Esophageal disorders: pathophysiology and therapy, New York, 1985, Raven Press, p. 257.

47. Orringer, M.B.: Surgical treatment of esophageal strictures resulting from gastroesophageal reflux. In Stipa, S., Belsey, R.H.R., and Moraldi, A., editors: Medical and surgical problems of the esophagus, New York, 1981, Academic Press, p. 165.

48. Ellis, F.H.: The surgical management of esophageal stricture. In Stipa, S., Belsey, R.H.R., and Moraldi, A., editors: Medical and surgical problems of the esophagus, New York, 1981, Academic Press, p. 181.

49. Skinner, D.B., Walther, B.C., Riddell, R.H., et al.: Barrett's esophagus: comparison of benign and malignant cases, Ann. Surg. **198:**554-556, 1983.

50. Belsey, R.H.R.: Reconstruction of the esophagus with left colon, J. Thorac. Cardiovasc. Surg. **49:**33-55, 1965.

51. Heimlich, H.J.: Reversed gastric tube esophagoplasty for failure of colon, jejunum and prosthetic interposition, Ann. Surg. **182:**154-160, 1975.

52. Anderson, K.D., and Randolph, J.G.: Gastric tube interposition: a satisfactory alternative to the colon for esophageal replacement in children, Ann. Thorac. Surg. **25:**521-525, 1978.

53. Polk, H.C., and Richardson, J.D.: Non-functional esophagogastric junction: treatment by jejunal interposition. In Stipa, S., Belsey, R.H.R., and Moraldi, A., editors: Medical and surgical problems of the esophagus, New York, 1981, Academic Press, p. 188.

54. Belsey, R.H.R.: Esophageal reconstruction with colon for benign disease. In Stipa, S., Belsey, R.H.R., and Moraldi, A., editors: Medical and surgical problems of the esophagus, New York, 1981, Academic Press, p. 195.

55. Skinner, D.B.: Functional effects of colon interposition in reconstruction of the esophagus. In Stipa, S., Belsey, R.H.R., and Moraldi, A., editors: Medical and surgical problems of the esophagus, New York, 1981, Academic Press, p. 193.

56. Payne, W.S., and Olsen, A.M.: The esophagus, Philadelphia, 1974, Lea & Febiger, p. 130.

57. Fekete, F.: Total duodenal diversion. In DeMeester, T.R., and Skinner, D.B., editors: Esophageal disorders: pathophysiology and therapy, New York, 1985, Raven Press, p. 135.

Management of reflux strictures

DISCUSSION

Lucius D. Hill

Dr. Watson presents a clear and succinct picture of the problem of management of reflux stricture. The sections on pathophysiology and diagnosis very nicely outline the problem. We take exception, however, with one point in the pathophysiology, and that is in regard to the question of esophageal shortening. This is an important point because esophageal shortening is cited as the reason for performing esophageal lengthening procedures or resection. If one is to base the selection of an operation on a given point such as esophageal shortening, the observations should be scientific and sound. As Dr. Watson points out, the mortality and morbidity rates for a straightforward antireflux procedure are far lower than for a resectional procedure and, in fact, are lower than for most reports of esophageal lengthening procedures. It follows, then, that if the surgeon makes the statement that the esophagus is short, it would be well to know just how long the esophagus is or how much shortening has occurred. There have been no experimental or clinical observations to support in a scientific manner the concept of the short esophagus. Only in those patients in whom the esophagus has been perforated or in whom the esophagus is virtually destroyed have we been able to demonstrate any shortening whatever. We have challenged those surgeons who constantly use this term to produce a scientific measurement of the esophagus and tell us precisely how much shortening has occurred. No such scientific measurement has been forthcoming. Watson's experience supports our observation that esophageal shortening is rare.

I agree completely that the indications for surgery should be very strict and the workup should be complete to rule out motility disorders, scleroderma, esophageal spasm, and other problems that may mimic the clinical picture of strictures. Dr. Watson makes the statement that manometry and pH recording are necessary to quantify reflux and categorize its type as well as to identify coexisting motility problems, all of which may have important therapeutic implications.

As far as nonoperative management of reflux stricture is concerned, we would agree that a trial of vigorous medical management, including H_2 blockers as well as a dietary regimen and elevation of the head of the bed, is important. We are concerned, however, with repeated dilatations over a long period of time. We reported 160 patients undergoing antireflux operations for peptic esophageal stricture.[1] The series now numbers 243 patients and appears to be larger than any series reported. The mean follow-up period in the reported group was 47 months. One hundred seven patients operated upon early in the course of the disease had better results (90% good, 9% fair, and only 1% poor) than 31 patients having a previous failed operation (52% good, 23% fair, 26% poor) and 22 patients having multiple dilatations (45% good, 23% fair, and 32% poor) ($p < 0.05$). This data indicates that the worst results are seen in those patients who have had repeated dilatations over a long period of time. The best group is the patients who have had a single dilatation. It is in this group of patients, who had only 1% poor results, that the esophagus is not damaged by repeated dilatations, and following surgery these same patients show a rather rapid healing of the stricture, and they become asymptomatic very soon after surgery. It is well to point out that many gastroenterologists persist in dilating strictures because they have had a bad experience with patients who have undergone surgery. Many of these patients have come back with complaints of gas bloat syndrome, dysphagia, or persistent reflux.

Two distinct patient groups treated by dilatation alone have been identified by Patterson, et al.[2] One group improved after an initial series of dilatations. The second group, comprising 46% of patients with stricture, required repeated dilatations. One can extrapolate from this report that if the patient does not have a good clinical result after a single course of dilatations, surgery should be considered rather than putting the patient through repeated dilatations, which may irreversibly damage the esophagus or lead to perforation. Overall good results were obtained in 84% of Patterson's patients, who were followed up for a mean of only 26 months. A nonrandomized trial of surgical and medical management found dilatation alone satisfactory in only 65% of 120 patients treated by Dr. Watson's group.[2a]

Surgical treatment of peptic esophageal stricture has evolved toward nonresectional techniques. When we first presented this concept before the American Surgical Association in 1970, our report created a great deal of controversy because the concept of the short esophagus and the need for resectional procedures had become ingrained in the surgical literature. Professor Conrad Lam[3] was one of the first to coin the phrase "the myth of the short esophagus." With the passage of time, more and more surgeons around the world have come to agree with the concept that a simplified antireflux procedure that corrects reflux will indeed allow a reflux stricture to heal. The problem that we see all too often is that an antireflux procedure is done but fails to correct reflux, the stricture persists, and the surgeon then becomes convinced that an antireflux procedure does not work in the presence of stricture. I am delighted, therefore, to see Dr. Watson's outstanding experience with 68 patients treated by an antireflux procedure for stricture. The technique that Dr. Watson describes consists of a transhiatal mobilization and fixation of a long intraabdominal segment of esophagus (thus the majority of the LES) to the posterior crura, producing an intraabdominal segment of esophagus with accentuation of the flutter valve at the cardia. This technique is consistent with the principles of the technique that we have employed for the past 20 years in dealing with esophageal reflux. Dr. Watson adds a 120-degree fundoplication to achieve reflux control, objectively demonstrated by 24-hour pH recording. He has performed this procedure in 248 patients with gastroesophageal reflux over an 11-year period, including 68 patients with reflux stricture. He states that he has used the procedure primarily as a transabdominal approach, using the thoracoabdominal approach only in the presence of marked periesophagitis. Ninety-seven percent of Dr. Watson's patients showed subjective improvement. Reflux control was obtained in 85% of patients, as evidenced by 24-hour pH monitoring. His manometric studies have shown

the range of resting LES pressure to be similar to that of asymptomatic controls, as distinct from the Nissen fundoplication, which, in many reports, results in supraphysiologic values of resting LES pressure, although success rates in patients with uncomplicated reflux are better. Dr. Watson is to be congratulated for achieving an 81% success rate with these more complicated patients with reflux stricture.

Our technique differs from the author's in that we do not include a fundoplication, although our procedure has been depicted as a fundoplication by those who do not understand the technique. We have refrained from using fundoplication because of the very complications that Dr. Watson so clearly outlines. Instead of performing a fundoplication, we utilize the phrenoesophageal bundles of tissue and simply imbricate these along the lesser curvature, which mimics the normal anatomy in that this places tension on the collarsling musculature and accentuates the flutter valve mechanism and calibrates the cardia.

We agree completely that the routine use of motility and pH studies, both before and after operation, is very helpful in order to define the problem initially and to determine whether the basic problem has been corrected. We go a step further and utilize additional available technology to obtain intraoperative pressure measurements. The most important single measurement that we take is the one during the operation, since we have never seen a preoperative or postoperative pressure measurement improve the patient's status in any way. If the postoperative pressure measurement shows a sphincter pressure of 0, the operation is a total failure, whereas if the intraoperative pressure measurement is 0 it alerts the surgeon to persist in calibrating the cardia until he or she can construct a measurable barrier to reflux. It has been a mystery to us why surgeons have resisted applying this effective and available technique to the operation itself, where the measurement is most critical. Intraoperative pressure measurements can be done quickly, adding only 10 to 15 minutes to the procedure. They have produced no complications and give the surgeon assurance that the barrier pressure is within a range that will allow the patient to swallow and yet is tight enough to prevent reflux. I will wager that if Dr. Watson added this to his armamentarium, the 15% of patients in whom reflux was not controlled and the 19% of patients with strictures who had less than a good result would be markedly improved. As long as there is any persistent reflux in these patients, we will continue to strive to do a better job. Calibrating the cardia is a safe, easy, and effective method of providing objective data that will lead to minimizing symptom recurrence resulting from technical operative error.

Dr. Watson states that when extensive periesophagitis and esophageal shortening preclude the easy conduct of a standard antireflux procedure, a transthoracic or thoracoabdominal approach enables greater mobilization of the esophagus to be achieved. He states that a Nissen fundoplication situated within the chest has been shown to effectively control reflux but that a disturbing incidence of gastric ulceration and even perforation has been reported in such circumstances. We would agree with this entirely, and in our experience the intrathoracic Nissen fundoplication creates a paraesophageal hernia, which is subject to life-threatening complications. We have seen deaths from perforation of the transthoracic Nissen in both infants and adults.

As Dr. Watson states, the most popular thoracoabdominal operation is the Collis gastroplasty, but it is difficult to tell from his discussion whether this procedure has been used by his group. In our series of 243 patients we have not found an esophageal lengthening procedure necessary. Only in those patients in whom the esophagus has been destroyed by multiple dilatations, particularly following perforation, and in whom there is no esophageal lumen, have we found it necessary to resort to resection.

Pearson[4] has reported the largest series of the Collis-Belsey procedure. One hundred sixty-six patients were treated by Pearson for reflux strictures, and he had a good result in 85%. This is probably the best record with the Collis-Belsey procedure achieved anywhere in the world. Having had the privilege of participating in an operation with Dr. Pearson, I can say from firsthand observation that he is one of the world's outstanding surgeons and is able to perform the Collis-Belsey procedure with very low mortality and morbidity, but in the hands of the surgeon who only occasionally deals with antireflux problems, this operation is a far more extensive procedure than that described by Dr. Watson.

Dr. Watson's experience with resection is in complete agreement with ours. Out of his entire experience, he has done only three resections for reflux stricture. We agree that resection should be reserved for those cases resistant to more conservative techniques. We, too, prefer stomach as the primary organ for replacement, with left colon as a second choice when stomach is not available.

In the illustrations in Dr. Watson's chapter, there are two patients shown with very severe fibrous strictures treated by antireflux surgery without dilatation. These strictures are very similar to examples presented in other studies that purport to show a shortened esophagus with an undilatable stricture. The fact that the antireflux procedure performed caused these strictures to completely disappear, resulting in a postoperative barium swallow that looks normal, is entirely consistent with our experience and demonstrates quite clearly the great healing capacity of the esophagus once reflux is controlled.

An important observation made by Dr. Watson's group is that no patient undergoing antireflux surgery subsequently developed carcinoma while four cases of carcinoma developed in medically treated patients. Our experience was the same until recently, when one patient with Barrett's esophagus developed adenocarcinoma following antireflux surgery, with postoperative pH and motility studies demonstrating correction of reflux. Review of his previous biopsies showed that insufficient material was taken to tell the degree of dysplasia.

Our policy at present for the management of Barrett's esophagus consists of endoscopy with generous biopsies in multiple sites. These are then studied carefully and if there is dysplasia, we have the patient examined by Dr. Haggitt and his associates, who have done the most sophisticated and advanced studies on Barrett's mucosa.[5] Dr. Haggitt's group takes 20 to 50 generous biopsies, which are then subjected to a variety of studies, including light and electron microscopy and flow cytometry. A battery of oncogenes are defined and cytogenetic studies are done. This group is now following 160 patients with columnar epithelium in the esophagus, 90 of whom have had this extensive study. From this experience they have been able to categorize Barrett's epithelium into nondysplastic and dysplastic columnar epithelium. The dysplastic columnar epithelium is further stratified into low-grade dysplasia and high-grade dysplasia. Haggitt's group has termed high-grade dysplasia "Barrett's specialized metaplasia," and, in fact, Haggitt's group reserves the diagnosis of Barrett's esophagus for patients whose biopsies show Barrett's specialized metaplastic epithelium (BSME) in the tubular esophagus. Available data indicate that it is this epithelium that is associated with an increased risk of adenocarcinoma.

For practical purposes, one needs guidelines for following patients with Barrett's epithelium. Haggitt's group suggests that it is the patients with BSME who need close follow-up. Since high-grade dysplasia in Barrett's esophagus refers to an unequivocally neoplastic transformation in the epithelium, it is these patients who need intense surveillance.

Haggitt and his associates do not believe that a patient with high-grade dysplasia is in need of a resection. Their group recommends early follow-up with endoscopy in order to take multiple biopsies of the area of dysplasia to determine its extent and to search for coexisting adenocarcinoma. Each patient with high-grade dysplasia must be evaluated individually, with the examiner weighing the usual clinical factors when considering surgery. Repeat biopsies in 3-month to 6-month intervals are recommended.

High-grade dysplasia in Barrett's esophagus is rare. Most pathologists do not have the opportunity to see many of these cases and therefore should seek a second opinion before surgical resection is considered. Adenocarcinomas may be so well differentiated that they can be distinguished from high-grade dysplasia only by demonstrating invasion below the muscularis mucosa. This may be difficult because endoscopic biopsies often do not obtain significant amounts of submucosal tissue and because ulceration may obliterate the muscularis mucosa, the landmark that must be traversed to prove submucosal invasion.

Although patients with low-grade dysplasia are not at as great a risk as those with high-grade dysplasia, they do merit more intense surveillance than patients without dysplasia.

Once adenocarcinoma is documented, the treatment is surgical resection in the patient who is an acceptable risk. Because high-grade dysplasia and adenocarcinoma are often multicentric and involve large areas of the columnar mucosa, all of the columnar-lined segment of the esophagus should be removed in patients undergoing surgery.

In conclusion, Dr. Watson is to be congratulated because this series of 68 patients with reflux strictures treated by antireflux surgery with no mortality and minimum morbidity represents the best results in any series of this size. It is noteworthy that he states he has confirmed the resolution of strictures in four patients treated by antireflux surgery alone. Each of these patients had true fibrous strictures impassible with an Olympus 11-mm endoscope. The remainder of the patients had the transabdominal repair described by Watson, which accentuates the flutter valve and restores the cardia with fixation of a long intraabdominal segment of esophagus to the crura. This type of transabdominal repair is very close to the repair we have used, except that we do not employ a fundoplication. We have employed our technique in 243 patients with reflux strictures, with 85% good results, which compares favorably with those of Dr. Watson. It is experiences like these that should lay to rest the notion that the esophagus is shortened in reflux strictures and that resections and esophageal lengthening procedures are necessary.

It is results such as Dr. Watson's that will restore the confidence of gastroenterologists, thereby providing surgeons earlier access to patients—before multiple dilatations have destroyed the esophagus. With improved technique and modern technology, we can relieve the stricture patient from a life of dilatations and risk of perforation, with a minimum of mortality and morbidity.

REFERENCES

1. Mercer, C.D., and Hill, L.D.: Surgical management of peptic esophageal stricture, J. Thorac. Cardiovasc. Surg. **91:**371-378, 1986.
2. Patterson, D.J., Graham, D.Y., Smith, J.L., et al.: Natural history of benign esophageal stricture treated by dilatation, Gastroenterology **85:**346-350, 1983.
2a. Watson, A.: The role of antireflux surgery combined with fiberoptic endoscopic dilatation in peptic esophageal structure, Am. J. Surg. **148:**346-349, 1984.
3. Lam, C.R., and Gahagan, T.H.: Special comment: the myth of the short esophagus. In Nyhus, L.M., and Harkins, H.N., editors: Hernia, Philadelphia, J.B. Lippincott, Co., p. 450.
4. Pearson, F.G.: Collis-Belsey procedure for peptic strictures: 5 to 15 year follow-up in esophageal disorders. In DeMeester, T.R., and Skinner, D.B., editors: Pathophysiology and therapy, New York, 1985, Raven Press, p. 257.
5. Reid, B.J., Haggitt, R.C., and Rubin, C.E.: Barrett's esophagus and esophageal carcinoma. In Hill, L.D., Castell, D.O., McCallum, R.W., Kozarek, R.A., and Mercer, C.D., editors: Management of esophageal disorders, Philadelphia, 1987, W.B. Saunders Co. (In press.)

18 Surgical management of caustic injuries to the upper gastrointestinal tract

Michel Jean Noirclerc, Jacques Di Costanzo,
Bernard Sastre, Jacqueline Jouglard, André Gauthier,
Jacques Figarella, and Bruno Berthet

Injuries to the upper digestive tract by swallowing of caustic substances such as alkalis (65% of cases), acids (16% of cases), or oxidizing agents, occur accidentally (two thirds of cases) or intentionally. In this part of the gut even relatively minor chemical burns can lead to the most severe consequences.

In the last 10 years the prognosis in cases of caustic burns has been considerably improved as a result of standardized regimens based on the initial endoscopic findings. This treatment calls for artificial feeding in the most serious cases, followed by surgery should sequelae develop during the healing phase.

NATURAL COURSE OF CAUSTIC BURNS IN THE UPPER DIGESTIVE TRACT

After ingestion of a caustic substance, two phases are observed. The first is the necrotic phase, and the second is the healing phase. The duration of the healing phase is variable.[1-3]

In some cases the wall of the digestive tube may be transgressed, resulting in injury to surrounding organs. Such burns usually result in immediate or delayed death. Emergency surgery must be undertaken with a view to removing the lesions before necrosis passes beyond the wall of the esophagus.

In all other cases healing time depends on the extent of the initial injury. For mild injuries, not involving the submucosa, the healing period generally lasts from 20 to 30 days. For deeper burns, involving the submucosa, healing takes between 90 and 120 days. In 50% of patients with deep burns in which mucosal necrosis is associated with edema and local infection, fibrosis and retraction occur. In 20% of cases fibrosis

leads to stricture formation. Such strictures are rarely short and often extensive.

Esophageal lesions occur in 70% of cases. In 65% of these cases the middle third of the esophagus is affected, in 15% it is the upper third, and in 18% the whole organ is involved. The stomach is affected in 17% of cases. The antral region is a predilection site for caustic burns (91% of cases); involvement of the whole stomach is rare (9% of cases). In 14% of cases lesions occur both in the esophagus and in the stomach.

ASSESSING THE GRAVITY OF A CAUSTIC BURN AND INITIAL TREATMENT

Two investigative techniques are essential to the assessment of the gravity of a caustic burn:
1. The patient and his family should be questioned to determine the nature and concentration of the caustic substance, the approximate amount ingested, the time of ingestion, and the circumstances.
2. Endoscopy should be carried out early to confirm the existence of lesions (present in 85% of cases), to determine their extent and location in the pharynx, esophagus, and stomach, and to assess the intensity of the burn (on the basis of mucosal erythema, ulceration, necrosis, hemorrhage, and so on).[4-7]

On the basis of the endoscopic findings, caustic lesions are staged as shown in Table 18-1. A review of the relevant literature shows that 10% of patients have no lesions, 30% have stage I lesions, 31% have stage II lesions, and 32% have stage III lesions. In the remaining cases classification is difficult. Endoscopic examination is

TABLE 18-1. Endoscopic stages

Stage	Characteristics
I	Inflammation of the mucosa
II	
A	Ulceration, little hemorrhage
B	Limited or circular necrosis
III	Extensive necrosis involving the whole organ and massive hemorrhage
IV	Characteristics of stage III plus intravascular disseminated coagulopathy and metabolic acidosis

crucial to early diagnosis and to determining those high-risk patients in whom urgent treatment must be undertaken. Endoscopy does not, however, allow assessment of the depth of the lesion in the acute phase. Patients with stage I lesions can resume eating immediately. For patients with stage II and stage III lesions, artificial nutrition should be instituted to allow the upper digestive tract time to heal. To counteract initial hypercatabolism, the caloric and nitrogen levels of the artificial diet should be high (30 to 50 kcal and 150 to 200 mg of nitrogen per kilogram per day). For patients with stage II lesions the average duration of artificial nutrition is 20 to 30 days, while for patients with stage III lesions it is 90 to 120 days. Artificial nutrition can be achieved either intravenously or enterally by a continuous flow through a nasoduodenal tube or a jejunostomy catheter.

Stage IV lesions pose the problem of whether emergency esophagogastrectomy is needed to save the patient. The decision to operate depends on the following factors[8-10]:

1. The nature of the caustic substance (lye, hydrochloric acid), the quantity ingested, the presence of autolysis
2. Bloody emesis, signs of gravity
3. Endoscopic observation of extension beyond the pylorus, and duodenal lesions. In serious cases hyperleukocytosis is a consistent finding but metabolic acidosis and DIC are delayed events
4. Secondary occurrence of toxic shock with hyperventilation, hypocapnia, and hypoxia

Median laparotomy allows assessment of the extent of abdominal damage. If the stomach is not completely necrosed but rather appears purplish with thrombosis of some epiploic vessels, the back side of the organ should be inspected. To achieve this inspection it is necessary to open the omental bursa; in so doing, great care should

be exercised to avoid damaging gastroepiploic vessels. If the stomach appears viable, the abdomen is closed after placement of a jejunostomy catheter. If, on the other hand, partial or total necrosis is observed, esophagectomy without thoracotomy and total gastrectomy must be carried out. At the end of the operation, the cervical esophagus is brought out the neck, a jejunostomy catheter is installed, and a large posterior mediastinal and submesenteric drain is placed. Digestive patency is reestablished at a second operation when healing is complete—that is, at least 3 months postoperatively.

In the first 2 or 3 weeks after ingestion of a caustic substance, a number of complications can occur. Respiratory complications, seen in 11% of patients, usually result from edema of the glottis or inhalation of the toxic agent. Tracheobronchial complications are fatal in 3% of cases. The life-threatening nature of these complications justifies early endoscopic inspection of the airways in all cases involving massive absorption or ingestion of a volatile substance. Secondary digestive complications, reported in 10% of cases, include digestive hemorrhage and occasionally organ perforation.

PATIENT SURVEILLANCE AND PREVENTION OF SEQUELAE

During the healing period, patients with caustic burns of the upper digestive tract treated by total parenteral nutrition must undergo regular endoscopic inspection. Given the remarkably precise course of healing in most cases, endoscopy can usually be scheduled on the 10th, 20th, 90th, or 120th day—that is, after 8 to 10 days for stage I lesions, after 20 to 30 days for stage II lesions, and after 90 to 120 days for stage III lesions.

Prevention of stricture formation is currently the main problem. This complication occurs in half the cases involving stage II or III lesions. The systematic use of corticoids, early dilatation, and Silastic stents has led to inconclusive results in the prevention of such stenosis.[11]

PREOPERATIVE WORKUP AND SURGICAL TREATMENT OF SEQUELAE

Endoscopy is mandatory before eating can be resumed. However, when it is carried out during the healing phase, this procedure does not allow assessment of the extent of esophageal stenosis or visualization of distal lesions in the esophagus and stomach. Endoscopy is nevertheless important at this stage to accurately locate the uppermost extension of the stenosis and confirm that healing is complete. If an esophageal lumen persists, an esophagogastroduodenal transit study using a hydrosoluble agent is useful to investigate the condition of the esophagus and stomach distal to the stenosis. In addition to x-ray and endoscopic data, the nutritional and overall status of these patients, who are fed artificially for 3 months, should be thoroughly checked. The surgical technique used to repair the upper digestive tract after caustic burns depends on the location(s) of the lesions.[12-18]

Lesions in the upper esophagus

Lesions in the upper esophagus can be managed by interposition of the transverse colon with a left pedicle. The colonic graft is placed in a retrosternal position. The cologastric anastomosis is made to the front side of the stomach after the pedicle is passed through the lesser omentum. To prevent reflux a trap is fashioned on the front side of the stomach, using a 5-cm segment of the colon.

The upper anastomosis is usually made via a left cervical approach between the heads of the sternocleidmastoid muscle. The configuration of this anastomosis depends on where the esophagus must be transected. If the length of the cervical esophagus remaining after transection is sufficient, a classic esophagocolonic anastomosis is made (a 15-mm split is made up the left edge of the esophageal stump to increase the surface of anastomosis). On the other hand, if the stenosis is located at the level of the hypopharynx, a pharyngocolonic anastomosis becomes necessary. In this case the surgeon continues dissection up to a point just below the jugulocarotid plexus behind the body of the thyroid. After transection of the esophagus at its commencement, the pharynx is split up the posterior aspect until the surface area is big enough to allow anastomosis. Two great advantages of this technique are that retraining the patient to swallow takes less than 2 weeks and that endoscopic checkups are easy. In the rare cases in which a lesion involving the larynx may require surgical repair in the hypopharynx, the translaryngeal approach gives an excellent operative field but in our experience necessitates a longer period of retraining.

Lesions in the lower esophagus

Lesions in the lower esophagus are relatively infrequent. This location is one of the rare indications for reconstruction by elevating the stomach into the thorax and making a leakproof, intrathoracic, esophagogastric anastomosis. This procedure can be carried out after left thoracophrenotomy, laparotomy, and right thoracotomy or by laparotomy and a transhiatal approach. After gastrolysis, pyloroplasty, and lower esophagectomy, a large gastric tube fashioned from the greater curvature of the stomach is brought up into the thorax through an enlarged hiatus and a careful leakproof anastomosis is made with the remaining thoracic esophagus.

Lesions involving only the stomach

Total stenosis of the stomach alone is rare after ingestion of a caustic substance. This condition can be treated by total gastrectomy followed by a Roux-en-Y jejunal loop procedure to restore digestive continuity. The antral region is the most common location of partial gastric stenosis after ingestion of caustic substances. Antral stenosis is frequently associated with destruction of the valve mechanism of the cardia. Such lesions can easily be corrected by antrectomy followed by a Roux-en-Y jejunal loop procedure to restore continuity. This operation not only cures the stenosis but also eliminates the risk of secondary esophagitis.

Combined stenosis

Two combinations are frequently encountered. The first is stenosis in the upper esophagus and total gastric stenosis. In these cases a small gastric lumen always persists. Such lesions can be managed by interposition of a long retrosternal colonic bypass anastomosed to a Roux-en-Y jejunal loop. The second combination is stenosis in the upper esophagus and stenosis of the gastric antrum. Such lesions can be managed by colonic interposition anastomosed distally to the front side of the stomach after resection of the subjacent antral stenosis. Gastrointestinal continuity is again restored by a Roux-en-Y jejunal loop.

Second-stage reestablishment of digestive continuity after emergency laparotomy

Restoration of digestive continuity is carried out 3 months after emergency laparotomy. The exact nature of the procedure depends on whether the stomach was resected. If the stomach was not resected, residual lesions may vary from simple antral stenosis to total esophagogastric stenosis. Surgical management is achieved as previously described. After total esophagogastrectomy a long colonic substitute anastomosed distally to the pharynx and proximally to a Roux-en-Y loop is the most appropriate surgical method.

The risk of cancer after fibrotic healing in a functioning digestive tube cannot be excluded. For this reason victims of serious burns in the upper digestive tract should be strongly advised to have regular life-long checkups. In our department patients undergo reexamination at 3 and 12 months in the first year and then yearly thereafter; this examination includes digestive fibroscopy with staged biopsy.

PSYCHIATRY AND CAUSTIC BURNS

The mental state of patients who ingest caustic substances as the climax to a transient period of acute depression generally improves during convalescence. This improvement can probably be attributed to the intercession of a supportive medical staff during the 3-month hospitalization, which helps the patient to work out his problems with his family or relations. When these suicide attempts are committed by chronic mental patients, improvement in the psychiatric condition is more unlikely. Furthermore, the fact that many such patients require heavy sedation hinders recovery because of the slowing effects of the drugs used on the motility of the digestive tract.

CAUSTIC BURNS IN CHILDREN

Swallowing of caustic substances by toddlers and small children is one of the most serious domestic hazards because the esophageal stenosis that may result can definitively compromise esophageal function. These accidents are twice as frequent in boys, whose average age at ingestion is 2.5 years. About 5000 such accidents are recorded annually in the United States. Liquid as opposed to granulated caustic agents (even if only a small quantity is ingested) cause the most severe lesions. Early esophagoscopy is the only way to detect the existence of an esophageal burn. In small children fibroscopy must be performed under general anesthesia with endotracheal intubation without local anesthesia. The proper therapeutic approach in the acute phase is a matter of controversy. Some authors recommend the use of steroids or placement of an intraluminal stent to prevent stricture formation, but such techniques carry risks of their own.

RESULTS
Operative mortality

Mortality after emergency surgery varies from 30% to 100% depending on the technique used. This high rate is explained by the adverse operating conditions created by extensive plurivisceral lesions, intense metabolic disturbances, major hemodynamic irregularities, sepsis, and hypercatabolism. Better results can probably be achieved by carrying out surgery as soon as possible after ingestion of the caustic substance and by the use of less traumatic techniques (esophagectomy without thoracotomy); this implies early detection of organ perforation on the basis of information obtained from the patient or family and from endoscopic and laboratory findings. Mortality after elective surgery is around 8% and should be zero.

Functional results at 3 months

At 3 months functional results are for the most part excellent. In 5% of cases, however, stenosis of the cervical anastomosis of the colonic substitute requires dilatation or, exceptionally, reoperation to enlarge the passage.

Fate of the unresected esophagus and long-term follow-up

The long-term risk of esophageal cancer after caustic burn is a controversial claim. Apparently, carcinoma develops only in patients with functional esophagi, especially if dilatation was practiced. As with other authors, we do not recommend that burns in the upper esophagus be bypassed without esophagectomy by means of retrosternal colonic interposition. In our experience second-stage esophagectomy was necessary in two cases as the result of compressive dilatation of a supple segment of esophagus distal to a total stenosis.

For deep burns we prefer to initiate artificial feeding to allow the esophagus to rest and to administer broad-spectrum antibiotics to prevent infection. Because of the progress made in pediatrics by using percutaneous central catheters for parenteral nutrition, we now use this technique. A second endoscopic and x-ray examination is performed on the twenty-first day to ascertain the subsequent therapy; if healing is uneventful, eating can be resumed, but if a stricture has formed, a gastrostomy tube must be placed for feeding. For a local stenosis, weekly dilatations are sometimes successful in keeping the esophagus open. If dilatation fails or in cases of extensive stenosis, surgery is mandatory 3 to 4 months after the insult. Esophageal reconstruction can be achieved either by retrosternal colonic interposition or by elevation of the stomach. The long-term risk of cancer if the bypassed esophagus is not resected is as yet uncertain. Statistics show cancer after caustic burns accounts for about 1% to 4% of all cases of adult esophageal cancer.[19-23]

CONCLUSION

Coordinated treatment of caustic burns in the upper digestive tract has led to better cooperation between the various specialists involved in the management of this injury. Several problems have not yet been satisfactorily solved. The most serious of these is stricture formation, which could possibly be avoided by controlling edema in the initial phase of injury. The outcome of severe upper-digestive-tract burns is tainted by the predisposition of patients to cancer, and it is for this reason that regular checkups are needed and justified.

REFERENCES

1. Noirclerc, M., Chauvin, G., Jouglard, J., Garbe, L., and Dicostanzo, J.: Les brûlures du tractus digestif supérieur. In Encycl. Med. Chir. Paris, Estomac Intestin 4, 9200 A10, 1978.
2. Leape, L.L., Ashcraft, K.W., Scarperlli, D.G., and Holder, T.M.: Hazard to health: liquid lye, N. Engl. J. Med. **284:**578-581, 1971.
3. Oakes, D., Sherck, J., and Mark, J.: Lye ingestion: clinical patterns and therapeutic complications, J. Thorac, Cardiovasc. Surg. **83:**194-204, 1982.
4. Dicostanzo, J., Cano, N., Martin, J., and Noirclerc, M.: Surgical approach to corrosive injuries of the stomach, Br. J. Surg. **68:**879-881, 1981.
5. Dicostanzo, J., Noirclerc, M., Drif, M., Lambert, H., Paris, J.C., Huncke, P., and Camboulives, J.: Conduite actuelle en présence d'ingestion de caustiques, Acta Endoscopica **15:**179-186, 1985.
6. Dicostanzo, J., Noirclerc, M., Jouglard, J., Escoffier, J.M., Cano, N., Martin, J., and Gauthier, A.: New therapeutic approach to corrosive burns of the upper gastro intestinal tract, Gut **21:**370-375, 1980.
7. Dilawari, J.B., Surjit Singh, M., Rao, P.N., and Anand, B.S.: Corrosive acid ingestion in man: a clinical and endoscopic study, Gut **25:**183-187, 1984.
8. Mislawski, R., and Chesquiere, F.: Exérèse large pour brûlure caustique gastro-duodénale, Presse Med. **13:** 1742-1744, 1984.
9. Pouyet, M., Bouletreau, P., and Morel, J.: Plaidoyer pour une chirurgie d'éradication d'urgence dans certaines brûlures caustiques majeures du tractus digestif supérieur, Lyon Chir. **76:**389-392, 1980.
10. Ribet, M., Ghisbain, H., and Chambon, J.P.: Brûlures caustiques gastro-intestinales, Med. Chir. Dig. **13:**255-256, 1984.
11. Hill, J.L., Norberg, H.P., Smith, M.D., Young, J.A., and Reyes, H.M.: Clinical technique and success of the esophageal stent to prevent corrosive strictures, J. Pediatr. Surg. **11:**433-450, 1976.
12. Chien, K.Y., Wang, P.Y., and Lu, K.S.: Oesophagoplasty for corrosive stricture of the oesophagus: an analysis of 60 cases, Ann. Surg. **179:**510-515, 1974.
13. Gutpa, S.: Total obliteration of oesophagus and hypopharyngus due to corrosives: a new technique of reconstruction, J. Thorac. Cardiovasc. Surg. **60:**264-268, 1970.
14. Noirclerc, M., Dicostanzo, J., Sastre, B., Drif, B., Durif, L., Fulachier, V., Botta, D., and Brun J.G.: Reconstructive operations for oesophagogastric corrosive lesions, J. Thorac. Cardiovasc. Surg. **87:**291-294, 1984.
15. Holt, C.J., and Large, A.M.: Surgical management of reflux esophagitis, Ann. Surg. **153:**555-562, 1961.
16. Thomas, A.N., Dedo, H.H., Lim, R.C., and Steele, M.: Pharyngo-oesophageal caustic stricture: treatment by pharyngo-gastrostomy compared to colon interposition combined with free bowel graft, Ann. J. Surg. **32:**195-203, 1976.
17. Mislawski, R., Brun, J.G., Ferry, J., Tran Ba Huy, P., Frachet, B., Beutter, P., and Celerier, M.: Sténoses digestives caustiques intéressant l'hypopharynx: l'oesophagoplastie par greffon iléo-colique droit, Nouv. Presse Med. **11:**2921-2924, 1982.
18. Tran Ba Huy, P., Assens, P., Mislawski, R., Brun, J.G., Frachet, B., Beutter, P., Brasnud, D., and Celerier, M.: L'oesopharyngoplastie par transplantation d'un greffon iléo-colique droit dans le traitement des séquelles des sténoses caustiques de l'oesophage et de l'hypopharynx, Ann. Otolaryngol. **99:**489-495, 1982.
19. Dor, J., Despieds, R., Humbert, P., Bouyala, S.M., and Guerinel, G.: La cancérisation des rétrécissements cicatriciels de l'oesophage par caustique, Mem. Acad. Chir. **86:**1193-1203, 1960.
20. Gaillard, J., Bouchayer, M., and Haguenauer, J.P.: Le risque de dégénerescence cancéreuse tardive dans les sténoses caustiques de l'oesophage, Ann. Otolaryngol. **87:**637-644, 1970.
21. Guivarc'h, M., and Zamora, A.: Cancérisation étendue d'une sténose caustique de l'oesophage: Récidive gastrique après exérèse et coloplastie, Chirurg. **108:**830-834, 1982.
22. Hopkins, R.A., and Postlethwait, R.W.: Caustic burns and carcinoma of the esophagus, Ann. Surg. **194:**146-148, 1981.
23. Ti, T.K.: Oesophageal carcinoma associated with corrosive injury: prevention and treatment by oesophageal resection, Br. J. Surg. **70:**223-225, 1983.

Surgical management of caustic injuries to the upper gastrointestinal tract

DISCUSSION

Ö.P. Horváth

The cause and incidence of corrosive esophageal and gastric burns vary geographically. In Eastern Europe and in the Middle East they occur more frequently than in Western countries.[1] Considering the number of suicides per 100,000 inhabitants, Hungary belongs to the leading countries in the world in this regard. This is shown clearly in the distribution of corrosive injuries resulting from human intention; the ratio between accidental injuries and those resulting from suicide attempts is 1 to 2, in contrast to Western societies, where it is 1 to 1.

In our experience the intention of the patient has a vital effect on the future outcome of the injury. In patients requiring surgical treatment after attempting suicide by deliberately drinking corrosive fluids seven of eight will have damaged the esophagus, while among victims of accidents who required surgery this ratio is only 1 to 3.

In the past few decades a varying tendency can be observed in the quality of corrosive materials. In Hungary between the two World Wars 90% of the corrosive injuries were caused by lye, but in the past 10 years in our clinic 70% have been caused by acid. Lye generally causes lesions in the esophagus, but acids cause serious damage to the stomach—either partly or wholly.

DIAGNOSIS

Diagnosis is based on a history of ingestion, burns of the mouth and larynx, endoscopy, and the subsequent course of events. We disagree with Noirclerc et al. that acute endoscopy should be performed, as it does not help us decide the most serious question of the acute period—the need for surgical intervention.

The extent of the corrosive trauma as a rule becomes evident in the third or fourth week, when the patient begins to suffer dysphagia and the first disturbances of gastric function can be observed. The results of swallowing tests with contrast materials, as well as of endoscopy, will provide useful and important information on the seriousness of injuries, the prognosis, and the nature of the therapy that is required.

If the patient is unable to swallow, then his stomach cannot be examined and a thin gastric tube should be placed in the stomach after careful dilatation for contrast studies, to obtain information on the present state of gastric emptying.

EMERGENCY TREATMENT

Corrosive materials cause very serious injuries to the tissues in a few seconds, injuries whose extent and depth cannot be influenced.[1] This is why there is no use in applying the method of neutralization. Acute treatment consists of shock prevention, fluid and electrolyte therapy, and appropriate doses of antibiotics.

If there is the slightest sign of peritoneal involvement, then laparotomy should be performed, since stomach necrosis will rarely seal off. Pain in the left shoulder indicates fundus necrosis. Damage to the stomach is generally observed in the antrum and fundus, but acute necrosis usually affects the major part of the stomach, and is only very rarely cured by partial resection. Surgical intervention requires total esophagogastrectomy, with cervical esophagostomy and jejunostomy for nutrition. The esophagus should be removed in case of total gastrectomy, even if it has not been seriously injured, since either immediate reconstruction or blind closing of its distal end is a very dangerous procedure. Continuity of the gastrointestinal canal is restored in 2 to 3 months by colon interposition.

During the past ten years we have been obliged to do emergency operations on five patients. One of these recovered after the acute esophagogastrectomy, but the other four died. Two of them were badly injured, and the other two were operated on too late. It is generally true that acute operation after the first 24 hours is either too late or useless.

DILATATION TREATMENT

As a rule the first dilatation is made in the fourth week, after preliminary radiography. This identifies three main groups:

1. The stricture can easily be dilated without any risk, and the interval between dilatations can be gradually increased. The stricture can be cured by bougienage.
2. The stricture can be dilated with medium difficulty and a little risk. The interval between dilatations can be very slowly increased, or it cannot be increased at all. The patient swallows quite well between dilatations. About 50% of these cases will require an operation on the esophagus, but this can be postponed to a more optimal time—6 months to 1 year.
3. The stricture can be dilated only with great difficulty and by taking great risks. Surgical intervention must be applied in these cases. The aim of the intervention is to wait for the development of the final stage and gain time for curing the occasional gastric outlet stenosis by way of operation.

In 64 corrosive-injured patients, 44 had a stricture demanding treatment, and 27 of these were successfully cured by dilatation or kept in a satisfactory state from the point of view of swallowing; 17 cases required surgical intervention.

DEFINITIVE TREATMENT

The final consequences of gastric and esophageal burns appear by 6 to 8 weeks. This is why surgical intervention with the aim of reconstruction can be first done at this time.[2] In case of injury to the stomach *and* the esophagus, the gastric emptying disturbances should be cured first, so the definitive treatment is performed in two stages. It is generally urgent to eliminate emptying disturbances, since the patient is unable to eat and esophagitis may aggravate the already strictured esophagus because of gastroesophageal reflux.

Two thirds of the cases will have an antral stenosis that can easily be cured by gastric resection (generally according to Billroth I).

If the injury occurs on the lesser curvature with shortening, then a bypass operation is performed such as esophagojejunostomy or gastroduodenostomy. If the injury to the stomach occurs with a stricture in the lower third of the esophagus, then the chances of successful dilatation can be improved by stenting the strictured part. In the 64 patients, 52 had injuries to the stomach, and of these, 32 had gastric injuries together with esophageal stricture.

None of our patients who had an operation on the stomach died.

Seventeen patients were operated on for corrosive esophageal stricture, after curing of gastric emptying disturbances and unsuccessful dilatation.

In cases of strictures in the lower third of the esophagus (seven cases) esophageal resection was performed through a left thoracolaparotomy, with jejunal replacement. With strictures in the middle third or in the whole of the esophagus (10 cases), a new esophagus was made from colon. In nine cases, after transthoracic resection, substernal or intrathoracic replacement was performed. In one case, the patient had a substernal bypass operation. Disagreeing with Noirclerc et al., because of the late unfavorable functional consequences, we have not used the stomach for replacement, and have always used a transthoracic resection, since there is a possible danger of serious inflammation and cicatrization around the esophagus 6 to 12 months following the injury.

In these seventeen patients two died after the surgical intervention.

LATE CONSEQUENCES

It is well known that the risk of development of esophageal cancer in corrosive strictures is 1000 times greater than in the normal population of the same age, presuming that more than 25 years have already passed since the injury.[3]

The factors that lead to the development of cancer are as follows:

1. Cicatrization
2. Repeated trauma caused during dilatation treatment
3. Stasis, since passage is slowed down by the stricture
4. Gastroesophageal reflux resulting from

traction-type hiatal hernia, which nearly always accompanies corrosive stricture[4]

In the 502 patients with esophageal cancer who were treated at our clinic, 36 suffered from a so-called scar cancer. This 7.2% incidence is considered to be the highest ratio in the literature.[5,6]

Esophageal resection may seem to be the best method of preventing cancer, and we were of the same opinion for a long time,[7] but we now understand that esophageal resection will not provide full safety for the patient against cancer.[6] As an example, we can mention two of our patients in whom scar cancer developed in the remaining part of the esophagus 14 and 4 years after resection, respectively. Some 10% to 15% of patients suffering from corrosive stricture will develop scar cancer, but this number corresponds to the average death rate from esophageal resection. There is therefore no use in performing preventive total esophagectomy.[8] On the other hand, the riskiest part of esophageal reconstruction is the anastomosis to the esophagus. Esophagectomy does not vitally increase this risk, so it is wise to perform esophageal resection if surgical intervention is necessary to restore the swallowing capability of the patient. Bypass operations should be performed only in very serious cases and if the patient is over 50 years of age.

REFERENCES

1. Belsey, R.: Corrosive stricture of the esophagus. In DeMeester, T.M., and Skinner, D.B., editors: Esophageal disorders, New York, 1985, Raven Press, pp. 261-269.
2. Dicostanzo, J., Cano, N., Martin, J., and Noirclerc, M.: Surgical approach to corrosive injuries of the stomach, Br. J. Surg. **68:**879-881, 1981.
3. Kiviranta, U.K.: Corrosion carcinoma of the esophagus: 381 cases of corrosion and nine cases of corrosion carcinoma, Acta Otolaryngol. **42:**89-95, 1952.
4. Imre, J., and Wooler, G.H.: Peptic ulceration of the esophagus following corrosive burns, Thorax **24:**762-764, 1969.
5. Appelqvist, P., and Salmo, P.: Lye corrosion carcinoma of the esophagus: a review of 63 cases, Cancer **45:**2655-2658, 1980.
6. Csíkos, M., Horváth, Ö., Petri, A., Petri, I., and Imre, J.: Late malignant transformation of chronic corrosive oesophageal strictures, Langenbecks Arch. Chir. **365:**231-238, 1985.
7. Imre, J., and Kopp, M.: Arguments against long-term conservative treatment of oesophageal strictures due to corrosive burns, Thorax **27:**594-598, 1972.
8. Siewert, J.R., and Bartels, H.: Oesophagusverätzung— "prophylaktische" Oesophagektomie? Langenbecks Arch. Chir. **365:**227-229, 1985.

CHAPTER **19** Drug-induced esophageal injuries

David D. Oakes and John P. Sherck

Chemical injury to the esophagus has long been a topic of interest to thoracic surgeons. Early in this century Chevalier Jackson developed the distally lighted esophagoscope in large part to aid in the management of patients with caustic strictures.[1] Even today few injuries are more devastating or more difficult to manage than those arising from the inadvertent or purposeful ingestion of potent caustic or corrosive agents.[2] This type of chemical injury is discussed in detail in Chapter 18. The following discussion will be limited to esophageal injuries that arise as the result of the intentional ingestion of commercially available medications being used for therapeutic purposes.

TYPES OF INJURY

Drug-induced esophageal injuries can be caused either directly (by retention of the offending medication within the esophagus) or indirectly (secondary to systemic effects of the ingested drug). Examples of indirect injuries include (1) reflux esophagitis caused by drugs that diminish pressure in the lower esophageal sphincter, (2) viral or fungal esophagitis in patients receiving immunosuppressive agents,[3] (3) intramural hematomas in patients receiving anticoagulants,[4] and even (4) esophageal rupture following the use of medications that induce vomiting.[5] The remainder of this chapter, however, will discuss injuries arising directly from the failure of orally ingested medications to pass uneventfully into the stomach.

The first reports of direct drug-induced esophageal injuries appeared in 1970. Knauer and colleagues, from our institution, discovered an esophagoesophageal fistula in a 62-year-old woman with advanced achalasia who was taking 2.4 g of aspirin per day for treatment of rheumatoid arthritis.[6] The esophagus was redundant and looped back upon itself just above the gastroesophageal junction (see Fig. 19-1). The authors speculated that "aspirin particles or tablets lodged in the dependent portion of the proximal loop could have been responsible for

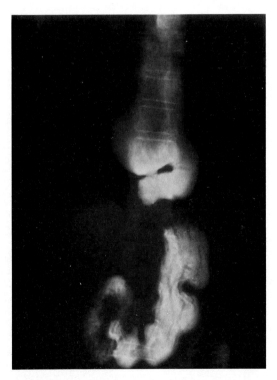

Fig. 19-1. Barium swallow demonstrating an esophago-esophageal fistula in the markedly redundant distal esophagus of a 62-year-old woman with advanced achalasia. The fistula presumably was caused by aspirin tablets or particles that lodged in this area, producing deep ulceration and eventual fistulization. The patient was treated by resection of the distal esophagus. (From Oakes, D.D., and Sherck, J.P.: Drug-induced esophagitis. In DeMeester, T.R., and Skinner, D.B., editors: Esophageal disorders: pathophysiology and therapy, New York, 1985, Raven Press. With permission.)

ulceration and eventual fistulization into the distal loop." The same year, Juncosa reported the case of a 75-year-old man who developed melena and anemia while taking phenylbutazone and prednisone for arthritis. A barium swallow demonstrated spasm and ulceration in the distal third of the esophagus.[7] The syndrome was particularly well described and documented by Pemberton; he reported a 44-year-old woman who complained of difficulty swallowing a large potassium supplement tablet (Slow-K) 9 days after undergoing mitral valve replacement.[8] She developed severe retrosternal pain and dysphagia. A barium swallow the following morning demonstrated a filling defect consistent with an impacted tablet in the lower third of the esophagus, just above the area where the esophagus was compressed by a massively enlarged left atrium (see Fig. 19-2). Esophagoscopy revealed mucosal ulceration, filled with and surrounded by white powder. Symptoms resolved after 5 days of tube feedings and substitution of a liquid potassium preparation.

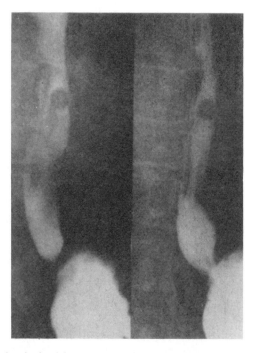

Fig. 19-2. Barium study obtained in a 44-year-old woman the morning after she complained of difficulty swallowing a large potassium supplement tablet (Slow-K). During the night she had developed intense retrosternal pain and dysphagia. Five hours later, esophagoscopy showed mucosal ulceration filled with and surrounded by white powder. The lesion occurred at the point where the esophagus was compressed and displaced by a markedly enlarged left atrium (secondary to long-standing mitral valvular disease.) (From Pemberton, J.: Esophageal obstruction and ulceration caused by oral potassium therapy, Br Heart J. **32:**267-268, 1970. With permission.)

EPIDEMIOLOGY

Drug-induced esophageal injury was rarely recognized in the early 1970s, but has been reported with increasing frequency since 1975 (see Fig. 19-3). As of February, 1985, 22 drugs had been implicated in the etiology of this disorder (see Table 19-1). Discussions in the rest of this chapter are based upon our analysis of 251 case reports published through February, 1985. These reports varied considerably in detail and documentation, but all seemed clearly representative of this syndrome. The reader is also referred to several excellent review articles.[9-14]

In our review there were 251 patients, ranging in age from 5 to 89 years (average, 37.7 years). The age profile varied according to the different drugs, probably reflecting differences in the population at risk. Thus, tetracycline (used for acne, urethritis, and minor infections) and emepronium (an anticholinergic agent used in Europe for the treatment of enuresis and bladder irritability) affected a younger age group than did potassium chloride and quinidine, generally used in older patients with heart disease. The age profile was as follows: tetracycline, 15 to 75 years (average, 31.5 years); emepronium, 5 to 89 years (average, 34.9 years); potassium chloride, 14 to 74 years (average, 51.2 years); and quinidine, 12 to 77 years (average, 59.4 years). There were 129 females and 63 males; in 59 cases gender was not specified. Although this may mean that females have an increased propensity to develop this disorder, it probably simply reflects the fact that more females than males use these medications, and hence that females represent a larger population at risk.

The classic symptom complex was progressively severe retrosternal pain followed by painful swallowing (odynophagia) and dysphagia developing minutes to hours after ingestion of a capsule or tablet. Only 20 patients complained of dysphagia without pain; eight of these had established strictures at the time of presentation. Hematemesis was rare, but carried a grave prognosis; of eight patients with this symptom, four died of exsanguination. Only 14% (35 of 251) developed a foreign-body sensation, making them aware that the medication had been retained in the esophagus.

Improper ingestion of tablets or capsules may predispose a person to esophageal injury (see Table 19-2). Eighty-six patients (34%) took their pills at bedtime or shortly before lying down; a like number used little or no water at the time of ingestion. In 107 cases (43%) one of these two conditions obtained (dry ingestion or early recumbency).

Preexisting esophageal pathology that might interfere with normal swallowing was identified in 31 patients (12%) (see Table 19-2). Nineteen had extrinsic compression of the distal esophagus secondary to left-atrial enlargement, usually associated with mitral valvular disease. One patient with tetralogy of Fallot and pulmonic atresia had compression of the esophagus by an enlarged

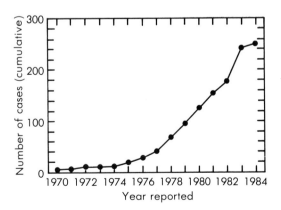

Fig. 19-3. Historical profile of the recognition and reporting of drug-induced esophageal injuries. By the end of 1975, only 19 cases had been reported; by 1985 the number exceeded 250.

TABLE 19-1. Drug-induced esophageal injury, 1970-1985 (251 reported cases)

Drug	No. of cases
Tetracycline	123
Emepronium	68
Potassium chloride	19
Quinidine	10
Pinaverium	6
Indomethacin	4
Clindamycin	3
Aspirin	2
Ferrous sulfate	2
Praxilene	2
Ascorbic acid	1
Aspirin-phenacetin-codeine	1
Co-trimoxazole	1
Cromolyn	1
Lincomycin	1
Mexiletine	1
Pantagar	1
Phenobarbital	1
Phenylbutazone-prednisone	1
Rhinasal	1
Theophylline	1
Tolmetin	1

TABLE 19-2. Drug-induced esophageal injury: predisposing factors (251 patients)

	No. of cases	Percent
Dry ingestion	86	34
Early recumbency	86	34
Either dry ingestion or early recumbency	107	43
Esophageal pathology (31 patients)		12
Left-atrial enlargement	19	
Hiatal hernia	4	
Dysmotility	3	
Carcinoma	2	
Multiple sclerosis	1	
Stricture	1	
Compression by enlarged bronchial artery	1	
Normal deglutition	220	88

TABLE 19-3. Drug-induced esophageal injury: results of barium swallow (134 patients)

Findings	No. of patients
Normal/nonspecific	81[*]
Abnormal (53 patients)	
Ulcer	34
Esophagitis	9
Stricture	8
Perforation	1
Fistula	1

[*]Endoscopy revealed: 73 ulcers; 5 cases of esophagitis; 2 resolved without further studies; 1 endoscopy normal 7 days later.

TABLE 19-4. Drug-induced esophageal injury: results of endoscopy

	No. of patients
Early examinations: 195 patients	
Positive findings	
Ulcer/erosion	165
Esophagitis	18
Stricture	11
"Inflammation"	1
Biopsies: 73 patients	
Inflammation	71
Carcinoma (remote)	1
Carcinoma in situ	1

bronchial artery. Other predisposing conditions included hiatal hernia (4), motility disorders (3), carcinoma (2), chronic stricture (1), and multiple sclerosis (one). *It is important to note that 88% of patients developed drug-induced esophageal injury in spite of apparently normal deglutition.*

DIAGNOSIS

The diagnostic evaluation of these patients utilized contrast roentgenography, endoscopy, or both. One hundred thirty-four patients had barium swallows (see Table 19-3). Eighty-one barium studies were felt to be normal or to show only nonspecific abnormalities. Definitive anatomic diagnoses were later established by endoscopy in 78 of these patients: 73 ulcers and 5 cases of esophagitis. These false-negative results illustrate the insensitivity of contrast roentgenography in the diagnosis of drug-induced esophageal injury. Recent reports, however, suggest that utilization of a double-contrast technique will increase the sensitivity of these studies and permit the detection of erosions, superficial ulcerations, and other subtle changes in the esophageal mucosa.[15] Fifty-three patients had the following lesions diagnosed by barium swallow: ulcer (34), esophagitis (9), stricture (8), perforation (1), and fistula (1) (see Table 19-3).

Esophagoscopy was the most definitive diagnostic study in the evaluation of patients with suspected drug-induced esophageal injury (see Table 19-4). Of 195 patients undergoing endoscopy within 5 days of the onset of symptoms, positive findings were present in every case: ulcer/erosion (165), esophagitis (18), stricture (11), and unspecified inflammation (ulcer/esophagitis) (1). Biopsies were performed in 73 patients; 71 revealed only ulceration, necrosis, and acute inflammation. All specimens were negative for evidence of fungal or viral lesions. One patient, with an ulcer in the midesophagus caused by a ferrous sulfate tablet, was serendipitously found to have a carcinoma in the proximal esophagus—unrelated to his acute injury.[16] Only one patient was found to have a malignancy in the area of acute inflammation: this was a 57-year-old male who had no esophageal symptoms until one morning when a bolus of solid food stuck in

TABLE 19-5. Drug-induced esophageal injury: diagnostic studies and anatomic diagnoses

Early studies:	221 patients
Barium swallow plus endoscopy	117
Endoscopy only	84
Barium swallow only	17
Postmortem only	3
Findings:	223 lesions
Ulcer/erosion	178
Esophagitis	27
Stricture	15
Perforation	2
Fistula	1
Late studies: 1 patient; negative examination at 7 days	
Not studied: 29 patients	

TABLE 19-6. Drug-induced esophageal injury: deaths

	Number
Mechanism	
Exsanguination	4
Perforation	2
Inanition	2
Unspecified	1
Medication	
Potassium chloride	6
Doxycycline	2
Indomethacin	1

DRUG-INDUCED ESOPHAGEAL INJURY: TREATMENT

Stop oral medications
Antacids
Analgesics
Topical anesthetics
Bland diet
Liquid diet
Feeding tubes
Intravenous hydration
Intravenous nutrition

---

his midchest.[12] He was taking quinidine for the treatment of ventricular ectopy. A barium swallow showed mucosal irregularity and multiple small polypoid filling defects just proximal to the gastroesophageal junction, but was otherwise normal. Endoscopy revealed friable, erythematous mucosa extending from 35 cm to 40 cm from the incisors and covered with a white exudate. The exudate formed two masses, which nearly occluded the lumen. The endoscope dislodged the exudate and revealed an area of inflammation and ulceration. Biopsies showed an acute inflammatory infiltration with ulceration and "an incidental lesion of squamous cell *carcinoma in situ.*"[12] Subsequent distal esophagectomy showed resolution of the acute inflammatory reaction and only a small focus of noninvasive squamous cell carcinoma.

Among the 251 patients reviewed, there was direct documentation of esophageal injury in 221—by barium swallow plus esophagoscopy (117), by esophagoscopy only (84), by barium swallow only (17), or by postmortem examination (3) (see Table 19-5). Two hundred twenty-three lesions were described in these 221 patients: ulcer/erosions, 178; esophagitis, 27; stricture, 15; perforation, 2; and fistula, 1. One patient had negative studies, but was not examined until 7 days after the onset of symptoms. Twenty-nine patients were not studied, and the diagnosis of drug-induced esophageal injury was made on clinical grounds only.

TREATMENT

The initial treatment of drug-induced esophageal injury is symptomatic and supportive (see box, above, at right). After stopping all oral medications, most authors recommend the liberal use of antacids. Analgesics, topical anesthetics (e.g., viscous lidocaine), bland or liquid diets, tube feedings, and intravenous hydration or nutrition were utilized as indicated for individual patients. Antibiotics were administered to only one patient, a 5-year-old girl who presented with fever, leukocytosis, and an elevated erythrocyte sedimentation rate.

RESULTS

Although most patients recovered completely after 5 to 7 days of supportive therapy, symptoms persisted in some cases as long as 3 to 4 weeks. Major complications developed in 26 patients: 15 strictures, 8 hemorrhages, 2 perforations, and 1 esophagoesophageal fistula. The strictures did not require resection, but periodic dilatations were needed for as long as 2 years in some cases. The patient with the esophagoesophageal fistula underwent resection.

Nine deaths were directly or indirectly related to the esophageal lesions (see Table 19-6). Four patients exsanguinated—two from large hemorrhagic ulcers, one from an esophagoaortic fistula, and one (with pulmonic atresia) from an esophagobronchial artery fistula (see Fig. 19-4). One patient died of mediastinitis and sepsis following the contained perforation of a deep esophageal ulcer (see Fig. 19-5, *A*). A 72-year-old woman with Ehlers-Danlos syndrome underwent esophagogastrectomy for treatment of a free perforation of her distal esophagitis. Fourteen days later she died of a pulmonary embolus. Two patients with advanced mitral valvular disease developed tight esophageal strictures and required feeding jejunostomies because of near-total dysphagia. Their conditions gradually deteriorated, and they died after 1 week and 8 months, respectively. No details are available regarding the death of the ninth patient. Six of the fatal lesions were produced by potassium chloride tablets, two by doxycycline, and one by indomethacin.

PATHOPHYSIOLOGY

The pathophysiology of drug-induced esophageal injury appears to be local chemical damage secondary to delayed passage of a tablet or capsule into the stomach. Prolonged contact between the medication and the esophageal mucosa produces a localized inflammatory lesion. Depending upon the nature of the chemical agent, the rate of dissolution, and the duration of contact, the result can range from mild esophagitis to deep ulceration and even perforation. Pressure alone will not cause these changes: chemically inert tablets of calcium lactate or barium sulfate are well tolerated when suspended in the esophagi of cats or dogs for 5 to 8 hours.[17,18] By contrast, inflammatory lesions are regularly produced when animals are exposed to a variety of oral medications under identical experimental conditions[17] (see Fig. 19-5, *B*). Drug-induced reflux esophagitis cannot account for these lesions, because most occur in the upper and middle thirds of the esophagus and characteristically are discrete areas of ulceration surrounded proximally and distally by normal mucosa (see Fig. 19-6).

Why do tablets or capsules become impacted in the esophagus? Anatomic or functional abnormalities (e.g., strictures or dysmotility) will obviously predispose a person to this condition,

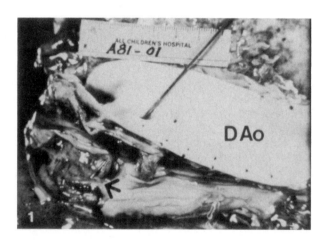

Fig. 19-4. Autopsy specimen from a 14-year-old girl with tetralogy of Fallot, complicated by atresia of the pulmonary valve and main pulmonary artery. She was taking potassium supplementation in the form of a wax-matrix tablet (Slow-K). While hospitalized for fever, anorexia, fatigue, and epigastric pain, she suddenly developed massive hematemesis and died. Autopsy revealed a deep esophageal ulcer (*arrow*), which had eroded into a large bronchial collateral artery. The aorta (*D Ao*) and esophagus are shown opened posteriorly. Demonstrating the course of the left bronchial collateral artery, the probe is seen entering the esophagus through the base of the ulcer (*arrow*). (From Henry, J.G., Skinner, J.J., Martino, J.H., and Cimino, L.E.: Fatal esophageal and bronchial artery ulceration caused by solid potassium chloride, Pediatr. Cardiol. **4:**251-252, 1983. With permission.)

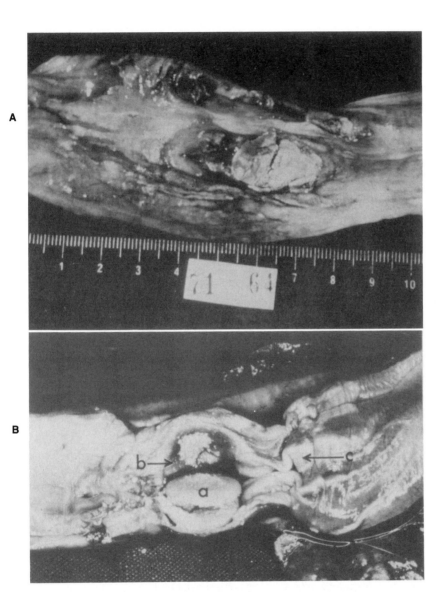

Fig. 19-5. A, Autopsy specimen showing a large ulcer with a necrotic base in the midesophagus of a 65-year-old woman who was receiving 500-mg noncoated potassium chloride tablets. The patient died of septic shock while being treated for substernal pain and dysphagia. Clumps of cocci were identified in the base of the ulcer. There was evidence of periesophagitis and localized mediastinitis—presumably resulting from a contained perforation. **B,** A similar lesion produced experimentally by exposing a cat's esophagus to one 200-mg tablet of alprenolol for 5 hours. The esophagus has been opened to reveal (*a*) the partially dissolved tablet, (*b*) deep ulceration of the adjacent mucosa, and (*c*) intense muscle spasm and edema of the nearby esophageal wall. (**A** from Rosenthal, T, Adar, R., Militanu, J., and Deutsch, V.: Esophageal ulceration and oral potassium chloride ingestion, Chest **65**(4): 463-465, 1974; **B** from Carlbourg, B., and Densert, O.: Esophageal lesions caused by orally administered drugs: an experimental study in the cat, Eur. Surg. Res. **12**:270-282, 1980, by permission of S. Karger AG, Basel, Switzerland.)

Delayed transit was noted in 157 swallowings (22%) and was commonly associated with a combination of a small amount of water (25 ml) and the recumbent position. When a pill was retained in the esophagus, only one of three subjects was aware of that fact. Oval tablets were more easily swallowed than round ones; high-density capsules more easily than low-density ones; and small, oval, coated tablets more easily than uncoated ones. The authors recommended that patients swallow tablets with at least 100 ml of water and remain standing for at least 90 seconds. Liquid medications were suggested for those who are bedridden or who have swallowing abnormalities. In a similar study, Channer and Virjee reported arrested transit in 52% of patients who swallowed standard gelatin capsules filled with barium sulfate.[21] If the capsules were swallowed with 60 ml of water in the upright position, however, all reached the stomach within 5 seconds.

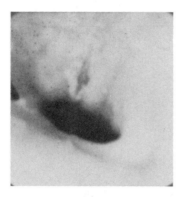

Fig. 19-6. Endoscopic photograph showing a typical discrete linear ulcer in the distal esophagus of a patient who awoke with retrosternal chest pain several hours after swallowing a 250-mg tablet of tetracycline. There is no inflammation of the surrounding mucosa or other evidence of reflux esophagitis. This endoscopy was performed 2 weeks after the onset of symptoms. (From Kikendall, J.W., Friedman, A.C., Oyewole, M.A., Fleischer, D., and Johnson, L.F.: Pill-induced esophageal injury: case reports and review of the medical literature, Dig. Dis. Sci. **28**(2):174-182, 1983. With permission.)

but even in individuals with normal deglutition, orally ingested drugs do not reach the stomach as rapidly and reliably as commonly assumed. This is particularly true when medications are taken without water or shortly before lying down. Evans and Roberts studied 98 patients who swallowed barium sulfate capsules identical in size and shape to commercial aspirin.[19] After swallowing the tablets with about 15 ml of water, the patients immediately lay down. Tablets were retained in the esophagus for more than 5 minutes in 57 of 98 patients and for more than 10 minutes in 14 patients. Thirty-six of these individuals had no roentgenographic abnormalities of the esophagus. The authors concluded that tablets should be taken before or during meals or with at least a full glass of water. Hey and colleagues studied 726 swallowings in 121 normal volunteers.[20] Subjects were given barium sulfate tablets or capsules in 6 commonly used sizes and shapes. They were studied both recumbent and standing, using either 25 ml or 100 ml of water. Normal esophageal transit time was considered to be 90 seconds.

SUMMARY

The following summarizes the points made in this discussion:
1. Localized chemical injury
2. Many potential agents
3. Characteristic symptoms
4. Diagnose by endoscopy
5. Biopsy persistent lesions
6. Withdraw medication
7. Antacids, bland or liquid diet
8. Prevent by adequate fluid, upright position
9. Avoid all pills if esophagus abnormal, left atrium enlarged, or patient bedridden

Drug-induced esophageal injury occurs when an orally ingested tablet or capsule becomes impacted in the esophagus and releases its chemical contents in high local concentration. Although many drugs have been associated with this condition, three (tetracycline, emepronium, and potassium chloride) account for 84% of reported cases. Patients characteristically complain of progressively severe retrosternal pain followed by odynophagia and dysphagia developing minutes to hours after ingestion of the offending tablet or capsule. A routine barium swallow will fail to diagnose most of these lesions, but double-contrast roentgenography may improve the sensitivity of this test. Endoscopy is the mainstay of diagnosis and should be performed promptly in patients with severe symptoms that persist in spite of antacid therapy. Biopsies are usually unrevealing and are not necessary unless the lesion fails to resolve or unless an infectious etiology is suspected (fungal or viral). After stopping of all oral medications, treatment is symptomatic and supportive. In most patients symptoms will resolve with 3 to 5 days of antacid therapy. Complete healing can be documented by follow-up endoscopy. A few patients will develop deep ulcerations, which can lead to hemorrhage, stricture, or perforation; nine deaths occurred among the 251 patients reviewed.

Drug-induced esophageal injury can be largely prevented if patients are instructed to take their medications in an upright position and to wash them down with adequate amounts of food or water. All tablets or capsules are best avoided in bedridden patients and in those with abnormalities of esophageal function or structure, including extrinsic compression from left-atrial enlargement.

REFERENCES

1. Jackson, C.: Esophageal stenosis following the swallowing of caustic alkalis, JAMA **77**:22-23, 1921.
2. Oakes, D.D., Sherck, J.P., and Mark, J.B.D.: Lye ingestions: clinical patterns and therapeutic implications, J. Thorac. Cardiovasc. Surg. **83**(2):194-204, 1982.
3. Hemstreet, M.P.B., Reynolds, D.W., and Meadows, J., Jr.: Oesophagitis: a complication of inhaled steroid therapy, Clin. Allergy **10**:733-738, 1980.
4. Smart, R.F., and Stone, A.R.: Intramural oesophageal haematoma complicating anticoagulant therapy, N.Z. Med. J. **87**:176-177, 1978.
5. Cochrane, P.: Spontaneous oesophageal rupture after carbachol therapy, Br. Med. J. **1**:463-464, 1973.
6. Knauer, C.M., McLaughlin, W.T., and Mark, J.B.D.: Esophago-esophageal fistula in a patient with achalasia, Gastroenterology **58**(2):223-228, 1970.
7. Juncosa, L.: Ulcus peptico yatrogeno del esopago, Rev. Esp. Enferm. Apar. Dig. **30**:457-458, 1970.
8. Pemberton, J.: Esophageal obstruction and ulceration caused by oral potassium therapy, Br. Heart J. **32**:267-268, 1970.
9. Carlborg, B., Densert, O., and Lindqvist, C.: Tetracycline-induced esophageal ulcers: a clinial and experimental study, Laryngoscope **93**(2):184-187, 1983.
10. Collins, F.J., Matthews, H.R., Baker, S.E., and Strakova, J.M.: Drug-induced oesophageal injury, Br. Med. J. **1**(6179):1673-1676, 1979.
11. Doman, D.B., and Ginsberg, A.L.: The hazard of drug-induced esophagitis, Hosp. Pract. **16**:17-25, 1981.
12. Kikendall, J.W., Freidman, A.C., Oyewole, M.A., Fleischer, D., and Johnson, L.F.: Pill-induced esophageal injury: case reports and review of the medical literature, Dig. Dis. Sci. **28**(2):174-182, 1983.
13. Mason, S.J., and O'Meara, T.F.: Drug-induced esophagitis, J. Clin. Gastroenterol. **3**:115-120, 1981.
14. Oakes, D.D., and Sherck, J.P.: Drug-induced esophagitis. In DeMeester, T.R., and Skinner, D.B., editors: Esophageal disorders: pathophysiology and therapy, New York, 1985, Raven Press, pp. 241-246.
15. Creteur, V., Laufer, I., Kressel, H.Y., et al.: Drug-induced esophagitis detected by double-contrast radiography, Radiology **147**(2):365-368, 1983.
16. Kobler, E., Nuesch, N.J., Buhler, H., et al.: Mediakamentos bedingte osophagusulzera, Schweiz. Med. Wochenschr. **109**(32):1180-1182, 1979.
17. Carlborg, B., and Densert, O.: Esophageal lesions caused by orally administered drugs: an experimental study in the cat, Eur. Surg. Res. **12**:270-282, 1980.
18. Walta, D.C., Giddens, J.D., Johnson, L.F., et al.: Localized proximal esophagitis secondary to ascorbic acid ingestion and esophageal motor disorder, Gastroenterology **70**:766-769, 1976.
19. Evans, K.T., and Roberts, G.M.: Where do all the tables go? Lancet **2**:1237-1239, 1976.
20. Hey, H., Jorgensen, F., Sorensen, K., et al.: Oesophageal transit of six commonly used tablets and capsules, Br. Med. J. **285**:1717-1719, 1982.
21. Channer, K.S., and Virjee, J.: Effect of posture and drink volume on the swallowing of capsules, Br. Med. J. **285**:1702, 1982.

Drug-induced esophageal injuries

DISCUSSION

Michael Atkinson

The steadily increasing incidence of drug-induced esophageal injuries may in part be the result of better diagnosis as a result of more widespread use of esophagoscopy, but it is undoubtably real. The pattern of offending drugs is continuously changing, and while potassium preparations are now seldom given in tablet form and potassium-sparing diuretic combinations have diminished the need for oral potassium supplements, the consumption of nonsteroidal anti-inflammatory drugs is rising sharply.[1] These are now believed to be a common cause of esophageal injury. It is perhaps surprising that so few patients reported by Drs. Oakes and Sherck had received nonsteroidal anti-inflammatory drugs. The more widespread use of antimitotic chemotherapy in the past decade predisposes patients to esophageal candidiases and herpetic infections.

Impairment of esophageal emptying, as Drs. Oakes and Sherck emphasize, frequently predisposes patients to drug-induced esophageal injury. Such impairment, resulting from peristaltic failure, is frequently so mild that it is acceptable without complaint by the patient and overlooked by the clinician, since it becomes apparent only in recumbency, when gravity is no longer operative. It is not surprising that in 88% of patients with drug-induced esophageal injury, deglutition was apparently normal. The elderly are particularly vulnerable, presumably because the mucosa is thinner and less resistant and because of presbyesophagus resulting in impairment of peristaltic amplitude and coordination.[2] Diseases such as systemic sclerosis[3] and diabetic autonomic neuropathy[4] are known to delay esophageal clearing in recumbency and would be expected to increase the risk of esophageal drug injury. Achalasia of the cardia causes gross delay in esophageal transit, and associated esophageal ulceration and fistula formation are recorded by Drs. Oakes and Sherck. However, such lesions are rare because of the protective action of the esophageal food and fluid residues often present in achalasia. The fluid residue provides a larger volume of distribution for irritant drugs and a lower local concentration at the mucosal surface. After successful cardiomyotomy, emptying improves and food residues are abolished or greatly reduced, yet peristalsis remains disrupted and esophageal delineation persists, as does the risk of drug-induced esophageal injury.

Drug combinations are frequently used, and when a drug that suppresses motility is given with an irritant drug, esophageal injury may result. Many drugs have inhibiting effects on esophageal motility—notably those with anticholinergic side effects, such as the tricyclic antidepressants, and those with a direct effect on smooth muscle, such as the calcium blockers (e.g., nifedipine).[5] It is therefore essential to review all medication being consumed by the patient to ensure that those which may affect esophageal motility are as far as possible avoided in the late evening and that they are not given at the same time as drugs which are potential esophageal irritants.

Gastroesophageal reflux and its consequences have several important bearings on drug-induced esophageal injury. A clear correlation has been found between the presence of hiatal hernia, gastroesophageal reflux, disordered peristalsis, and tablet sticking,[6] and patients with reflux esophagitis are thought to be particularly vulnerable to esophageal injury from nonsteroidal anti-inflammatory drugs. Nevertheless, this was not apparent from the data reported in Table 19.4, which showed 18 patients with gross evidence of esophagitis and 71 patients with histologic changes of inflammation, among 195 patients examined endoscopically. However, in these circumstances it is difficult to distinguish injury caused by reflux from that caused by drugs. Similarly, strictures may be caused by drug damage or by gastroesophageal reflux. In one study, a group of 76 patients with long-standing symptoms of gastroesophageal reflux showed a significantly greater consumption of nonsteroidal anti-inflammatory drugs during the 3 months before the appearance of dysphagia from a developing stricture than did a control population.[7] After discontinuation of the nonsteroidal anti-inflammatory drugs the esophagitis often persisted and a number of the strictures recurred after dilatation, suggesting that the drug may not have been the sole cause of esophageal damage. It seems probable that acid reflux and drug-induced irritation have an additive effect in causing esophageal injury. There is now increasing evidence that such is the case in peptic ulceration of the stomach and duodenum, because drug histories from patients presenting with bleeding[8] or perforation[1] have revealed a significantly greater consumption of nonsteroidal anti-inflammatory drugs than in a matched control population. Drug-induced esophageal injury often occurs at points of narrowing, such as the aortic indentation,[9] and it was found by Drs. Oakes and Sherck to be commonest in the upper esophagus and midesophagus, whereas reflux esophagitis is maximal in the lower esophagus. It seems probable that in the presence of reflux esophagitis the lower esophageal mucosa may be more susceptible to drug damage than that elsewhere. Under these circumstances the importance of iatrogenic injury may go unrecognized.

When the offending medication is stopped, drug-induced esophageal lesions do not always disappear rapidly, and it is of interest that the need for dilatation in some drug-induced strictures persisted for as long as 2 years. Recurrent re-stricturing suggests continuous inflammation, and other factors, such as gastroesophageal reflux, should be sought in such circumstances. Obviously, the possibility of other esophageal disease must be kept in mind, and deep ulceration with luminal narrowing might have a neoplastic basis, as in one of the cases reported.

Being alert to the possibility of drug-induced esophageal injury is a crucial aspect of diagnosis, and the importance of obtaining a full history of all present and recent medication must be emphasized. The elderly and those with arthritic or bladder disorders are particularly at risk, as are those with preexistent esophageal disease. In the diagnosis of drug-induced esophageal injury, endoscopy has advantages over radiology in detecting superficial ulceration and providing histologic material, which, even if it shows nonspecific changes, is helpful in excluding other disorders such as neoplasm. If stricturing has occurred, dilatation can be done then and there. However, the ultimate diagnostic criterion is that the lesions resolve after discontinuation of the drug in question.

In the management of drug-induced esophageal injuries, Drs. Oakes and Sherck emphasize the value of simple adjustments in the times and the way tablets are taken. Upright posture and drink volume correlate directly with rate of transit of capsules through the esophagus.[10] The possibility of using another, nonirritant, drug must be examined. Patients with arthritic pains are sometimes reluctant to give up a drug that is providing relief of symptoms in favor of one that may be less effective. Administration in suppository form may sometimes overcome this problem. Difficulty may arise in patients with bladder problems who are reluctant to swallow enough fluid to wash down their tablets because of fear of nocturnal incontinence. Follow-up examination, preferably with repeat endoscopy, is essential to confirm healing esophageal lesions and to detect any additional disease.

REFERENCES

1. Walt, R., Katschinsky, B., Logan, R., Ashley, J., and Langman, M.: Rising frequency of ulcer perforation in elderly people in the United Kingdom, Lancet **1**:489-492, 1986.
2. Soergel, K.H., Zbralske, F., and Amberg, J.R.: Presbyesophagus: esophageal motility in nonagenarians, J. Clin. Invest. **43**:1472-1479, 1964.
3. Cohen, S., Fisher, R., Lipshutz, W., Turner, R., Myers, A., and Schumacher, R.: Pathogenesis of esophageal dysfunction in scleroderma and Raynaud's disease, J. Clin. Invest. **51**:2663-2668, 1972.
4. Stewart, I.M., Hosking, D.J., Preston, B.J., and Atkinson, M.: Oesophageal motor changes in diabetes mellitus, Thorax **31**:278-283, 1976.
5. Blackwell, J.N., Holt, S., and Heading, R.C.: Effect of nifedepine on oesophageal motility and gastric emptying, Digestion **2**:50-56, 1981.
6. Evans, K.T., and Roberts, G.M.: The ability of patients to swallow capsules, J. Clin. Hosp. Pharm. **6**:207-208, 1981.
7. Heller, S.R., Fellows, I.W., Ogilvie, A.L., and Atkinson, M.: Non-steroidal anti-inflammatory drugs and benign oesophageal stricture, Br. Med. J. **285**:167-168, 1982.
8. Somerville, K., Faulkner, G., and Langman, M.: Non-steroidal anti-inflammatory drugs and bleeding peptic ulcer, Lancet **1**(8479):462-464, 1986.
9. Collins, F.J., Matthews, H.R., Baker, S.E., and Strakova, J.M.: Drug induced oesophageal injury, Br. Med. J. **1**(6179):1673-1676, 1979.
10. Hey, H., Jørgensen, F., Sørensen, K., Hasselbalch, H., and Wamberg, T.: Oesophageal transit of six commonly used tablets and capsules, Br. Med. J. **285**:1717-1719, 1982.

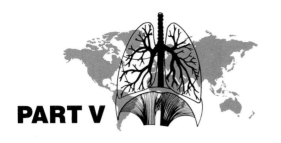

PART V MOTILITY DISORDERS

CHAPTER 20

Reflux control in operations for achalasia

Geoffrey M. Graeber and Roy K.H. Wong

Reflux has long been a problem associated with procedures employed to correct achalasia. In this chapter the historical basis for the current surgical procedures used to treat achalasia will be examined. The results of therapy and the incidence of reflux occurring after surgical correction will be reviewed for each of the two major schools of thought. Strengths and weaknesses of current published results will be synthesized and analyzed to present our current level of understanding of this perplexing problem. Some new material that represents a compromise between the two techniques will be presented and discussed. Finally, the anticipated avenues of future research will be explored in anticipation of better analysis of existing modalities and new methods of therapy.

HISTORICAL PERSPECTIVE

The lineage of today's procedures used to treat achalasia may be traced to the work of Heller, who reported his double myotomy in 1913.[1] As described, his procedure consisted of both an anterior and a posterior myotomy conducted through a transperitoneal approach. Obviously, the gastroesophageal junction had to be mobilized sufficiently to conduct myotomies far enough onto the esophagus to relieve the obstruction. With such dissection, the potential for reflux was great. Heller's concepts underwent revisions as attempts were made to find ways to relieve the obstruction to swallowing while not producing unacceptable reflux. Two other surgeons, Groeneveldt and Zaaijer, are credited with modifying Heller's original technique to a single

myotomy conducted through a transperitoneal approach.[2,3] Although the single myotomy was able to relieve the obstruction to swallowing caused by achalasia, the dissection required in order to obtain a complete myotomy and ensure success led to reflux in a significant number of cases. The transthoracic approach to a single myotomy was adopted subsequently, since this allowed precise visualization of the distal esophagus without extensive dissection of the gastroesophageal junction and would, theoretically, hold subsequent reflux to a minimum. Ellis and his colleagues are recognized for presenting the physiologic foundations for this approach and for popularizing the technique.[4]

Controversy today centers around how much myotomy should be conducted and whether or not an antireflux procedure should be added to diminish the incidence of reflux disease. Two major positions exist. One, as proposed by Ellis and his colleagues, states that a precise myotomy, extending onto the stomach less than 1 cm, should be conducted through a transthoracic approach. Only enough dissection of the gastroesophageal junction is conducted to allow adequate visualization of the gastric wall where the caudad extent of the myotomy will be terminated. According to this view, further dissection of the gastroesophageal junction is not warranted and may prove detrimental, particularly in the hands of inexperienced surgeons. Furthermore, the antireflux procedure required after such an extensive dissection may defeat the purpose of the myotomy by producing distal esophageal obstruction.

The other major position states that the entire gastroesophageal junction needs to be mobilized in order to conduct an adequate myotomy. Proponents of this view usually carry the myotomy farther distally onto the stomach than those who perform the previously described technique. Adequate visualization of the stomach is necessary, they feel, to ensure that the myotomy is carried far enough onto the stomach to divide the ob-

The opinions and assertions contained herein are the private views of the authors and are not to be construed as official or as reflecting the views of the Department of the Army or the Department of Defense.

structing muscle fibers. A modified antireflux procedure is conducted after completion of the myotomy, to reduce the chance of postoperative reflux.

ANALYSIS OF CURRENT RESULTS

Since no generally accepted, reliable animal model of achalasia exists, most data have been generated by analyses of patient series. Obviously, the results obtained from each of the two approaches need to be examined for strengths and weaknesses, both when reported by major proponents and when reported by other surgeons practicing the procedure. The major proponents of each view have adopted their position on the basis of the favorable results they have obtained. To be valid, these results have to be reproducible in the hands of other experienced as well as less experienced surgeons.

The favorable results of the limited myotomy without mobilization of the entire gastroesophageal junction and proximal stomach are best represented by the work of Ellis and his colleagues.[5,6] Their continuing experience with 113 patients shows that 91% had good results with myotomy alone while only nine patients had poor results (see Table 20-1). In four of the nine, the poor results were due to reflux esophagitis; in all four the condition was controlled with medical therapy. The amplitude of the lower esophageal sphincter pressure dropped from 32.5 ± 1.6 (SEM) mm Hg to 14.5 ± 1.4 mm Hg postoperatively. The length of the lower esophageal sphincter decreased from 3.7 ± 0.1 cm to 2.2 ± 0.1 cm after the myotomy. These data suggest that significant reduction in the length of and pressure in the lower esophageal sphincter can be achieved with a very low incidence of reflux.

Equally good results have been reported from the Mayo Clinic's experience. This is not surprising, since much of Ellis' early work was conducted at that institution. In a report that compared the results of treatment for both esophagomyotomy and forceful dilatation, Okike and associates reviewed the success of surgical correction in 456 patients.[7] Excellent or good results were obtained in 85% of this group, while only 3% had clinically significant reflux (see Table 20-1). Sixteen patients had hiatal hernias associated with their achalasia and underwent some type of diaphragmatic hernia repair at the time of myotomy. Twelve of these patients had good or excellent results, while only two had poor results. One of the patients with a poor result had reflux and a stricture. No mention is made of any esophageal obstruction resulting from the hiatal herniorrhaphy in any of the 16 cases.

Further support for the conduct of a limited myotomy alone was advanced recently by members of the staff at the Medical College of Georgia.[8] Two groups of patients were compared —those who had the esophagomyotomy alone and those who had the myotomy in association with some type of hiatal hernia repair. Sixteen patients had the myotomy alone. Seventeen had an associated repair: 14 had a Belsey, two had an Allison, and one had a Nissen. Of the patients with the myotomy alone, 15 (94%) had good results and none had symptomatic reflux (see Table 20-1). In the patients who had a hiatal herniorrhaphy associated with the myotomy, 12 (70%) had good results while two developed symptomatic reflux and three had distal esophageal obstructions that were due to the hiatal herniorrhaphies and not to incomplete myotomies. These data, the authors felt, supported the position that myotomy alone is sufficient therapy for achalasia. Earlier reports arrived at similar conclusions as long as the normal relationship of the esophagus to the hiatus was preserved and appropriate repair of preexisting hiatal hernias was conducted.[9]

Belsey was far less enthusiastic with his results when he used only the transthoracic Heller myotomy to correct the distal obstruction caused by achalasia.[10] In the 64 patients he treated with myotomy alone, 13 had what would be classified as poor results. Ten of these patients suffered from reflux and required subsequent operative repair. Indeed, seven of the patients had strictures. After this initial experience he performed a modified Mark IV repair in all patients who had myotomies for achalasia. This modified repair had two rows of sutures, as did the standard Mark IV, but the stitches that normally would have been placed in the middle (at the site of the myotomy) were omitted. The remaining four sutures were placed so that they not only created the valve mechanism and returned the gastroesophageal junction below the diaphragm but also tended to draw the two edges of the myotomy apart. Belsey's results with the myotomy and the modification of the Mark IV repair showed improvement over those obtained with the myotomy alone. Distal esophageal obstruction was relieved in all cases, with no evidence of esophagitis or fibrous stenosis in 62 patients (see Table 20-1).

Other authors have documented similar experiences. Jara and associates in their series emphasized the increasing incidence of reflux

TABLE 20-1. Analyses of results of operations for achalasia

Author	Year	Procedure	Patients	Excellent results (%)	Poor results (%)	Reflux (%)	Obstruction resulting from antireflux procedure (%)
Ellis et al.[6]	1984	Myotomy	113	94 (91)	9 (8)	4 (3)	—
Okike et al.[7]	1979	Myotomy	456	388 (85)	27 (6)	14 (3)	—
Okike et al.[7]	1979	Myotomy and hernia repair	16	12 (75)	2 (12.5)	1 (6)	—
Pai et al.[8]	1984	Myotomy	16	15 (94)	1 (6)	0	0
Pai et al.[8]	1984	Myotomy and hernia repair	17	12 (70)	3 (18)	2 (12)	3 (18)
Ferguson and Burford[9]	1960	Myotomy	44	35 (81)	8 (19)	4 (10)	—
Belsey[10]	1966	Myotomy	64	51 (80)	13 (20)	10 (16)	—
Belsey[10]	1966	Myotomy and Mark IV	62	62 (100)	0	0	None mentioned
Jara et al.[11]	1979	Myotomy	121	97 (80)	—	63 (52)	—
Peyton et al.[12]	1974	Myotomy and Mark IV	8	—	—	2 (29)	None mentioned
Bjorck et al.[13]	1982	Long myotomy	63	33/41 (80)	8/41 (20)	8/41 (20)	—
Bjorck et al.[13]	1982	Long myotomy	11				None mentioned
		Long myotomy and hernia repair	11	22 (100)	0	0	

with time.[11] They performed myotomies in 145 patients; 121 were located for long-term follow-up. Ninety-eight percent of their patients had transthoracic myotomies performed by a technique in which the diaphragm was opened away from the hiatus and a gastrostomy was created. A finger was introduced into the stomach through the gastrostomy, and the myotomy was conducted over the finger. Eighty percent of the patients had relief of dysphagia, but 52% of the entire group had reflux if followed to 13 years after surgical correction. Furthermore, the authors found that extension of the myotomy onto the stomach for more than 2 cm was associated with a 100% incidence of reflux. For these reasons they suggested that an antireflux procedure be performed at the time of the initial esophagomyotomy.

Peyton and his associates evaluated fourteen patients with achalasia, using intraesophageal manometry and standard acid reflux testing.[12] Seven of the 14 patients exhibited gastroesophageal reflux. Repair consisting of a Heller esophagomyotomy and a Belsey Mark IV hiatal herniorrhaphy was conducted in eight patients. Standard acid reflux testing revealed reflux on preoperative evaluation in five of the seven patients treated surgically. Two of the seven patients evaluated postoperatively still had reflux. These authors concluded that the significant incidence of preoperative gastroesophageal reflux necessitated the hiatal herniorrhaphy to ensure functional integrity of the lower esophageal sphincter. The low incidence of true hiatal hernia with achalasia was stressed and has been supported by others.[14]

One report from Sweden has emphasized the necessity of evaluating existing reflux disease and hiatal hernia before correcting distal esophageal obstruction resulting from achalasia.[13] This study divided patients into two groups: those who did not have preoperative evaluation for conditions that predisposed them to reflux and those who did have such evaluation. In the first group, 63 patients underwent long myotomies (12 cm) with 2-cm incisions carried down onto the gastric wall. Forty-one patients were not evaluated preoperatively. Eight patients developed severe reflux complications from 1 to 5 years after operation. In the second group (total of 22 patients) 11 were found to have conditions that would predispose them to reflux: hiatal hernia (4), gastroesophageal reflux (5), and megaesophagus (2). All 11 had hiatal herniorrhaphies: Husfeldt repairs were conducted in five and Belsey Mark IV repairs in the remaining six. In the remaining 11 patients, who had neither gastroesophageal reflux nor hiatal hernia, only the esophagomyotomy was performed. Special care was taken in these 11 patients to fix the previously narrowed portion of the esophagus below the diaphragm after the myotomy. After follow-up (mean, 4 years), 14 patients were without symptoms and eight had occasional, slight dysphagia. All were evaluated radiographically, and 15 were evaluated by intraesophageal pH monitoring. Slight reflux was observed on provocation in only three patients on pH testing, and no reflux was observed radiographically. This study emphasizes the importance of preoperative evaluation of patients with achalasia for coexisting esophageal disease. The importance of tailoring the patient's operative repair to the existing disorders cannot be overemphasized. Appropriate continued surveillance using objective criteria in the postoperative period is mandatory in order to assess relief of obstruction and evaluate reflux. Other centers have also attempted to identify conditions that would predispose patients to postoperative reflux.[15] These indications for an antireflux procedure include, in addition to those already stated, pulmonary complications associated with aspiration and repeat operative procedures.

Two other reports deserve mention. One group that still performs the myotomy through an abdominal approach found strong evidence in favor of a hiatal repair after their procedure.[16] Fifty-five of 108 patients who had a formal repair after dissection of the hiatus had no evidence of reflux disease, whereas 20 patients who did not have a formal repair did have symptoms of reflux. Another study, which examined results of surgical therapy in 65 patients with diffuse esophageal spasm, found that results differed with the type of hiatal herniorrhaphy conducted.[17] Interestingly, this study suggests that total fundoplication after a long myotomy may be associated with obstruction.

In summary, the literature suggests that the surgical procedure selected for a given patient with achalasia must take into account not only the primary condition but associated disorders. If reflux is present, a hiatal hernia is documented, or megaesophagus is confirmed, the addition of an antireflux procedure to the myotomy is strongly indicated. If the hiatus is dissected extensively or the distal myotomy is extended more than 2 cm onto the stomach, an antireflux procedure is indicated. If the myotomy may be conducted with minimal hiatal dissection and is limited to 1 cm or less of the gastric wall, no adjunctive procedure may be necessary.

TECHNIQUE OF ESOPHAGEAL MYOTOMY AS CURRENTLY PERFORMED AT WALTER REED ARMY MEDICAL CENTER

The major problem with many of the previous reports on reflux after operations for achalasia is that most of the work has centered on subjective findings from patients. Very few objective data have been offered to evaluate reflux occurring either before surgical intervention or after the correction of distal esophageal obstruction. Neither the approach of the minimal dissection to effect the longitudual myotomy nor the approach of complete dissection of the hiatus followed by a myotomy and an antireflux procedure has been evaluated thoroughly by esophageal manometry or 24-hour pH monitoring. Ideally, the results of both surgical techniques should be evaluated by a prospective study utilizing esophageal manometry and 24-hour reflux testing to evaluate the patient preoperatively and after corrective surgery. The study should not be limited to the immediate postoperative period but should be conducted over a period of years after surgical correction, since reflux can develop as the inflammation and scarring around the repair undergo modification.

Our institution is currently conducting an evaluation of patients with achalasia that includes both esophageal manometry and 24-hour pH monitoring. In this study, patients are evaluated preoperatively to establish the diagnosis of achalasia and to assess existing reflux. After surgical correction, 24-hour pH monitoring and esophageal manometry are conducted at the time of discharge from the hospital and at subsequent yearly intervals to evaluate the effectiveness of the correction and to determine whether gastroesophageal reflux is present.

The operative procedure that we are currently using is a synthesis of the two schools of thought on the type of correction that should be done. In essence, it attempts to combine the anticipated better aspects of both types of repair in that most of the gastroesophageal junction is not mobilized, a precise myotomy is conducted onto the stomach for only 1 cm, and two sutures are placed at the end of the procedure, which create an anterior gastroesophageal ridge and replace the stomach beneath the diaphragm. In essence, this allows for a precise myotomy and return of the distal esophagus and stomach into the peritoneal cavity without a major antireflux repair.

A thoracotomy is performed through the left seventh intercostal space using an adequate incision to ensure appropriate visualization of the distal esophagus. The parietal pleura over the esophagus is opened laterally, and the esophagus is dissected from surrounding areolar tissue using sharp and blunt dissection. Localization of the esophagus and the dissection are facilitated by the placement of a no. 42 bougie in the esophagus prior to the thoracotomy. The parietal pleura is opened only in the most anterolateral portion of the esophageal hiatus. The central tendon of the diaphragm is then grasped with a Kocher clamp, and tension is directed anteriorly and laterally to open the anterolateral portion of the hiatus. Limited dissection is carried out underneath the diaphragm to allow placement of a Richardson retractor at the very antrolateral portion of the hiatus. With the bougie being used as a stent, the myotomy is conducted only over the segment of the esophagus that corresponds to that portion identified by manometry to be the segment that does not relax. We have found that this segment may vary in length between patients; hence, appropriate measurement of the myotomy must be conducted and the myotomy individualized for each patient. The myotomy is carried down onto the stomach so that the gastric mucosa is visualized for less than 1 cm. One of the landmarks that is most helpful in defining the inferior limits of the myotomy is the very cephalad portion of the peritoneum, where it reflects onto the stomach. Once this glistening membrane and the veins of the anterior gastric seromuscular wall are reached, the caudad extent of the myotomy is delineated. The bougie in the esophagus helps to determine the segmental extent of the myotomy in that the portion of the esophagus that does not relax generally is quite tight on the bougie. The gastric wall and the wall of the esophagus above the segment that does not relax are loose and move over the bougie easily. The incision is, therefore, carried 1 cm down onto the stomach beyond this constricting portion of the esophagus and approximately 1 cm onto the dialated esophagus above the afflicted segment.

Once the myotomy has been completed, the anterior repair that reestablishes the gastroesophageal junction in the peritoneal cavity (high-pressure zone) underneath the diaphragm is conducted. This repair is shown in the accompanying diagrams. The first of two stitches is positioned anteriorly by using a pledgeted 3-0 braided synthetic suture placed in a horizontal mattress fashion first through the esophagus approximately 1 cm above the gastroesophageal junction, then through the gastric wall 1 cm beyond the gastroesophageal junction. This suture is then passed in

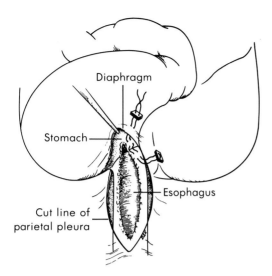

Fig. 20-1. The completed esophageal myotomy with the edges oversewn by a 4-0 chromic suture. The length of the myotomy has been exaggerated slightly in these drawings to allow better diagrammatic presentation. The first stitch to position the gastroesophageal junction below the diaphragm has been placed anteriorly. The no. 42 bougie used to stent the esophagus for the myotomy remains in place.

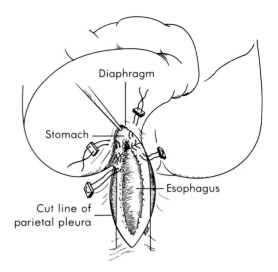

Fig. 20-2. With the no. 42 bougie remaining in place, a second stitch is placed posterior to the myotomy. Note that most of the gastroesophageal junction has not been dissected from surrounding tissues.

a parallel fashion through the diaphragm and through a second pledget. The suture is positioned through the diaphragm in such a manner that the gastroesophageal junction will be reestablished in its former anatomic position when the suture is tied. The pledgets are used so that these stitches do not tear through the frail tissues when tied. These stitches are exactly analogous to the type described by Belsey in his Mark IV repair (see Fig. 20-1). A second stitch is then placed, in a similar fashion, posterior to the myotomy and approximately 90 to 120 degrees in rotation on the esophagus away from the anterior stitch (see Fig. 20-2). As can be seen from the diagram, this pledgeted suture is brought down through the esophagus first, into the stomach, through the diaphragm, and then pledgeted. The esophagus and stomach, which have been partially exposed through the opening in the hiatus anteriorly, are then reduced down to their normal anatomic position by the surgeon, and each of the two sutures is tied in place by the assistant, who ensures that just enough pressure is placed on both sutures to return the esophagus and stomach to the position they occupied prior to dissection. Once these two sutures have been tied (Fig. 20-3), it is apparent that a portion of the myotomy then lies below the diaphragm. It may be seen that these sutures not only return this portion

below the diaphragm, but also, by their placement 90 to 120 degrees from each other, ensure that the edges of the myotomy do not lie in close proximity to one another. Once this maneuver has been completed, the surgeon inserts his or her index finger into the posterior portion of the hiatus. If the index finger fits into the hiatus snugly with a no. 42 bougie in place, the repair is appropriate (see Fig. 20-4). If the index finger of the surgeon does not fit down into the hiatus behind the no. 42 bougie, the repair is too tight and appropriate correction should be made. In our experience, however, the closure of the hiatus is usually appropriate with placement of only the two anterior stitches. On occasion, a single posterior stitch has been placed in order to narrow the hiatus slightly.

After the hiatus has been checked, the remaining exposed myotomy is covered by the parietal pleura, which is reconstructed using a running chromic suture. It should be noted that before the placement of the two stitches to position the esophagus and stomach under the diaphragm, the muscular edges of the myotomy have been oversewn with a running 4-0 chromic suture and the esophagus itself has been checked for possible perforations of the mucosa by introducing 10 ml of methylene blue dye through a separate nasogastric tube passed down next to the bougie.

After the patient has had sufficient time to recover from the surgery, manometry and 24-hour pH testing are conducted. This usually occurs at

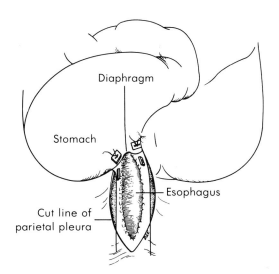

Fig. 20-3. Note that both of the stitches have been tied, causing the gastroesophageal junction to return to the position it occupied before the anterolateral dissection. The stitches are placed so that the caudad edges of the myotomy are drawn away from each other.

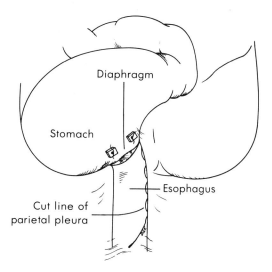

Fig. 20-4. The cut edges of the pleura have been reconstructed over the myotomy to complete the procedure. Before the pleura is closed, the adequacy of the hiatal opening is checked against the bougie. While the bougie is in place, methylene blue is injected into the esophageal lumen through a nasogastric tube to confirm that the mucosa has not been violated.

7 to 10 days postoperatively. Patients are often able to eat successfully between 3 and 5 days after the procedure. Most are discharged after the 24-hour pH monitoring study.

In a very limited series of patients studied in this manner, we have achieved correction of the achalasia with no evidence of recurring reflux. So far we have evaluated five patients for more than 2 years after repair. Only one patient has shown any evidence of recurrence of his achalasia. He was treated by a second myotomy and a fundoplication. The distal end of his myotomy had healed with fusion of the fibers underneath the diaphragm. Since his second operation he has had no reflux disease and has had complete relief of his achalasia. The other four patients have had complete relief of their achalasia and on 24-hour pH monitoring have shown no evidence of reflux.

SUMMARY

Gastroesophageal reflux is a recognized complication of most operations used to treat achalasia. Proper preoperative assessment is mandatory if an appropriate procedure is to be conducted for a given patient. Preoperative manometry and 24-hour pH monitoring not only aid in diagnosis but also determine a baseline for comparison of similar postoperative studies. Prospective studies are in progress to evaluate the adequacy of correction and the incidence of reflux. The objec-

tive data obtained will allow better evaluation of the various procedures and selection of methods that produce superior results.

ACKNOWLEDGEMENTS

The authors wish to thank SP4 John L. MacDonald and PFC Kelly A. Mittelstaedt for obtaining the references. Our gratitude is extended to Mrs. Linda G. Ellis and Miss Sylvia A. Burch for preparation of the manuscript. We are also indebted to David S. Kern of the Division of Medical Audiovisual Services, Walter Reed Army Institute of Research, for the illustrations.

REFERENCES

1. Heller, E.: Extramukose cardioplastik beim chronischen cardiospasmus mit dilatations des oesophagus, Mitt. Grenzgeb. Med. Chir. **27**:141, 1913.
2. De Bruine Groeneveldt, J.R.: Over cardiospasmus, Ned Tijdschr. Geneeskd. **54**:1281, 1918.
3. Zaaijer, J.H.: Cardiospasm in the aged, Ann. Surg. **77**:615, 1923.
4. Ellis, F.H., Jr., Kiser, J.C., Schlegel, J.F., et al.: Esophagomyotomy for esophageal achalasia: experimental, clinical, and manometric aspects, Ann. Surg. **166**:640, 1967.
5. Ellis, F.H., Jr., Gibb, S.P., and Crozier, R.E.: Esophagomyotomy for achalasia of the esophagus, Ann. Surg. **192**:157, 1980.

6. Ellis, F.H., Jr., Crozier, R.E., and Watkins, E., Jr.: Operation for esophageal achalasia: results of esophagomyotomy without an antireflux operation, J. Thorac. Cardiovasc. Surg. **88:**344, 1984.

7. Okike, N., Payne, W.S., Neufeld, D.M., et al.: Esophagomyotomy versus forceful dilation for achalasia of the esophagus: results in 899 patients, Ann. Thorac. Surg. **28:**119, 1979.

8. Pai, G.P., Ellison, R.G., Rubin, J.W., et al.: Two decades of experience with modified Heller's myotomy for achalasia, Ann. Thorac. Surg. **38:**201, 1984.

9. Ferguson, T.B., and Burford, T.H.: An evaluation of the modified Heller operation in the treatment of achalasia of the esophagus, Ann. Surg. **152:**1, 1960.

10. Belsey, R.: Functional disease of the esophagus, J. Thorac. Cardiovasc. Surg. **62:**164, 1966.

11. Jara, F.M., Toledo-Pereyra, L.H., Lewis, J.W., and Magilligan, D.J.: Long-term results of esophagomyotomy for achalasia of esophagus, Arch. Surg. **114:**935, 1979.

12. Peyton, M.D., Greenfield, L.D., and Elkins, R.C.: Combined myotomy and hiatal herniorrhaphy: a new approach to achalasia, Am. J. Surg. **128:**786, 1974.

13. Bjorck, S., Dernevik, L., Gatzinsky, P., and Sanberg, N.: Oesophagocardiomyotomy and antireflux procedures, Acta Chir. Scand. **148:**525, 1982.

14. Binder, H.J., Clemett, A.R., Thayes, W.R., et al.: Rarity of hiatus hernia in achalasia, N. Engl. J. Med. **272:**680, 1965.

15. Murray, G.F., Battaglini, J.W., Keagy, B.A., et al.: Selective application of fundoplication in achalasia, Ann. Thorac. Surg. **37:**185, 1984.

16. Black, J., Vorbach, A.N., and Collis, J.L.: Results of Heller's operation for achalasia of the esophagus: the importance of hiatal repair, Br. J. Surg. **63:**949, 1976.

17. Henderson, R.D., and Ryder, D.E.: Reflux control following myotomy for diffuse esophageal spasm, Ann. Thorac. Surg. **34:**230, 1982.

Reflux control in operations for achalasia

DISCUSSION

R.E. Lea

Since achalasia has been treated there has been concern about the incidence of postoperative esophageal reflux. Early operations such as esophagogastrectomy had a high incidence of reflux.[1] In 1913 Heller described his double myotomy, which was subsequently modified to the now-standard single myotomy.[2,3] The operation was originally described as being done through an abdominal approach but is now usually performed through the chest. Although reflux can occur after a successful modified Heller's operation and even after balloon dilatation, it is not an inevitable consequence. The incidence in various series has been from 1.1%, as reported by Ellis et al.,[4] to 62%, reported by Acheson and Hadley.[5] Because of this wide variation in reflux, the place of antireflux surgery after myotomy remains controversial. If reflux always occurred, there would be no question that an antireflux procedure was indicated. The disadvantage of a repair is the risk of producing dysphagia in a poorly functioning esophagus.

The reason for the variation in incidence of reflux is that the operation, as practiced by surgeons, although essentially the same, does have important differences. These small differences in surgical technique may influence the results of surgical treatment.

The points that should be considered are as follows:

1. Thoracic approach or abdominal approach
2. Amount of mobilization of the hiatus
3. Length of the myotomy
4. Extent of the myotomy onto the stomach
5. Whether any type of antireflux procedure has been done

Because of these differing technical details it is difficult to compare results, since many authors do not give precise details of their operations. Nevertheless, it is apparent that some techniques are more likely to produce postoperative reflux than are others.

An abdominal approach certainly requires more extensive mobilization of the esophagus and the hiatus. This method was used by Black et al.,[6] Hawthorne et al.,[7] Barlow,[8] and Douglas and Nicholson,[9] all of whom described a high incidence of reflux.

That the amount of mobilization is important, whether from above or below, is shown in the series by Jara et al.[10] In their cases the stomach was opened and the myotomy done with a finger in the esophagus. One year after the operation 24% had reflux; this increased to 48% at 10 years.

Although the length of the myotomy does not appear to be important, provided the incision extends proximally onto thy hypertrophied muscle, the lower extent of the incision does appear to be crucial. Jara et al. found that if this distance was more than 2 cm, reflux always occurred. This finding confirms the experimental work of Ellis et al.[11] in studies of the effects of (1) a classic Heller; (2) a long Heller, which meant extension onto the stomach for 3 cm; and (3) a short Heller, in which the incision just extended onto the stomach. Only the short Heller was not associated with reflux.

The abnormality in achalasia is confined to the esophagus, with no involvement of the stomach. The only reason for extending the incision onto the stomach is to ensure that all the circular muscle fibers are divided. The best way to identify stomach is by the veins in the submucosa. Once these are reached there is no reason to extend the incision. If the incision is extended well onto the stomach, there is little doubt that the incidence of reflux is increased.

To overcome the problem of reflux, fundoplication and repair of the hiatus have been recommended. The disadvantage of an antireflux procedure is the possibility of causing dysphagia. Peristalsis in the proximal esophagus is abnormal, and the propulsive power may be too poor to overcome the resistance of the repair. This is particularly apparent in a Nissen 360-degree fundoplication. To overcome the problem of dysphagia, surgeons have used either the Belsey operation with a 270-degree wrap or a short Nissen, the one-stitch Nissen as described by Henderson and Ryder.[12]

From the published series it is apparent that good results are obtained in 75% to 85% of patients. The poor results are due to a variety of factors, but in some they are secondary to gastroesophageal reflux. What is not known is the incidence of gastroesophageal reflux after a modified Heller's operation, and, if reflux is present, whether it is causing symptoms. Another difficulty in assessing results is the variable length of follow-up. It is apparent that many patients who have had surgical treatment remain well for 4 or 5 years and then relapse. It is therefore important that patients be followed for an adequate length of time. When a patient returns with recurrent symptoms, it is essential that there be full investigations with esophageal manometry and pH studies to elucidate the cause of the problem. Only after this has been done can the correct remedial measures be taken.

It remains unclear what is the best surgical treatment in achalasia. This can only be resolved by an accurate preoperative assessment, an exact description of the operative technique, and a long period of postoperative assessment. A major problem is that the incidence of the disease is low—approximately 0.7 cases per 100,000 persons—and any one surgeon's experience will be fairly small.

Drs. Graeber and Wong describe a protocol for the management of patients in the future. Their technique is simple and should ensure that the gastroesophageal junction remains within the abdomen. In following Ellis's guidelines and just extending the myotomy onto the stomach, they ensure that the incidence of reflux should be minimal. If more surgeons used a similar approach, the incidence of reflux after surgery might soon be known. This treatment is similar to the approach in our unit, and our results suggest that reflux is not a major problem, provided the hiatal dissection is minimal and the incision onto the stomach is only far enough to

identify stomach. In 1981, 100 consecutive cases were reviewed (personal series) for a minimum 5 years postoperatively; 75% could be classed as good results. In the moderate and poor groups, failure was mainly due to recurrent dysphagia, but in only three cases was this related to reflux.

From the published evidence it would appear that provided a modified Heller's operation is done through the chest with the myotomy confined to the esophagus, an antireflux procedure is not necessary. If the operation is performed transabdominally and the incision is extended onto the stomach, an antireflux procedure would be wise although a standard Nissen should be avoided.

REFERENCES

1. Heller, E.: Extramukose Cardioplastik beim chronischen Cardiospasmus mit Dilatations des Oesophagus, Mitt. Grenzgeb. Med. Chir. **27:**141, 1913.
2. Zaaijer, J.H.: Cardiospasm in the aged, Ann. Surg. **77:**615, 1923.
3. Groeneveldt, deB., Jr.: Over cardiospasmus, Ned. Tijdschr. Geneeskd. **54:**1281, 1918.
4. Ellis, F.H., Gibb, S.P., and Crozier, R.E.: Esophagomyotomy for achalasia of the esophagus, Ann. Surg. **192:**157, 1980.
5. Acheson, E.D., and Hadley, G.D.: Cardiomyotomy for achalasia of the cardia, Br. Med. J. 1,549, 1958.
6. Black, J., Vorbach, A.N., and Collis, J.L.: Results of Heller's operation for achalasia of the oesophagus, Br. J. Surg. **63:**949, 1976.
7. Hawthorne, H.R., Frobese, A.S., and Nemir, P., Jr.: The surgical management of achalasia of the oesophagus, Ann. Surg. **144:**653, 1956.
8. Barlow, D.: Problems of achalasia, Br. J. Surg. **48:**642, 1961.
9. Douglas, K., and Nicholson, F.: The late results of Heller's operation for cardiospasm, Br. J. Surg. **47:**250, 1959.
10. Jara, F.M., Toledo-Pereyra, L.H., Lewis, J.W., and Magilligan, D.J.: Long term results of esophagomyotomy for achalasia of the esophagus, Arch. Surg. **114:**935, 1979.
11. Ellis, F.H., Jr., Kisser, J.C., Schlegel, J.F., et al.: Esophagomyotomy for esophageal achalasia: experimental, clinical and manometric aspects, Ann. Surg. **166:**640, 1967.
12. Henderson, R.D., and Ryder, D.E.: Reflux control following myotomy for diffuse esophageal spasm, Ann. Thorac. Surg. **34:**230, 1982.

CHAPTER 21 Management of failed Heller's operation

François Fekete

The treatment of idiopathic megaesophagus by Heller's operation gives good results in 85% to 96% of cases.[1,2] In the remaining cases of recurrent or persistent dysphagia, a distinction should be made between unsuccessful Heller's operations and undesirable postoperative complications, especially esophagitis.

In France, the abdominal route is usually undertaken, sufficient to perform a long myotomy of 8 to 10 cm on the esophagus and 1 cm on the stomach, below the vessels crossing the cardia. An antireflux procedure, an easy surgical procedure in the abdomen, must be associated. A diaphragmatic crura suture is performed behind the esophagus, and at the narrowing of the His angle a suture is placed from the left side of the myotomy to the right wall of the fundus of the stomach. The anterior wall of the stomach is folded over the front of the myotomy.[1,3]

PREOPERATIVE CHECKUP

Before any therapeutic decision, a complete appraisal is undertaken to explain the reason for failure of Heller's operation.

X-ray examination of the esophagus and stomach confirms the absence of other lesions, such as diverticula or tumor. It must be noted that on the barium esophagogram the criteria for a satisfactory Heller's operation are decreased esophageal diameter, absence of stasis, a hernia of the mucosa, good esophageal clearance, reappearance of the gastric air pocket, and absence of reflux.

Fiberoptic endoscopy verifies the absence of tumor and looks for reflux esophagitis and/or a stricture.

The pH reflux tests may indicate gastroesophageal reflux. Manometry is absolutely necessary for the study of these patients and can measure the lower esophageal sphincter pressure and possibly ascertain the reality of diffuse spasm associated with achalasia.

Finally, the precise psychologic makeup of the patient must be evaluated.

Thus, of 21 reoperations, Patrick et al.[4] made a correct diagnosis in 17 cases (nine out of 13 achalasia, and eight out of eight esophagitis). This problem is important, since it can determine the surgical approach: left thoracotomy is suggested in cases of uncertain diagnosis.

MATERIAL AND METHODS

We have treated 86 patients who underwent one or more Heller's operations: out of these, 59 were initially operated on in other centers and referred to us for reintervention and 27 were operated on in our center, giving a reintervention rate of 6% of a series of 446 initial Heller's operations performed between 1950 and 1985 with the same technique.

The types of initial operations performed are listed in Table 21-1. All 86 patients underwent at least one Heller's operation, and in some patients who were referred to us, this was followed by a

TABLE 21-1. Initial procedures in 86 patients

Procedure	No. of patients
1 Heller's operation	64
2 Heller's operations	7
3 Heller's operations	1
Heller's + cardiopolasty or Heyrowski	8
Heller's + splanchnisectomy	2
Heller's + second antireflux procedure	2
2 Heller's + second antireflux procedure	1
2 Heller's + cardiopolasty + colonic interposition (Belsey)	1

cardioplasty or an esophagogastric anastomosis (Heyrowski). In our own practice, some patients were submitted to several reoperations—for example, Heller's through the abdominal route, extended myotomy through the thoracic route, and total duodenal diversion for esophagitis.

CAUSES OF FAILURE

The analysis of the data shows several, sometimes complex, reasons for failure after Heller's operations. In Table 21-2, the causes of failure are shown; a defective surgical technique appears to be the most common cause.

In Heller's operation, the muscle fibers at the lower end of the esophagus are dissected so as to eliminate permanent hypertonia of the lower esophageal sphincter. In this way, a dysfunction is counteracted by the creation of an unphysiologic condition,[5] and the major causes of failure stem from this—for example, continued achalasia in cases of inadequate myotomy, or reflux esophagitis in cases of incompetent cardioesophageal junction.

Persistent or recurrent spasm from motility disorders

Signs indicating a poor result usually appear fairly soon, if not immediately, and only seven patients out of 47 showed an improvement lasting longer than 2 years. Clinical manifestations include the persistence or early recurrence of the

TABLE 21-2. Causes of failure after Heller's operation

Defective surgical technique:
    Inadequate myotomy
    Periesophageal sclerosis
    No antireflux procedures (esophagitis)
Correct myotomy:
    Antireflux not efficient (esophagitis)
Antireflux procedure:
    Interstitial sclerosis
    "Diverticulization" of the mucosa
    Progressive dyskinesia
Defective indication:
    Diffuse esophageal spasm
    Dolichomegaesophagus
    Unrecognized carcinoma in the megaesophagus
    Unrecognized reflux ulcer with secondary
        megaesophagus
Others:
    Excessive antireflux procedure
    Gastric volvulus
    Secondary development of cancer

preoperative problems (dysphagia, regurgitation). The clearest indication of failure is the failure to regain weight. However, since some patients were reluctant to undergo further surgery, reoperation was performed from 1 to 29 years later.

The x-ray film in Fig. 21-1 reveals that the size of esophagus is unchanged, stasis is persistent, and there are difficulties of barium passage into the stomach as well as an absence of gastric air pocket. The signs of a mucosal hernia, indicating the presence of an anterior myotomy, are nonexistent or very scarce. Manometry reveals any remaining portion of the suprahiatal lower esophageal sphincter.

These signs have led us to suspect the inadequacy of Heller's operation in 47 cases. This finding is comparable to findings reported in other series.[4,6] Among these cases, six etiologic circumstances can be identified (see Table 21-3).

Inadequate myotomy

An inadequate myotomy is usually due to an imperfect surgical technique; this is evident at reoperation, when the unexpectedly few postoperative adhesions allow the esophagus to be approached very easily. The initial myotomy can

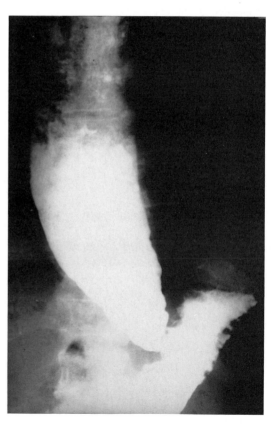

Fig. 21-1. Failure of the myotomy.

usually be found again, and seems too short upward or downward and/or too shallow with respect to the internal circular layer of muscle. Several of these defects can often be found simultaneously; this is probably due to an insufficient exposure of the hiatal area and fear of damaging the mucosa (see Table 21-4).

The transabdominal approach has been cited as a cause of the high frequency of inadequate

TABLE 21-3. Reasons for unsuccessful Heller's operation (persistent or recurrent spasm) in 47 patients

Reason	No. of patients
Standard cardiospasm (technical imperfection)	30
Dolichomegaesophagus	8
Atypical megaesophagus; diffuse spasm	2
Secondary extension of spasm	3
Interstitial esophageal sclerosis	3
Diffuse idiopathic intestinal pseudoobstruction	1

myotomies,[4] but our own findings in a series of 446 initial Heller's operations do not support this view.

Treatment. Treatment of inadequate myotomy is generally a second myotomy. In elderly patients or before reoperation (see Fig. 21-2), endoscopic pneumatic dilatation has been used; our experience shows this to be relatively ineffective. In cases of persistent cardiospasm—without esophageal asystole, in which situation it is bound to fail—repeated cardiomyotomy is necessary. All that remains to be decided is whether a transab-

TABLE 21-4. Results of preoperative evaluation of myotomy defect in 30 cases of standard cardiospasm*

Finding	No. of cases
Heller too short upward	15
Heller too short downward	10
Heller insufficient in depth	11

*Several defects can be associated.

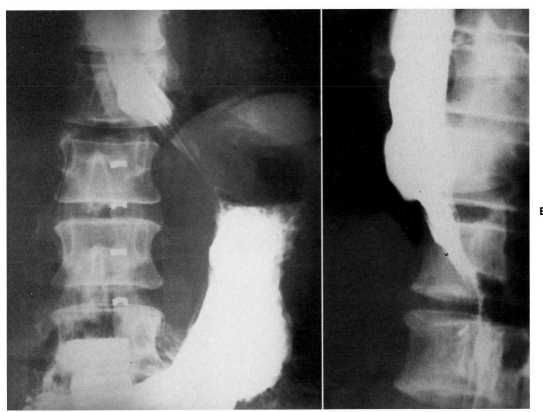

A

B

Fig. 21-2. A, After second myotomy (abdominal approach). **B,** Same patient; note the hernia of the mucosa.

dominal or transthoracic approach is to be used. On the basis of our experience, we tend to repeat the laparotomy if the information in the initial operation report, or the barium meal, leads us to suspect a technical error. In this route, the operation is easy in most cases, and it is possible to perform a longer myotomy in the same site as the former one, or on the opposite side.

We have had to abandon the transabdominal approach in only three out of 30 cases, in which access to the esophagus was impeded by periesophageal sclerosis. The only disadvantage of this method is the risk of damaging the mucosal membrane, although in our experience, this does not produce any serious consequences if it is immediately repaired by suture. This operation should always be accompanied by repair of the antireflux mechanism. Several North American authors[4,6,7] recommend the left thoracic approach, which allows the myotomy to be performed on the posterior part of the esophagus, minimizing the risk of mucosal damage. We use this approach only when we are sure that the initial myotomy was performed correctly, and when we need to extend the myotomy in cases of diffuse spasm.

The results were excellent in 86% of cases (26 of 30). The symptoms disappeared, and the patients regained weight and were able to resume their normal activities.

Interstitial esophageal sclerosis

Interstitial esophageal sclerosis is an unforeseeable cause of failure, since it can be diagnosed only by the anatomopathologist on biopsy of the resected wall of the myotomy. We have encountered it three times; in these cases repeated myotomy gave two failures that required resection and one unsatisfactory result. There are no preoperative radiologic or endoscopic diagnostic criteria. This lesion is seldom discussed in the literature and is possibly only a scarring of the initial myotomy, as was suggested[4,6,8] or a result of associated esophagitis. In these cases it would again be a case of poor operative technique producing an insufficient separation of the muscle and the mucosa.

Dolichomegaesophagus

Certain dolichomegaesophagi can more correctly be identified as esophageal asystole (see Fig. 21-3); a large tortuous esophagus with a low base and folds over the dome of the diaphragm allows the contents to stagnate and creates a definite risk of failure for Heller's operation (see Fig. 21-4). We have observed eight cases of unsuccessful Heller's operation performed on this kind of dolichomegaesophagus. The initial myotomy, in seven of these cases, was performed in our center. Attention should therefore be focused on the reasons for failure.

Technically, it is more difficult to perform a cardiomyotomy in these cases than in cases of normal achalasia, even though a long tract of muscle is divided. However, it is usually impossible to straighten the esophageal flexure through an abdominal approach, so that a cul-de-sac below the level of the cardia remains. The appearance of the symptoms can be immediate or late (11 years). Relapse may not always appear in the form of dysphagia but may appear as hemorrhage, regurgitation, or a feeling of thoracic oppression. We have performed three consecutive myotomies, all of which were unsuccessful. Until now, the indication for a primary or repeated Heller's operation has been an unwillingness to perform a resection on a patient with a benign condition. However, the excellent results obtained with mechanical esophagogastric anastomoses[9] and with esophagectomy without thoracotomy at present encourage us to use resection after failure with an initial myotomy.

Diffuse spasm of esophagus

In certain atypical cardiospasms, such as diffuse spasm of the esophagus, routine myotomy is inadequate. This rare disease, described by Lortat-Jacob in 1950,[10] gives specific manometric readings that differentiate it from achalasia, allowing an effective, appropriately long transthoracic myotomy to be performed immediately. However, the length of the myotomy is still under discussion. Ellis prefers to respect the lower esophageal sphincter,[11] whereas we support the work of Vantrappen,[12] who finds sphincter hypertonia in a third of cases, and we perform a complete myotomy upward but extended in length downward because of similarities with idiopathic megaesophagus.

Neuropathic involvement

Cases with neuropathic involvement are to be differentiated from ones with delayed dysphagia after several years of good results (see Fig. 21-5). Manometry shows a gradual involvement of the esophageal body by the neuropathy.

Endoscopic pneumatic dilatations have been useless in the three cases that we have observed. A large myotomy by thoracotomy was undertaken successfully.

Other disorders

We have also observed one case of idiopathic intestinal pseudoobstruction as a manifestation of

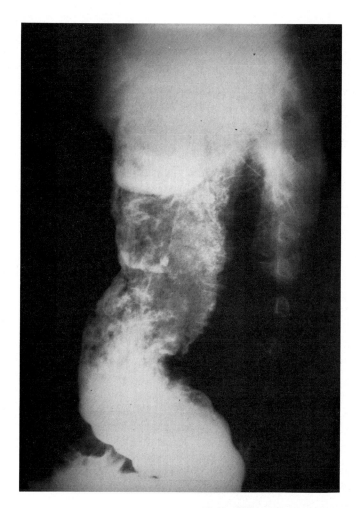

Fig. 21-3. Dolichomegaesophagus.

Fig. 21-4. Persistent stasis after efficient Heller's operation.

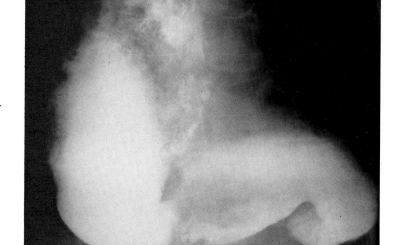

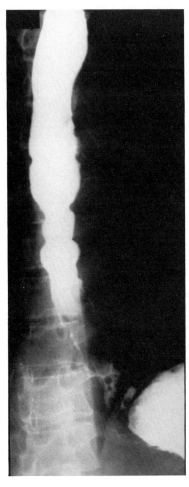

Fig. 21-5. Extensive dyskinesia 20 years after Heller's operation and esophagitis. Manometry demonstrated an advanced megaesophagus in the body of the esophagus and hypertonia of the lower esophageal sphincter.

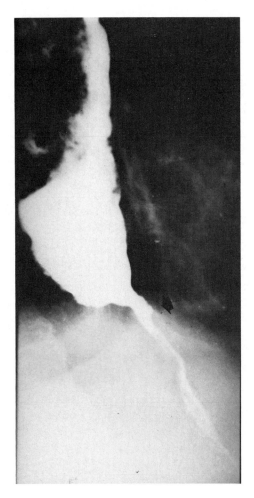

Fig. 21-6. Reflux stenosis with ulcer *(arrow)* after Heller's operation.

TABLE 21-5. Pathologic conditions caused by Heller's operation (39 cases)

Condition	No. of cases
Reflux esophagitis	32
Periesophageal sclerosis	3
"Diverticulization"	2
Extensive hiatal repair	1
Gastric volvulus	1

atypical megaesophagus. Here the abnormal esophageal disorder is comparable to achalasia,[13,14] but our case would lead us to conclude that the failure of the Heller's operation was due to poor gastric emptying, which was corrected by a gastrectomy.

Esophagitis

The success of Heller's operation can sometimes be obscured by the development of severe reflux esophagitis (see Table 21-5), which presents with pain, pyrosis, dysphagia, and sometimes profuse hemorrhaging (see Fig. 21-6). Thirty-two cases of severe esophagitis required a reintervention.

This condition is due to the destruction, during cardiomyotomy, of the fibers of the lower esophageal sphincter and the division of the esophageal attachments to expose the esophagus. Furthermore, it is the usual consequence of side-to-side esophagogastric anastomoses or cardioplasties, which have been abandoned for this reason. Esophagitis may occur in the first couple of years after the myotomy or subsequently up to 21 years, perhaps because of a progressive neuropathy leading to the decrease of esophageal clearance.

TABLE 21-6. Surgical treatment of esophagitis after Heller's operation (32 cases)

Procedure	No. of cases
Hiatal repair	3
Esophagogastric resection	21
Total duodenal bypass	8

This is particularly serious, since the reflux stagnates in the aperistaltic and often still dilated esophagus. Reflux is even more serious if it is alkaline or mixed as a result of pyloroplasty.

Jara et al.[5] have correlated the incidence of gastroesophageal reflux with the length of myotomy performed on the stomach: if this is greater than 2 cm, then reflux is always present.

A diagnosis of reflux esophagitis or esophageal ulcer should be based on the clinical picture; x-ray findings, which can reveal a stricture and/or an ulcer; and endoscopy. But above all, manometry demonstrates any atony of the sphincter and pH studies reveal cardial incompetence and the grade and nature of the reflux.

Treatment

Treatment of reflux esophagitis after Heller's operation is difficult (see Table 21-6). Medical treatment is always necessary but not sufficient in cases of stenosis or ulcer.

Endoscopic dilatation is difficult and dangerous after Heller's operation and, if efficient, cannot prevent recurrence of reflux esophagitis. Until recent years, esophagogastric resection was usually performed in such cases (21 cases). The technique varies with time: esophagogastric resection (Sweet), resection with continent anastomosis (esophagogasric resection with circular gastric valve,[15] or resection with jejunal interposition[16] or colonic interposition.[17]

Since 1978 we have used total duodenal diversion in 8 cases; an antrectomy with Roux-en-Y jejunal anastomosis, 70 cm long, avoids any alkaline biliopancreatic reflux.[18] The truncal vagotomy necessary to avoid stomal ulcer on the gastrojejunal anastomosis is difficult and dangerous by the abdominal approach, because the mucosa in the case of esophagitis is very fragile and can be torn open by a simple pulling during the approach.[4-8] This is the reason why vagotomy is performed by the transthoracic approach.

Results of eight duodenal diversions were excellent in seven cases of reflux esophagitis after Heller's operation. Patients were free of symptoms: x-ray, endoscopic, and pH studies demon-

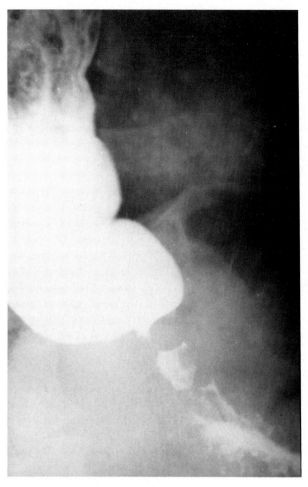

Fig. 21-7. Periesophageal sclerosis after Heller's operation.

strated the total healing of esophagitis and the disappearance of reflux. One patient developed an ulcer on the gastrojejunal anastomosis after antrectomy without vagotomy. Therefore, this technique avoids any resection. Prevention of esophagitis after Heller's operation requires a routine antireflux procedure, but this is still sometimes unable to prevent late esophagitis.

Periesophageal sclerosis

Sclerosis (Fig. 21-7) prevents easy access to the anterior myotomy during reintervention. We have encountered 15 such cases, and in five of these the formation of a pseudocartilaginous sheath made esophageal dissection extremely difficult. In two cases, it was necessary to abandon the transabdominal approach and operate transthoracically. This kind of sclerosis is not associated with esophagitis, nor is it a consequence of an initial mucosal wound. We, like Patrick et al.,[4] believe that it is related to imperfect hemostasis during the initial Heller's operation. In fact, we also found this kind of lesion during reintervention after a hiatal hernia repair. Postoperative sclerosis was not mentioned as being one of the causes of failure in the Mayo Clinic series,[4] but it appeared to us to be the real cause in three cases of extrinsic stenosis of the esophagus; these were resolved by freeing the hiatal area. This type of complication can be prevented by draining the low mediastinum and the hiatal area with a suction tube.

Cancer

Usually cancer that has developed in the megaesophagus is identified before Heller's operation. Thirty-two cases were observed in our department.

We also observed five cases of cancer after Heller's operation. The incidence is reported as being between 1% and 10%.[19] The development of cancer can occur in two forms, each of which gives the impression of an unsuccessful operation:
1. Dysphagia may reappear several years after an effective Heller's operation; this is not common.
2. Dysphagia may persist despite a correctly performed Heller's operation, the benefit of which has been to eliminate the stasis that obscured the cancer.

Only three curative esophagogastric resections were possible out of the five cases of cancer observed after Heller's operation. (See Fig. 21-8.)

Miscellaneous causes

In certain cases, the causes of failure of Heller's operation were the following:
1. Failure of initial diagnosis. One patient was referred to us after an unsuccessful Heller's operation. In fact, he suffered from a reflux esophageal ulcer with secondary megaesophagus and was cured by esophagogastric resection.
2. Extensive hiatal repair, which was encountered in one case. Local reintervention was necessary.
3. Gastric volvulus resulting from postoperative adhesions. This occurred once.
4. Mucosal stenosis after Heyrowski's operation. This was treated by the Thal procedure.
5. "Diverticulization" of the mucosa through the myotomy (Fig. 21-9). This occurred in two cases without any functional or organic stenosis of the cardia. Two esophagogastric resections were performed for these patients.

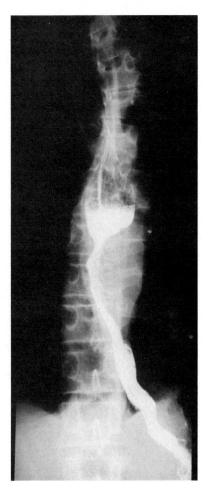

Fig. 21-8. Carcinoma developing 14 years after Heller's operation.

TREATMENT

Ninety-five operations were performed on 86 patients (see Table 21-7). Forty-one were repeat myotomies (see Tables 21-7 and 21-8). Of these, 34 were performed transabdominally and all but one in the same operative site as the initial myotomy. The antireflux mechanism was always reconstructed and pyloroplasty performed because of possible vagal trauma.

Thirty-seven resections were necessary, although the type of resection used changed with time (see Table 21-7). Resection was performed for reflux esophagitis in 21 of these cases (13 after Heller's operation, and eight after Heller's operation with cardioplasty or Heyrowski's operation). The remaining 16 cases requiring resection are listed in Table 21-9.

Eight duodenal bypasses were performed in recent years for severe reflux esophagitis, with or

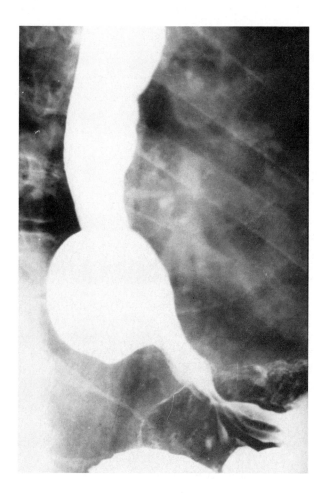

Fig. 21-9. "Diverticulization" of the mucosa after Heller's operation.

TABLE 21-7. Management of the 86 patients in whom reoperations were performed (95 operations)

Procedure	No. of operations
Repeat myotomy	41
Resection (37)	
Esophagojejunostomy	5
Sweet or Lewis	16
Continent anastomosis	11
Belsey colonic interposition	5
Total duodenal bypass	8
Hiatal reconstruction	3
Various	6

TABLE 21-8. Causes of 41 repeat myotomies

Cause	No. of operations
Cardiospasm	30
Interstitial sclerosis	3
Megadolichoesophagus	3
Diffuse spasm	2
Secondary extended spasm	3

TABLE 21-9. Causes of 37 esophagogastric resections after Heller's operation

Cause	No. of operations
Reflux esophagitis	21
Periesophageal stricture	2
Unsuccessful repeated myotomies (interstitial sclerosis)	2
Megadolichoesophagus	4
Mucosal stenosis after Heyrowski	1
Perforated esophagus resulting from dilatation	1
Cancer	3
Ulcer with secondary megaesophagus	1
Diverticulization of myotomy	2

without stenosis, Barrett's mucosa, bleeding esophagitis, and so on. One patient underwent several unsuccessful Heller's operations followed by Belsey's colonic interposition and developed a severe reflux esophagitis on the esophagocolic anastomosis with bile reflux.

We find that a total duodenal diversion makes it possible to avoid resection in patients with

TABLE 21-10. Results in 95 post-Heller reoperations

Operation	Number	Deaths	Excellent (%)	Fair (%)	Poor (%)	Mean follow-up
Repeat myotomy	41	0	31 (75)	4 (10)	5 (12)	12 yr
Resection	37	3	28 (83)	4	2	10 yr
Duodenal bypass	8	0	7	1	0	2 yr
Hiatal repair	3	0	3	0	0	—
Various	6	—	—	—	—	—

reflux esophagitis after a Heller's operation.

The remaining operations performed were antireflux mechanism reconstruction, surgery to free the esophageal hiatus, and palliative operations for cancer.

RESULTS

The mortality was 3%: there were three deaths out of 95 reoperations (one fistula after resection, one pulmonary embolism, and one diffuse hemorrhagic syndrome), all occurring after resection. There were no deaths resulting from the 41 repeat myotomies, and the morbidity consisted of seven discharging wounds, all without serious consequences.

Long-term results, after a mean follow-up of over 10 years (see Table 21-10) were 31 excellent (75%), four fair (10%), and five poor (12%). The patients in the last group required resection (three for dolichomegaesophagus and two for interstitial sclerosis).

The functional results for esophagogastric resection (see Table 21-10) were excellent in 26 of the 34 surviving patients.

Two patients with severe esophagitis after resection required esophagoplasty and colonic interposition (Belsey), respectively; two complained of reflux symptoms, which were treated medically. Two patients have slight dysphagia (after continent anastomosis). Two more suffer from thoracic oppression after resection for asystole of the esophagus.

Excellent results were observed in seven patients who had undergone a duodenal bypass, but one, with antrectomy and no vagotomy, developed an ulcer on the gastrojejunal anastomosis.

SUMMARY

A correct analysis of causes of failure after Heller's operation is necessary in order to suggest an appropriate treatment.

Usually a second myotomy is performed through an abdominal approach if the initial Heller's operation proves to be incorrect, or through a thoracic approach if the initial Heller's operation was well done or if extensive dyskinesia is discovered at manometry.

Until 1978, esophagogastric resection was performed for severe reflux lesions after Heller's operation. Antrectomy with Roux-en-Y gastrojejunostomy avoids resection. Vagotomy may be performed through a thoracic approach or through a transdiaphragmatic approach.

Esophageal resection is reserved for major asystolies of the esophagus, certain cases of sclerosis, and carcinomas occurring or discovered after Heller's operation.

ACKNOWLEDGMENT

I wish to thank Brice Gayet for his assistance in the preparation of the final draft of the manuscript for this chapter.

REFERENCES

1. Fekete, F., Breil, P., and Tossen, J.C.: Reoperation after Heller's operation for achalasia and other motility disorders of the esophagus: a study of eighty-one reoperations, Int. Surg. **67**:103, 1982.
2. Maillet, P., Micol, P., Parsal, J.P., et al.: Les résultats du traitement chirurgical du méga-oesophage (72 observations), Ann. Chir. **27**(6):579, 1973.
3. Menguy, R.: Management of achalasia by transabdominal cardiomyotomy and fundoplication, Surg. Gynecol. Obstet. **133**:482, 1971.
4. Patrick, D.L., Payne, W.S., Olsen, A.M., and Ellis, E.H.: Reoperation for achalasia of the esophagus, Arch. Surg. **103**:122, 1971.
5. Jara, F.M., Toledo-Pereyra, L.H., Lewis, J.W., and Magilligan, D.J.: Long term results of esophagomyotomy for achalasia of the esophagus, Arch. Surg. **114**:935, 1979.
6. Ellis, E.H., and Gibb, S.P.: Reoperation after esophagomyotomy for achalasia of esophagus, Am. J. Surg. **129**:407, 1975.

7. Okike, N., Payne, S.W., et al.: Esophagomytomy versus forceful dilatation for achalasia of the esophagus: results in 889 patients, Ann. Thorac. Surg. **28:**119, 1979.

8. Saubier, E., Chalencon, J.F., and Beaulieux, J.: Réintervention chirurgicales après opérations de Heller pour méga-oesophage essentiel, Lyon Med. **223:**883, 1970.

9. Fekete, F., Breil, P.H., Ronsse, H., et al.: EEA stapler and omental graft in esophago gastrectomy, Ann. Surg. **193**(6):825, 1981.

10. Lortat-Jacob, J.L.: Peut-on envisager le démembrement des syndromes fonctionnels de l'oesophage, Sem. Hop. Paris **26:**117, 1950.

11. Ellis, F.H.: Surgical management of esophageal motility disturbance, Am. J. Surg. **139:**752, 1980.

12. Vantrappen, G., Janssens, J., Hellemans, U., et al.: Achalasia, diffuse oesophageal spasm and related motility disorders, Gastroenterology **76:**450, 1978.

13. Schuffer, M.D., and Charles, E.P.: Esophageal motor dysfunction in idopathic intestinal pseudobstruction, Gastroenterology **70:**677, 1976.

14. Sullivan, M.A., Snape, W.J., et al.: Gastrointestinal myoelectrical activity in idiopathic intestinal pseudo-obstruction, N. Engl. J. Med. **207:**233, 1977.

15. Lortat-Jacob, J.L., Maillard, J.L.N., and Fekete, F.: A procedure to prevent reflux after esophagogastric resection, Surgery **50:**600, 1961.

16. Allison, P.R., Wooler, G.H., and Gunning, A.J.: Esophagojejunogastrostomy, J. Thorac. Surg. **33:**738, 1957.

17. Belsey, R.H.R.: Reconstruction of the esophagus with left colon, J. Thorac. Cardiovasc. Surg. **49:**33, 1965.

18. Holt, C.J., and Large, A.M.: Surgical management of reflux esophagitis, Ann. Surg. **153:**555, 1961.

19. Viard, H., Favre, J.P., Paupert, A., et al.: Méga-oesophage et cancer: six observations; arguments pour l'opération de Heller précoce et une stricte surveillance post opératoire, Ann. Chir. **34:**81, 1980.

Management of failed Heller's operation

DISCUSSION

Robert E. Condon

Symptomatic failure following Heller's myotomy for the treatment of achalasia is, fortunately, not a common event. It is because of his extensive experience in the treatment of achalasia that Professor Fekete is able to review in this chapter one of the largest experiences in the world with this difficult problem.

Professor Fekete nicely outlines the various causes of failure. Several points deserve emphasis. First, the most common cause of failure is an inadequate initial myotomy. I agree that complete transection of the esophagogastric sphincter is essential to success and that the myotomy needs to be carried across the gastroesophageal junction into the muscle of the stomach. The transabdominal approach is preferred to accomplish this objective.

If the gastric portion of the myotomy is short enough, postoperative reflux esophagitis may not ensue. But, because of variability from patient to patient, it is nearly impossible to arrange the length of the gastric myotomy with sufficient precision to ensure complete sphincter transection and the absence of reflux postoperatively. If the myotomy is incomplete, obstruction persists postoperatively; if the myotomy is too long, florid reflux ensues. We have, therefore, preferred the approach advocated by Fekete, and in both primary and secondary cases combine esophagogastric myotomy with a "floppy" fundoplication. In our 30 cases, the results have been quite satisfactory.

Second, adenocarcinoma arising at the gastroesophageal junction may clinically mimic achalasia, and is the most common cause of an erroneous diagnosis. A high index of suspicion concerning the possible presence of cancer needs to be maintained in evaluating every patient with a disorder thought to be achalasia. Appropriately deep biopsy specimens should be obtained preoperatively and intraoperatively if there is any mucosal lesion or undue thickening or firmness of the esophagus in the area of the gastroesophageal junction.

Third, the totally decompensated esophagus associated with achalasia, an entity termed "dolichomegaesophagus" by Fekete, usually does not recover sufficient function after myotomy to prevent esophageal stasis and resultant symptoms. We have always advocated resection of the thoracic esophagus and cervical esophagogastrostomy in such cases, even though we are treating a benign disease. The function of a thoracic gastric tube is better than that of a noncontractile esophagus. Placing the esophagogastric anastomosis in the neck obviates postoperative reflux.

Finally, the occurrence of a large mucosal hernia ("diverticulization") following myotomy is unusual (see Fig. 21-9). Such an event may indicate incomplete transection of the esophagogastric sphincter, leading to persistence of a high-pressure zone below the diverticulum; the etiology of this event following myotomy is similar to that of a primary suprahiatal esophageal diverticulum. Such patients should be investigated with this possibility in mind, and a repeat myotomy should be conducted if indicated.

CHAPTER 22 Extended esophageal myotomy in the management of diffuse esophageal spasm

Robert D. Henderson

Extended esophageal myotomy is used in the management of diffuse esophageal spasm (DES) and related esophageal primary motor disorders.

In 1889, Osgood[1] described a patient with esophagismus, and in 1934 Moersch and Camp[2] more clearly described an esophageal motor spastic disorder considered to be DES. Both reports are vague and lack investigative support; however, these authors are generally credited with the original description of DES. A more accurate and scientific description followed the development of esophageal manometric studies. The first surgical myotomy was reported by Lortat-Jacob[3] in 1950.

ETIOLOGY AND PATHOLOGY

The etiology of DES is unknown; however, it is generally accepted as being a primary neurogenic disorder. Pathologic studies have demonstrated vagal nerve degeneration with intact ganglia. In addition, there is smooth muscle hyperplasia involving the circular muscle bundles of the lower two thirds of the esophagus.[4,5] Circular muscle hyperplasia is the most striking feature of DES, and the muscle thickness ranges from 0.4 cm to greater than 1 cm (see Fig. 22-1). Longitudinal muscle is normal in thickness. Muscle hyperpla-

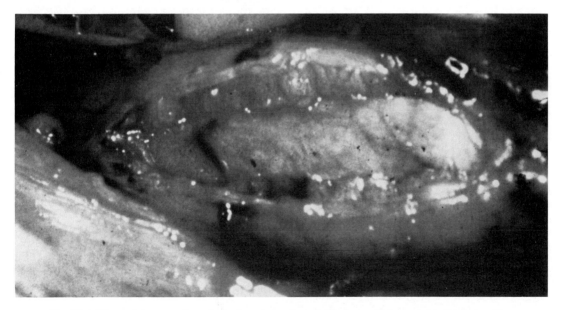

Fig. 22-1. The early stages of esophageal myotomy. Longitudinal muscle is normal in thickness. The circular muscle is gathered in large muscle bundles and is 0.75 cm thick.

sia does not involve the high-pressure zone (HPZ), indicating that either the muscle type or the nerve supply is different. There is controversy as to the proximal extent of muscle involvement; however, most likely all proximal circular muscle is involved.

CLINICAL EVALUATION

Esophageal motor disorders must all be investigated by history, radiology, manometry, and endoscopy. Each of these studies is necessary to accurately determine the specific disorder and to exclude alternate pathology.[6]

History

The general history in DES (Table 22-1) is similar to that obtained from patients with gastroesophageal reflux. Many of these patients have reflux as a component part of their symptom complex. There are some specific aspects of the DES history that merit emphasis.

Almost all patients with DES have both pain and dysphagia as dominant symptoms. Pain may be related to eating, food obstruction, and postural change; however, in 25%[7] of patients pain is unrelated to eating. This type of spontaneous pain may mimic cardiac disease, particularly if pain is referred to the arm and fingers.

Dysphagia is commonly present in patients with gastroesophageal reflux; however, with DES almost all patients have dysphagia, and frequently this is severe and associated with weight loss.

Radiology

There are certain features in a barium swallow that radiologically suggest DES.[8] Frequently there is a hiatal hernia or radiologic reflux (see Fig. 22-2). Motor spasm is usually demonstrable

at least below the aortic arch; occasionally, spasm is present to the apex of the chest. In advanced DES the lower esophagus may be tortuous or spastic, and the proximal esophagus can dilate with food and air retention (see Fig. 22-3). Esophageal wall thickening may be demonstrated through the use of rotational views to display the esophagus away from the thoracic spine. The best demonstration of mural thickening is on the lateral aspect of the esophagus, since on the medial esophagus mediastinal pleura and fat can give a misleading picture of wall thickening.

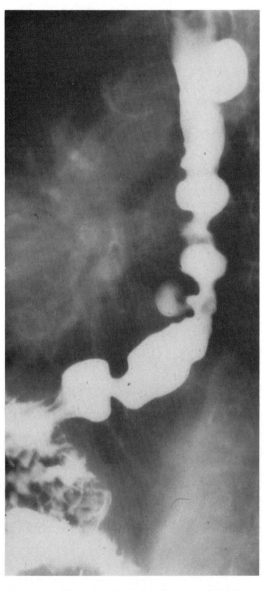

Fig. 22-2. Typical radiologic features of DES are present. Severe motor spasm is present in the body of the esophagus. In this patient a small hiatal hernia is also present.

TABLE 22-1. Diffuse esophageal spasm symptoms (65 patients)

	Number	Percent
Pain	64	98.5
Reflux	34	52.3
Aspiration	5	7.7
Eructation	31	47.7
Hiccough	9	13.8
Waterbrash	20	30.7
Nausea	33	50.8
Vomiting	16	24.6
Motor dysphagia	59	90.8
Stricture	4	6.1

The combination of wall thickening and esophageal motor spasticity is almost diagnostic of DES.

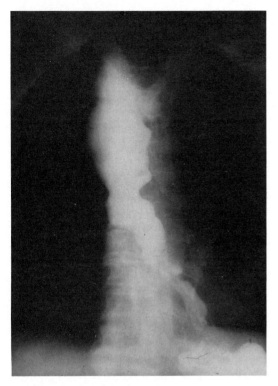

Fig. 22-3. The radiologic appearance of advanced DES shows severe lower esophageal motor spasm and some dilatation of the proximal esophagus with food retention.

Reviewing the radiologic accuracy in 65 patients whose conditions were treated surgically as DES, I found that a definite diagnosis was made in 40%, an incorrect diagnosis of achalasia was made in 10.3%, an incomplete diagnosis of hiatal hernia or reflux was made in 29.2%, and 20% were called normal.[7]

Esophageal manometry

The classic manometric features of DES[9] are easily described; however, many variations in the manometry are possible, and there is some overlap between the disorders of hypertonic HPZ,[10] "nutcracker" esophagus,[11] achalasia,[12] and DES.

To understand better these variations, it is helpful to use the PRV[13] system of classification: P is peristalsis; p no peristalsis; R is HPZ relaxation; r no relaxation; V is high-amplitude disordered motor activity (DMA); and v is low-amplitude DMA.

Classic DES consists of a normally functioning HPZ, some residual peristalsis, and high-amplitude DMA. This would be recorded as PRV (Fig. 22-4). Several variations are compatible with a diagnosis of DES, including inducing the absence of peristalsis or relaxation and the presence of low-amplitude DMA (see Fig. 22-5).

Table 22-2 shows an analysis of the manometric data in the 65 patients treated surgically for DES. The most characteristic features of the motor waves are their prolonged duration and multipeaked form, which all patients had, rather than their high amplitude.

Differentiation of DES from achalasia is occa-

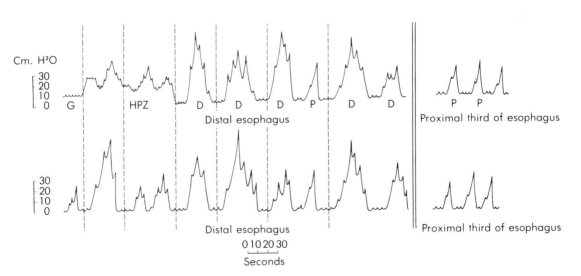

Fig. 22-4. The classic manometric features of DES, type PRV. In this study, *G* is stomach and *HPZ* is high-pressure zone. This is a diagrammatic representation of a classic PRV type of DES. More than 30% of motor waves in the distal esophagus are greater than 50 cm H_2O in amplitude. In the proximal esophagus well-formed peristaltic motor waves are present.

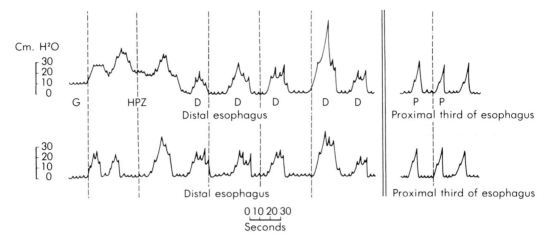

Fig. 22-5. The classic manometric features of DES, type PRV. The symbols used are identical to those in Fig. 22-4. Although motor waves greater than 50 cm H$_2$O can occur, they do not account for 30% of total motor waves and as such are considered to represent a low-amplitude DES.

TABLE 22-2. Manometric classification of DES (65 patients)

	Number	Percent
PRV	24	36.9
PRv	30	46.2
pRV	2	3.1
pRv	4	6.2
Prv	2	3.1
prv	1	1.5
Pv	1	1.5
PV	1	1.5

sionally difficult. Achalasia does not have lower esophageal peristalsis, HPZ relaxation is reduced or absent, and in achalasia, unlike DES, the esophageal basal pressure is usually elevated to a range of 12 to 20 cm H$_2$O.

The "nutcracker"[11] esophagus may be a variation of DES; however, the high-amplitude motor waves that characterize this disorder are predominantly peristaltic.

Hypertonicity[14] of the HPZ can occur in conjunction with DES, but this is also described as occurring independently.

Esophageal stimulation by Mecholyl[15] or ergonovine[16] has been reported as having some diagnostic value. Both medications may stimulate further motor spasm and may reproduce typical chest pain; however, since both DES and achalasia respond to the medications, these tests are of limited value in precise diagnostic differentiation.

Esophageal scintigraphy

Scintigraphic[17] studies are reported as showing delayed esophageal emptying in patients with DES. Unfortunately, although these studies are of value in quantitating emptying time and of value in assessing the results of therapy, the finding of delayed emptying is nonspecific and cannot be used to establish a diagnosis.

Endoscopic evaluation

Endoscopic evaluation should be conducted with fiberoptic flexible instruments. Stomach and duodenum must be examined. It is of particular importance to examine the gastric fundus, since an obstructing malignancy can mimic both DES and achalasia. An incompetent HPZ is commonly present in DES, and there may be associated reflux pathology of inflammation, ulceration, or stricture. In the 65 patients studied, only one had a peptic stricture and this patient had had previous surgery. Esophageal hypermotility can be observed endoscopically; however, this finding cannot be quantitated and although suggestive is not diagnostic of DES. The prime value of endoscopy in DES is to exclude malignancy and other pathology that might affect diagnostic accuracy.

Diagnostic accuracy of investigation

No single method of investigation is totally diagnostic of DES; however, the combined evaluation allowed an accurate preoperative diagnosis in 61 of the 65 patients treated surgically. In four the diagnosis was made because of typical intraoperative pathology. The most strongly diagnostic features are radiologic spasm with a visible wall thickening and the presence of high- or low-amplitude prolonged-duration multipeaked motor waves.

I regard the intraoperative pathology[17] as being specific and a necessary finding before the diagnosis is confirmed; however, this is controversial. Intraoperatively the esophagus can be mobilized and carefully palpated. The HPZ should be normal in diameter and wall thickness. Between the proximal end of the HPZ and the arch of the aorta the esophagus can be palpated and should demonstrate both mural thickening and spasticity. Thickening by itself is not diagnostic, since similar woody nonspastic changes are associated with reflux-induced panmural esophagitis. Spasticity is easily recognized by the esophagus changing from a flaccid state to one of firm sausage-like consistency. Without this intraoperative finding I am not prepared to accept the diagnosis of DES and at the time of surgery would not proceed to an extended myotomy.

TREATMENT

Several forms of management have been tried with varying success. These include medical control of reflux, use of nitrites or calcium blockers,[18,19] indirect bougienage,[20] and bag dilatation[21] of the esophagus.

The prime indication for surgery is failure of medical or other management in the patient with severe symptoms and good general health. In a few patients dysphagia is so severe that the disease presents as a life threat, and alimentation is necessary before surgery.

Medical management

Medical control of reflux is generally ineffective in patients with established DES. Severe degrees of secondary motor spasm can be produced by reflux, and this may well respond to medical management; however, in those with established DES a primary motor abnormality is present and the success rate with reflux control is low. In the selection of appropriate reflux management, diet, antacids, and H_2 blockers are appropriate. Cholinergic medication should be avoided, since DES is probably secondary to nerve degeneration and as such may be aggravated by cholinergics.

Short- and long-acting nitrates[22] have proved of limited value. These can be shown to decrease esophageal motor spasm as recorded manometrically; however, their effect clinically seems to be

marginal, and even in patients who get a satisfactory clinical response it is usually of short duration.

Calcium-blocking[19] medications have been described as being of value both in DES and achalasia. These medications are certainly not universally effective, and their role has not been fully established.

Esophageal dilatation[20]

The passage of a no. 60 Fr. mercury bougie should not, and usually does not, benefit the patient. I have, however, seen three patients with classic DES who had substantial clinical improvement following dilatation.

Bag dilatation[21,23] has been reported as effective occasionally, although it is difficult to see why destruction of the HPZ should be beneficial to a disorder in the body of the esophagus.

Surgical management of DES

With surgery the best chance of success is the first operation. If this fails, the chance of success with anything short of interposition surgery is very reduced. The surgical literature on this subject is limited, and many opinions expressed are controversial. The two major areas of controversy are the extent of esophageal myotomy and whether a hiatal hernia repair should be added for reflux control. Each of these areas must be examined before I describe my particular approach to extended myotomy.

Extent of myotomy

In general, there are three possible methods of esophageal myotomy:

1. Myotomy from the aortic arch to the lower end of the HPZ[24]
2. Esophageal myotomy with preservation of the HPZ[14]
3. Myotomy from the apex of the chest to the lower end of the HPZ[25]

Although many authors subscribe to the lower esophageal myotomy, all agree that when indicated by preoperative investigation, the myotomy may be extended to the apex of the chest. There is a general opinion expressed that the proximal extent of motor spasm can be determined by radiologic and manometric investigation, so that when more proximal spasm is noted this can be included in the myotomy.

Preservation of the HPZ is a relatively new concept.[14,26,27] Evaluations of the motor defect in DES have shown that in most patients the HPZ functions normally. In a few patients a hypertonic HPZ is present, and under these circumstances should be myotomized.

Preservation of the HPZ, in the absence of a hiatal hernia, and in the absence of hypertonicity, totally avoids the problem of myotomy-induced reflux. As noted later in the discussion, reflux following myotomy of the HPZ is an important problem and worth avoiding if possible. I do not have personal experience with sphincter-saving myotomy; however, I have had experience with six patients who had had proximal myotomy with an intact HPZ prior to consultation, all of whom presented with severe esophageal obstruction. Similar experience is reported by McGiffen et al.,[26] who noted that 25% of their patients treated by a sphincter-sparing myotomy developed progressive dysphagia. The original series, reported by Leonardi et al.,[14] has a short-duration follow-up, which needs updating before it can be fully evaluated.

The proximal extent of the myotomy is equally controversial. Two studies we have done assist in evaluating this problem. In the first study we determined the proximal extent of esophageal smooth muscle,[5] and in the second examined the accuracy of manometric and radiologic studies in determining the extent of proximal motor spasm.[9]

There is general acceptance of the fact that the proximal third of the esophagus is striated muscle and that the distal two thirds is smooth muscle. To determine more accurately the distribution, we studied 10 autopsy esophagi from patients who died from unrelated problems. The esophagus was marked in situ at the level of the HPZ, the inferior pulmonary vein, the lower margin of the aorta, the upper margin of the aorta, the mid–upper esophagus, the apex of chest, and below the cricopharyngeus. Muscle biopsies were examined by light microscopy and a cell count was conducted to determine the proportions of smooth and striated muscle cells. The distribution of smooth muscle was 100% below the aortic arch, 85% above the arch, 65% in the mid–upper esophagus, 18% at the apex of chest, and 3% in the cervical esophagus.

DES is a disorder of smooth muscle, and as with other primary lower esophageal motor disorders it should involve the entire smooth-muscle esophagus.

The second study was conducted in seven patients with DES who were treated by surgical myotomy. In each patient preoperative radiologic and manometric studies were conducted to determine the extent of proximal esophageal motor spasm.

Manometric studies used a water-perfusion system. The manometric catheters were marked with a radiopaque marker. After completion of a diagnostic study, the catheters were passed again to the stomach and withdrawn in stages until the middle of three openings was located at the proximal limit of esophageal motor spasm. The catheters were fixed in place, and the location of the radiologic marker was identified by chest x-ray film.

Following this study an independent radiologist did a standard barium esophagogram and located the level of proximal spasm in both the horizontal and vertical positions.

There was considerable variation in the level of spasm located manometrically and radiologically, and, in addition, the level of spasm radiologically varied according to whether the patient was in the horizontal or vertical position. This study showed that manometry and radiology are inaccurate in determining the level of proximal esophageal motor spasm.

Evaluating the data available, and accepting the fact that there is considerable controversy, I believe that the most reliable myotomy extends from the distal end of the HPZ to the apex of the chest. Such a myotomy avoids the problem of distal motor obstruction, and guarantees myotomy of all involved smooth muscle. As will be noted in the operative description, extending the myotomy to the apex of the chest is not technically difficult and does not add to the operative morbidity or mortality.

Reflux control

There is controversy as to whether it is necessary to add a hiatal hernia repair for reflux control. Myotomy reduces but does not obliterate HPZ tone, and there is still a preserved relaxation-contraction deglutition response.[25]

In achalasia the addition of a hernia repair is also controversial; however, the reported experience is of longer duration, and there are several studies using comparative series with and without hernia repair. In achalasia Heller myotomy without hernia repair has a reported incidence of reflux of 16% to 18%[28] and 0% with hernia repair. In achalasia the problems of reflux are less severe, since 50%[29] of patients have a low gastric acid, and many also continue to have esophageal secretions that dilute the reflux bolus.

Using myotomy without hernia repair, Ellis reported reflux in 16.6%[16] and a peptic stricture in 6.6% of 30 patients with radiologic follow-up. This figure is similar to that reported in achalasia. In my personal series of 65 patients treated by extended myotomy, reflux was an early problem and has only been corrected by adding more competence to the type of hernia repair used.[7]

These data favor the addition of hernia repair;

however, there are valid counterarguments that must be considered. The arguments used would include avoidance of HPZ mobilization, myotomy to the most proximal gastric veins, and the risk of producing overcompetence when hernia repair is added.

Mobilization is an essential part of hernia repair, and, clearly, once mobilized the HPZ does require an antireflux procedure for protection.

Myotomy to the most proximal gastric veins is a generally accepted principle and important whether or not hernia repair is added. Overcompetence in the hernia repair must be avoided. The greatest risk of overcompetence lies in the application of a long Nissen fundoplication procedure. Overcompetence would be rare following a partial fundoplication procedure.

Extended myotomy: surgical description

In the management of DES all my patients have been treated by extended myotomy from the distal HPZ to the apex of the chest (6 to 10 cm above the aortic arch). During a 15-year experience all have had a hiatal hernia repair; however, this has progressed from a standard 270-degree Belsey fundoplication to a partial fundoplication gastroplasty[25] (PFG; Belsey gastroplasty[30]) and later to a short fundoplication total fundoplication gastroplasty (TFG; Nissen gastroplasty[31]). In the past 5 years, reflux control has been achieved by a short Nissen fundoplication. The use of a TFG, and more recently a short Nissen fundoplication, has given excellent results, and this will be described as the procedure of choice.

A left thoractomy is used through the bed of the sixth rib. The relatively high incision is used to give optimal exposure both to the esophagogastric hiatus and to the apex of the chest and aortic arch. Preferably the lung is collapsed using a divided-lumen endotracheal tube, although this is not essential.

The inferior pulmonary ligament is now divided. Sharp and blunt dissection is used to mobilize the esophagus circumferentially below the inferior pulmonary vein.

A Babcock clamp is placed on the anterior aspect of the esophageal hiatus and lifted forward. With the esophagus held under slight tension, the phrenoesophageal ligament can be opened anteriorly and medially, exposing proximal fundus, gastroesophageal fat pad, and the anterior surface of the peritoneal coverings of the lesser sac and caudate lobe of the liver.

To preserve the vagus, a finger is passed along the medial aspect of stomach, and the vagus can then be palpated above and below the diaphragm.

Dissecting scissors can now be passed medial and posterior to the vagus to enter the lesser sac of the peritoneum.

With the gastroesophageal junction mobilized anteriorly and medially, the gastric fundus can be rolled up into the chest, exposing the short gastric veins attached to stomach and fat pad. One or two short gastric veins can be divided with digital control of the vagus to prevent injury.

At this stage the esophagogastric fat pad is removed. Posterior no. 1 silk crural sutures are placed, to be tied following completion of the hernia repair.

Attention is now turned to mobilizing the remaining subaortic esophagus. A finger can be easily passed behind and medial to the esophagus as far as the aortic arch. Pleura is divided between aorta and lung, exposing the surface of the esophagus. Most of the aortic blood supply to esophagus is preserved except for one large branch 1 cm below the aortic arch, which must be divided prior to myotomy to avoid bleeding.

The subaortic esophagus is now well exposed and can be inspected and palpated. It has been my practice to continue with myotomy only when the classic pathologic features of DES are present. Recently some authors[14] have stated that the visible and palpable pathology does not have to be present to make a diagnosis of DES. In my experience with six cases diagnosed as DES preoperatively, since the pathology was not found they were not myotomized, a hiatal hernia repair only was performed, and the preoperative symptoms of pain and dysphagia were satisfactorily eliminated. Had a myotomy been performed, credit for the clinical outcome would have been given to the myotomy. On the basis of this experience, I firmly believe that specific pathology should be present before a conclusive diagnosis is made.

Pathologic features are easily recognized. The HPZ is normal in diameter and consistency. From the HPZ to the aorta the esophagus is thickened and motor spastic. If the esophagus is held gently, it will be flaccid and gentle manipulation will produce a visible and palpable contraction. A lesser degree of motor spasticity can be elicited occasionally from the esophagus in patients with reflux; however, this is not as dramatic and is not associated with muscle thickening.

When eventually the myotomy is complete, the HPZ is normal in appearance.[30] In the thickened esophagus the longitudinal muscle layer is normal. Hyperplasia of the circular muscle is clearly visible, and the muscle is gathered in large circular bundles. After myotomy the muscle bundles can be noted to contract in response to palpation.

Muscle thickening above the aortic arch is difficult to demonstrate, since the smooth muscle content decreases, and, also, using a left thoracotomy circumferential mobilization above the arch is difficult and unnecessary.

Esophageal mobilization from below the arch to the apex of the chest is now carried out, if the presence of DES pathology is confirmed.

The first step in mobilization behind the aortic arch is to use fingertip blunt dissection below the arch and protrude the finger above the arch and behind pleura. It is now safe to open the pleura over the fingertip and continue the opening as a pleural window to the apex of the chest. Rarely is it necessary to divide intercostal arteries or veins. The one structure of concern is the thoracic duct, which may appear in the left lateral angle between aorta, esophagus, and vertebrae. Unrecognized damage to the duct can result in a chylothorax.

The esophagus is now ready for myotomy (see Fig. 22-6). A no. 40 Fr. Maloney bougie is passed into the stomach. This allows the operator to stretch mucosa over the bougie and reduce the risk of mucosal incision. My preference is to use blunt-tipped Allison dissecting scissors and to begin the myotomy at the level of the inferior pulmonary vein. Dissection can easily be carried to the mucosal level and then extended proximally and distally. In the body of the esophagus there is little difficulty; however, at the lower HPZ the proximal gastric veins are easily damaged. Recognition of the lower margin of dissection depends on the presence of transverse veins; however, the phrenoesophageal ligament and the mucosal expansion into stomach are also recognizable.

At the aortic arch, dissection is carried under the arch and a small tunnel made between mucosa and muscle. A finger can now be passed under the arch, and muscle will open fairly easily. With the finger in place, the proximal margin of myotomy can be recognized above the arch and dissection then continued to the apex of the chest. This is the most difficult portion of the myotomy; however, with care the mucosa should not be injured. After completion of the myotomy, the muscle is spread gently back from mucosa to give 180 degrees of mucosal exposure. Hemostasis by cautery is used sparingly on the muscle surface, but pressure only is used on the mucosal surface. In the 65 reported cases the mucosa was never penetrated during myotomy; 1 patient developed a transient leak 5 days postoperatively, which was probably related to mucosal ischemia.

Hiatal hernia repair

The method of fundoplication used was initially developed for the management of patients with the adynamic esophagus of scleroderma. It was recognized that the standard fundoplication of 1 cm created overcompetence and risked the development of fundoplication-related dysphagia. The initial fixation of fundus to esophagus is by three mattress sutures of 0-0 silk incorporating the distal 4 cm of esophagus. This creates the intraabdominal segment. Fundus is now rotated medially and laterally around the esophagus, and the fundoplication is with one mattress 0-0 silk suture over a maximum distance of 0.5 cm. The fundoplication is done without a bougie in place, and a finger easily passes between esophagus and gastric wrap. Supporting medial and lateral sutures are added for stability (see Fig. 22-7).

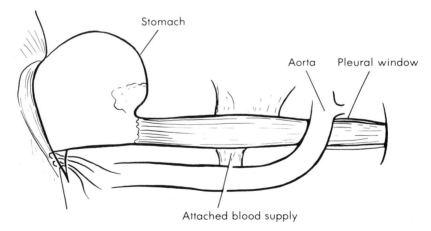

Fig. 22-6. The esophagus is mobilized to the aortic arch level, and the anterolateral surface above the arch is exposed through a pleural window. Mobilized gastroesophageal junction is drawn up into the chest at the time of myotomy. The myotomy is from the apex of the chest to the distal margin of the HPZ.

Finally, three mattress sutures are passed from the apex of the fundoplication through everted diaphragm, to be tied following abdominal reduction of the repair. With the repair reduced below the diaphragm, the posterior crural sutures are tied and finally the fundodiaphragmatic sutures are tied.

The chest is closed in a standard fashion, and a chest drain placed to the apex of the chest.

Results of surgery

The number of reported series of surgical myotomy for DES is very small, and many have short-term follow-up. Also, there are enough variations in the extent of myotomy and the presence and type of hernia repair that comparison has limited value. There is also controversy as to which patients should be included in a study as having DES. As previously stated, I believe that wall thickening and motor spasticity must be present before a diagnosis of DES can be made. This statement is based on my experience with six patients who would fit the clinical, radiologic, and manometric criteria of DES but who did not have the pathology; they were treated by hernia repair only and had excellent symptomatic results. In contradistinction, within the series of 65 patients there are seven patients previously treated by only hernia repair who did have pathology and who did not improve clinically.

Literature review. There are several major series in the literature; however, the methods of reporting results vary, most series are small, and none describe 5-year review. As a further difference, there is a variation in the proximal and distal extent of myotomy and whether or not a hiatal hernia repair is added. In seven major series, totalling 148 patients, excellent results are noted in 100 patients (68%), moderate in 22 (15%), and poor results in 25 (17%).* In Table 22-3 myotomy of the HPZ, lower esophagus, or total thoracic esophagus is marked for each series; however, there are exceptions within each series. Hernia repair is universal in some series, and selective in the presence of a hernia in other series. Esophageal wall thickening was universal in some series and present on average in 83.1% of patients. The reported results show wide variation, which may in part depend upon the method of reporting.

It should be noted that myotomy below the arch was performed in 66 patients, below the arch with HPZ intact in 11, above the arch in 63, and above the arch with HPZ intact in 8. Hernia repair was universally added in three series and added selectively in the remaining five series. Classic pathology of wall thickness and spasticity was universally present in four series. Wall thickness is recorded in 123 (83.1%) of 148 patients. With so much variation in technique, and argument also about the definition of the disease, there can be no clear statement as to the most appropriate surgical technique. At best the results of a series can be reported and compared with the average quality of result already quoted. From my own experience with 65 previously reported cases of diffuse spasm, all have

---

*References 7, 14, 24, 26, 27, 32, and 33.

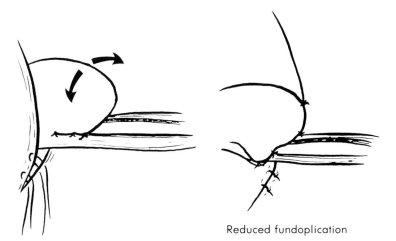

Reduced fundoplication

Fig. 22-7. After completion of the myotomy, reflux control is achieved by a short fundoplication Nissen. With this technique 4 cm of esophagus is included in the fundoplication; however, the complete fundoplication is reduced to less than 0.5 cm.

TABLE 22-3. Review of surgical results

Author	Year	No. of patients	Follow-up	Myotomy HPZ	Myotomy Lower esophagus	Myotomy Thoracic esophagus	Hiatal hernia repair	Wall thickness	Results (percent) Asymptomatic	Results (percent) Minor residual problems	Results (percent) Major residual problems
Ellis et al.[24]	1964	40	1-6 yr	+	+	−	22	22	67	11	22
Leonardi et al.[14]	1977	11	3.2 yr	−	+	−	2	6	82	9	9
Craddock et al.[32]	1966	5	—	+	+	−	—	3	80	20	0
Nicks[33]	1969	7	—	+	+	−	7	7	85.7	14.3	0
McGiffen et al.[26]	1982	8	0.5-6 yr	−	−	+	0	8	75	0	25
Ferguson[27]	1969	14	0.5-12 yr	+	+	−	4	14	69.2	23.1	7.7
Henderson[7]	1982	29	9.3 yr	+	−	+	29 Belsey	29	48.2	13.9	37.9
Henderson[7]	1982	34	3.1 yr	+	−	+	34 Nissen	34	73.5	23.5	2.9

been treated by myotomy to the apex of the chest; however, the method of reflux control has varied.[7]

Initially, with a standard Belsey repair, eight patients were asymptomatic and two much improved; however, 10 developed significant reflux. This problem was partially corrected by adding a gastroplasty tube with Belsey fundoplication. In this second group of nine patients, six are asymptomatic, two have minor residual problems, and one has persistent major symptoms.

Five-year follow-up is available in 34 patients with a short Nissen fundoplication and total thoracic myotomy. In the first 16 a gastroplasty was added, and in the last 17 a short total fundoplication only.

With gastroplasty, 12 are asymptomatic, three have minor residual symptoms, and one has major symptoms. In the group with short fundoplication only, all are asymptomatic. One was lost to follow-up.

The overall result at 5 years is as follows: asymptomatic, 29 (87.9%); minor residual symptoms, 3 (9.1%); and major persistent symptoms, 1 (3%). The results are clearly better than the average results previously reported and now approximate those achieved in hiatal hernia repair for reflux.

Summary

The surgical management of DES remains controversial; however, the results have been and should continue to be improved. There are too many short-term reports and too few long-term follow-up studies in the literature, and this urgently requires follow-up assessment. The key to success lies in a more precise surgical definition of the disease, clarification of the gross and microscopic pathology, and careful attention to detail in its operative management.

REFERENCES

1. Osgood, H.: A peculiar form of esophagismus, Boston Med. Surg. J. **120**:401, 1889.
2. Moersh, H.J., and Camp, J.D.: Diffuse spasm of lower part of esophagus, Ann. Otol. Rhinol. Laryngol. **43**:1165, 1934.
3. Lortat-Jacob, J.L.: Myomatoses localisées et myomatoses diffuses de l'esophage, Arch. Mal. App. Digest. **39**:519, 1950.
4. Cassella, R.R., Ellis, R.H., and Brown, A.: Diffuse spasm of the lower part of the esophagus, JAMA **191**:107, 1965.
5. Friesen, D.L., Henderson, R.D., and Hanna, W.: Ultrastructure of esophageal muscle in achalasia and diffuse esophageal spasm, Am. J. Clin. Path. **79**:319, 1983.

6. Henderson, R.D.: The esophagus: reflux and primary motor disorders, Baltimore, 1980, The Williams & Wilkins Co.

7. Henderson, R.D.: Diffuse esophageal spasm, Surg. Clin. North Am. **63**:951, 1983.

8. Henderson, R.D., and Ryder, D.E.: Reflux control following myotomy in diffuse esophageal spasm, Ann. Thorac. Surg. **34**:230, 1982.

9. Henderson, R.D.: Esophageal manometry in clinical investigation, New York, 1983, Praeger Publishers.

10. Code, C.F., Schlegel, J.F., Kelley, M.L., Jr., Olsen, A.M., and Ellis, F.H., Jr.: Hypertensive gastroesophageal sphincter, Mayo Clin. Proc. **35**:391, 1960.

11. Zaino, C., and Beneventano, T.C.: Radiologic examination of orohypopharynx and esophagus, New York, 1977, Springer-Verlag.

12. Olsen, A.M., and Creamer, B.: Studies of esophageal motility, with special reference to the differential diagnosis of diffuse spasm and achalasia (cardiospásm), Thorax **12**:279, 1957.

13. Vantrappen, G., Janssens, J., Hellemans, J., and Coremans, G.: Achalasia, diffuse esophageal spasm and related motility disorders, Gastroenterology **76**:450, 1979.

14. Leonardi, H.K., Shea, J.A., Crozier, R.E., and Ellis, F.H., Jr.: Diffuse spasm of the esophagus: clinical, manometric and surgical considerations, J. Thorac. Cardiovasc. Surg. **74**:736, 1977.

15. Kramer, P., and Ingelfinger, F.J.: Esophageal sensitivity to Mecholyl in cardiospasm, Gastroenterology **19**:242, 1951.

16. Koch, K.L., Curry, R.C., Feldman, R.L., Pepine, C.J., Lowa, A., and Methias, J.R.: Ergonovine induced esophageal spasm in patients with chest pain resembling angina pectoris, Dig. Dis. Sci. **27**:1073, 1982.

17. Taillefer, R., and Beauchamp, G.: Scintigraphy: radionuclide esophagogram, Clin. Nucl. Med. **9**:465, 1984.

18. Gelford, M., Rozen, P. and Gilat, T.: Isosorbide dinitrate and nifedipine treatment of achalasia: a clinical, manometric and radionuclide evaluation, gastroenterology **83**:963, 1982.

19. Schwartz, M.L., Rotmensch, H.H., Viasses, P.H., and Ferguson, R.K.: Calcium blockers in smooth muscle disorders: current status, Arch. Intern. Med. **140**:403, 1984.

20. Vinson, P.P.: Diagnosis and treatment of cardiospasm, South. Med. J. **40**:387, 1947.

21. Plummer, H.S.: Cardiospasm, with a report of forty cases, JAMA **51**:549, 1908.

22. Dunlop, D.M., Davidson, S., and Alstead, S.: Textbook of medical treatment, London, 1958, E & S Livingston, Ltd., p. 478.

23. Ebert, E.C., Ouyang, A., Wright, S.H., Cohen S., and Lipshutz, W.H.: Pneumatic dilatation in patients with symptomatic diffuse esophageal spasm and lower esophageal sphincter dysfunction, Dig. Dis. Sci. **28**:481, 1983.

24. Ellis, F.H., Jr., Olsen, A.M., Schlegel, J.F., and Code, C.F.: Surgical treatment of esophageal hypermotility disturbances, JAMA **188**:862, 1964.

25. Henderson, R.D., and Pearson, F.G.: Reflux control following extended myotomy in primary disordered motor activity (diffuse spasm) of the esophagus, Ann. Thorac. Surg. **22**:278, 1976.

26. McGiffen, D., Lomas, C., Gardner, M., McKeering, L., and Robinson, D.: Long oesophageal myotomy for diffuse spasm of the oesophagus, Aust. N.Z. J. Surg. **52**:193, 1982.

27. Ferguson, T.B.: Diffuse esophageal spasm (editorial), Ann. Thorac. Surg. **18**:431, 1974.

28. Black. J., Vorbach, A.N., and Collis, J.L.: Results of Heller's operation for achalasia of the oesophagus: the importance of hiatal repair, Br. J. Surg. **63**:949, 1976.

29. Dooley, C.P., Taylor, T.L., and Venezuela, J.E.: Impaired acid secretion and pancreatic polypeptide release in some patients with achalasia, Gastroenterology **84**:809, 1983.

30. Pearson, F.G.: Surgical management of acquired short esophagus with dilatable peptic stricture, World J. Surg. **1**:463, 1977.

31. Henderson, R.D.: The gastroplasty tube as a method of reflux control, Can. J. Surg. **21**:264, 1978.

32. Craddock, D.R., Logan, A., and Walbaum, P.R.: Diffuse esophageal spasm, Thorax **21**:511, 1966.

33. Nicks, R.: The surgery of oesophageal dysrhythmias, Aust. N.Z. J. Surg. **39**:167, 1969.

Extended esophageal myotomy in the management of diffuse esophageal spasm

DISCUSSION

F. París and M. Tomas-Ridocci

The excellent report of Dr. Henderson is very important in our view because it is related to a controversial problem, namely the extended esophageal myotomy as treatment for primary vigorous motor disorders of the esophagus.[1-3]

Following the Vantrappen and Hellemans criteria,[4] we have classified esophageal motor disorders as follows: (1) primary—classic achalasia, vigorous achalasia (VA), symptomatic diffuse esophageal spasm (SDES), and symptomatic esophageal peristalsis (SEP) (or "nutcracker" esophagus), and other related disorders and (2) secondary—to gastroesophageal reflux (GER), tumors, and other generalized neural, muscular, metabolic, or systemic diseases.

This discussion is based on our own experience of extended esophageal myotomy performed in 21 patients in whom clinical, radiologic, and manometric studies were carried out preoperatively and postoperatively; 9 had SDES, 10 had VA, and 2 had SEP.

Some clinical differences with the Henderson series have been noted. Retrosternal pain, dysphagia, weight loss, and active or passive esophageal regurgitation were the predominant symptoms in our series, but symptoms of GER were not present. In our opinion, the symptoms of patients with diffuse spasm secondary to GER are milder than those with primary SDES (less severe dysphagia and no weight loss), and they disappear.

Manometrically we have classified our disorders according to the PRV system,[5] as in the Henderson report. The capital letters P and R indicate the presence of peristaltic contractions (P) and lower esophageal sphincter relaxations (R) after some swallows. The small letters p and r indicate their absence. Swallowing waves may be vigorous (V) or nonvigorous (v). From our studies, according to this classification, some manometric differences with the Henderson series

have been found: PRV in seven patients and PrV in two patients corresponding to SDES; prV in 10 patients corresponding to VA; and PRV in two patients corresponding to SEP. From our preoperative manometric studies we would emphasize the following points: increase in the percentage of tertiary waves in SDES; increases in the lower esophageal sphincter pressure (LESP) and basal body esophageal pressure without peristaltic waves in VA; and a great increase in amplitude of the peristaltic waves in SEP (see Table 22-4).

We agree with Henderson with regard to the significance of the endoscopy. Endoscopic findings should exclude other associated pathologic conditions, especially reflux esophagitis and malignancy. Furthermore, through radionuclide esophageal emptying of a solid meal it is possible to find significant differences between normal subjects and patients suffering from primary motor disorders of the esophagus. It is our opinion that the differential diagnosis of the different types of primary esophageal motor disorders must be done by manometry. Nevertheless, radionuclide studies should help in the evaluation of the therapeutic efficacy of calcium antagonists[6] or myotomy[7] employed in the management of these patients (see Fig. 22-8).

The indications for surgery depend on the severity of symptoms and not on the radiologic or manometric findings. Many patients suffering from esophageal motor disorders do not need surgical treatment. Following Belsey,[1] we propose extended esophageal myotomy in the following circumstances: severe pain and/or dysphagia, and presence of esophageal diverticula. We agree with Henderson that these patients should be treated medically first, especially with calcium antagonists.[6] If this treatment has failed, surgery should be considered. We must emphasize that treatment with long-acting nitrites or calcium

TABLE 22-4. Preoperative and postoperative values (mean $\pm$ SD) in our patients

	Preoperative			Postoperative		
	SDES	**VA**	**SEP**	**SDES**	**VA***	**SEP†**
LESP (mm Hg)	20.1 $\pm$ 7.7	42.4 $\pm$ 21.1	27.5 $\pm$ 10.6	7.11‡ $\pm$ 2.66	10.1‡ $\pm$ 6.2	12.5 $\pm$ 3.5
Basal body esophageal pressure (mm Hg)						
Inspiratory	-5 ± 4.4	-0.6 ± 4	Normal	-7.1 ± 2.4	-5 ± 2.9§	Normal
Expiratory	2 ± 3	5.4 ± 3	Normal	0.7 ± 1.7	-1 ± 3.4	Normal
Amplitude of swallowing waves (distal third, mm Hg)	63.3 $\pm$ 15.7	33.5 $\pm$ 11.7	335 $\pm$ 123	11.4‡ $\pm$ 4.06	11.9‡ $\pm$ 7.92	12.5 $\pm$ 3.5
Peristaltic waves (percent)	25 $\pm$ 17	0	100	—	—	—

*In three patients (10%) the esophageal peristalsis disappeared.
†Paired data studies were not performed (two cases).
‡p < 0.001.
§p < 0.01 (paired data).

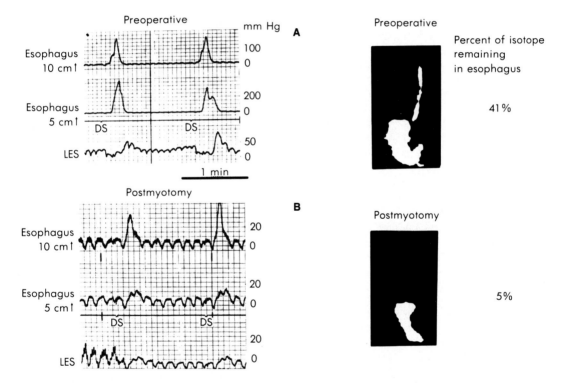

Fig. 22-8. Preoperative and postoperative studies in a patient with symptomatic esophageal peristalsis (**A**) and in a patient with vigorous achalasia (**B**). After myotomy, the amplitude of peristaltic waves decreased significantly in the patient with SEP, and radionuclide esophageal emptying improved significantly in the patient with VA.

antagonists is contraindicated in patients with diffuse spasm secondary to GER,[8,9] because these drugs decrease LESP and favor the GER.

In this study we have included only patients with 3 years of clinical follow-up after the surgical procedure. The mean of this follow-up was 7 $\pm$ 2 years (range, 3 to 11 years). Our extended esophageal myotomy is similar to that described by Henderson, but we have added some modifications. Concerning the surgical approach, a left thoracotomy through the sixth intercostal space was carried out. Proximally the esophageal myotomy was extended to the level of the aortic arch in 20 patients. Only in one case was the myotomy continued to the apex of the chest, because the manometric preoperative studies showed important abnormalities in the upper intrathoracic esophagus. Distally the myotomy was carried to the stomach, where the gastric veins were exposed. With this technique, the LES is divided. This policy differs from that used by some authors, who exclude the LES from the myotomy.[10]

We do not use Maloney bougies. Our preference is to avoid mucosal damage by using gentle traction on the muscular layer, placing two 0-0 silk traction sutures through the muscle on each side of the exposed esophagus. To perform the myotomy, the use of dissecting clamps and scissors rather than a knife decreases the risk of esophageal mucosal damage. At the gastroesophageal junction the risk of opening the mucosa is greatest. In none of the 21 cases in our series was the mucosa perforated. In our opinion the presence of a Maloney tube "in situ" during myotomy may increase the risk of perforation.

Submucosal vessels must be carefully treated by diathermy or, better, by forceps, pressure, or ligation. The myotomy must be complete. Any residual circular fibers may require division. After the myotomy, the muscular layer is dissected from the mucosa so that it will remain free over 180 degrees. In one of four cases with esophageal diverticula a diverticulopexy was performed.

At thoracotomy direct inspection and palpation of the esophagus will show the degree of muscle thickening. We do not believe that the presence of visible or palpable esophageal contractions at thoracotomy is a pathognomonic sign of DES. The diagnosis of SDES must be done preoperatively by clinical history, radiologic studies, and esophageal manometry.

The next step aims toward the restoration of the gastroesophageal junction. In our series we have used the Belsey Mark IV repair, modified for the myotomized esophagus, and we have not had postoperative problems of GER in any patient. We must emphasize that our series consists of primary motor disorders without GER, involving a bad peristaltic pump on the esophageal body, in which the aim was only to repair the LES submitted to myotomy. In these cases the use of a tight Nissen repair is contraindicated because it will produce an overcompetence, which is not desirable. For similar reasons the gastroplasty is not recommended.

In our opinion the mini-Nissen procedure using one mattress 0-0 silk suture will have the same effect as a Belsey Mark IV repair, or another partial plication, if it is well performed.

The myotomy provides a significant decrease in LESP in all groups of patients; an important decrease in the basal pressure of the esophageal body in VA; and a drastic decrease in the amplitude of esophageal contractions in SEP (see Fig. 22-8), which is similar to that reported by other authors[4] (see Table 22-4). These effects cause an improvement in esophageal emptying (see Fig. 22-8) and are correlated with the clinical recovery observed in our patients. We consider the clinical results to be as follows: excellent in 6 SDES, 7 VA, and 2 SEP; good in 2 SDES and 2 VA; moderate in 1 SDES; and poor in 1 VA.

We conclude that with extended esophageal myotomy we cannot correct the nature of functional disorders, but by reducing the amplitude of the waves and lowering the LESP, we can relieve the patient's symptoms and obtain excellent clinical results in 15 of 21 (72%) patients.

REFERENCES

1. Belsey, R.: Disorders of function of the esophagus. In Smith, A., and Smith, R.E., editors: Surgery of the esophagus: the Coventry Conference, London, 1972, Butterworths, pp. 193-207.
2. Payne, W., Ellis, F.H., and Olsen, A.M.: A follow-up study in patients undergoing esophagomyotomy, Arch. Surg. **81:**411-418, 1960.
3. Tummala, V., Traube, M., and McCallum, R.W.: Surgical myotomy in nutcracker esophagus: manometric and clinical effects (abstract), Gastroenterology **88:**1619, 1985.
4. Vantrappen, G., and Hellemans, J.: Esophageal motor disorders. In Cohen, S., and Soloway, R.D., editors: Diseases of the esophagus, New York, 1982, Churchill Livingstone, pp. 161-179.
5. Vantrappen, G., Janssens, J., and Hellemans, J.: Achalasia, diffuse esophageal spasm and related motility disorders, Gastroenterology **76:**450-457, 1979.
6. Tomas-Ridocci, M., Mora, F., Romero de Avila, C., et al.: Efecto de la nifedipina sobre la respuesta esofagica a la ingesta de alimentos sólidos en pacientes con trastornos motores esofagicos primarios: estudio manometrico y isotopico, Gastroenterol. Hepatol. (Barcelona). (In press.)
7. Holloway, R.H., Krosin, G.A., Lange, R.C., et al.: Radionuclide esophageal emptying of a solid meal to quantitate results of therapy in achalasia, Gastroenterology **84:**771-776, 1983.
8. Swamy, N.: Esophageal spasm: clinical and manometric response to nitroglycerine and long acting nitrites, Gastroenterology **72:**23-27, 1977.
9. Benages, A., Paris, F., Tomas-Ridocci, M., et al.: Lesser curvature tubular gastroplasty with partial plication for gastroesophageal reflux: manometric and pH-metric postoperative studies, Ann. Thorac. Surg. **26:**574-580, 1978.
10. Leonardi, H.K., Shea, J.A., Crozier, R.E., and Ellis, F.H.: Diffuse spasm of the esophagus: clinical, manometric, and surgical considerations, J. Thorac. Cardiovasc. Surg. **74:**736-743, 1977.

CHAPTER 23 Diffuse esophageal spasm and related disorders

F. Henry Ellis, Jr.

Esophageal manometry has alerted the medical profession to the fact that esophageal motility disorders are a frequent cause of symptoms in patients with noncardiac chest pain. Achalasia and diffuse esophageal spasm (DES) represent well-recognized clinical entities that may cause chest pain, but there are other motility disorders associated with chest pain that are less easily classifiable. Some of the latter, which are now being increasingly recognized, have been categorized under such headings as vigorous achalasia, hypertensive lower esophageal sphincter (LES), high-amplitude peristalsis (nutcracker esophagus), dyschalasia, and nonspecific esophageal motility disorders. No unanimity of opinion exists, however, regarding their interrelationship.

In a recent study from England, an esophageal disorder was found to be the cause of pain in 60% of patients with angina-like symptoms and negative findings on coronary arteriography.[1] Vantrappen and associates[2] observed that about 24% of patients with motility disorders severe enough to require treatment did not fit the diagnostic criteria for achalasia or DES. Katz and Castell[3] reported that 60% to 75% of esophageal disorders associated with chest pain were the result of nonspecific motor disorders or high-amplitude peristalsis rather than the more commonly recognized classic DES and achalasia.

In this chapter, emphasis is placed on the diagnosis and management of DES, and discussion of other conditions that either are associated with DES or have some features in common with it is included. Because the specific neuromuscular defects responsible for achalasia, DES, and related motility disorders are unknown, the question of whether these various syndromes constitute separate entities or are interrelated is unlikely to be answered soon.

DIFFUSE ESOPHAGEAL SPASM

Esophageal spasm was first described clinically in 1889 by Osgood,[4] but the term "diffuse spasm of the lower part of the esophagus" was not introduced until 1934 by Moersch and Camp[5] of the Mayo Clinic. This condition, which is characterized by symptoms of intermittent chest pain with or without dysphagia, has been described by various names, such as localized esophageal spasm, segmental spasm, curling of the esophagus, corkscrew esophagus, and pseudodiverticulosis. Some of these terms are descriptive of the abnormal appearance on esophagograms. Findings on esophagography are normal, however, in the majority of patients.[6] The diagnosis depends on esophageal manometry, which shows nonperistaltic deglutitory contractions of increased amplitude and duration that are often repetitive and sometimes spontaneous. Usually only the lower third to two thirds of the intrathoracic esophagus is involved. The LES itself functions normally, although resting pressures are sometimes in the hypertensive range.

Demography

The disease is much less common than achalasia and can occur at any adult age, although it is usually seen in persons more than 50 years of age. There is no sexual predilection. In contrast to patients with achalasia, those with DES tend to be high-strung individuals, and symptoms are often accentuated during periods of stress. The relationship between psychiatric illness and contraction abnormalities of the esophagus was emphasized by Clouse and Lustman,[7] who determined that hypermotile esophageal disorders were of psychiatric origin in 21 of 25 patients (84%).

Pathology

Hypertrophy of the muscular coat of the esophagus, although by no means always present, has been observed in this disease. Auerbach's plexus is preserved, but electron microscopic examination has shown wallerian degeneration in the esophageal branches of the vagus nerve, thus suggesting a possible abnormality of the afferent nerve supply of the esophagus.[8]

Diagnosis
Symptoms

The characteristic pain experienced by patients with DES is substernal, intense, and cramping and may radiate to the neck, jaw, and arm, mimicking cardiac pain. It occurs intermittently, not necessarily during deglutition, and may awaken the patient from a sound sleep at night. Vagovagal syncopal episodes during eating have been described.[9]

Dysphagia may also be present, usually occurring during episodes of pain. The ingested bolus usually passes with relaxation of the episode of spasm, however, and endoscopic removal is rarely required. Dysphagia was present in 31 of 46 patients with DES, a hypertensive LES, or both, reported on by my associates and me[6] from the Mayo Clinic. In all but seven of these 46 patients, however, severe pain was also present. Symptoms of reflux, regurgitation, vomiting, and weight loss are uncommon in this disease, in contrast to achalasia, in which regurgitation (especially nocturnal) and weight loss are common.

Radiography

Fewer than one half of the patients treated surgically by my associates and me[6] exhibited radiographic findings suggestive of DES. These findings, which vary widely, include diffuse narrowing of the lower half of the esophagus with mild proximal dilatation (Fig. 23-1, *A*) and segmental spasm, a radiographic appearance that has prompted use of the terms "pseudodiverticulosis" and "corkscrew esophagus" (Fig. 23-1, *B*). An epiphrenic diverticulum (Fig. 23-1, *C*) is a rare but recognizable associated finding, as is a hiatal hernia, which presumably results from longitudinal muscle spasm. Careful examination may disclose thickening of the esophageal wall in some patients.[10]

Roentgenoscopic examination discloses abnormalities of transport characterized by a lack of peristalsis and the simultaneous development of contraction rings in response to swallowing. Even in the presence of a hiatal hernia, LES tone is usually maintained, and gastroesophageal reflux is rare.

Esophageal manometry

Creamer and associates[11] were the first to describe the characteristic motility pattern of DES. The deglutitory contractions in the body of the esophagus tend to be simultaneous in its lower third to two thirds. The contractions are of increased amplitude (mean, greater than 80 mm Hg), often prolonged (more than 4 seconds), and repetitive (see Fig. 23-2). Not always are these abnormal contractions associated with pain, however. In addition, spontaneous contractions of the esophagus may occur.

The LES usually relaxes normally and is characteristically of normal amplitude, although some patients with DES also have a hypertensive LES. DiMarino and Cohen[12] found that relaxation was impaired in ten of 27 patients with DES and that a hypertensive LES was present in nine.

When results of esophageal manometry are normal and symptoms are still suggestive of DES or a related abnormality, provocative tests are a valuable adjunct to routine manometric examination of the esophagus. An acid-infusion study may disclose characteristic findings of DES in patients with an acid-sensitive esophagus. The intravenous administration of edrophonium (Tensilon), 80 mg per kilogram of body weight, before performance of the motility study is an extremely safe provocative test, and it does not produce coronary spasm or chest pain in normal individuals.[13] In many patients with chest pain of esophageal origin the typical pain syndrome is reproduced with the occurrence of prolonged high-amplitude contractions in response to these provocative tests.

Treatment
Medical

The treatment of chest pain secondary to esophageal hyperactive disorders is difficult and disappointing. Because of the associated neuropsychiatric aspects of these disorders, reassurance and medications to relieve anxiety, such as diazepam (Valium), play an important therapeutic role. Convincing the patient that he does not have coronary artery disease is an important aspect of therapy. Smooth-muscle relaxants and vasodilators, such as nitroglycerin and long-acting nitrates, have been found to be effective in some patients.[14] Hydralazine has also been shown to be useful.[15] Calcium channel blockers, such as diltiazem (Cardizem) and nifedipine (Procardia), are promising agents because they have been shown to decrease the amplitude of contractions in the esophageal body and LES.[16] Some or all of these medical approaches should be initiated before surgical therapy is considered. Rarely, a trial of psychotherapy may be beneficial, particularly if the pain seems to be initiated by identifiable situations.

Surgical

A long esophagomyotomy for "diffuse nodular myomatosis of the esophagus" was reported by Lortat-Jacob[17] in 1950. The procedure was later

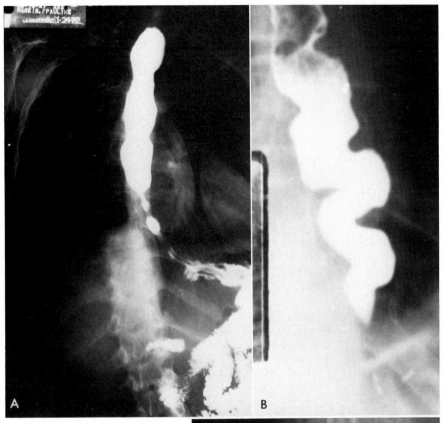

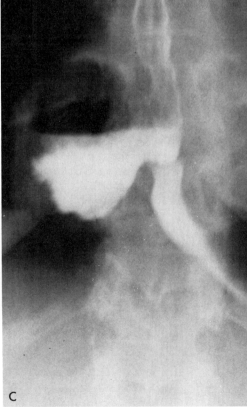

Fig. 23-1. Esophagograms in three patients with diffuse spasm of the esophagus. **A,** Diffuse spasm. **B,** Segmental contractions. **C,** Epiphrenic diverticulum. (From Leonardi, H.K., Shea, J.A., Crozier, R.E., et al.: Diffuse spasm of the esophagus, J. Thorac. Cardiovasc. Surg. **74:**737, 1977. With permission.)

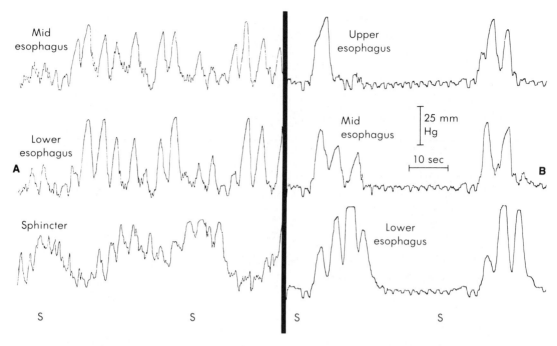

Fig. 23-2. Typical preoperative deglutitory responses of LES and body of esophagus in two patients with DES. Note normal sphincteric relaxation (**A**). Both records demonstrate simultaneous repetitive contractions of high amplitude in response to swallowing. In **A** these contractions also occur spontaneously. In **B** note the repetitive and long-duration contractions throughout the esophagus. *S* indicates a swallow. (From Leonardi, H.K., Shea, J.A., Crozier, R.E., et al.: Diffuse spasm of the esophagus, J. Thorac. Cardiovasc. Surg. **74:**738, 1977. With permission.)

applied by my associates and me[18] to selected patients with manometrically proven DES, and it has continued to be used with only slight technical modifications.[6,19] Results of esophagomyotomy for DES have been less successful than for achalasia, and therefore careful selection of patients is required. The best results are achieved in patients with marked manometric abnormalities coupled with an abnormal appearance on esophagograms. In this group the esophageal muscular wall is often found to be abnormally thick. Why better results seem to be achieved in these patients than in those with less characteristic findings is unclear, but the large psychologic overlay to symptoms in most of these individuals may be a pertinent factor.

Long esophagomyotomy is performed using a left thoracotomy through the bed of the unresected eighth rib. The distal thoracic esophagus is then gently elevated from the mediastinum. The length of the myotomy depends on the manometrically determined extent of the disease, and the LES is spared when it is normal. The longitudinal and circular muscles are incised down to the mucosa, which is allowed to pout through the incision after lateral mobilization of the overlying musculature (see Fig. 23-3). The

incision may extend as high as the aortic arch when necessary. I have encountered only one patient in whom the disease involved the entire thoracic esophagus; a right-sided approach is preferable when such an extensive myotomy is required. In those few patients with an associated hiatal hernia, the gastroesophageal junction is returned to its intraabdominal position using nonabsorbable mattress sutures through esophageal muscle above the gastroesophageal junction, passed through the hiatus, and tied to the undersurface of the diaphragm. The crura are approximated if the hiatus is patulous.

In the 46 patients reported on by my associates and me[6] the length of follow-up was sufficient to warrant analysis of 40. Surgery was considered to have resulted in improvement in 31 patients (78%). Symptomatic gastroesophageal reflux developed in three of the patients who had a poor outcome. As a result the technique was subsequently modified so that the LES was included in the myotomy only when hypertensive. The conditions of ten of 11 patients (91%) who were managed with this approach were considered to have been improved by operation, which eliminates the abnormal deglutitory contractions (see Fig. 23-4) and restores the esophagus to a more

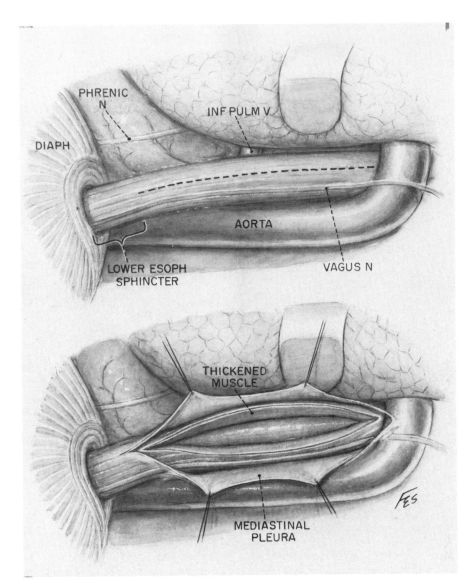

Fig. 23-3. Technique of extended esophagomyotomy. Note that the incision spares the LES. (From Leonardi, H.K., Shea, J.A., Crozier, R.E., et al.: Diffuse spasm of the esophagus, J. Thorac. Cardiovasc. Surg. **74:**739, 1977. With permission.)

normal appearance (see Fig. 23-5).[19] Comparable results have been reported by others.[20-22]

Because of a high incidence of postoperative esophagitis when a long myotomy was combined with a Belsey antireflux procedure, Henderson and Pearson[23,24] modified the operation, first including a Collis gastroplasty with the myotomy and later adding a Belsey maneuver. Henderson and co-workers[25,26] currently prefer a long myotomy and a short total fundoplication without the gastroplasty, which has resulted in an improvement rate of 88% over a 5-year follow-up period. In my opinion these complicated maneuvers are unnecessary if the LES is not incised. Further-

more, any wrapping procedure provides the potential for postoperative dysphagia when esophageal peristalsis is absent.

ASSOCIATED ESOPHAGEAL DISORDERS
Esophageal diverticulum

Almost all patients with an epiphrenic diverticulum have an underlying esophageal motility disorder, usually either DES or achalasia. Fifteen percent to 20% of patients who undergo long esophagomyotomy for DES and related disorders

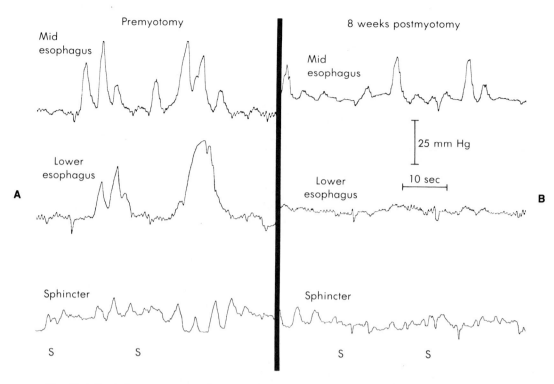

Fig. 23-4. Deglutitory pressures in lower esophagus and sphincter before operation (**A**) and 8 weeks after myotomy (**B**) in patient with DES treated by long myotomy. Note reduction in amplitude and repetitiveness of deglutitory contractions in body of esophagus and normal function of LES both before and after operation. (From Leonardi, H.K., Shea, J.A., Crozier, R.E., et al.: Diffuse spasm of the esophagus, J. Thorac. Cardiovasc. Surg. **74:**740, 1977. With permission.)

have an associated epiphrenic diverticulum.[6,19] The lesion is characterized by protrusion of the esophageal mucosa through the circular and longitudinal muscle of the esophagus, usually several centimeters above the level of the hiatus and presumably at a level above the LES (see Fig. 23-1, *C*). The diverticulum can project to either the right or the left. Symptoms are more reflective of the underlying motility disorder than the diverticulum itself because the pouch usually drains reasonably well, although its neck may be narrow.

Preoperative esophageal motility studies should be performed in all patients with an epiphrenic diverticulum, because simple diverticulectomy may fail to relieve symptoms and may predispose patients to complications associated with leakage at the suture line. These complications can be avoided if the underlying disorder is corrected when diverticulectomy is performed through a left thoracotomy. After dissection of the mucosal pouch to its neck, a stapler is applied to the neck and activated. Narrowing of the esophageal lumen must be avoided. The suture line is covered by suture approximation of the

overlying muscle layers. The myotomy is then performed at another point on the circumference of the esophagus.

Although an epiphrenic diverticulum is the most common condition associated with DES, such lesions can occur at other levels. Midesophageal diverticula are most often associated with granulomatous involvement of mediastinal and carinal lymph nodes, resulting in traction diverticula. However, some diverticula in this location are associated with an underlying motility disorder of the spastic type.[27] Rarely, multiple diverticula may develop in association with an underlying disorder, such as DES (see Fig. 23-6).

Hypertensive LES

Code and associates[28] were the first to describe hypertension of the LES as determined by pressure measurements with open-tipped catheters or balloon-covered transducers. Using perfused catheters, resting LES pressures greater than 25 to 30 mm Hg are considered hypertensive. Relaxation of the LES in the cases reported by Code and associates[29] was normal. The condition may

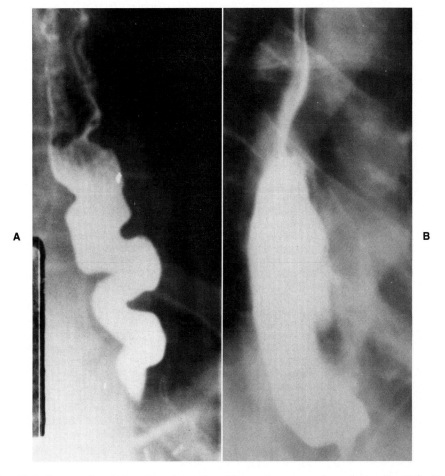

Fig. 23-5. Preoperative **(A)** and postoperative **(B)** esophagograms in patient with DES. Note elimination of corkscrew appearance of esophagus by operation. (From Leonardi, H.K., Shea, J.A., Crozier, R.E., et al.: Diffuse spasm of the esophagus, J. Thorac. Cardiovasc. Surg. **74**:739, 1977. With permission.)

occur as an isolated finding but is more commonly associated with DES or achalasia. Of 32 patients reported by Berger and McCallum,[28] 14 had achalasia and seven had DES. In another report,[6] eight of 39 patients operated on for DES had a hypertensive LES. The condition known as hypercontracting LES has also been described,[30] although its relationship to a hypertensive LES is unclear. Why symptoms of dysphagia can accompany a fully relaxing LES regardless of its resting pressure is undetermined. Symptoms of pain are more easily explained on the basis of "spasm" with or without elevated contraction pressures of the LES.

Bougienage may benefit some patients with an isolated hypertensive LES.[29] Rarely is it necessary to advise operative correction. When, as is more common, a hypertensive LES is associated with DES, the sphincter should be included in the long esophagomyotomy in an effort to return the resting LES pressures to normal levels.

Diffuse muscular hypertrophy of the lower esophagus

Muscular hypertrophy of the lower half of the esophagus was first described in 1954 by Sloper.[31] Since all but two of the cases he reported were based on necropsy findings, the relationship of this disorder to DES is unclear. In my opinion, muscular hypertrophy is a common associated finding in patients with DES undergoing long esophagomyotomy; this belief is also supported by Ferguson and associates.[21] The first patient to undergo a long esophagomyotomy was said to have had diffuse myomatosis of the esophagus,[17] but I suspect that the underlying disorder was actually DES. Not all patients with DES will be found at pathologic examination to

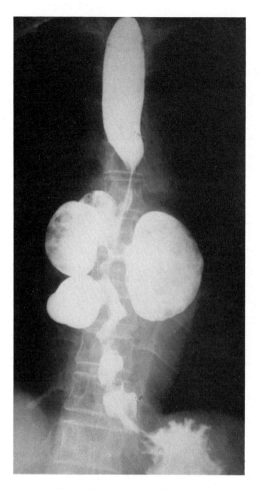

Fig. 23-6. Unusual appearance of esophagogram in patient with multiple midesophageal diverticula. (Courtesy Dr. Robert A. Berendson.)

have muscular hypertrophy of the esophagus, but this was true of 23 of 29 patients who underwent long esophagomyotomy at the Lahey Clinic.[32] As previously indicated, such patients are more apt to achieve a good response to surgery than those in whom the esophageal wall is found to be of normal thickness at the time of myotomy.

RELATED ESOPHAGEAL MOTOR DISORDERS

As indicated at the outset of this chapter, a number of motility disorders are not easily classified according to any classic pattern. Some patients with achalasia may have occasional peristaltic waves, relaxation of the LES, or both.[2] Recurrence of peristalsis after treatment has been reported[2,33] in some patients with achalasia.

Furthermore, patients with all of the manometric characteristics of DES may present with peristaltic waves of high amplitude, a condition to which a variety of names have been applied.[34] Although the relationship among these various entities has not been defined as yet, it is tempting to consider them as part of a spectrum of disorders of esophageal motility, all of which are interrelated, rather than as constituting totally separate entities. Some of these presumably related disorders are discussed here.

Vigorous achalasia

Vigorous achalasia was a term first applied in 1957 by Olsen and associates[35] to a small group of patients who had the clinical features and the abnormalities of motility characteristics of both achalasia and DES. Sanderson and co-workers[36] later reported 72 such cases. Although pain was a frequent symptom, nearly one fourth of the patients complained only of dysphagia and regurgitation. In some patients the appearance on esophagography was similar to that described for DES. This syndrome is seen early in patients with achalasia, and esophageal manometry discloses deglutitory contractions that are simultaneous but of high amplitude, in contrast to findings in patients with classic achalasia, in whom deglutition is accompanied by simultaneous low-amplitude contractions. Presumably, early in the course of the disease, before marked dilatation has occurred, the esophageal musculature can still generate high-pressure waves. Only after esophageal dilatation and "decompensation" of the esophageal musculature have occurred does the classic low-amplitude simultaneous deglutitory contraction phase occur. Failure of LES relaxation distinguishes the condition from DES.

The specific relationship between DES and vigorous achalasia is obscure. Before the development of esophageal manometry, vigorous achalasia might easily have been diagnosed incorrectly as DES and, with progression of the disease, the faulty conclusion drawn that a transition to achalasia had occurred. Such a transition can indeed take place, however, as has been documented by Vantrappen and associates[2] as well as others.[37] I have treated two such patients; the esophagograms of one are presented in Fig. 23-7. About 3% to 5% of cases of DES are estimated to progress to achalasia,[2] a figure that seems high to me.

Treatment of the patient with vigorous achalasia is surgical. A long myotomy is not required. Rather, these individuals, like other achalasia patients, should be treated with a short esophagomyotomy involving the LES and extending to

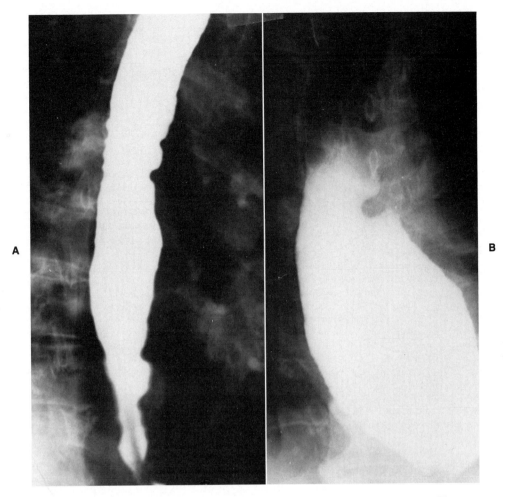

Fig. 23-7. Esophagograms demonstrating transition from DES (**A**) to achalasia (**B**).

the stomach for only a few millimeters and a short distance up onto the thick-walled part of the esophagus to ensure complete incision of the encircling musculature of the LES. With relief of the distal esophageal obstruction, the stimulus for the development of excessively high deglutitory contractions in the body of the esophagus is eliminated, and pain usually disappears.

High-amplitude peristalsis

A related disorder being recognized with increasing frequency in patients with angina-like chest pain is caused by deglutitory peristaltic contractions of increased amplitude. A number of terms have been applied to this condition, including symptomatic esophageal peristalsis,[2] nutcracker esophagus,[38] and hypertensive peristalsis.[39] The condition possesses all of the clinical and manometric features of DES except that the high-amplitude deglutitory contractions are for the most part peristaltic rather than simultaneous. Therefore, the condition in all likelihood is but a variant of DES. It is much more common, however, than classic DES, and it accounted for pain of esophageal origin in one third of patients studied by Katz and Castell.[3] Medical treatment is often effective, and I have rarely found it necessary to employ long esophagomyotomy in such patients.

Nonspecific esophageal motor disorders

In 1958, Moersch and associates[40] coined the term "dyschalasia" to describe an esophageal disorder that did not coincide with any classic description. Other terms subsequently applied to this group of abnormalities include atypical motility disorders, intermittent motiity disorders, and nonspecific esophageal motility disorders.[41] The last term seems to be the most descriptive, and in the experience of Katz and Castell[3] this diagnosis accounted for one third of all patients they studied with chest pain of esophageal origin. Any combination of disorders of esophageal contraction may be present, including repetitive contractions, contractions of prolonged duration, and nontransmitted contractions. The LES is usually normal. Treatment is medical. Goldin and coworkers[42] observed improvement in 83% of patients after bougienage, but their study included some patients with high-amplitude peristalsis. Surgery plays no role in the management of patients with this diagnosis.

REFERENCES

1. de Caestecker, J.S., Blackwell, J.N., Brown, J., et al.: The oesophagus as a cause of recurrent chest pain: which patients should be investigated and which tests should be used? Lancet **2:**1143-1148, 1985.
2. Vantrappen, G., Janssens, J., Hellemans, I., et al.: Achalasia, diffuse esophageal spasm, and related motility disorders, Gastroenterology **76:**450-457, 1979.
3. Katz, P.O., and Castell, D.O.: Review: esophageal motility disorders, Am. J. Med. Sci. **290:**61-69, 1985.
4. Osgood, H.: A peculiar form of oesophagismus, Boston Med. Surg. J. **120:**401-405, 1889.
5. Moersch, H.J., and Camp, J.D.: Diffuse spasm of the lower part of the esophagus, Ann. Otol. Rhin. Laryn. **43:**1165-1173, 1934.
6. Ellis, F.H., Jr., Schlegel, J.F., Code, C.F., et al.: Surgical treatment of esophageal hypermotility disturbances, JAMA **188:**862-866, 1964.
7. Clouse, R.E., and Lustman, P.J.: Psychiatric illness and contraction abnormalities of the esophagus, N. Engl. J. Med. **309:**1337-1342, 1983.
8. Cassella, R.R., Ellis, F.H., Jr., and Brown, A.L., Jr.: Diffuse spasm of the lower part of the esophagus: fine structure of esophageal smooth muscle and nerve, JAMA **191:**379-382, 1965.
9. Kopald, H., Roth, H.P., Fleshler, B., et al.: Vagovagal syncope: report of a case associated with diffuse esophageal spasm, N. Engl. J. Med. **271:**1238-1241, 1964.
10. Johnston, A.S.: Diffuse spasm and diffuse muscle hypertrophy of lower esophagus, Br. J. Radiol. **33:**723, 1960.
11. Creamer, B., Donoghue, E., and Code, C.F.: Patter of esophageal motility in diffuse spasm, Gastroenterology **34:**782-796, 1958.
12. DiMarino, A.J., Jr., and Cohen, S.: Characteristics of lower esophageal sphincter function in symptomatic diffuse esophageal spasm, Gastroenterology **66:**1-6, 1974.
13. Richter, J.E., Wu, W.C., Blackwell, J.N., et al.: The edrophonium response: use in diagnosis and possible understanding of mechanism of esophageal chest pain (abstract), Gastroenterology **5:**1285A, 1983.
14. Swamy, N.: Esophageal spasm: clinical and manometric response to nitroglycerin and long acting nitrates, Gastroenterology **72:**23-27, 1977.
15. Mellow, M.H.: Effect of isosorbide and hydralazine in painful primary esophageal motility disorders, Gastroenterology **83:**364-370, 1982.
16. Richter, J.E., Dalton, C.B., Buice, R.G., et al.: Nifedipine, a potent inhibitor of contractions in the body of the human esophagus: studies in healthy volunteers and patients with the nutcracker esophagus, Gastroenterology **89:**549-554, 1985.
17. Lortat-Jacob, J.L.: Myomatoses localisées et myomatoses diffuses de l'oesophage, Arch. Mal. Appl. Digest. **39:**519-524, 1950.
18. Ellis, F.H., Jr., Code, C.F., and Olsen, A.M.: Long esophagomyotomy for diffuse spasm of the esophagus and hypertensive gastroesophageal sphincter, Surgery **48:**155-169, 1960.
19. Leonardi, H.K., Shea, J.A., Crozier, R.E., et al.: Diffuse spasm of the esophagus: clinical manometric and surgical considerations, J. Thorac. Cardiovasc. Surg. **74:**736-743, 1977.
20. Craddock, D.R., Logan, A., and Walbaum, P.R.: Diffuse oesophageal spasm, Thorax **21:**511-517, 1966.
21. Ferguson, T.B., Woodbury, J.D., Roper, C.L., et al.: Giant muscular hypertrophy of the esophagus, Ann. Thorac. Surg. **8:**218-236, 1969.
22. Flye, M.W., and Sealy, W.C.: Diffuse spasm of the esophagus, Ann. Thorac. Surg. **19:**677-687, 1975
23. Henderson, R.D., Ho, C.S., and Davidson, J.W.: Primary disordered motor activity of the esophagus (diffuse spasm): diagnosis and treatment, Ann. Thorac. Surg. **18:**327-336, 1974.
24. Henderson, R.D., and Pearson, F.G.: Reflux control following extended myotomy in primary disordered motor activity (diffuse spasm) of the esophagus, Ann. Thorac. Surg. **22:**278-283, 1976.
25. Henderson, R.D., and Ryder, D.E.: Reflux control following myotomy in diffuse esophageal spasm, Ann. Thorac. Surg. **34:**230-236, 1982.
26. Henderson, R.D., Ryder, D., and Marryatt, G.: Extended esophageal myotomy and short total fundoplication hernia repair in diffuse esophageal spasm: five year review in 34 patients, Ann. Thorac. Surg. **43:**25-31, 1987.
27. Kaye, M.D.: Oesophageal motor dysfunction in patients with diverticula of the mid-thoracic oesophagus, Thorax **29:**666-672, 1974.
28. Code, C.F., Schlegel, J.F., Kelley, M.L., Jr., et al.: Hypertensive gastroesophageal spincter, Mayo Clin. Proc. **35:**391-399, 1960.
29. Berger, K., and McCallum, R.W.: The hypertensive lower esophageal sphincter: a clinical and manometric entity (abstract), Gastroenterology **80:**1109, 1981.
30. Garrett, M.D., and Godwin, D.H.: Gastroesophageal hypercontracting sphincter: manometric and clinical characteristics, JAMA **208:**992-998, 1969.
31. Sloper, J.C.: Idiopathic diffuse muscular hypertrophy of lower oesophagus, Thorax **9:**136-146, 1954.
32. Ellis, F.H., Jr.: Unpublished data, 1986.
33. Mellow, M.H.: Return of esophageal peristalsis in idiopathic achalasia, Gastroenterology **70:**1148-1151, 1976.
34. Benjamin, S.B., Gerhardt, D.C., and Castell, D.O.: High amplitude, peristaltic esophageal contractions associated with chest pain and/or dysphagia, Gastroenterology **77:**478-483, 1979.

35. Olsen, A.M., Ellis, F.H., Jr., and Creamer, B.: Cardiospasm (achalasia of the cardia), Am. J. Surg. **93:**299-307, 1957.

36. Sanderson, D.R., Ellis, F.H., Jr., Schlegel, J.F., et al.: Syndrome of vigorous achalasia: clinical and physiologic observations, Dis. Chest **52:**508-517, 1967.

37. Kramer, P., Harris, L.D., and Donaldson, R.M., Jr.: Transition from symptomatic diffuse spasm to cardiospasm, Gut **8:**115-119, 1967.

38. Benjamin, S.B., and Castell, D.O.: The "nutcracker esophagus" and the spectrum of esophageal motor disorders, Curr. Concepts Gastroentrol. **5:**3-6, 1980.

39. Orr, W.C., and Robinson, M.G.: Hypertensive peristalsis in the pathogenesis of chest pain: further exploration of the "nutcracker" esophagus, Am. J. Gastroentrol. **77:**604-607, 1982.

40. Moersch, H.J., Code, C.F., and Olsen, A.M.: Dyschalasia of the esophagus. In Gambill, C.M., Eckman, J.R., Smith, M.K., et al., editors: Collected papers of the Mayo Clinic and Mayo Foundation, vol. 49, Philadelphia, 1957, W.B. Saunders Co., pp. 19-27.

41. Castell, D.O.: The spectrum of esophageal motility disorders, Gastroenterology **76:**639-640, 1979.

42. Goldin, N.R., Burns, T.W., and Herrington, J.P.: Treatment of nonspecific esophageal motor disorders: beneficial effects of bougienage (abstract), Gastroenterology **82:**1069, 1982.

Diffuse esophageal spasm and related disorders

DISCUSSION

Toni Lerut

This chapter is written by an expert in the field of functional disorders of the esophagus. He provides the reader with a clear overview of a matter that is very complex and for which the physiopathology is not sufficiently known.

Diffuse esophageal spasm and related motor disorders are dealt with in this chapter, while achalasia is not considered. However, it must be stressed that there is an increasing amount of evidence that disorders of hypermotility and hypomotility are the reflection of one affection with one and the same etiologic origin. In this hypothesis achalasia, vigorous achalasia, diffuse esophageal spasm, and nonspecific esophageal motility are all different expressions of the same underlying disorder. The change from one type of motility disorder to another during the natural course of the different mixed forms, as demonstrated by Vantrappen,[1] endorses this concept.

Because of the complex aspect of the various motility disorders, it is of primary importance to make a good diagnosis in the first place, certainly in the prospect of a possible surgical treatment. So one cannot stress enough the importance of a correct differential diagnosis with other diseases causing a similar symptomatology. Upon this matter, the author very properly brought to our attention a number of recent papers in which motility disorders proved to be the cause of the symptoms in different patients investigated initially for "typical" angina pectoris.

One should also differentiate the primary motility disorders of the esophagus from the secondary ones. This can prove to be difficult. As mentioned by the author, there is a frequent association between diffuse esophageal spasm and hiatal hernia. This is ascribed to esophageal shortening of the longitudinal muscle by the massive contraction. However, this picture can be completely identical to tertiary contractions provoked by gastroesophageal reflux. It is clear that the therapeutic consequences of these will be different.

Tertiary contractions may also be observed in asymptomatic elderly patients, patients with carcinoma of the cardia, and so forth. Therefore, in making the differential diagnosis, one must use all available modern techniques for investigation of the esophagus—for example, x-ray investigation, endoscopy, manometry (eventually with provocational tests), 24-hour pH monitoring, and scintigraphy.

As already put forward by the author, the treatment of diffuse esophageal spasm and related motility disorders is less successful than the treatment of achalasia; this applies to medical as well as surgical treatment.

Ellis was one of the first to underline the importance of a long extramucosal myotomy up to the aortic arch in the treatment of diffuse esophageal spasm.

For the related esophageal disorders, however, he proposed to restrict the myotomy to the distal part of the esophagus, as in vigorous achalasia, or up to the level of involvement, as determined by manometry. In our opinion it is better not to make this differentiation and to extend the myotomy all the way up to the aortic arch, since, probably, most of these affections are mixed forms or, as already stated, expressions of one and the same underlying disease, so that an evolution in one or the other way is still possible.

Indeed, failure of surgery is often due to an insufficiently highly extended myotomy. Recently we have experienced an exceptional example of this. A patient, who had had a long myotomy (up to the aortic arch) performed for diffuse spasm, presented with high dysphagia and pain a few months after the operation. Manometry showed significant residual motility disturbances finally requiring a myotomy up to the cricopharyngeus muscle.

Whether the myotomy should be completed with an antireflux procedure and, if so, what type should be performed remain points of controversy. The author is known as defending a simple myotomy without incision of the LES and hence without an antireflux procedure. This attitude seems perfectly acceptable to us in the pure form of DES (without hiatal hernia or dysfunction of the LES).

In the presence of a hiatal hernia or of related esophageal motor disorders with dysfunction of the LES—as, for example, in vigorous achalasia—one is forced to extend the myotomy up to the level of LES. As a consequence in these cases, the risk of gastroesophogeal reflux and peptic esophagitis increases. Very few surgeons manage to perform this operation in such a way that the incidence of postoperative reflux esophagitis is restricted to about 5%, as in Ellis' series.

In the literature one regularly finds incidences of postoperative reflux esophagitis up to 50%. The cause of this is probably a lack of experience with this kind of intervention on the part of the surgeon. For this reason we think that these surgeons should add an antireflux procedure to the myotomy whenever it is extended to the LES or when there is an associated hiatal hernia. The type of antireflux procedure used is of some importance. A Nissen fundoplication, if not per-

formed meticulously, carries a greater risk of postoperative dysphagia, especially when there is a hypomotility disorder of the esophagus or when the esophageal disorder evolves. For this reason, we prefer the Belsey Mark IV type of antireflux procedure with a 240-degree fundoplication. This operation ensures a sufficient control of the reflux and carries less risk of postoperative dysphagia. The classical technique of this operation needs a modification in the sense that only two mattress sutures (one on either side of the myotomy) instead of three can be placed. One has to remark, however, that, since the muscular wall is thickened, it is possible to take deeper bites so that these sutures hold better. In our, be it limited, experience with surgery for esophageal motility disorders in 16 patients with dysfunction of the LES or with associated hiatal hernia, as well as in cases of achalasia, the results were very satisfying, with an incidence of postoperative reflux of 6% and no single patient having symptomatic dysphagia. This policy is confirmed by a number of recent publications.

REFERENCE

1. Vantrappen, G., Janssens, J., Hellemens, I., et al.: Achalasia, diffuse esophageal spasm, and related mobility disorders, Gastroenterology **76:**450-457, 1979.

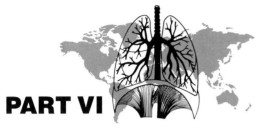

PART VI **THE UPPER ESOPHAGUS**

24 Pharyngeal dysphagia

Edwin Lafontaine

The subjective awareness that something has gone wrong with the act of swallowing is called *dysphagia;* this is not a diagnosis but only a general symptom. Classification of dysphagia is based on the location of the swallowing difficulty. *Transfer* or *pharyngeal dysphagia* is caused by a disturbance in the coordinated neuromuscular events during the initiation of swallowing and the propulsion of the swallowed material from the oropharynx to the cervical esophagus. *Transport dysphagia* results from a problem in the passage of material through the body of the esophagus. *Delivery* or *esophagogastric dysphagia* occurs when the bolus has difficulty entering the stomach. In an individual case, overlapping of these types may exist, but such a classification is convenient for the purposes of discussion because patients commonly localize their complaints to one of these three areas. Ten percent of patients with esophageal dysphagia may localize the site of the obstruction to the neck, whereas patients with oropharyngeal, or "preeosophageal," dysphagia rarely localize the site of obstruction in the chest.[1] A review of the preesophageal causes of dysphagia—excluding Zenker's diverticulum, which is discussed in another chapter—will follow (see box, p. 336).

Patients with dysphagia resulting from preesophageal causes experience difficulty with swallowing within a few seconds of deglutition. The neuroregulation of normal swallowing involves the complex interplay of cortical, medullary, and peripheral sensorimotor tracts and receptors. The signals are coordinated to produce a seemingly simple action that normally takes less than 1 second. The most common neuromuscular cause of esophageal dysphagia is central nervous system disease.[2]

NORMAL DEGLUTITION

Structures participating in pharyngeal deglutition are the tongue, soft palate, pharyngeal musculature, larynx, and faucial pillars. The act of deglutition can be divided into four phases. During the *oral preparatory phase,* food is manipulated in the mouth and masticated if necessary. Food introduced into the mouth cannot be prepared for swallowing unless it is mixed with saliva. The soft palate is normally pulled actively anteriorly and rests against the back of the tongue, which is elevated to keep the material in the oral cavity. The major portion of the bolus is pulled together into a cohesive mass and held between the anterior tongue and the palate. The larynx and pharynx are at rest, and nasal breathing may continue until the voluntary swallow is initiated.

The *oral* or *voluntary stage* of swallowing is initiated with the tongue squeezing the bolus against the hard palate and moving it posteriorly. This involves an intact labial musculature to prevent leakage from the oral cavity and lingual movement to propel the bolus posteriorly.

The *pharyngeal phase* begins with triggering of the swallowing reflex. In normal individuals this occurs when the bolus stimulates the anterior faucial arch. From this moment voluntary control and respiration cease. Posterior movement of the bolus is not interrupted. This reflex causes a number of physiologic events important to successful swallowing. Elevation and retraction of the soft palate are essential to ensure closure of the nasopharynx and prevent oronasal regurgitation. Initiation of pharyngeal peristalsis by the squeezing action of the pharyngeal constrictors ensures passage of the bolus through the pharynx to the top of the cricopharyngeus muscle. Tracheal aspiration is prevented by elevation and closure of the larynx. Passage of the bolus into the esophagus is assured by relaxation of the cricopharyngeus muscle. This occurs when the bolus reaches the posterior pharyngeal wall. Pharyngeal transit time is usually 1 second or less. During this transit there is no hesitation anywhere in the pharynx. When this phase is over, there is normally very little food left in the pharynx.

Gravity and peristalsis ensure passage of the

CLASSIFICATION OF PHARYNGEAL DYSPHAGIA

A. Neuromuscular diseases
  1. Central nervous system or upper motor neuron
     (a) Congenital
        (1) Riley-Day syndrome
        (2) Friedreich's ataxia
        (3) Olivopontocerebellar degeneration
     (b) Acquired
        (1) Cerebrovascular accident
        (2) Brainstem tumors
        (3) Parkinson's disease
        (4) Huntington's chorea
        (5) Amyotrophic lateral sclerosis
        (6) Multiple sclerosis
        (7) Poliomyelitis
        (8) Tabes dorsalis
  2. Peripheral neuropathy or lower motor neuron
     (a) Alcoholic
     (b) Diabetic
  3. Disease of the motor endplate
     (a) Myasthenia gravis
     (b) Botulism
  4. Disorders of striated muscle
     (a) Polymyositis, dermatomyositis
     (b) Muscular dystrophy (myotonic, oculopharyngeal)
     (c) Metabolic myopathy (steroid, hypothyroidism or hyperthyroidism)

B. Mechanical defects
   (a) Oropharyngeal carcinoma
   (b) Congenital webs of the pharynx and upper esophagus (Plummer-Vinson syndrome)
   (c) Postsurgical (resection, tracheostomy)
   (d) Extrinsic compression
      (1) Thyromegaly
      (2) Cervical lympadenopathy
      (3) Hyperostosis of the cervical spine
   (e) Inflammatory disorders
      (1) Pharyngitis, epiglottitis
      (2) Pharyngeal abscess
      (3) Gastroesophageal reflux
C. Idiopathic dysfunction
   (a) Pharyngoesophageal diverticulum (Zenker)
   (b) Cricopharyngeal dysfunction
      (1) Abnormalities of resting pressure
      (2) Abnormalities of relaxation (achalasia)
      (3) Cricopharyngeal bar
   (c) Psychogenic: globus hystericus

TABLE 24-1. Sensory innervation of swallowing

Innervation	Sensory function
Lingual, trigeminal (V)	General sensation of texture and temperature, anterior two thirds of tongue
	Salivation
Chorda tympani, facial (VII)	Taste, anterior two thirds of tongue
Glossopharyngeal (IX)	Taste and general sensation, posterior two thirds of tongue
	Salivation
	Sensation to soft palate, pharynx
	Sensory component to pharyngeal (gag) reflex
Vagus (X)	Sensation of pharynx, larynx

bolus into the stomach during the *esophageal phase*. Respiration resumes during this longer period. The upper esophageal sphincter (UES) remains closed and at rest. Its major functions are to prevent esophageal distention during respiration and to protect against esophagopharyngeal reflux with subsequent tracheobronchial aspiration. The sensory portion of swallowing is carried by cranial nerves V, VII, IX, and X and the major motor function by cranial nerves IX, X, and XII[3] (see Tables 24-1 and 24-2).

TABLE 24-2. Motor innervation of swallowing

Innervation	Motor function
Trigeminal (V)	Mastication
	Muscles, floor of mouth
Facial (VII)	Muscles of lip and facial expression
Glossopharyngeal (IX)	Pharyngeal constrictors
Vagus (X)	Palate, pharynx, larynx
	Pharyngeal (gag) reflex
Hypoglossal (XII)	Tongue

Any defect in the complex mechanism of the preesophageal phase of swallowing may cause dysphagia. In addition, associated symptoms such as leaking of the bolus from the oral cavity, oronasal regurgitation, aspiration, and dysphonia may be present. Patients with neurologic disorders have greater difficulty swallowing liquids than solids. Postdeglutitive coughing is not specific for aspiration secondary to incoordinate swallowing; a tracheoesophageal fistula or gastroesophageal reflux must be ruled out. Weight loss may be a prominent complaint and provides an excellent parameter to measure the severity of the process and improvement following treatment. Dysphagia characterized by a swallow, then a gag, cough, oral or nasal regurgitation, or a sensation of blockage within a few seconds is typical of preesophageal dysphagia. Repeated attempts to initiate a swallow are frequently observed. Neuromuscular diseases affecting different levels of the neuraxis are the main causes of this clinical disorder. Mechanical lesions are less frequently implicated, as are idiopathic dysfunction of the cricopharyngeus muscle. The box on p. 336 offers a classification of diseases presenting with dysphagia, based primarily on the level of pathology along the complex neuraxis.

Non–food-related dysphagia, classically called globus hystericus, is the most common complaint in relation to the swallowing mechanism. Affected patients may feel a constant lump, pressure, or fullness in the throat. This sensation worsens with time and is not necessarily associated with meals. These patients should still have a thorough workup to rule out other causes.[4]

INVESTIGATION

Evaluation of the patient with disordered deglutition begins with careful history taking and thorough bedside examination. It should be considered a team evaluation, since no one discipline can assess in detail all phases of swallowing. Presentation may be acute or chronic, a manifestation of a variety of neuromuscular diseases or an isolated symptom in an otherwise stable patient. Associated symptoms may help to eliminate certain diagnoses and identify the physiologic abnormality. Neurogenic dysphagia occurs more frequently with liquids and is rarely associated with odynophagia. Preesophageal painful swallowing is usually a manifestation of inflammation of the oropharyngeal mucosa.

Examination of the patient includes assessment of nutritional status and mental status. The muscles of mastication and facial expression, as well as the range of movement of the tongue, are inspected. The pharyngeal phase of deglutition is evaluated by observing for an adequate elevation of the larynx and the presence of a gag reflex. Careful oral and pharyngeal inspection is essential to rule out a mechanical obstruction and to assess sensitivity of the mucosa. Indirect laryngoscopy should be performed to visualize the base of the tongue, vallecula, epiglottis, piriform sinuses, vocal and vestibular folds, and infraglottic area. Vocal cord function is essential in airway protection during the pharyngeal stage of swallowing. Suspicious mucosal lesions should be biopsied. The presence of food debris or pooling of secretions in the vallecula or piriform sinuses is an indication of a poor swallowing reflex.

Radiographic studies are essential in the evaluation of preesophageal dysphagia. Frontal and lateral soft-tissue neck films are particularly useful for acute dysphagia. Soft-tissue edema, such as that associated with epiglottitis or retropharyngeal abscess, and foreign bodies such as bone may be detected. Nonopaque foreign bodies such as meat can be suspected by the trapped air that is almost invariably associated with them. Hyperostosis of the cervical spine may be visualized. Double-contrast laryngopharyngography may demonstrate pharyngeal tumors that otherwise would be obscured by the density of the barium-filled pharynx. Cineradiography of deglutition will demonstrate functional and structural abnormalities. It is necessary to detect motor dysfunction of the successive phases of deglutition, such as abnormal movements of the tongue and nonpropulsive and asymmetric pharyngeal contractions. Misdirection of the bolus is visualized and classified as buccal regurgitation, nasopharyngeal reflux, or tracheal aspiration. Observation of the cricopharyngeus may reveal incomplete relaxation or poor coordination, with pharyngeal contraction manifested as premature closure or poor opening. A posterior cricopharyngeal bar denotes a physiologic abnormality of relaxation, although lesser degrees of it are usually not associated with clinical symptoms. Webs and diverticula may also be observed. Cineradiography currently is the most accurate objective test to evaluate pharyngeal contraction, the dynamics of airway protection, and the function of the UES.[5,6]

Manometric evaluation of the pharynx and UES is extremely difficult. The rapidity of the oropharyngeal events, the mobility of the larynx and cricopharyngeus, and the asymmetry of the UES are obstacles to accurate and reproducible data.[7,8] However, abnormalities in the resting tone and relaxation of the UES—manifested by incomplete relaxation, premature closure, or delayed relaxation—may be detected. Upon deglutition the UES resting pressure normally drops to baseline pharyngeal pressure to allow a bolus to pass from the pharynx into the esophagus without having to cross a pressure gradient. Cricopharyngeal achalasia refers to incomplete relaxation of the UES. Asherson has defined it as a failure or a delay in relaxation of the cricopharyngeus.[9] This may occur as an isolated phenomenon or secondary to an underlying disease such as poliomyelitis or bulbar paralysis. Premature closure of the UES plays a major role in the pathogenesis of Zenker's diverticulum.[10] Delayed relaxation has been observed in patients with familial dysautonomia.[11] Manometry also rules out motility disorders of the esophageal body.

Endoscopy should be performed routinely in the workup of dysphagia. Mucosal folds at the cricopharyngeus or difficulties in negotiating a way through it have been described in association with dysfunction of the UES. Endoscopy will eliminate obstructive benign and malignant lesions of the esophageal body, which may cause dysphagia referred to the neck.

Isotopic assessment of pharyngoesophageal transit may prove in the future to be a more accurate test to evaluate dysphagia. Quantification of the deficit may be used to evaluate objectively the therapeutic results. When gastroesophageal reflux is clinically suspected, pH monitoring should be done to rule it out.

NEUROGENIC CAUSES OF DYSPHAGIA

A variety of neuromuscular disorders may cause dysphagia. Oropharyngeal and cricopharyngeal abnormalities have been described in cerebrovascular accidents, brainstem tumors, and degenerative diseases of the nervous system such as amyotrophic lateral sclerosis, Parkinson's disease, and multiple sclerosis. Clinically, these patients are identified through such factors as the duration of the swallowing process, dysphagia experienced with liquids and solids, and the usual absence of odynophagia. Associated drooling, nasal regurgitation, dysarthric speech, and aspiration may be present, because of the intimate relationship of the last four cranial nerves. A neurologic cause of dysphagia is more likely if the anatomy is normal without any deformity.

Stroke disorders, trauma, and tumors affecting the brainstem will cause severe dysphagia resulting from bilateral representation in the brainstem. The mechanism of dysphagia is primarily cricopharyngeal dysfunction. Wallenberg's syndrome is a typical brainstem syndrome secondary to occlusion of a dominant vertebral artery or the posterior inferior cerebral artery. Typically, dysphagia is accompanied by nausea, vomiting, ataxia, vertigo, and nystagmus. Unilateral hemispheral or cortical lesions affect swallowing less severely. The main cause of dysphagia is the absence or severe delay in triggering of the swallowing reflex. Lingual hemiparesis results in a disturbed propulsion of the bolus during oral transit. Unilateral pharyngeal paralysis induces a decrease in the peristaltic activity on the affected side. This results in debris remaining in the vallecula and piriform sinus on the diseased side.[6,12,13]

Parkinson's disease and Huntington's chorea are the main representatives of extrapyramidal diseases causing dysphagia. Motor function is disturbed, resulting in muscular rigidity, tremor, and involuntary movements. Evaluation of these patients reveals hesitancy in bolus formation and weakness of mastication. Most have pharyngeal motility problems associated with stasis, aspiration, and nasal regurgitation, and 50% will demonstrate cricopharyngeal sphincter dysfunction.[14-16] There may be improvement in swallowing with treatment of the underlying disease. The use of L-dopa in parkinsonism has been associated with improvement in pharyngeal deglutition.[17] The use of neuroleptic drugs to treat choreas rarely improves the dysphagia.

Disturbances of swallowing are not unusual in multiple sclerosis. Dysphagia develops with demyelination of cranial nerves participating in the act of swallowing. The most frequent abnormalities are a reduction in pharyngeal peristalsis and a delay in the swallowing reflex secondary to involvement of the ninth cranial nerve. Patients in advanced stages of the disease will manifest poor lingual control of the bolus and tracheal aspiration.[6,18]

Amyotrophic lateral sclerosis is a progressive disease involving upper and lower motorneurons. It causes spastic and atrophic symptoms in the cranial, spinal, and peripheral musculature. It may progressively affect all phases of swallowing. Dysphagia often begins with reduction in tongue mobility. Oral control of the bolus is absent and mastication inadequate. Progression of the disease results in poor pharyngeal peristalsis, delay of the swallowing reflex, and discoordination of the cricopharyngeus.[6,13,19]

Myasthenia gravis, a neurologic disease affecting the myoneural junction, usually presents with fatiguability first observed in the ocular muscles. With bulbar involvement, dysphagia occurs. Swallowing becomes more difficult with repeated use of the musculature of deglutition. Typically, function improves with rest. One third of patients with myasthenia gravis have dysphagia secondary to fatigue. Oral abnormalities are hesitancy in initiating deglutition, inefficiency in forming a bolus, and slow, inefficient tongue movements that become progressively weaker with continued attempts at swallowing. Pharyngeal abnormalities include pooling in the pharynx itself, and as a result of weakness of pharyngeal peristalsis, stasis in the pharyngeal recesses. When suspected, the diagnosis should be confirmed by electromyography and response to cholinergic drugs. Dysphagia usually responds to appropriate therapy.[6,12,20]

Peripheral neuropathy resulting from alcohol, diabetes, or trauma may produce oropharyngeal dysphagia by damage to the afferent and efferent nerves involved in swallowing. The most frequent cause is involvement of the vagus nerve as a result of trauma, neoplasm, or surgical division. Dysphagia reflects damage to the innervation of the cricopharyngeus. These conditions may render the musculature needed for swallowing either weak or paretic. Several nerves may be involved. The swallowing reflex is absent or very weak, and the intellect is usually intact.[21]

Congenital diseases, such as Friedreich's ataxia and familial dysautonomia (Riley-Day syndrome), may present with pharyngeal dysfunction secondary to tissue destruction in the motor nucleus of the ninth and tenth cranial nerves. Familial dysautonomia is inherited as an autosomal recessive trait occurring almost exclusively in Jewish families of East European extraction. The clinical features are episodic hypertension, excessive perspiration, disordered swallowing, marked diminution in sensory modalities, and decreased or absent tendon reflexes. Radiographic studies in these patients have demonstrated delayed opening of the UES with swallowing.[11]

Palliation of neurogenic dysphagia is complex. Ethical considerations posed by the fatal outcome in patients with degenerative brain disease are problematic. Dysphagia, in many cases, is secondary to pathologic changes affecting multiple phases of deglutition. Palliation at one level may not improve the whole process.

Initially, the underlying disease should be treated. Significant clinical improvement may be obtained in myasthenia gravis and Parkinson's disease. Scant information is available on the pattern of recovery of normal swallowing in patients with cerebrovascular accidents or cerebral trauma. However, most patients who require a nasogastric tube after the incident because of a reduced or absent swallowing reflex and who recover from the injury will regain normal swallowing within 3 months. The prognosis for recovery is good, and therefore recommendations for a more permanent type of therapy, such as a cricopharyngeal myotomy, should be deferred for at least 3 months.

Cricopharyngeal myotomy should be considered in patients who have recovered but still have incapacitating dysphagia manifested by weight loss, food incarceration, and tracheal aspiration. This procedure will improve the conditions of 60% of patients with neurogenic dysphagia. Most studies have failed to describe objective criteria for selecting patients who will be likely to respond. When the criteria used for selection of patients in these studies are carefully examined, it is often clear that patients with swallowing disorders other than cricopharyngeal dysfunction have been treated by myotomy. The success rate increases with careful selection of patients after a complete evaluation. Patients most likely to respond have maintained the motor ability to move the bolus through the oral and pharyngeal phases of deglutition and an intact sensation of the oropharynx to trigger the swallowing reflex. Cricopharyngeal dysfunction must be the predominant problem. Results of cricopharyngeal myotomy for neurogenic dysphagia are described in Table 24-3. Most of these studies include a variety of diseases. The study of Lebo et al. describes the results in amyotrophic lateral

TABLE 24-3. Results of cricopharyngeal myotomy for neurogenic dysphagia

Author	Number of patients	Length of follow-up (mo)	Results (%)			Operative mortality (%)
			Excellent	Satisfactory	Poor	
Akl and Blakely[22]	5	0-36	20		80	—
Bonavina et al.[23]	11	30	81		19	—
Gay et al.[24]	13	—	84			—
Lebo et al.[19]	38	5-6	0	64	36	5
Loizou et al.[25]	25	0-24	52	8	20	20
Mills[26]	17	3-24		94.2	5.8	5.8

sclerosis. Cricopharyngeal myotomy is far from resulting in uniform success in these patients, probably because of the severity of the abnormalities affecting all aspects of deglutition.[19]

Patients with peripheral neuropathy will respond to cricopharyngeal myotomy when cricopharyngeal dysfunction has been demonstrated and is the main mechanism causing dysphagia.[21] Otherwise, efforts at rehabilitation consist of strengthening of the oral and pharyngeal muscles and selection of an appropriate diet most likely to stimulate an absent or weak swallowing reflex. No definite long-term reports are available on the indications for and results of cricopharyngeal bougienage for neurogenic dysphagia.

DISORDERS OF STRIATED MUSCLE

Primary muscle disorders may involve the pharyngeal musculature. Myopathies are characterized by weakness that is not due to emotional or neurogenic causes. The dystrophies are a subgroup of myopathy characterized by a history of progressive weakness and a heritable transmission. These patients present with manifestations of weak muscles. With involvement of the cranial muscles they may complain of dysarthria, dysphagia, diplopia, or ptosis. Cineradiography of deglutition in these patients reveals a prolongation of muscular activity and shallow, weakened pharyngeal contractions. In the advanced cases residual barium may be found in the pharyngeal recesses. The cricopharyngeal sphincter is usually not affected and opens normally.

Myotonic muscular dystrophy differs from other types of dystrophy in that the cranial muscles are frequently affected and limb weakness is initially more marked in distal muscles. Ptosis, facial weakness, dysphagia, and dysarthria are signs not seen in other forms of dystrophy. The swallowing abnormality is characterized by prolonged contraction and difficulty in relaxation of the involved muscles. The cricopharyngeal sphincter will not relax rapidly during swallowing. Loss of the normal high resting pressure of the UES has also been described. These patients present with excessive aspiration. The motor defect is present at all times and does not vary with fatigue.[27,28] These patients may respond dramatically to procainamide.

Certain forms of dystrophy are named after the prominent manifestations. Oculopharyngeal muscular dystrophy is a slowly progressive disorder in which ptosis of the eyelids and progressive dysphagia are the cardinal features. First described by Hutchinson in 1879 and studied in depth by Taylor in 1915, it is most common in French Canadian families and is transmitted as an autosomal dominant gene.[29,30] Manometric studies reveal low pharyngeal contraction pressures, and abnormalities of cricopharyngeal relaxation may be observed. Peristaltic activity is reduced in the upper third of the esophagus, with the distal third being relatively normal. An isotopic deglutition scan demonstrates the problems associated with poor pharyngeal contraction and stasis in the pharyngeal recesses (see Fig. 24-1). Results of cricopharyngeal myotomy for the relief of dysphagia are satisfactory. In one study of 15 patients, myotomy reduced UES resting and contracting pressures by more than 50%; pharyngeal contractions were unchanged. Clinically all patients were significantly improved.[31,32]

Polymyositis is an inflammatory disease of skeletal muscle characterized by symmetric weakness of the limb girdles, neck, and pharynx. Dysphagia, dysphonia, and dysarthria may occur with involvement of the pharynx. Cineradiographic abnormalities of deglutition include retention of barium in the vallecula, nasal reflux, hypomotility, and flaccidity of the pharynx and upper esophagus. Manometry and isotopic deglutition studies have confirmed the decrease in the contraction pressures of the pharynx, cricopharyngeus, and upper third of the esophagus. A radionuclide pharyngoesophagogram demonstrates these findings (see Fig. 24-2). A few cases of abnormal relaxation of the UES have been described.[33] About 10% of patients with polymyositis have coexistent malignancy. Myositis precedes the diagnosis of malignancy in 70% of cases. Therapy consists of steroids or cytotoxic drugs. Deaths from muscular weakness are relatively rare. A heliotrope rash occurs on the upper eyelids and face in 15% and is highly suggestive of the diagnosis of dermatomyositis.[34]

Other acquired myopathies may cause dysphagia in a similar way by involvement of the striated muscle of the upper portion of the digestive tract. Metabolic myopathies may occur, and thyroid function tests should be obtained. Muscular weakness may complicate both hyperthyroidism and hypothyroidism. Thyrotoxic myopathy is usually insidious in onset and occurs most often in men.[35] These patients usually respond to the treatment of the underlying disease.

MECHANICAL DEFECTS OF SWALLOWING

Acute inflammations resulting from bacterial, viral, or fungal agents may cause dysphagia. The

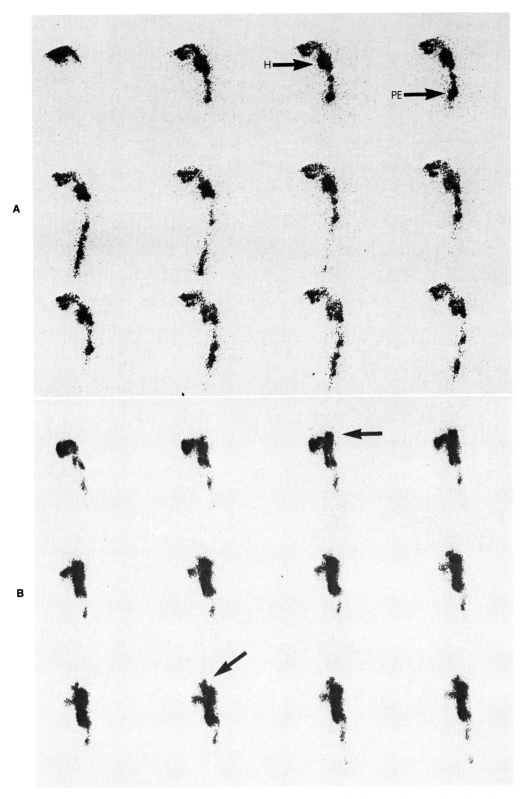

Fig. 24-1. Radionuclide studies of four patients with oculopharyngeal muscular dystrophy, demonstrating different complications of this myopathy. **A,** This study, performed with scrambled eggs labeled with technetium 99m sulfur colloid, demonstrates a delayed clearance of the solid bolus in the hypopharynx *(H)* and proximal esophagus *(PE)*. **B,** Significant hypopharyngeal stasis of the liquid radionuclide bolus with concomitant nasopharyngeal regurgitation *(arrow)*.

Continued.

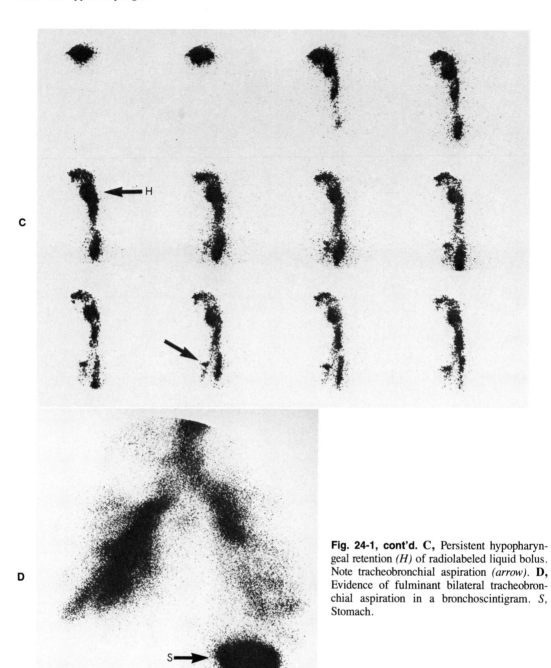

C

D

Fig. 24-1, cont'd. C, Persistent hypopharyngeal retention *(H)* of radiolabeled liquid bolus. Note tracheobronchial aspiration *(arrow)*. **D,** Evidence of fulminant bilateral tracheobronchial aspiration in a bronchoscintigram. *S, Stomach.*

buccal mucosa and, to a lesser extent, the pharyngeal mucosa are at least partly of ectodermal origin. Certain skin diseases such as Behçet's syndrome, pemphigus, lichen planus, and epidermolysis bullosa may affect the oropharynx, resulting in severe dysphagia and malnutrition.[36] Carcinoma of the structures involved in the deglutition process or surgical procedures for such tumors may cause dysphagia. It can be potentiated by preoperative or postoperative irra-

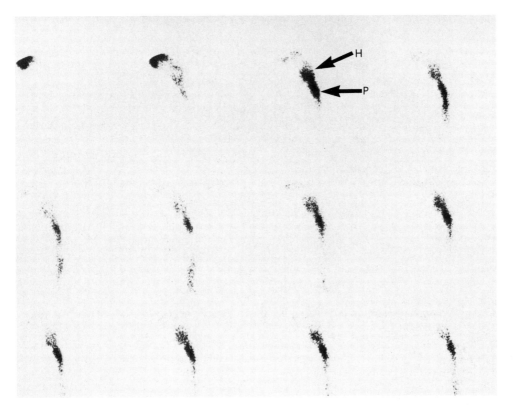

Fig. 24-2. Radionuclide pharyngoesophagogram from a patient with polymyositis following ingestion of 15 ml of water labeled with technetium 99m sulfur colloid. Dynamic images are obtained at 2-second intervals. Note the delayed clearance of the radioactivity in the striated muscular portion of the upper digestive tract. *H,* Hypopharynx; *P,* proximal esophagus.

diation, which produces oral and pharyngeal inflammation with subsequent pain in the soft tissues and bone. Other complications include a drying effect on the mucosal tissues, a diminished volume and thicker consistency of saliva, changes in taste sensation, and loss of appetite. Cricopharyngeal myotomy should be considered as an ancillary procedure to certain types of major oropharyngeal resections that would otherwise result in significant dysphagia. It has been recommended in cases in which the vagus nerve is injured or resected high in the neck, resections of half or more of the base of the tongue, resections of the oropharynx or hypopharynx, and epiglottectomies and laryngectomies. Resections that impair the oral phase of swallowing do not benefit from a cricopharyngeal myotomy.[37] A tracheostomy tube restricts normal laryngeal elevation by mechanical interference. It anchors the trachea to the strap muscles and the skin of the neck, thus limiting anterior elevation and rotation. This compromises glottal protection and interferes with relaxation of the cricopharyn-geus.[38] Once the tube is removed, normal function should resume.

Extrinsic compression from cervical lymph-adenopathy, thyromegaly, or hyperostosis of the cervical spine may cause dysphagia. Osteophytic changes in the cervical spine may be seen radiographically. Patients complain of dysphagia at the cricopharyngeal level, probably resulting from pressure of osteophytes, which are more frequently encountered at the C5-6 level. Other mechanisms of dysphagia have been proposed, such as local inflammation, edema, and spasm of the cricopharyngeal muscle. Dysphagia may be intermittent or exacerbated by neck flexion. Initial therapy may consist of anti-inflammatory drugs. Bone spur resection gives the most satisfactory results. Recurrence of the osteophytes has been observed after resection.[39,40]

Webs, located most frequently in the cervical esophagus, may occasionally be found in the hypopharynx between the piriform sinuses and the cricopharyngeus muscle. They are located mostly on the anterior wall but could be circular.

Their presence is rare compared to cervical esophageal webs.[41] They never occur on the posterior hypopharyngeal wall, and are easily differentiated from an incompletely relaxed cricopharyngeus, which always arises posteriorly—the so-called cricopharyngeal bar.

Patients with gastroesophageal reflux may experience cervical dysphagia. Hunt et al.[42] have reported increased pressures in the UES in these patients. The increased pressure serves as a protective mechanism to prevent pharyngeal regurgitation and aspiration. Belsey[43] described the presence of spasm of the cricopharyngeus in 3.5% of a large series of patients with hiatal hernia and gastroesophageal reflux. In less than 1% it was the patient's primary complaint. Control of reflux eliminated spasm of the UES and the attendant dysphagia. Belsey[43] has warned against the performance of a cricopharyngeal myotomy in these patients. In the presence of uncontrolled gastroesophageal reflux it could predispose patients to recurring aspiration pneumonitis. Henderson and Marryatt[44] have reported a 50% incidence of cervical dysphagia in 200 patients treated surgically for gastroesophageal reflux. Their manometric data, contrary to the data of Hunt and colleagues,[42] demonstrate a normal tone in the cricopharyngeus and premature closure similar to that described in patients with a cricopharyngeal diverticulum.[10] Abnormal relaxation of the UES was not present in all patients and could not be used to determine the presence or severity of dysphagia. In the experience of Henderson et al. approximately 10% of patients with major pharyngoesophageal dysphagia will not respond to operative correction of reflux.[45] Two percent will have major problems with coughing and aspiration. Cricopharyngeal myotomy relieved dysphagia and tracheal aspiration in 88% of patients. In Orringer's experience 50% of patients with residual cervical dysphagia after successful antireflux repair responded favorably to cricopharyngeal myotomy.[46] Contrary to Belsey's experience, Henderson and Marryatt have performed successful cricopharyngeal myotomy for relief of cervical dysphagia in patients too ill to have an antireflux procedure.[44]

IDIOPATHIC DYSFUNCTION

A number of symptoms appear to be attributable to disorders of the cricopharyngeus. The main clinical manifestation is cervical dysphagia. Tracheopulmonary aspiration may develop as well as a fear of eating. The severity of the process

may be measured by weight loss. The UES is in a state of tonic contraction during rest. Abnormalities of UES functions may be related to changes in resting tone and/or abnormalities in sphincter relaxation.

Above-normal UES pressure may be a clinical entity by itself or may be secondary to lesions in the pharynx or nervous system. Increases in the resting pressure may also be found in reflux esophagitis. The increased pressure serves as a protective mechanism to prevent pharyngeal regurgitation and aspiration.[42] Globus sensation, a feeling that something is always stuck in the throat without dysphagia, may be associated with a hypertensive sphincter.[47] It is important to rule out an organic basis for the dysphagia. In one review of patients given the diagnosis globus hystericus, 75% had demonstrable organic disease.[4]

Asherson in 1950 labeled as achalasia failure of relaxation of the cricopharyngeus in the absence of mechanical obstruction or neurogenic causes.[9] Sutherland in 1962 published the clinical features of the syndrome and the results of cricopharyngeal myotomy in eight patients. Follow-up results at 1 year were satisfactory.[48] With swallowing, respiration is halted, and the cricopharyngeus must relax as the bolus approaches. To ensure a smooth passage of the bolus from the pharynx into the cervical esophagus, UES relaxation must be complete and coordinated to accommodate the oncoming pharyngeal peristaltic wave. Three types of abnormalities of UES relaxation have been described. Incomplete relaxation is most frequently associated with achalasia. Premature closure of the UES plays a major role in the pathogenesis of Zenker's diverticulum.[10] Delayed UES relaxation with swallowing has been described in patients with familial dysautonomia.[11]

Patients with cricopharyngeal dysfunction may complain of a sensation of food hanging up in the back of the throat or the need for multiple swallows to completely pass food into the esophagus. The diagnosis is suggested by the patient's history and by observing his attempts to drink. The onset may be acute, and its severity may be assessed by weight loss. The diagnosis is confirmed by cineradiography, manometry, and endoscopy. A cricopharyngeal bar may be present on barium swallow and is accompanied by pooling of contrast medium in the vallecular folds and distention of the hypopharynx with delay of the passage of barium into the esophagus. Endoscopy is required in order to rule out other disease in the area. The cricopharyngeus may present as a posterior transverse, rather unyielding bar to the

A   B

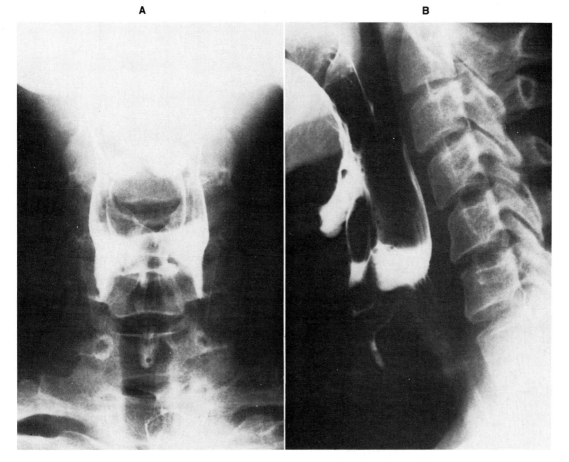

Fig. 24-3. Preoperative esophagograms from a female patient with cricopharyngeal achalasia. **A,** Anteroposterior film showing retention of the contrast medium at the level of the vallecula and piriform recesses, with no barium passing into the esophagus. **B,** Lateral film, taken opposite the C5-6 vertebrae, showing posterior indentation of the cricopharyngeus, retention in the hypopharynx, and tracheal aspiration.

passage of the endoscope into the proximal esophagus. The clinical significance of the presence of a cricopharyngeal bar is not well established. It may occur in patients without swallowing related symptoms. Achalasia of the UES affects patients over 40 years of age and most commonly those over 60. Bougienage rarely relieves dysphagia significantly. Patients with primary dysfunction of the UES respond more favorably to cricopharyngeal myotomy.[43,46] The radiologic appearance of UES achalasia is shown in Fig. 24-3. This patient underwent successful cricopharyngeal myotomy with excellent palliation of her dysphagia. Radionuclide studies of the hypopharyngeal clearance demonstrate the improved emptying after cricopharyngeal myotomy (see Fig. 24-4).

REFERENCES

1. Edwards, D.A.W.: Discrimination value of symptoms in the differential diagnosis of dysphagia, Clin. Gastroenterol. **5:**49, 1976.
2. Hurwitz, A.L., Nelson, J.A., and Haddad, J.K.: Oropharyngeal dysphagia: manometric and cine esophagraphic findings, Am. J. Dig. Dis. **20:**313, 1975.
3. Atkinson, M., Kramer, P., Wyman, S.M., et al.: The dynamics of swallowing. I. Normal pharyngeal mechanisms, J. Clin. Invest. **36:**581, 1957.
4. Slater, E.: Diagnosis of "hysteria," Br. Med. J. **1:**1395, 1965.
5. Donner, M.W.: Swallowing mechanism and neuromuscular disorders, Semin. Roentgenol. **9:**273, 1974.
6. Silbiger, M.L., Pikielney, R., and Donner, M.W.: Neuromuscular disorders affecting the pharynx: cineradiographic analysis, Invest. Radiol. **2:**442, 1967.
7. Gerhardt, D.C., Shuck, T.J., Bordeaux, R.A., and

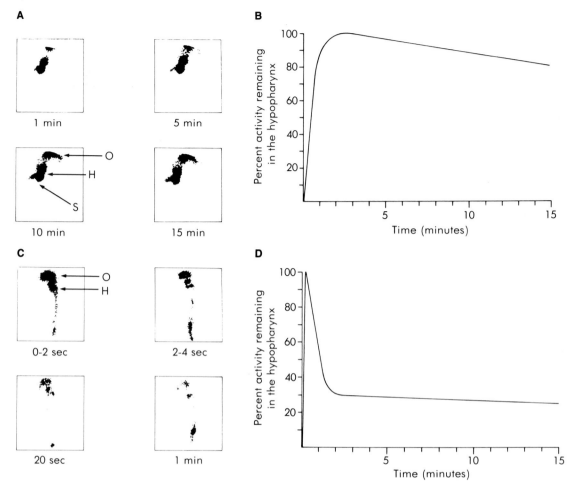

Fig. 24-4. Preoperative and postoperative radionuclide studies of hypopharyngeal clearance. The patient was standing in front of a scintillation camera interfaced to a computer. She swallowed 15 ml of water labeled with 0.5 mCi of technetium 99m sulfur colloid. Digital data acquisition was performed at 0.5-second intervals for 2 minutes and then at 5-second intervals for a total duration of 15 minutes. **A,** Preoperative analog images of the radionuclide pharyngoesophagogram. Anterior analog images. There is a significant hypopharyngeal radionuclide stasis, which persisted throughout the study. *O,* Oral activity; *H,* hypopharynx; *S,* level of upper esophageal sphincter. **B,** Preoperative radionuclide hypopharyngeal clearance. Time activity curve derived from a region of interest placed over the hypopharynx. At 15 minutes, only 20% of the initial ingested activity has cleared from the hypopharynx. **C,** Postoperative analog images of the radionuclide esophagogram. One week after a cricopharyngeal myotomy there was an increased hypopharyngeal emptying of the radionuclide bolus. **D,** Postoperative radionuclide hypopharyngeal clearance. Quantitative data obtained from a hypopharyngeal time-activity curve showed a clearance at 15 minutes of more than 75% of the initial activity. (Nuclear medicine studies courtesy Dr. R. Taillefer, Dept. of Nuclear Medicine, Hôtel-Dieu, Montreal.)

Winship, D.H.: Human upper esphageal sphincter: response to volume, osmotic and acid stimuli, Gastroenterology **75:**268, 1978.

8. Winans, C.S.: The pharyngoesophageal closure mechanism: a manometric study, Gastroenterology **63:**768, 1972.

9. Asherson, N.: Achalasia of the cricopharyngeal sphincter: a record of cases, with profile pharyngograms, J. Laryngol. **64:**747, 1950.

10. Ellis, F.H., Schlegel, J.F., Lynch, V.P., and Payne W.S.: Cricopharyngeal myotomy for pharyngoesophageal diverticulum, Ann. Surg. **170:**340, 1969.

11. Margulies, S.I., Brunt, P.W., Donner, M.W., and Silbiger, M.L.: Familial dysautonomia, Radiology **90:**107, 1968.

12. Kilman, W.J., and Goyal, R.L.: Disorders of pharyngeal and upper esophageal motor function, Arch. Intern. Med. **136:**592, 1976.

13. Fischer, R.A., Ellison, G.W., and Thayer, W.R.: Esophageal motility in neuromuscular disorders, Ann. Intern. Med. **63:**229, 1965.

14. Calne, D.B., Shaw, D.G., Spiers, A.S.D., and Stern, G.M.: Swallowing in Parkinsonism, Br. J. Radiol. **43:**456, 1970.

15. Nowack, W.J., Hatelid, J.M., and Sohn, R.S.: Dysphagia in Parkinsonism, Arch. Neurol. **34:**320, 1977.

16. Leopold, N.A., and Kagel, M.C.: Dysphagia in Huntington's disease, Arch. Neurol. **42:**57, 1985.

17. Cotzias, G.C., Papavasiliou, P.S., and Gellene, E.: Modification of Parkinsonism: chronic treatment with L-dopa, N. Engl. J. Med. **280:**337, 1969.

18. Daly, D.D., Code, C.F., and Anderson, H.A.: Disturbances of swallowing and esophageal motility in patients with multiple sclerosis, Neurology **12:**250, 1962.

19. Lebo, C.P., Sang, K., and Norris, F.H.: Cricopharyngeal myotomy in amyotrophic lateral sclerosis, Laryngoscope **86:**862, 1976.

20. Carpenter, R.J., McDonald, T.J., and Howard, F.M.: The otolaryngologic presentation of myasthenia gravis, Laryngoscope **89:**922, 1979.

21. Henderson, R.D., Boszko, A., and van Nostrand, A.W.P.: Pharyngoesophageal dysphagia and recurrent laryngeal nerve palsy, J. Thorac. Cardiovasc. Surg. **68:**507, 1974.

22. Akl, B.F., and Blakeley, W.R.: Late assessment of results of cricopharyngeal myotomy for cervical dysphagia, Am. J. Surg. **128:**818, 1974.

23. Bonavina, L., Khan, N.A., and DeMeester, T.R.: Pharyngoesophageal dysfunction: the role of cricopharyngeal myotomy, Arch. Surg. **120:**541, 1985.

24. Gay, I., Chisin, R., and Elidan, J.: Myotomy of the cricopharyngeus muscle: a treatment of dysphagia and aspiration in neurological disorders, Rev. Laryngol. Otol. Rhinol. (Bord.) **105:**271, 1984.

25. Loizou, L.A., Small, M., and Dalton, G.A.: Cricopharyngeal myotomy in motor neurone disease, J. Neurol. Neurosurg. Psychiatry, **43:**42, 1980.

26. Mills, C.P.: Dysphagia in pharyngeal paralysis treated by cricopharyngeal sphincterotomy, Lancet **1:**455, 1973.

27. Pierce, J.W., Creamer, B., MacDermot, V.: Pharynx and esophagus in dystrophia myotonica, Gut **6:**392, 1965.

28. Siegel, C.I., Hendrix, T.R., and Harvey, J.C.: The swallowing disorder in myotonia dystrophica, Gastroenterology **50:**541, 1966.

29. Hutchinson, J.M.: On ophtalmoplegia externa or symmetrical immobility (partial) of the eyes with ptosis, Trans. Med. Chir. Soc. Edinb. **62:**307, 1879.

30. Taylor, E.W.: Progressive vagus-glossopharyngeal paralysis with ptosis: a contribution to the group of family diseases, J. Nerv. Ment. Dis. **42:**129, 1915.

31. Duranceau, A., Forand, M.D., and Fauteux, J.P.: Surgery in oculopharyngeal muscular dystrophy, Am. J. Surg. **139:**33, 1980.

32. Montgomory, W.W., and Lynch, J.P.: Oculopharyngeal muscular dystrophy treated by inferior constrictor myotomy, Trans. Am. Acad. Ophthalmol. Otolaryngol. **75:** 986, 1971.

33. Dietz, F., Logemann, J.A., Sahgal, V., and Schmid, F.R.: Cricopharyngeal muscle dysfunction in the differential diagnosis of dysphagia polymyositis, Arthritis Rheum. **23:**491, 1980.

34. Metheny, J.A.: Dermatomyositis: a vocal and swallowing disease entity, Laryngoscope **88:**147, 1978.

35. Branski, D., Levy, J., Globus, M., Aviad, I., Keren A., and Chowers, I.: Dysphagia as a primary manifestation of hyperthyroidism, J. Clin. Gastroenterol. **6:**437, 1984.

36. Brookes, G.B.: Pharyngeal stenosis in Behçet's syndrome, Arch. Otolaryngol. **109:**338, 1983.

37. Mladick, R.A., Horton, C.E., and Adamson, J.E.: Cricopharyngeal myotomy: application and technique in major oral-pharyngeal resections, Arch. Surg. **102:**1, 1971.

38. Bonnano, P.C.: Swallowing dysfunction after tracheostomy, Ann. Surg. **174:**29, 1971.

39. Gamache, F.W., and Voorhies, R.M.: Hypertrophic cervical osteophytes causing dysphagia, J. Neurosurg. **53:**338, 1980.

40. Lambert, J.R., Tepperman, P.S., Jimenez, J., and Newman, A.: Cervical spine disease and dysphagia, Am. J. Gastroenterol. **76:**35, 1981.

41. Ekberg, O., and Nylander, G.: Webs and web-like formations in the pharynx and cervical esophagus, Diagn. Imag. Clin. Med. **52:**10, 1983.

42. Hunt, P.S., Connell, A.M., and Smiley T.B.: The cricopharyngeal sphincter in gastric reflux, Gut **11:**303, 1970.

43. Belsey, R.: Functional disease of the esophagus, J. Thorac. Cardiovasc. Surg. **52:**164, 1966.

44. Henderson, R.D., and Marryatt, G.: Cricopharyngeal myotomy as a method of treating cricopharyngeal dysphagia secondary to gastroesophageal reflux, J. Thorac. Cardiovasc. Surg. **74:**721, 1977.

45. Henderson, R.D., Woolf, C., and Marryatt, C.: Pharyngoesophageal dysphagia and gastroesophageal reflux, Laryngoscope **86:**1531, 1976.

46. Orringer, M.B.: Extended cervical esophagomyotomy for cricopharyngeal dysfunction, J. Thorac. Cardiovasc. Surg. **80:**669, 1980.

47. Watson, W.C., and Sullivan, S.N.: Hypertonicity of cricopharyngeal sphincter: cause of globus sensation, Lancet **2:**1417, 1974.

48. Sutherland, H.D.: Cricopharyngeal achalasia, J. Thorac. Cardiovasc. Surg. **43:**114, 1962.

Pharyngeal dysphagia

DISCUSSION

Adolfo Benages and F. Mora

Dr. Lafontaine's excellent review updates the clinical, diagnostic, and therapeutic problems of oropharyngeal dysphagia (OD), and we agree with him in his analysis of the physiologic mechanisms of swallowing, and with his evaluation of clinical inspection, endoscopy, and radiology as diagnostic tools.

An interesting aspect of the study of oropharyngeal emptying is the utilization of isotopes, since this permits one to quantify the efficiency of the oropharyngeal pump and its coordination with the relaxation of the upper esophageal sphincter; it also shows the behavior of the intraluminal content by visual images. Radionuclide studies of hypopharyngeal clearance demonstrate the deterioration of oropharyngeal emptying but do not permit a pathophysiologic or precise diagnosis. Their main value could be to control the therapy of patients suffering from OD.

In our opinion, esophageal manometry is an excellent method for the study of OD, especially when it is of the motor type. Lafontaine's objections about the reproducibility of manometric data are obviated with current techniques: (1) The hydropneumocapillary infusion system (low compliance) allows the exact recording of rapid pressure variations in this zone,[1,2] and the same results are obtained with use of the microtransducers, which do not require liquid perfusion, an additional advantage. (2) The radial disposition of three, four, or six orifices in the current catheters enables us to analyze the radial asymmetry of the UES and to obtain mean values for each withdrawal.

Esophageal manometry allows the quantification of static and dynamic motor phenomena with reproducible data if adequate techniques are used. This method also quantifies the oropharyngeal motor power (deglutition wave amplitude), the relaxation of the UES, and the coordination between them, as well as the sphincteric tone; that is; it analyzes the behavior of the muscular wall at this level. The coordination between pharyngeal contraction and sphincteric relaxation is the most difficult parameter to analyze. To do this we have used the "pharyngosphincteric synergic ratio" (PSSR); in physiologic conditions it will be equal to or greater than 1.[3]

Manometric data also allow the pathophysiologic classification of pharyngocricopharyngeal motor disorders (see box below) and provide a good understanding of the pathology of this digestive segment.

Esophageal manometry indicates the type of motor disorder in each patient with OD of functional origin. Thus, in patients with Wallenberg's syndrome, whose pathology is precisely reported by Lafontaine, only the manometry shows the motor disorders that produce dysphagia (see Table 24-4). In these patients, the dynamic parameters are most affected, while UES tone lies in the normal range.

The relationship between gastroesophageal reflux (GER) and the UES is complex, and since the reports of Hunt et al.[4] and Belsey[5] there has been increasing interest in this subject. Our work has confirmed the existence, in some of these patients, of sphincteric hypertony, which normalizes after surgical correction of GER.[6] It has already been demonstrated that patients with

---

MOTOR DISORDERS OF THE UES AND HYPOPHARYNX (MANOMETRIC CLASSIFICATION)

A. Resting:
  1. Hypotonic UES
  2. Hypertensive UES
B. Deglutition:
  1. Insufficient pharyngeal contraction
  2. Insufficient UES relaxation
  3. Pharyngocricopharyngeal incoordination

TABLE 24-4. Manometric data and clinical results after cricopharyngeal myotomy in patients with oropharyngeal dysphagia

	UES tone	Pharyngeal contraction	UES relaxation	Incoordination (pharyngeal-UES)	Clinical results after myotomy
Wallenberg's syndrome					
Case 1	Normal	Normal	↓	Yes	Good
Case 2	Normal	↓	↓	Yes	Bad
Case 3	↓	Normal	None	—	Acceptable
Case 4	Normal	↓	↓	Yes	Good
Case 5	Normal	↓	↓	Yes	Good
Zenker's Diverticula					
Case 6	Normal	Normal	Normal	Yes	Good
Case 7	↓	Normal	Normal	Yes	Good
Cricopharyngeal Achalasia					
Case 8	Normal	Normal	None	—	Good
Case 9	Normal	Normal	None	—	Good
Case 10	Normal	Normal	None	—	Good

TABLE 24-5. UES pressure (mean ± SE) in patients with reflux esophagitis (RE)

	Control group (A)	RE with regurgitation (B)	RE without regurgitation (C)
Patients	10	14	18
UES pressure (mm Hg)	84.6 ± 5.35	55.7 ± 3.6	76.2 ± 5.04

A versus B: p < 0.05; B versus C: p < 0.05; A versus C: NS

GER and regurgitation show UES hypotony, while patients without regurgitation show a UES tone similar to that of normal subjects,[7] and our data[8] are in agreement with this hypothesis (see Table 24-5).

In addition to disorders of tone in these patients, we have also observed incoordination between pharyngeal contraction and sphincter relaxation, as described by Henderson and Marryatt.[9] From our series of 100 patients with reflux esophagitis who were subjected to antireflux surgery, incoordination was observed before surgery in 15% of these patients; this decreased to 5% after surgical treatment, and none of these patients needed cricopharyngeal myotomy.

Idiopathic dysfunction of the UES groups together a series of motor disorders without specific cause. We reserve the denomination of cricopharyngeal achalasia[9] to define the insufficient relaxation of the UES in the absence of any known pathologic condition. We have studied three newborn babies with serious OD who needed prolonged nasogastric intubation but had no other pathology; they were diagnosed, by esophageal manometry, as having cricopharyngeal achalasia (see Table 24-4). The lack of specific

maturation could be the pathogenic basis of the dysfunction in these babies.

The pharyngosphincter motor disorders that appear in subjects with Zenker's diverticula cannot be included in the concept of cricopharyngeal achalasia, since there is adequate UES relaxation. The incoordination between pharyngeal contraction and sphincter relaxation, demonstrated by esophageal manometry (PSSR < 1), could be the pathogenic basis.

Although, as reported by Lafontaine, we agree that cricopharyngeal myotomy is indicated in some patients with OD, we must add that it should not be performed if GER is present, since myotomy facilitates regurgitation and the possibility of tracheal aspiration. Thus, we must add to these criteria the demonstration of a normal gastroesophageal junction.

Table 24-4 shows the clinical results of a personal series of 10 patients with OD of different causes who were submitted to cricopharyngeal myotomy. The clinical follow-up was performed 1 year after surgical treatment, with good results when dysphagia completely disappeared; acceptable results when dysphagia improved but persisted sporadically; and poor results when dysphagia was unaltered, with deterioration of the general condition. According to our data, in 80% of the patients with motor OD who are submitted to cricopharyngeal myotomy, dysphagia disappears; the worst results are observed in patients with neurogenic dysphagia (Wallenberg's syndrome).

REFERENCES

1. Dodds, W.J., Stef, J.J., and Hogan, W.J.: Factors determining pressure measurement accuracy by intraluminal esophageal manometry, Gastroenterology **70:**117-123, 1976.
2. Tomas-Ridocci, M., Mora, F., Molina, R., et al.: Manometria esofagica: sistema de infusion continua por jeringas frente a sistema hidroneumocapilar, Gastroenterol. Hepatol. (Barcelona), **7:**181-187, 1984.
3. Benages, A., Tomas-Ridocci, M., Civera, R.G., et al.: Estudio de la funcion motora del esofago y sus esfinteres: tecnica y analisis de trazados manometricos, Rev. Esp. Enferm. Apar. Dig. **41:**1-20, 1973.
4. Hunt, P.S., Connell, A.M., and Smiley, T.B.: The cricopharyngeal sphincter in gastric reflux, Gut **11:** 303-306, 1970.
5. Belsey, R.: Functional disease of the esophagus, J. Thorac. Cardiovasc. Surg. **52:**164-188, 1966.
6. Mora, F., Benages, A., Molina, R., et al.: El esfinter cricofaringeo y sus modificaciones tras la cirugia de la hernia hiatal, Gastroenterol. Hepatol. (Barcelona) **3:**15-19, 1980.
7. Gerhardt, D.C., Castell, D.O., Winship, D.H., and Shuck, T.J.: Esophageal dysfunction in esophago-pharyngeal regurgitation, Gastroenterology **78:**893-897, 1980.
8. Benages, A., and Mora, F.: Unpublished data.
9. Henderson, R.D., and Marryatt, G.: Cricopharyngeal myotomy as a method of treating cricopharyngeal dysphagia secondary to gastroesophageal reflux, J. Thorac. Cardiovasc. Surg. **74:**721-725, 1977.
10. Asherson, N.: Achalasia of cricopharyngeal sphincter: a record of cases, with profile pharyngograms, J. Laringol. Otol. **64:**747-758, 1950.

CHAPTER **25** Cricopharyngeal myotomy for pharyngoesophageal diverticula

Toni Lerut, J. Vandekerkhof, Guido Leman,
Paul J. Guelinckx, R. Dom, and Jacques A. Gruwez

A pharyngoesophageal diverticulum (Zenker's diverticulum) is a protrusion of the hypopharyngeal mucosa posteriorly between the oblique fibers of the inferior pharyngeal constrictor and the transverse fibers of the cricopharyngeus muscle. Its origin still remains unclear. For a long time this condition was considered as a strictly mechanical entity, with the diverticulum obstructing the esophagus by its volume and dependent position. Manometric studies, however, revealed the delicate and coordinated sequence of the swallowing act, in which the relaxation of an upper esophageal sphincter seems to play a major role. In this respect, several theories have been proposed to explain the genesis of a diverticulum. Ellis and Crozier in 1981[1] stated that premature contraction of the upper sphincter is one of the mechanisms that might account for upper esophageal dysphagia and pharyngoesophageal diverticula. According to Knuff et al. in 1982,[2] however, there is no incoordination at all, the sphincter pressure being normal in patients with pharyngoesophageal diverticula. So the basic mechanism responsible for the genesis of these diverticula remains unsolved, partly because of the lack of accurate manometric techniques used in this particular field.

Several different studies also mention the association between pharyngoesophageal diverticula and gastroesophageal reflux. Smiley in 1972[3] found gastroesophageal reflux in 28 of 30 patients with a pharyngoesophageal diverticulum. Hunt et al. in 1970[4] demonstrated a higher basal upper sphincter pressure in patients with gastroesophageal reflux, returning to normal values after antireflux surgery, suggesting that pharyngoesophageal pouches result from cricopharyngeal dysfunction caused by reflux. Henderson in 1976[5] showed an incoordination at the upper sphincter in the sense of a premature contraction in patients with gastroesophageal reflux complaining of upper dysphagia. In a study of 200 patients with reflux he noticed the presence of pharyngoesophageal dysphagia in 100 patients, disappearing in 90% of them after antireflux surgery.

Belsey in 1972[6] made a clear distinction between diverticula resulting from primary dysfunction of the upper sphincter and diverticula resulting from spasm secondary to gastroesophageal reflux. In this second group, when a small diverticulum occurs, the correction of the reflux can be sufficient to solve the problem of the diverticulum and leads to its disappearance.

MATERIAL AND METHODS

In order to evaluate the role of the upper esophageal sphincter in the treatment of Zenker's diverticulum, a retrospective study of our patients was performed, dealing with 95 patients divided into two groups (see Table 25-1). Some additional information will be used from a study performed on behalf of the Groupement Européen d'Etude des Maladies de l'Oesophage (GEEMO), dealing with 390 cases treated in 15 different European centers. Group I patients were treated by a simple diverticulectomy, whereas in group II the chosen treatment was an extramucosal myotomy with diverticulopexy. In all patients the diagnosis was made on clinical history confirmed by x-ray studies.

Endoscopic examination was performed in all patients in group II. However, an examination of the whole esophagus and stomach was possible in

TABLE 25-1. Pharyngoesophageal diverticulum, 1955-1984: 95 patients

Group I (1955-1975):	1 dilatation, 36 diverticulectomies
Group II (1976-1984):	58 diverticulopexies + myotomy

only 11 patients. Usually the scope will be unable to pass the cricopharyngeus muscle and will instead pass into the pouch. Although there is theoretically some risk of perforation, endoscopy is performed in every patient in order to exclude the presence of a carcinoma within the diverticulum. Indeed, carcinoma in Zenker's diverticulum has been reported occasionally (for example, by Kuwano et al. in 1982[7]) and should be ruled out especially when diverticulopexy will be performed. Equally, preoperative manometric studies of the upper sphincter are difficult to perform and were only possible in eleven patients. Twenty-four hour pH studies to confirm the diagnosis of associated gastroesophageal reflux were performed in 16 patients since 1982 either preoperatively or postoperatively.

Biopsies for microscopic examination were taken in eight patients. In order to evaluate the role of the cricopharyngeus as the genesis of pharyngoesophageal diverticulum, enzyme histochemistry (NADH-Tr-ATP pH 4.9, pH 4.65, pH 4.3) and contractile properties testing according to the method of Faulkner et al.,[8] were performed. Biopsy material for enzyme histochemistry was obtained from 10 patients with a Zenker diverticulum and from three patients with no history of cricopharyngeal pathology (organ donor patients). Contractile properties were studied on material obtained from three patients with Zenker's diverticulum and two patients with no cricopharyngeal pathology.

RESULTS

Dysphagia and regurgitation are typical symptoms present in all our patients, regardless of the

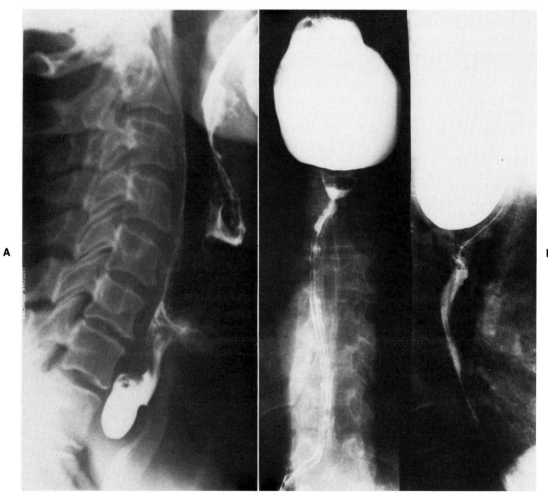

Fig. 25-1. Examples of a classic diverticulum **(A)** and a giant diverticulum **(B),** showing anterior and posterior and lateral views. Note in the lateral view the anterior deviation of the esophagus caused by the diverticulum.

size of the diverticulum (see Fig. 25-1). The average duration of symptoms was 25 months. The combination of old age (the average age was 70.5 years [ranging from 38 to 92 years]) and the high incidences of associated cachexia (29%) and severe pulmonary infection (36%) resulting from regurgitation and aspiration clearly illustrates the catastrophic situation to which Zenker's diverticulum may lead (see Table 25-2, group II).

Surgery was performed under general anesthesia in all patients. As already mentioned, our actual technique of choice is an extramucosal myotomy of the upper esophageal sphincter combined with a diverticulopexy. This operation is performed through a left cervical incision. The

TABLE 25-2. Incidences of associated pathologic conditions (percent)

	Group I	Group II
Cachexia	10	29
Pulmonary infections	28	36
Perforated diverticulum	3	1.7
Gastrointestinal		
Hiatal hernia and/or		
reflux	8	23
Achalasia	8	0
Gastric diverticulum	8	0
Gastroduodenal ulcer	8	11
Colonic diverticulosis	0	5
Spastic colon	0	1.7
Pancreatitis	0	1.7
Cholecystitis	0	1.7
Thyroid goiter	0	3
Cancer	0	0

pouch is completely freed up to its neck. The extramucosal myotomy incision is carried out over the anterolateral aspect of the upper esophagus, starting at the cricopharyngeus muscle and extending upward for 1 to 2 cm through the inferior constrictor of the pharynx above the neck of the pouch and downward for 4 to 5 cm into the upper esophagus. Only a very small pouch (less than 2 cm) will be left untouched. All other diverticula will be inverted behind the pharynx and, with sufficient tension to eliminate any prolapse of the pouch below the neck of the sac, firmly sutured to the anterior vertebral ligament with a series of interrupted mattress monofilament 4-0 sutures. These sutures are passed through the flattened diverticulum, right through its lumen, near its periphery, in the form of an inverted horseshoe, and serve to obliterate the pouch as well as to maintain its inversion and dependent drainage (see Fig. 25-2).

In the first group, three patients died. There was no fatal outcome with myotomy and diverticulopexy, probably merely as a result of better reanimation techniques and postoperative care in the second period rather than as a result of switching to another surgical technique.

The early postoperative complications in our patients were higher in group I and are related to the more extensive dissection and opening of the esophageal lumen in cases in which diverticulectomy was performed. This also was noticed in the GEEMO study, in which the most important complications, such as fistulas, abscesses, and hematomas, were found when a diverticulectomy was performed (see Table 25-3). It is interesting to notice that in cases in which a diverticulec-

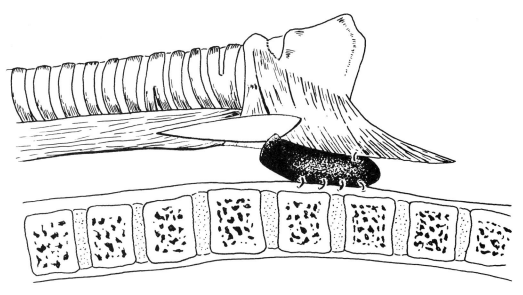

Fig. 25-2. Extramucosal myotomy of the upper esophageal sphincter zone and diverticulopexy.

TABLE 25-3. Complications* of operations for pharyngoesophageal diverticulum (GEEMO study, 390 patients)

	Diverticulectomy (184/390)	Diverticulectomy + extramucosal myotomy (121/390)	Diverticulopexy + extramucosal myotomy (55/390)	Extramucosal myotomy (26/390)	Diverticulopexy (4/390)	Total (%)
Fistula	8	4	0	0	0	12 (3)
Abscess	11	3	0	0	0	14 (3.5)
Hematoma	3	2	2	0	0	7 (1.8)
Recurrent nerve paralysis	5	1	1	0	0	7 (1.8)
Phonetic troubles	6	2	2	0	0	10 (2.5)
Claude-Bernard-Horner	0	0	1	0	0	1
Other	7	1	1	0	0	9 (2.3)
	40/184 (21.7%)	13/121 (10.7%)	7/55 (12.7%)	—	—	60/390 (15.4%)

Perioperative: 1% (4/390); Postoperative: 15.4% (60/390).

TABLE 25-4. Morbidity

	Group I (36 patients)	Group II (58 patients)
Mean duration of hospitalization	12.8 days	8.3 days
Mean duration of nasogastric tube	8.2 days	1.5 days
Mean duration of wound drainage	5.2 days	3.3 days

tomy was performed, the incidence of fistulas was twice as high if no extramucosal myotomy was added to the resection. This may suggest that the cricopharyngeus plays an obstructing role favoring a fistula formation.

Besides resulting in a lower complication rate, avoiding the opening of the esophageal lumen also allows the patient to eat almost immediately after the operation, without the need for a nasogastric tube, reducing morbidity, which is of the utmost importance for geriatric patients (see Table 25-4). In fact, we now remove the nasogastric tube immediately after the operation, and hospitalization usually lasts about 4 days. A nasogastric tube is always gently introduced before operation in order to prevent sudden aspiration from the pouch during intubation. In the long-term follow-up (the average follow-up being 4 years, and ranging from 6 mo to 8½ years), patients were evaluated clinically and by radiocinematography. In group II the follow-up was 100%; 95% of the patients were considered as excellent to very good (see Fig. 25-3), and 82% were judged completely asymptomatic. One patient required a second intervention—a second myotomy on the controlateral side—to solve the problem of persistent dysphagia. A possible primary muscle disease might explain the unsatisfactory result of the first operation.

Recently, routine biopsies of the cricopharyngeus for pathologic examination have been taken. Great care has been taken to obtain these biopsies without damaging the muscle tissue. No clear evidence of an underlying neurogenic or muscular pathology was found in any of the eight specimens. Some signs of muscular involution—for example, some minor degree of muscle damage and fibrosis, probably related to old age—were incidentally noticed. Such minor degrees of muscle damage, however, were also described by Cruse et al. in 1979[9] in postmortem specimens obtained from patients without any dysphagia or esophageal pathology during life. Therefore it cannot be concluded that these minor pathologic findings are a possible cause of the

A   B

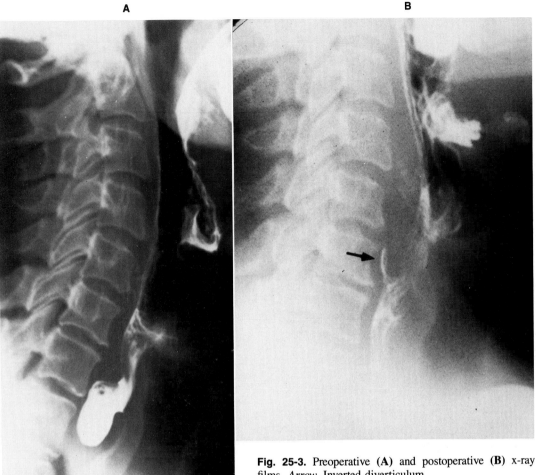

Fig. 25-3. Preoperative **(A)** and postoperative **(B)** x-ray films. *Arrow,* Inverted diverticulum.

onset of cricopharyngeal dysphagia or contribute to the genesis of a pharyngoesophageal diverticulum. In addition, it cannot be assessed whether these changes are occurring before or after and secondary to the onset of the diverticulum

Enzyme histochemistry shows that in the normal cricopharyngeus a type II fiber predominance exists. By contrast, in all cases with Zenker's diverticulum a type I fiber predominance was noticed, sometimes with a large variation in diameter, the latter suggesting a neurogenic disorder. For evaluation of contractility properties, the contraction time or time to peak twitch tension (PTT), one-half relaxation time (½ RT), amplitude (AMP), and velocity of force increment ($\Delta P/\Delta T$) were measured.

Despite the small number of examined specimens, the results indicate a tendency to less absolute force in Zenker's diverticulum, compared with the normal cricopharyngeus muscle.

Muscle contraction also seems to be slower in Zenker's muscle specimens.

Radiologic examination showed that one patient had an insufficient diverticulopexy but without any consequence since the operation 9 years previously. This illustrates the important role of the extramucosal myotomy.

Finally, a third patient had disturbances of deglutition with aspiration of contrast material persisting after operation because of a meningioma with involvement of the glossopharyngeal nerve.

Special attention has been paid to the possible association of gastroesophageal reflux and cricopharyngeal dysfunction. Associated reflux was detected in only 8% of the patients in group I but in 23% of the patients in group II (see Table 25-2). This latter percentage was confirmed in the GEEMO study, in which 25.5% of the patients had an associated hiatal hernia and/or

TABLE 25-5. Manometric results: rapid pull-through (maximal pressures ± SD, mm Hg), 11 patients

	Posterior	Anterior	Left	Right
Preoperative	98.3 ± 48.5	73.1 ± 67.1	25.4 ± 13.4	33.6 ± 16.7
Postoperative	74.8 ± 36.9	68.7 ± 34.2	22 ± 8.2	24.4 ± 12.5

reflux. The diagnosis of an associated hiatal hernia and/or reflux was made mainly on the clinical and x-ray findings. Perhaps the true incidence of reflux is lower than the above-mentioned figures. Additional information from the more recently performed 24-hour pH studies will be necessary to confirm these data. However, it is well known that the incidences of hiatal hernia and reflux are increasing in the elderly population. Consequently, the question remains whether this high percentage is not just a coincidence without any correlation with the genesis of pharyngoesophageal diverticula, since 56% of the patients in our series were older than 70 years and 30% older than 80 years. One third of those patients with associated reflux were asymptomatic, which also is consistent with the fact that elderly people frequently suffer from severe esophagitis without any symptoms.

After performance of a myotomy and diverticulopexy, it seems logical to add an antireflux procedure in those patients who present with an associated hiatal hernia and/or reflux, since the destruction of the upper sphincter abolishes the last barrier protecting the patients against aspiration pneumonitis caused by the refluxing gastric juice. However, as already mentioned, 56% of our patients were older than 70 years, one third having a severe pneumonitis and another one third being cachectic, seriously increasing the operative risk of a simultaneous antireflux operation. So eventually only two patients underwent a simultaneous operation for the diverticulum and reflux.

Although the purpose was to perform this antireflux operation in a second stage for the remaining patients, no patient, in contrast to what one could expect, developed an important or fatal pulmonary complication that could be related to aspiration during the long-term follow-up. Consequently, no further antireflux surgery has been performed. These findings are clearly in disagreement with the statement of Hurwitz et al. in 1979[10] that in the absence of adjuvant antireflux surgery, there is a high risk of serious or fatal pulmonary complications after myotomy of the cricopharyngeus. The explanation probably lies in the fact that the myotomy of the upper sphincter only diminishes the upper sphincter pressures without abolishing them, as has been shown in the preoperative and postoperative manometric studies performed in 11 of our patients (see Table 25-5 and Fig. 25-4).

In the long-term follow-up of patients treated with a simple diverticulectomy (group I), seven of the surviving patients were reexamined; one patient had a symptomatic partial stenosis at the operative site. Six other patients were asymptomatic, but all of them showed on x-ray film a recurrence or a spastic-like ring at the level of the upper sphincter. Four out of these six had proven esophageal reflux. Manometric studies performed in two of these patients did not reveal any significant abnormality in the sphincter pressure or any incoordination.

CONCLUSIONS

Pharyngoesophageal diverticulum frequently occurs in geriatric patients. Associated aspiration pneumonitis and cachexia may result in a catastrophic deterioration of their general condition. Diverticulopexy combined with extramucosal myotomy of the upper esophageal sphincter zone is our treatment of choice, with no mortality and minimum of morbidity.

The long-term follow-up results are excellent in more than 90% of the patients. With this treatment the absence of a simultaneous or late correction of associated reflux does not result in a higher incidence of aspiration pneumonitis. This can be explained by the fact that the sphincter pressure after myotomy is not completely abolished.

The myotomy is believed to play an essential role in the relief of the dysphagia. This is based on clinical grounds and on the results of the enzymehistochemistry and contractility studies.

Enzyme histochemistry of the cricopharyngeus muscle reveals a change from type II to type I muscle fibers in Zenker's diverticulum, with features suggesting a neurogenic disorder. The preponderance of type I fibers with tonic postural function capable of sustained contraction might explain local hypertony causing cricopharyngeal dysphagia and/or Zenker's diverticulum. Contractility studies seem to support the idea of a change from quickly activated, powerful contraction capacity (type II fibers), toward a more slowly

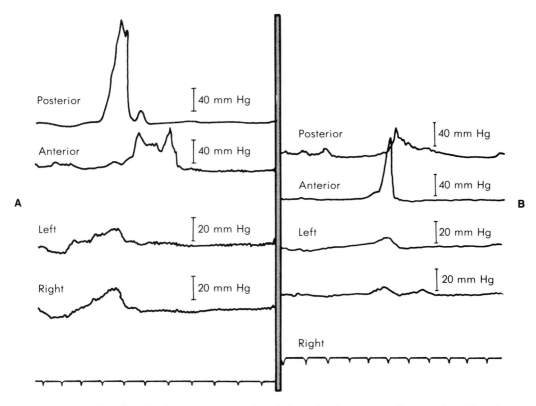

Fig. 25-4. Four-directional manometric study of the cricopharyngeous. Preoperative (**A**) and postoperative (**B**) studies after myotomy and diverticulopexy. Sphincter pressure is decreased but not abolished.

activated, less powerful but more sustained contraction pattern (type I fibers). The slower contraction pattern may also indicate a possible incomplete relaxation of the sphincter and some incoordination during swallowing. Nevertheless no major muscle changes were found at pathologic examination, and preoperative manometric studies did not reveal any incoordination or any abnormalities in resting pressures or length of the upper esophageal sphincter compared with the values in a normal population as measured by Pelemans in 1983.[11]

Despite a high incidence of associated gastroesophageal reflux, there is still no proof that reflux might be responsible for the pathogenesis of pharyngoesophageal diverticula. The etiology of the pharyngoesophageal diverticulum therefore remains unclarified.

REFERENCES

1. Ellis, F.H., Jr., and Crozier, R.E.: Cervical oesophageal dysphagia, Ann. Surg. **194:**279-289, 1981.
2. Knuff, T.E., Benjamin, S.B., and Castell, D.O.: Pharyngo-esophageal (Zenker's) diverticulum: a reappraisal, Gastroenterology **82:**734-736, 1982.
3. Smiley, T.B.: Pressure studies in the upper oesophagus in relation to hiatus hernia. In Smith, R.A., and Smith, R.E., editors: Surgery of the oesophagus, London, 1972, Butterworths, pp. 152-158.
4. Hunt, P.S., Connell, A.M., and Smiley, T.B.: The cricopharyngeal sphincter in gastro-esophageal reflux, Gut **11:**303-306, 1970.
5. Henderson, R.D.: Motor disorders of the esophagus, Baltimore, 1976, the Williams & Wilkins Co., p. 188.
6. Belsey, R.H.R.: Disorders of function of the oesophagus. In Smith, R.A., and Smith R.E., editors: Surgery of the oesophagus, London, 1972, Butterworths, pp. 193-216.
7. Kuwano, H., Sugimachi, K., and Inokuch, K.: Squamous cell carcinoma in a middle esophageal (parabronchial) diverticulum, Jpn. J. Surg. **12:**266-269, 1982.
8. Faulkner, J.A., Claflin, D.R., Mac Cully, K.K., and Jones, D.A.: Contractile properties of bundles of fiber segments from skeletal muscles, Am. J. Physiol. **243** (Cell Physiol. 12): C66-C73, 1982.
9. Cruse, J.P., Edwards, D.A., Smith, J.F., and Wyllie, J.H.: The pathology of cricopharyngeal dysphagia, Histopathology **3:**223-232, 1979.
10. Hurwitz, A.L., Duranceau, A., and Haddad, J.K.: Disorders of esophageal motility, Philadelphia, 1979, W.B. Saunders Co., pp. 67-84.
11. Pelemans, W.: Functie van de pharyngo-esophagale overgangszone en dysfunctie bij bejaarden, thesis, Leuven, 1983, p. 58.

Cricopharyngeal myotomy for pharyngoesophageal diverticula

DISCUSSION

André Duranceau and Glyn G. Jamieson

The work presented by Dr. Lerut and associates underlines a number of important aspects concerning the diagnosis and treatment of pharyngoesophageal diverticulum. The review of our retrospective experience with this condition will serve as a basis for discussion.

One hundred and twenty patients were evaluated and treated in our institution between 1949 and 1984. Sixty-four percent were males and 36% were females. The mean age of the group was 62 years and the peak incidence (34%) of the condition was seen in the sixth decade, while 28% of the patients were over 70. All patients were symptomatic, and the duration of symptoms was less than 3 years in 48% of the group and over 3 years for 42%. In order of frequency, symptoms were oropharyngeal dysphagia (98%), fresh food regurgitation (85%), aspiration (61%), cervical bruit on swallowing (32%), halitosis (25%), respiratory complication (17%), and voice change (13%). On physical examination 36% of patients had lost weight, and in 26% a bruit could be elicited on neck palpation.

The evaluation of the patient with a pharyngoesophageal diverticulum was mostly radiologic. The esophagogram was observed in all patients and showed a diverticulum smaller than 1 cm in 4% of the patients, between 1 and 2 cm in 20%, and over 2 cm in 76% of the group. The diverticulum was located on the midline in 67% of the examinations. For 22% of the patients it was median and protruded toward the left neck,

while in 10% of the group it was seen to protrude to the right. Eleven percent showed an associated hiatal hernia. The chest x-ray film revealed a 4% incidence of pneumonia and 4% of accompanying atelectasis.

Esophagoscopy was performed in 25% of all cases of diverticula evaluated and treated. In these patients the proximal esophageal opening was considered narrowed in 16% of the cases, while 3% showed a distal stricture with ulcerative esophagitis.

During the past 10 years, manometric evaluation of the proximal esophageal sphincter has been performed in all patients in whom the procedure was made possible by easy intubation. A detailed report on the initial 10 patients evaluated before and after surgical treatment[1] shows a normal relaxation of the upper esophageal sphincter (UES) in 88% of swallows and a premature contraction of the UES against the pharyngeal contraction in 28% of the swallows. The resting pressure of the sphincter and the closing pressure of the UES are significantly lower than in controls.

Treatment changed between the initial period of the study and the last 15 years (see Table 25-6). Between 1949 and 1969, 40 patients underwent a diverticulectomy and only one had a myotomy with a diverticulopexy. During the last 15 years, 54 had a myotomy with a diverticulum suspension while 25 had a diverticulectomy with or without a myotomy. During the past 9 years only

TABLE 25-6. Pharyngoesophageal diverticulum: treatment

	1949-1969	1970-1984	Total
Divertculectomy	40	11	51
Myotomy and suspension	1	54	55
Diverticulectomy and myotomy	—	14	14

358

two patients required a diverticulectomy with the upper sphincter myotomy. All the other patients had a myotomy with a diverticulum suspension. One hundred and ten of 120 patients had an uneventful recuperation after surgery (see Table 25-7). A wound infection was observed in six patients. Half of these were associated with a fistula, which was documented in a total of three patients. One fistula occurred following a myotomy and diverticulum suspension. Four patients suffered cardiorespiratory complications, and two patients showed a recurrent laryngeal nerve paralysis. Mortality resulted from cardiac complications and occurred in two patients.

The diagnosis of a pharyngoesophageal diverticulum is usually made from the patient's history and then confirmed radiologically. Patient populations may vary, as shown from the series presented: 56% of the patients of Lerut and associates are over 70 years of age, and more than 30% of his group are older than 80. Our group shows a mean age of 63, with only 28% of the patients over 70 and 3% over 80. This is certainly one factor that can influence morbidity and mortality.

Dysphagia well localized to the neck region and regurgitations of undigested food are by far the most common presenting symptoms. It is noteworthy that acute respiratory symptoms are not common in our group while they are predominant in the European study. While 61% of our patients had symptoms of aspiration, 17% of the group showed respiratory complications in their evaluations. Despite the short duration of symptoms, the Belgian group shows a high incidence of cachexia with an equally high incidence of severe pulmonary infection resulting from regurgitation and aspiration. This difference might be related to later consultation and diagnosis, with a higher incidence of significant complications caused by dysfunction and obstruction at the upper esophageal sphincter level in an older and weaker population.

The dysphagia present in patients with a pharyngoesophageal diverticulum may be related to the mechanical factor imposed by the presence of the diverticulum or by the dysfunction of the pharyngoesophageal junction. Lahey and Warren[2] regarded phase I diverticula as small and relatively asymptomatic. However, these small pouches can be associated with disproportionate dysphagia,[3,4] and this can only be explained by incoordination of the swallowing mechanism. Undoubtedly enlargement of the diverticulum with forward pressure on the proximal esophagus adds a mechanical obstruction factor to the dysfunction. The large diverticulum in fact replaces the esophagus in its normal axis, and most of the material swallowed will transit into the diverticulum before being propelled toward the stomach or being regurgitated.

Radiology is the most important way of providing a definitive diagnosis for a pharyngoesophageal diverticulum. Cineradiography or videoradiography, when used, provides objective evidence of junctional derangements of the upper esophageal sphincter, when present. It is the only means of diagnosis of minute diverticula that can be observed only transiently in oropharyngeal dysphagia patients. These small outpouchings of mucosa that come and go at the posterior pharyngoesophageal region have been reported in 4% to 5% of normal people.[5,6] That these transient diverticula develop into permanent pouches remains logical but unproven. A smaller pouch probably causes fewer symptoms as a whole, since only 4% of patients consult a physician when they have a diverticulum smaller than 1 cm. In this group of patients an associated hiatal hernia was not specifically looked for. Eleven percent of the patients were found to have a sliding type of hernia present. In our experience when it was investigated prospectively, five out of 10 patients had a hiatal hernia. A number of reports have quoted an incidence ranging from

TABLE 25-7. Management of 120 patients with pharyngoesophageal diverticula

	1949-1969	1970-1984	Total	Percent
Morbidity				
None	38	72	110	91.6
Recurrent nerve	0	2	2	1.6
Wound infection	1	5	6	5
Esophagocutaneous fistula	0	3	3	2.5
Retropharyngeal hematoma	0	2	2	1.6
Intervertebral discitis	0	1	1	.8
Cardiopulmonary	2	2	4	3.3
Mortality	1	1	2	1.6

22% to greater than 90% of cases.[7,8,9] Endoscopy was advocated by Chevalier Jackson and Shallow[10] to diagnose the pharyngoesophageal diverticulum. However, today most regard this procedure as unnecessary and even dangerous. Lerut and associates report endoscopic examination of the diverticulum in all 58 patients who eventually underwent a myotomy and a diverticulopexy. No carcinoma was found in any of the patients. With the very low incidence of carcinoma occurring in a diverticulum, this examination should be used only when an attendant malignancy is suspected on radiology or at surgery. Despite this policy, esophageal problems frequently accompany a diverticulum of the pharyngoesophageal junction and may require endoscopic documentation of the condition. Our attitude is to perform esophagoscopy at the time of surgery if any malignancy or ulcer is suspected in the diverticulum. Full endoscopic evaluation of the esophagus is performed later, after correction of the diverticulum, if any esophageal condition requiring endoscopy accompanies the pharyngoesophageal problem.

Most authors regard pharyngoesophageal diverticulum as an acquired disorder with a pulsion origin—that is, developing because of forces from within the pharynx and esophagus. It was initially thought from endoscopic and cineradiographic studies that the cricopharyngeus failed to relax in front of the oncoming peristaltic wave in the pharynx. However, other theories on the dysfunction were developed, suggesting premature UES contraction, delayed relaxation, or simple spasm of the cricopharyngeus muscle. The development of manometric techniques since the 1950s helped to clarify the abnormalities present in association with a pharyngoesophageal diverticulum. However, as emphasized by Lerut and his colleagues, these studies are dependent on the accuracy of the manometric techniques and on the interpretation criteria. It becomes evident that the reported studies do not record all of the abnormalities present.

Kodicek and Creamer[11] reported normal resting pressures of relaxation and coordination in five patients with a pharyngoesophageal diverticulum. Pederson et al.[12] showed similar results and Lerut and co-workers report normal resting pressures when using a rapid-pull-through technique. In contrast, Ellis et al.[7] and Ellis and Crozier[13] report lower resting pressures in the sphincter, with an abnormal temporal relationship in 14% to 90% of swallows for seven patients initially and later in 10 more patients. The abnormality was interpreted as a premature relaxation of the sphincter so that the closing sphincter works against pharyngeal contraction. Duranceau et al.[1] reported similar observations in 10 patients, showing 28% of the swallows resulting in a premature sphincter closure against pharyngeal contraction (see Fig. 25-5). Lichter[14] observed a premature relaxation of the upper sphincter in 50% of swallows, and repetitive pharyngeal contractions were present in his patients. Knuff et al.[15] reported lower resting pressures in the sphincter but normal coordination. Hunt et al.[16] reported elevated sphincter pressures without observations on the relaxation and the coordination.

It seems reasonable to suppose that the differences in these numerous observations relate to technical factors associated with the actual recording techniques. When abnormalities are recorded, it is still unknown whether they are caused by sphincter dysfunction or by the excursion of the sphincter zone around the recording catheter. The mechanical effects of the diverticulum itself on the recording are not known. In some ways compression by the diverticulum could result in the various recording abnormalities reported. The process of diverticulum formation is probably very slow, with only a proportion of all swallows showing abnormal temporal

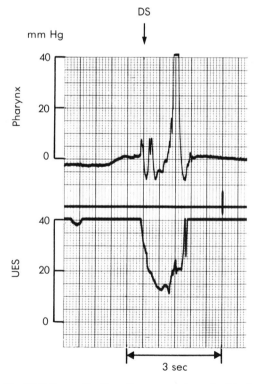

Fig. 25-5. Incoordination of upper esophageal sphincter closure against pharyngeal contraction in a patient with pharngoesophageal diverticulum.

relationships between the pharynx and the UES. Einharssen[17] observed no change in three small diverticula and a slow increase in size in five more patients. His patients were observed for 8 or more years after their initial diagnoses.

Despite the reported high incidence of oropharyngeal dysphagia in reflux disease,[18] other studies mention a 3% to 9% incidence of active reflux accompanying this condition.[3,19]

Treatment of pharyngoesophageal diverticula has changed over the years. This change took place possibly on the basis of the physiologic abnormalities reported, even if these remain open to discussion. The recurrence rate of the diverticulum following diverticulectomy may be another reason why such change has taken place. In our experience, diverticulectomy was initially the preferred method of treatment. A cricopharyngeal myotomy was subsequently added to the diverticulectomy, and in most recent years, cricopharyngeal myotomy with diverticulum suspension has become the preferred form of treatment. It seems that the same evolution has occurred in the experience of Dr. Lerut and associates. Interestingly, the GEEMO group of patients follows a different route, with a large majority undergoing a diverticulectomy with or without a myotomy.

Lahey[20] reported 82 patients treated by a first-stage operation in which the diverticulum was isolated and suspended; 3 weeks later the second stage of the operation consisted of removing the sac. This approach permitted the sealing of the mediastinum and a decrease in septic complications at a time when antibiotics were not easily available. When reporting a series of 365 patients so treated, Lahey and Warren[2] described twelve recurrences in 250 patients followed for more than 2½ years.

The one-stage operation was described by Chevalier Jackson and Shallow.[10] Later, Sweet[21] reported his results in 77 patients, with no mortality, one fistula, and two patients with persistent dysphagia. The Mayo Clinic reported its results with the one-stage operation.[22] In 888 patients treated between 1944 and 1978, the mortality was 1.2% and the recurrence rate 3.6%. A wound infection was seen in 3% of the patients, and more than half of these were associated with a fistula. Vocal cord paralysis was the other significant complication, occurring in 3.2% of the group. Long-term results observed after 5 to 14 years in 135 patients showed good to excellent control of symptoms in over 93% of patients. In parallel, it is very appropriate that Dr. Lerut and associates report a very similar morbidity through the GEEMO study: 3.5% abscess formation, 3% fistula formation, 1.8%

recurrent nerve paralysis, and 1.8% hematoma formation. Three deaths occurred in the 37 patients of the diverticulectomy group. Our experience with diverticulectomy correlates well with these observations.

These results need to be looked at with the notion that a recurring diverticulum possibly takes a long time to develop. Four long-term radiologic follow-up studies report a much higher recurrence rate than those just mentioned, following diverticulectomy alone. Nicholson[23] reported 13 recurrent pouches in 20 patients. Hansen et al.[24] showed a radiologic recurrence in three of 19 cases, while Holinger and Schild[25] and Einharssen[17] respectively reported 14 of 68 cases and 17 of 20 cases that recurred. In the Einharssen study, 12 of the pouches were small and five showed evidence of food retention. In all these series, although a radiologic recurrence was evident, the incidence of significant symptoms was much lower than before the initial operation.

When the one-stage diverticulectomy is compared with treatment by myotomy and diverticulum suspension, Dr. Lerut and associates suggest a global morbidity that is significantly less (12.7%) than that of diverticulectomy alone (21%). However, when a myotomy is added to the diverticulectomy, the resulting morbidity falls to 10%.

Myotomy of the upper esophageal sphincter for pharyngoesophageal diverticulum was initially reported by Aubin.[26] He described the diversion of the muscle and the excision of the diverticulum. Escher[27] modified the technique by opening the diverticulum and using his finger as a stent for the dissection of the cricopharyngeus. Kramer et al.[28] suggested that, although the manometric characteristics of the cricopharyngeus might be normal, it could still "get in the way" of the pharyngeal contraction and result in functional obstruction. These concepts resulted in a different approach toward the pharyngoesophageal diverticulum. The diverticulum became a complication of the muscular dysfunction, and the important gesture was to remove the abnormally functioning sphincter while either ignoring or suspending the diverticulum. Another approach is to follow the recommendations of Aubin and remove the diverticulum at the same time the myotomy is completed. Cricopharyngeal myotomy alone without attention to the diverticulum will bring permanent control of symptoms in only 78% of patients.[22] Ellis et al.[7] and Ellis and Crozier[13] reported two failures in patients who had a simple myotomy. It is very appropriate of Dr. Lerut and colleagues to underline the importance of suspending all visible diverticula with enough tension to eliminate any prolapse of the pouch below the neck of the sac. The only pouches that should be left untouched are those that are seen on cineradiology but are not identifiable after dissection or myotomy. Cricopharyngeal myotomy with diverticular suspension should be followed by very good to excellent results in 95% of patients operated on, as in the series of Dr. Lerut and associates and in our experience with this operation.

The technical aspects of surgery may vary. General anesthesia is not an absolute necessity. Hiebert[29] used local anesthesia to obtain a better evaluation of pharyngoesophageal function during surgery and to ensure the completeness of the myotomy. We use general anesthesia with a left cervical approach. After dissection of the diverticulum, a no. 36 mercury-filled bougie is passed within the esophagus to serve as a stent for the myotomy; at the same time it locates the exact position of the neck of the diverticulum and protects the integrity of the esophageal lumen if a diverticulectomy is performed. For the diverticulum suspension three or four silk stitches will anchor the peripheral limits of the diverticulum to the posterior wall of the pharynx. Transdiverticulum stitches and fixation of the diverticulum on the prevertebral fascia may result in contamination and acute fasciitis or discitis in the postoperative period. This is the reason why we now fix the diverticulum on the posterior pharynx. If the diverticulum is larger than 4 cm, the retropharyngeal space may not be able to accommodate its bulk and it will need to be resected. A standard stapler resection is then used, with care being taken to suspend the remaining collar behind the pharynx as for a smaller diverticulum. The myotomy is left wide open despite the thin mucosal and submucosal closure.

We agree with the initial conclusion proposed by Dr. Lerut and colleagues. Diverticulopexy with myotomy is our treatment of choice, with the technical details added as just noted. If a diverticulectomy must be added to the myotomy, the myotomy is left wide open to remove any functional abnormality that would persist with a closed cricopharyngeus. This, then, becomes a treatment philosophy more than anything. It is quite evident from this discussion that strong data favoring one treatment over the other are not available. Despite more than five decades of evolution in the evaluation of this pathologic condition, we still lack a good knowledge of its etiology and we still need simple and good prospective evaluation of the diverticulum, its associated conditions, and their treatment. Most reports (including ours) present with the weakness of a retrospection and poorly planned long-term follow-up. Manometric recordings, with their technical limitations, can only suggest that functional abnormalities may be present. No documentation clearly compares the long-term effect of a suspended diverticulum with the evolution of the diverticulectomy patient. Both forms of surgery result in good to excellent control of all symptoms. Large cooperative and long-term prospective studies showing the incidence of morbidity and recurrent diverticulum formation will be the only way to obtain clear answers to these questions. Pathology and electromyography still need extensive investigation before any result can be related to a precise etiology. The role of reflux in the diverticulum formation and following diverticulum treatment needs to be assessed in the same manner.

REFERENCES

1. Duranceau, A., Rheault, M.J., and Jamieson, G.G.: Physiological response to cricopharyngeal myotomy and diverticulum suspension, Surgery **96:**655-662, 1983.
2. Lahey, F.H., and Warren, K.W.: Esophageal diverticula, Surg. Gynecol. Obstet. **98:**1-28, 1954.
3. Belsey, R.: Functional disease of the esophagus, J. Thorac. Cardiovasc. Surg. **52:**164-188, 1966.
4. Harrington, S.W.: Pulsion diverticulum of the hypopharynx at the pharyngoesophageal junction: surgical treatment in 140 cases, Surgery **18:**66-81, 1945.
5. Gray, E.D.: Radiological demonstration of potential pharyngeal diverticulum, Br. J. Radiol. **5:**640-642, 1932.
6. Holmgren, B.S.: Inkonstante hypopharynx divertikel: eine rontgenologische untersuchung, Acta Radiol. **61**(Suppl.):129-136, 1946.
7. Ellis, F.H., Jr., Schlegel, J.F., Lynch, V.P., and Payne, W.S.: Cricopharyngeal myotomy for pharyngoesophageal diverticulum, Ann. Surg. **170:**340-349, 1969.
8. Smiley, T.B., Caves, P.K., and Porter, D.C.: Relationship between posterior pharyngeal pouch and hiatus hernia, Thorax **25:**725-732, 1970.
9. Worman, L.W.: Pharyngoesophageal diverticulum: excision or incision, Surgery **87:**236-237, 1980.
10. Jackson, C., and Shallow, T.A.: Diverticula of the esophagus: pulsion, traction, malignant and congenital, Ann. Surg. **83:**1-19, 1926.
11. Kodicek, J., and Creamer, B.: A study of pharyngeal pouches, J. Laryngol. Otol. **75:**406-411, 1961.
12. Pedersen, A.S., Hansen, J.B., and Alstrup, P.: Pharyngoesophageal diverticula: a manometric follow-up study of ten cases treated by diverticulectomy, Scand. J. Thorac. Cardiovasc. Surg. **7:**87-92, 1973.
13. Ellis, F.H., and Crozier, R.E.: Cervical esophageal dysphagia: indications for and results of cricopharyngeal myotomy, Ann. Surg. **194:**279-289, 1981.
14. Lichter, I.: Motor disorder in pharyngoesophageal pouch, J. Thorac. Cardiovasc. Surg. **76:**273-275, 1978.
15. Knuff, T.E., Benjamin, S.B., and Castell, D.O.: Pha-

ryngoesophageal (Zenker's) diverticulum: a reappraisal, Gastroenterology **82:**734-736, 1982.

16. Hunt, P.S., Connell, A.M., and Smiley, T.S.: The cricopharyneal sphincter in gastric reflux, Gut **11:**303-306, 1970.

17. Einharssen, S.: On the treatment of esophageal diverticula, Acta Otolaryngol. (Stock.) **64:**30-36, 1967.

18. Henderson, R.D., Woolf, C., and Marryatt, G.: Pharyngoesophageal dysphagia and gastroesophageal reflux, Laryngoscope **86:**1531-1539, 1976.

19. Bonavina, L., Khan, N.A., and DeMeester, T.R.: Pharyngoesophageal dysfunctions: the role of cricopharyngeal myotomy, Arch. Surg. **120:**541-549, 1985.

20. Lahey, F.H.: The management of pulsion esophageal diverticulum, JAMA **109:**1414-1419, 1937.

21. Sweet, R.H.: Excision of diverticulum of the pharyngoesophageal junction and lower esophagus by means of the one-stage procedure, Ann. Surg. **143:**433-438, 1956.

22. Payne, W.S., and King, R.M.: Pharyngoesophageal (Zenker's) diverticulum, Surg. Clin. North Am. **63:**815-824, 1983.

23. Nicholson, W.F.: Late results of operations for pharyngeal pouch, Br. J. Surg. **49:**548-552, 1962.

24. Hansen, J.B., Jagt, T., Gundtoft, P., and Sørensen, H.R.: Pharyngoesophageal diverticula, Scand. J. Thorac. Cardiovasc. Surg. **7:**81-86, 1973.

25. Holinger, P.H., and Schild, J.A.: The Zenker's (hypopharyngeal) diverticulum, Ann. Otol. **78:**679-688, 1969.

26. Aubin, A.: Un cas de diverticule de pulsion de l'oesopage traité par la résection de la poche associée à l'oesophagotomie extramuqueuse, Ann. Otolaryngol. **2:**167-177, 1936.

27. Escher, F.: Zur Therapie der zenkerschen Divertikel, Schweiz. Med. Wochenschr. **84:**1073-1078, 1954.

28. Kramer, P., Atkinson, M., Wyman, S., and Ingelfinger, S.J.: The dynamics of swallowing: neuromuscular dysphagia of the pharynx, J. Clin. Invest. **36:**589-595, 1957.

29. Hiebert, C.A.: Surgery for cricopharyngeal dysfunction under local anesthesia, Am. J. Surg. **131:**423-427, 1976.

CHAPTER 26 Proximal esophageal strictures

Alex G. Little and Keith S. Naunheim

Information about strictures of the proximal esophagus is limited compared to information about strictures of the midesophagus and distal esophagus. Strictures of the distal esophagus are typically due to reflux of gastric contents, particularly acid and pepsin. The majority of these patients can be treated with antireflux surgery if the stricture is dilatable. A small number will have undilatable strictures and require resection and reconstruction with either colon or jejunum. A few, who either are judged to be poor surgical candidates or who have good results from medical treatment, can be treated with serial dilatations and medical management of the reflux. Strictures of the midesophagus are typically due to Barrett's stricture at the junction of squamous epithelium with the metaplastic columnar or Barrett's epithelium. Again, experience has shown that, in the absence of dysplasia or frank carcinoma, these patients can be managed with a combination of dilatation, effective antireflux surgery, and/or medical management of the gastroesophageal reflux.

Very few reports focusing on strictures of the proximal or cervical esophagus exist. Nonetheless, this clinical problem occurs with sufficient frequency to be of importance to the thoracic surgeon who deals with problems of the esophagus. It is the purpose of this chapter to review the considerations of prevalence, clinical presentation, diagnosis, and, particularly, treatment of proximal esophageal strictures. By "proximal," we refer to strictures of the cervical and upper thoracic esophagus. Endoscopically this is roughly the region between 16 and 24 cm from the incisor teeth, assuming the average gastroesophageal junction to be at 40 cm. Radiographically the landmarks of the proximal esophagus are, again roughly, the C6 vertebra as the cephalad limit and the top of the aortic arch caudally.

PREVALENCE AND ETIOLOGY

One indication of the uncommon nature of these proximal esophageal strictures is the infrequency with which they are detected. A review of an endoscopic experience over a 7½-year period at a single institution showed that 20 of 238 endoscopically recognized esophageal strictures were in the upper esophagus.[1] This was only 8.4% of all their strictures. In fact, seven of these 20 lesions were due to clinically evident carcinoma of the cervical esophagus, so in only 13 (or 5.5%) of all stricture patients was there a true cervical stricture, as distinguished from an obvious carcinoma. This detection of 13 patients in a 7½-year period is very similar to our experience at The University of Chicago Medical Center.[2] A review of hospital discharge diagnoses of all patients between 1970 and 1982 detected 10 patients with strictures of the proximal esophagus. These data do not allow speculation about the prevalence of this condition. It can be assumed that, on the average, one new patient with a cervical stricture may be diagnosed yearly in a typical university hospital.

Table 26-1 shows the etiologies of proximal esophageal strictures in the only two reported series. Because the problem of clinically evident carcinoma of the proximal esophagus is different than the problem we are focusing on here, we have excluded six such patients from the Phoenix report, leaving a total of 24 patients in the combined series. The stricture in nine (or 38%) of the patients was due to surgery, usually laryngectomy, in combination with postoperative, high-dose radiation therapy. There were two patients with lye ingestion, two patients with lung cancer metastatic to mediastinal nodes, and two with occult esophageal carcinoma. All the other diagnoses occurred once each. It should be stressed that although clinically evident esopha-

TABLE 26-1. Proximal esophageal stricture

Etiology	Treatment
The University of Chicago:	
Congenital fibrous band	Resection
Iatrogenic (endoscopic perforation)	Resection
Laryngectomy + radiation	Resection
Plummer-Vinson syndrome	Resection
Occult esophageal carcinoma	Resection
Esophagogastric anastomotic stricture	Resection
Laryngectomy + radiation	Dilatation
Idiopathic (? Crohn's disease)	Dilatation
Occult bronchogenic carcinoma	Dilatation
Lye ingestion	Colon bypass
Phoenix Veterans Administration Medical Center:	
Laryngectomy + radiation	Puestow dilatation
Laryngectomy + radiation	Puestow dilatation
Laryngectomy + radiation	Puestow dilatation
Laryngectomy + radiation	Puestow dilatation
Laryngectomy + radiation	Maloney dilator
Laryngectomy + radiation	Maloney dilator
Palate resection + radiation	Maloney dilator
Lye ingestion	Retrograde Puestow-Maloney dilator
Firecracker trauma	Puestow dilator
Intramucosal diverticulosis	Puestow dilator
Barrett's esophagus	Maloney dilator
Benign mediastinal adenopathy	Maloney dilator
Occult esophageal carcinoma	Puestow dilator
Occult bronchogenic carcinoma	Maloney dilator + stent

geal carcinoma is not included in this review, there were two patients who had esophageal carcinoma that eventually proved to be producing their strictures.

In addition to the stricture etiologies that were present, one etiology that was not found should also be mentioned; in no patient is a proximal stricture caused by gastroesophageal reflux. This is in striking contrast to strictures of the lower esophagus, which are routinely due to the effects of chronic gastroesophageal reflux.

DIAGNOSIS

Dysphagia, frequently subjectively localized to the cervical region, is the symptom leading to evaluation and diagnosis. As in all patients with dysphagia, a barium swallow esophagogram is the appropriate initial evaluation to be performed. Fig. 26-1 shows several representative barium swallow examinations of patients with proximal strictures. Variable appearances can be seen, and the esophagogram serves primarily to localize the problem to the proximal esophagus, and to allow evaluation of the anatomy of the remainder of the

upper gastrointestinal tract, rather than to provide a definitive diagnosis.

Endoscopy is required in all patients to establish a histologic diagnosis. A flexible endoscopic instrument may suffice for the examination. However, visualization of a very proximal lesion may be difficult because of its proximity to the cricopharyngeus. Furthermore, the biopsy channel of many flexible scopes does not permit passage of an instrument large enough to obtain deep (i.e., submucosal) biopsies. Accordingly, if either of these two potential limitations is encountered, then rigid endoscopy should be employed. This ensures a clear view of the cervical esophagus and allows passage and use of generously sized biopsy forceps so that sufficient material to allow a histologic diagnosis is obtained. Since occult carcinoma is a possible diagnosis, the requirement for adequate tissue sampling is clear.

TREATMENT
Dilatation

The treatments employed in the patients from The University of Chicago and The Phoenix

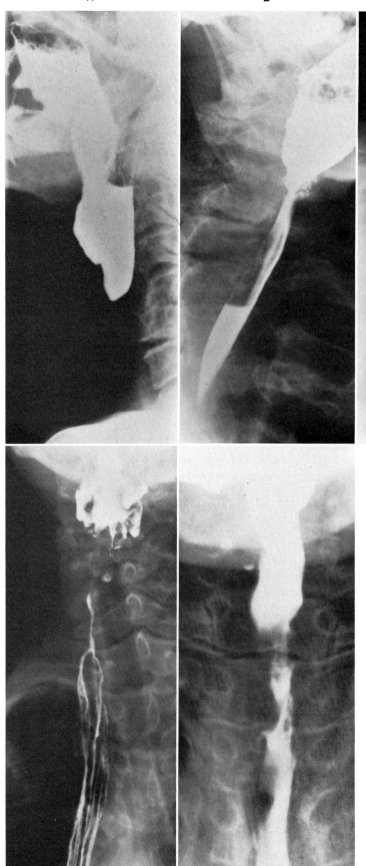

Fig. 26-1. A, Barium swallow esophagogram showing complete obstruction of the cervical esophagus by a radiation stricture. **B,** Barium swallow esophagogram showing a radiation-induced stricture at the hypopharyngeal-esophageal junction. **C,** Barium swallow esophagogram showing a short stricture associated with the Plummer-Vinson syndrome. **D,** Barium swallow esophagogram showing a strictured proximal esophagus above a gastric interposition. **E,** Barium swallow esophagogram showing a proximal esophageal stricture that was proved by sleeve resection to be an esophageal carcinoma.

Veterans Administration Medical Center are shown in Table 26-1. Multiple therapeutic strategies are possible, and treatment for each patient should be individualized. Dilatation is a reasonable starting point for all patients. If the stricture does not respond to Maloney or Hurst dilators, then bougienage with Puestow dilators after endoscopic guidewire placement is appropriate.

Following the initial dilatation, definitive therapy must be selected. Long-term dilatation is possible, as shown by the Phoenix experience, but is not ideal unless only few or intermittent dilatations are required or the patient's overall status does not allow more aggressive intervention. When dilatation is required more frequently than every 3 to 6 months, more definitive treatment, as outlined below, should be considered. Otherwise the patient is subjected to the very real discomfort of continued, frequent dilatations as well as the constant risk of perforation. More definitive forms of treatment are available and will be separately described.

Sleeve resection

For selected patients, a sleeve resection of the strictured area with a primary anastomosis is a valid alternative. We had six such patients at The University of Chicago. All patients underwent multiple dilatations of their strictures before surgery, but in each case the stricture recurred, so that operative intervention was chosen. The longest length of resected esophagus was approximately 5 cm, but most resections were closer to 3 cm in length. Results were variable. The patient with a congenital fibrous band in the lumen of the esophagus was completely relieved of dysphagia, had no operative complications, and has not required any further treatment. The woman with a stricture at the site of an endoscopic perforation has not developed a recurrent stricture and has not required postoperative dilatations. She did develop mild, new, heartburn during convalescence, and repeat pH monitoring of the distal esophagus showed that acid reflux had increased from before the operation. Only mild reflux was present, however, and she has been successfully treated medically. Two patients required esophageal dilatations following their sleeve resections. The patient with Plummer-Vinson syndrome required four series of dilatations prior to his death from unrelated causes 18 months later. At the time of his death he had not had a dilatation for 6 months and had no dysphagia. He also developed symptoms of gastroesophageal reflux following his operation, and abnormal reflux was documented by esophageal pH monitoring. Again, this was mild reflux and was adequately treated medically.

The fourth patient developed a recurrent stricture following resection of his radiation stricture at age 88. There was improvement in his status, however, as the recurrent stricture could be dilated whereas the original stricture was undilatable.

The fifth patient deserves additional discussion. After extensive preoperative evaluation, including multiple endoscopies with biopsy, a sleeve resection was uneventfully performed. Pathologically, however, invasive squamous cell carcinoma, the major portion of which was extralumenal, was found. The patient was well for several months thereafter but required total esophagectomy with gastric interposition for a documented local recurrence 8 months later. The patient had no operative complications from the second procedure and had unrestricted oral intake until death occurred as a result of widespread metastatic disease.

Our final patient having resection was a 33-year-old woman who had had an esophagectomy at age 5 for lye ingestion; reconstruction was with gastric interposition and a cervical esophagogastrostomy. She required dilatation of an anastomotic stricture at age 18 but was then asymptomatic for 12 years. At age 30 the dysphagia recurred and attempted dilatations were unsuccessful. She had resection of her strictured esophagogastric anastomosis through a cervical incision with construction of a new esophagogastrostomy. Histologic examination of the resected tissue showed only chronic fibrosis. She did have the operative complication of a left recurrent nerve palsy. A few dilatations were required during the first 6 months after surgery, but it is now 5 years since her last dilatation and she is having no dysphagia.

Principles of sleeve resection are the following. The possibility of an occult esophageal carcinoma should be eliminated, as far as is feasible, by obtaining multiple endoscopic biopsies, using a rigid endoscope if necessary. All abnormal tissue must be included in the resection, and the final anastomosis must be without undue tension. Finally, excessive esophageal shortening, resulting from overly generous esophageal mobilization and resection, may lead to gastroesophageal reflux, as seen in two of our patients. On the basis of our experience, resection of 3 to 5 cm of esophagus can be consonant with these surgical principles.

Colon interposition

One patient who ingested lye in a suicide attempt suffered severe burns of the posterior pharynx and upper esophagus. After the acute injury resolved, dilatations were attempted but were unsuccessful. The proximal esophagus was severely contracted and, because of its fibrotic nature, was not an acceptable site for anastomosis. Accordingly, bypass with a segment of isoperistaltic left colon was performed, with the proximal anastomosis to the pharynx at the level of the piriform sinus. A simultaneous esophagectomy was performed because of the risk of development of late carcinoma in the injured esophagus. Postoperatively the patient had difficulty with occasional aspiration while eating, for a period of approximately 3 months. After adaptation, he recovered the ability to eat and drink without any restrictions or difficulty, and he is now completely asymptomatic.

Presumably, few patients will require this major surgical intervention, but it should certainly be considered for the younger patient with severe injury to the area of the hypopharynx and cricopharyngeus. A period of adaptation may be required, but complete recovery of the ability to eat normally can be expected. This is obviously preferable to a life of tube feedings!

Plastic operations

Finally, two recently described surgical procedures for addressing proximal strictures should be mentioned. Although we have not had personal experience with them, they should be in the surgeon's armamentarium for consideration. The first procedure is a two-stage approach that leads to a permanent enlargement of the strictured area.[3] In the first stage the stricture is exteriorized with an extended cervical esophagostomy. The second stage, in 4 or 6 weeks, requires trapdooring the adjacent skin to the stoma over the defect. This provides a significant amount of skin to augment the esophageal lumen. The reported experience shows excellent results in a small number of patients. This approach, however, is clearly only applicable to patients with benign strictures who have not had radiation therapy. Radiation effects on the skin would make it a poor substitute and would interfere with healing.

A more attractive and widely applicable procedure, which uses an island cheek flap to repair cervical esophageal strictures, has also been described.[4] This technique would be applicable to all patients, including those with radiation injury, and should be considered for those in whom a sleeve resection, a less complicated and technically easier operation, is not applicable. The technique is described in detail in the article by Sasaki et al. and has the real advantage of bringing well vascularized tissue from afar into an area of radiation damage.

CONCLUSIONS

Our recommendations for treatment are as follows. First, a definitive diagnosis must be established; particularly, the possibility of an occult malignancy should be excluded. If an esophageal cancer is found, then treatment should be based on staging results. All patients with strictures of a benign etiology should have dilatation initially. If long-term dilatation is indicated, because of patient preference or poor medical status, this can be undertaken. However, if frequent dilatations are required, then alternative, definitive treatment should be considered. Sleeve resection is clearly a viable consideration. If a long segment must be resected or if the proximal esophagus, including the cricopharyngeus, is totally destroyed, then colon interposition to the posterior pharynx above the vocal cords works surprisingly well. Finally, there are plastic techniques available, which also can provide satisfactory results when their use is required.

REFERENCES

1. Kozarek, R.A.: Proximal strictures of the esophagus, J. Clin. Gastroenterol. **6:**505-511, 1984.
2. Little, A.G., DeMeester, T.R., and Skinner, D.B.: Strictures of the proximal esophagus. In DeMeester, T.R., and Skinner, D.B., editors: Esophageal disorders: pathophysiology and therapy, New York, 1985, Raven Press, pp. 277-284.
3. Pierce, M.K.: Cervical esophageal strictures: a surgical approach, Laryngoscope **90:**95-97, 1980.
4. Sasaki, T.M., Standage, B.A., Baker, H.W., McConnell, D.B., and Vetto, R.M.: The island cheek flap: repair of cervical esophageal stricture and new extended indications, Am. J. Surg. **147:**650-653, 1984.

Proximal esophageal strictures

DISCUSSION

K. Moghissi

The management of proximal esophageal stricture is problematic, partly because of the infrequency with which such lesions are encountered, and also because of the multiplicity of their etiology. It therefore follows that experience with this type of lesion is scanty and limited to a few cases, even for those centers that usually manage a large number of patients with esophageal pathology. This is well illustrated by Little and Naunheim, who could find no more than two publications concerned with proximal esophageal strictures in the literature. The definition of terminology is an important aspect of any discourse, and this is particularly true in regard to the term relevant to "proximal esophageal stricture," which might convey different connotations to different individuals.

Little and Naunheim's definition accords perfectly with ours. On the basis of this definition, the incidence of proximal stricture in one series of 238 patients with esophageal stricture quoted by the authors was 5.5%; interestingly, this is similar to our own series. Over a period of 15 years (1970 to 1985) 449 esophageal strictures were seen in our center. Twenty-two of these were "proximal strictures"—an incidence of 4.9%.

The etiologies of the strictures in our patients are listed in Table 26-2, which indicates also a general similarity to cases presented by Little and Naunheim.

In all our cases the diagnosis of proximal stricture was established by contrast radiology and endoscopy. We believe that a barium swallow recorded on a videocassette is particularly useful in these cases and that it is superior to standard barium swallow "films," which on rare occasions fail to demonstrate a proximal stricture. We do share Little and Naunheim's opinion with respect to the use of the rigid esophagoscope in diagnosing this type of stricture, not only because it allows a larger biopsy specimen to be obtained but also because it provides a better general view

TABLE 26-2. Management of proximal esophageal stricture in 22 patients

Etiology	No. of patients	Treatment
Humberside Cardiothoracic Surgical Center:		
Fibrous membrane	2	Dilatation (rigid esophagoscopy)
Radiation	4	Repeated dilatation
Anastomotic		
Esophagocoloplasty	3	1 excision, 2 repeated dilatation (1 by pull-through technique)
Esophagoesophageal (esophageal atresia)	2	Repeated dilatation
Lye stricture	1	Repeated dilatation
Reflux stricture (Barrett-type esophagus)	4	Intraoperative dilatation + antireflux operation
Foreign body + caustic (flashlight battery lodged in esophagus)	1	Repeated dilatation + gastrostomy (pull-through technique)
Unknown etiology (postoperative)	2	1 resection + reconstruction (gastric) 1 exploration + conservative operation (incision + transverse resuture)
Postoperative following excision of pharyngeal pouch	2	Conservative operation (incision + transverse resuture)
Occult carcinoma	1	Resection + reconstruction (gastric)

and gives the "feel" of the stricture. The fact that every series of proximal stricture appears to include at least one case of "occult" carcinoma indicates the difficulty in diagnosing an early carcinoma from a simple stricture at or near the pharyngoesophageal junction.

My overall policy with respect to the management of proximal esophageal strictures has been geared toward conservative treatment, one reason being that failure of radical surgery in this type of stricture has a serious consequence because of limitation in the choice of a substitute for reconstruction of the esophagus at that level. Also, many proximal strictures are secondary to pathologic conditions that affect the vascularization of the esophagus at or around the stricture.

As can be seen from Table 26-2, in 10 of our patients simple dilatation of the stricture was used as the sole method of therapy, with good results. Among these were two infants who previously had reconstruction of the esophagus for congenital esophageal atresia and tracheoesophageal fistula. In these the dilatation had to be carried out repeatedly and at frequent intervals for a period of 1 year, but the outcome was satisfactory. Now aged 12 and 8 years respectively, they are both well and free from obstructive symptoms.

In one child who developed a stricture following retention of a pocket light battery (with leakage of the contents) in the cervical esophagus, a more sophisticated (pull-through) technique of dilatation was undertaken. The technique employed was to carry out a gastrostomy (which was used for feeding) and then to pass a fine thread through the mouth. The end of this thread was then recovered through the gastrostomy and the abdominal wall, and the mouth end of it was then attached to bougies of increasing diameter, which were drawn via the gastrostomy end of the thread into the stricture. This procedure was repeated several times, and the result was excellent.

This guided dilatation was also very successfully used in another child, who developed a stricture following esophagocoloplasty for a complicated type of esophageal atresia and tracheoesophageal fistula. This child is now aged 7 and has remained well and without dysphagia for 2 years.

Retrograde dilatation of the stricture coupled with an antireflux procedure (total fundoplication) was carried out in four patients in whom the esophageal mucosa was lined by columnar epithelium (Barrett-type esophagus) and whose strictures were situated at the root of the neck. All these have remained symptom free for 6 to 9 years following their operations.

Vertical incision of the stricture followed by transverse suturing was undertaken in three patients. Two of these had previous operations for the excision of a pharyngeal pouch, and in the third patient the etiology was uncertain. The outcome was successful in all three, and there were no postoperative complications.

Excision of a stricture at the site of the previous esophagocoloplasty and reanastomosis were necessary in one patient. The procedure was simple, involving cervical incision and an esophagocolonic reanastomosis. In two patients only, in our series, resection of the stricture and esophagogastric anastomosis were carried out. One of these was a case of occult carcinoma that became apparent some 6 months after repeated dilatation. At each occasion a biopsy of the stricture area had shown no evidence of malignancy. This patient died 3 months after the operation. In the second patient the etiology was not established. The stricture appeared 18 months after open-heart surgery for valve replacement.

CONCLUSIONS

As with Little and Naunheim, our experience with proximal esophageal stricture has been limited. My overall policy is one of conservatism. The etiology and the type of stricture should be determined. Repeated bougienage is particularly suitable for short strictures and those following surgery or radiotherapy. Dilatation of the stricture coupled with an antireflux operation, we believe, is the treatment of choice in Barrett-type strictures with gastroesophageal reflux.

Plastic repair or local excision of the stricture is a suitable method in postoperative (iatrogenic) cases. Only exceptionally is radical surgery with resection of the stricture and reconstruction of the upper alimentary tract necessary (e.g., when the etiology is obscure and neoplasia cannot be ruled out).

We believe that dilatation of these strictures is best carried out through a rigid esophagoscope using the Chevalier Jackson and Gum elastic types of bougies at the start of a dilatation session, then followed by Maloney mercury-filled bougies.

Occasionally in difficult cases the use of the "pull-through" technique of bougienage, particularly when a feeding gastrostomy is needed, can save the patient from a radical operation.

Index